Surgical Technology

Principles and Practice

Surgical Technology

Principles and Practice

Third Edition

Joanna Ruth Fuller, CST
Former Department Head, Surgical Technology
College of California Medical Affiliates
San Francisco, California

Technical and Professional Consultant:
Linda K. Groah, RN, MS, CNOR

W.B. SAUNDERS COMPANY
A Division of Harcourt Brace & Company
Philadelphia ○ London ○ Toronto ○ Montreal ○ Sydney ○ Tokyo

W.B. SAUNDERS COMPANY
A Division of
Harcourt Brace & Company

The Curtis Center
Independence Square West
Philadelphia, Pennsylvania 19106

Library of Congress Cataloging-in-Publication Data

Fuller, Joanna Ruth.

Surgical technology: principles and practice / Joanna R. Fuller : technical and professional consultant, Linda K. Groah.—3rd ed.

    p.   cm.

Includes bibliographical references and index.

ISBN 0-7216-4064-8

    1. Surgical Technology.   I. Title. [DNLM: 1. Operating Room Nursing.   2. Operating Room Technicians.   WY 162 F966s]

RD32.3/F84   1994

617′.9—dc20

DNLM/DLC   92-49085

SURGICAL TECHNOLOGY: PRINCIPLES AND PRACTICE   ISBN 0-7216-4064-8

Printed in the United States of America

Last digit is the print number: 9   8   7   6

Preface

· ·

The technologic changes in medicine during the last decade have occurred more rapidly than any educator, practitioner, or student could have predicted. Surgery, traditionally a conservative field, has not been left behind. Advances in imaging techniques, diagnostics, and molecular biology have extended to the operating room and produced new procedures and more efficient ways to perform them.

Along with these technologic advances we have witnessed the birth and spread of a tragic and devastating disease. AIDS has touched every medical discipline. No matter what our connection with AIDS—professional or personal—nearly all of us have known someone who lost his or her life to this disease. Let us hope that through increased awareness, education, and research, we can halt its grim advance.

I have had two goals throughout the writing of these three editions. The first goal has been to teach technically correct and ethically sound techniques in a manner that *enlightens* rather than confuses. The second goal has been to impart a sense of *humanity* and *compassion* to a profession that sometimes gets caught up in technology and loses sight of its original purpose—to offer aid and comfort to the patient. It is my sincere hope that this purpose, above all others, has been achieved.

JOANNA RUTH FULLER, CST
Petaluma, California

Acknowledgments

. . . .

The third edition of *Surgical Technology: Principles and Practice* would not have been possible without the unending support and professional guidance of Linda K. Groah, RN, MS, CNOR. Her technical assistance has been flawless and her enthusiasm unmatched. I thank her deeply.

I would also like to thank Selma Ozmat, Editor of Health Related Professions at W.B. Saunders, for her confidence and support throughout the project.

United States Surgical Corporation and Ethicon, Inc. have been extremely cooperative during the project. Their contributions, in both materials and information, have been invaluable.

Finally, for his help and untiring patience, I wish to lovingly thank my husband, Peter Axelrod.

Contents

· ·

THE PRINCIPLES OF SURGERY

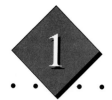

The Surgical Technologist—Past, Present, and Future

Learning Objectives

After reading this chapter you should be able to

♦ *Understand* the development of the surgical technologist after World War II.
♦ *Discuss* why there was a shortage of nurses during World War II and the Korean War.
♦ *Describe* the role of the Association of Operating Room Nurses in the establishment of the Association of Operating Room Technicians.
♦ *Understand* the significance of certification.
♦ *Describe* how medical economics has played a role in the development of surgical technology as a profession.
♦ *Discuss* the value of teamwork in a changing profession.

HISTORICAL DEVELOPMENT: 1900–1945

Since the development of effective anesthesia and antisepsis in the late 19th century, the role of the nurse in surgery has been easily defined and tracked. In the late 1800s she prepared instruments for surgery, and in the early 1900s she assisted in surgical procedures and in the administration of ether, called "etherizing" (Fig. 1–1). Her duties from about the 1920s to the 1940s were those of a circulating nurse. She also instructed student nurses in their surgical education (Fig. 1–2). Frequently the operating room supervisor was the only graduate nurse in surgery, and it was her duty to oversee the student nurses as they completed their rotation in the operating room (Fig. 1–3).

The need for assistive personnel in surgery did not arise until World War II. During World War I, army corpsmen were present on the battlefield to offer aid and comfort to the wounded; they had no role in surgery. World War II dramatically changed that. With the development of antibiotics such as penicillin and sulfa, war surgeons were able to operate on and save the lives of many more patients than was previously possible. The increase in battlefield survivors created a drastic shortage of nurses. In addition to those nurses

2

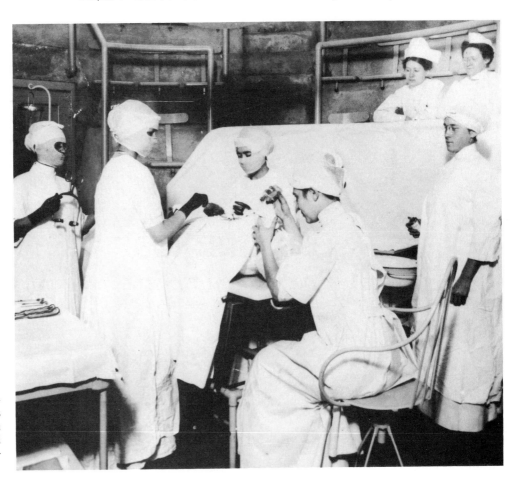

Figure 1–1. "Etherizing," circa 1900. (Courtesy of Archives and Special Collections on Women in Medicine, Medical College of Pennsylvania, Philadelphia, Pennsylvania.)

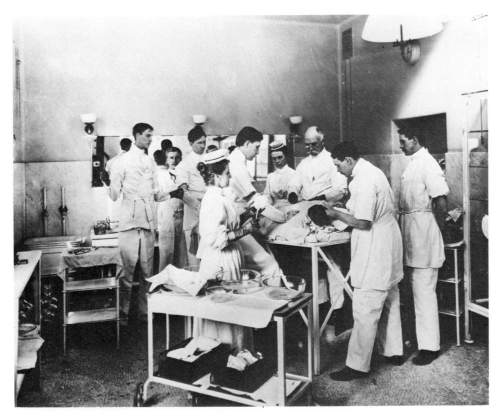

Figure 1–2. Roosevelt Hospital, New York, circa 1913. (Courtesy of Archives and Special Collections on Women in Medicine, Medical College of Pennsylvania, Philadelphia, Pennsylvania.)

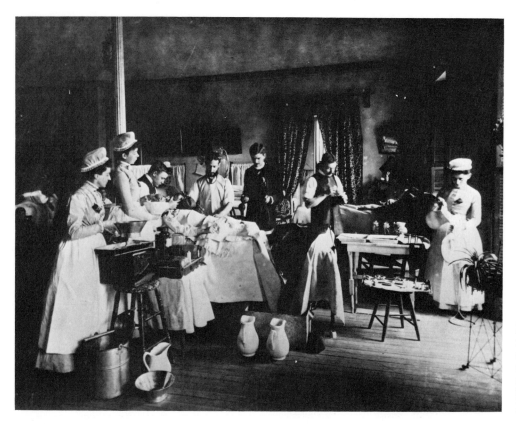

Figure 1–3. The operating room at Bellvue Hospital, circa 1870. (Courtesy of Archives and Special Collections on Women in Medicine, Medical College of Pennsylvania, Philadelphia, Pennsylvania.)

needed to staff the base hospitals, many more were needed at home to attend to the needs of the wounded who were returned from battle. To supply the field hospitals in the Pacific and European theaters, the army began training corpsmen to assist in surgery, a role that had previously been filled only by nurses. During that era, corpsmen were expected to administer anesthesia and also act as first assistant to the surgeon. When nurses were not available, such as on combat ships where women were not allowed, corpsmen worked under the direct supervision of the surgeon. Thus, a new profession was born, which the army called *surgical technicians.*

WORLD WAR II TO THE PRESENT

Following World War II, the Korean War caused a continued shortage of operating room nurses, and the need for fully trained nurses in the operating room was questioned. It was at this time that operating room supervisors began to recruit ex-corpsmen for work in civilian surgery. Their primary function was as circulating nurses. Registered nurses continued to fill the scrub or "instrument nurse" role until about 1965, when the roles were reversed.

Prompted by the need for guidelines and standards in training paramedical surgical personnel, the Association of Operating Room Nurses (AORN) published a book entitled *Teaching the Operating Room Technician* in 1967. Soon after this, the *Association of Operating Room Technicians* (AORT) was created in 1968 by the AORN

Board of Directors. In its early years the AORT was governed by the joint AORN-AORT advisory board. During this time, the operating room technician received his or her training only on the job.

Along with organizational independence came steps toward formalizing the technologist's education. The AORT formed two new committees: the Liaison Council on Certification and the Joint Review Committee on Education. The first certifying examination was held in 1970, and those technologists who passed the examination were given a new title—certified operating room technician. In 1973, the AORT became independent of the AORN and soon afterward changed the name of its professional organization to its current title, the Association of Surgical Technologists (AST).

Current Educational Standards

After certification, the surgical technologist is required to obtain continuing education credits to maintain certification. The current requirement is 72 hours of continuing education over a 6-year period. Although certification is not mandatory for employment, few hospitals hire noncertified technologists. In addition, certified technologists generally receive higher wages than those who are not certified.

Accreditation

Surgical technology programs are accredited by the American Medical Association's Committee on Allied

Health Education and Accreditation (CAHEA). CAHEA grants or denies accreditation after the Accreditation Review Committee of AST (ARC/AST) reviews the curriculum and the qualifications of each program's instructors. Currently there are more than 100 accredited surgical technology programs in the United States.

The Technologist's Future

A future role for technologists that will require further education—the role of the surgical technologist/first assistant—is in the developmental stage. In the past, technologists have been routinely required to retract tissue, sponge blood and fluids from the surgical wound, cut sutures, assist in wound irrigation, and apply wound dressings. The Association of Surgical Technologists now seeks to broaden the role of the technologist as surgical first assistant. The proposed role requires that the technologist work under the direct supervision of the surgeon and perform procedures that have traditionally been reserved for the surgical first assistant. However, not all state laws currently allow this practice. A further discussion of the legal aspects of the role of the technologist is provided in Chapter 3.

Economic Influences

For the past decade, the exact role of the technologist has been influenced by changes in medical economics. Hospital administrators are faced with the dilemmas of increased health care costs and decreased benefits from governmental support systems such as Medicare and state-supported programs.

As a result of these economies, health care providers are seeking new ways to apply the technologists' professional knowledge to help perform traditional nursing functions. This has led to the concept of the "nurse extender." Within this definition, the technologist's activities and functions are broadened but remain under the supervision of the registered nurse. A similiar concept is that of "assistive personnel."

These ideas have raised questions concerning the educational and professional level of those who provide patient care. Although there are no easy answers to these questions, one fact remains unchanged: the ability of all those involved in patient care depends on *teamwork*. Teamwork means that all share a common goal and that all work to their fullest ability to meet that goal. No matter what professional challenges confront them, the surgical team members must never lose sight of the fact that the goals of medicine, including surgery, are to relieve pain, ease suffering, and preserve the patient's dignity.

Questions for Study and Review

1. When did the need arise for assistive personnel in the operating room?

2. Why was there a sharp increase in the number of surgical patients during World War II?

3. When and why did the Association of Operating Room Nurses publish its first manual on operating room technology?

4. When was the Association of Operating Room Technicians formed?

5. When did the Assocation of Operating Room Technicians split off from AORN?

6. Who accredits surgical technology programs?

7. How does medical economics affect the role of the surgical technologist?

8. Why is teamwork so important in surgery?

References

Association of Surgical Technologists: An Introduction to the Association of Surgical Technologists. Englewood, CO, 1990.

Association of Surgical Technologists: History of the Surgical Technologist. Englewood, CO, 1979.

Litsky W, et al: Frances Ginsberg: Educator and advocate of surgical technologists. J Assoc Surg Technologists, July/August, 36–41, 1983.

Phippen ML, et al: Assistive personnel in the perioperative setting: Changing the paradigm. Semin Periop Nurs 1:2, 1992.

Surgical Conscience and Ethics in the Operating Room

Learning Objectives

After reading this chapter you should be able to

♦ *Discuss* "surgical conscience."
♦ *List* situations in operating room work that are affected by surgical conscience.
♦ *Recognize* situations that can undermine surgical conscience.

SURGICAL CONSCIENCE

Ethical behavior in the operating room involves many different types of activities. All, however, share a common principle: *There is a consequence for every act performed.* When a team member chooses behavior that places the patient's well-being above all else, he or she demonstrates a strong *surgical conscience.* The team member whose surgical conscience determines his or her actions always chooses alternatives that favor the patient's safety, even though these alternatives may be more strenuous or difficult.

Surgical conscience and ethical behavior in the operating room affect the patient in two distinct ways: physically and mentally.

Physical Protection of the Patient

Patients can be harmed in the operating room setting in many ways. It is the responsibility of all who care for

the patient to protect him or her against these injuries. In almost every case, this requires *constant* vigilance. While in the operating room during the preoperative, intraoperative, or postoperative period, the patient is frequently without complete sensibility. That is, he or she may be partially or completely unable to respond to physical sensations. Hence, the surgical technologist must "feel" for the patient.

Surgical conscience requires that the technologist *assess* the immediate danger to the patient and *remedy* the situation immediately whenever possible or *report* it *immediately* to someone who can. For example, it is within the technologist's ability to remove his or her contaminated glove during surgery. However, missing sponges must be reported to the surgeon so that the wound can be searched.

The technologist must never take the attitude that a certain situation is not his or her responsibility. Patient protection in the operating room is the responsibility of everyone. *The primary motivation for action in the operating room is the patient's safety and well-being.* It is the responsibility of everyone to at least report possible dangers, such as breaks in aseptic technique, to an appropriate staff member, who can then take action.

Common Physical Dangers

Electrical hazards are a major risk in the operating room. Cords that are frayed or plugs that appear defective must never be used. This seems like common sense, but there is a constant temptation to use such equipment "one more time" before sending it for repair. "One more time" may turn into tragedy.

Electrocautery units (discussed fully in Chapter 13) require careful patient grounding. Incomplete or faulty patient grounding may cause burns or electrocution.

Positioning the patient (discussed in Chapter 10) requires meticulous care to protect bony surfaces, prominent nerves, and blood vessels. Improper positioning may result in nerve damage, paralysis, bruising, or inadequate blood flow to a portion of the body.

Falls in the operating room are inexcusable. Patients may arrive in the operating room under sedation. The transfer of a patient under sedation or emerging from a general or light anesthetic requires specific protocol and a prescribed number of persons to help. Side rails must be raised and safety straps applied as soon as the transfer is complete. Surgical conscience dictates that protocol be followed and the patient be protected during any transfer (see Chapter 10).

Unnecessary time spent under anesthesia because of poor planning shows poor surgical conscience. One of the major risks to the surgical patient is anesthesia. Attention to detail before surgery will prevent delay of the procedure. The technologist should anticipate as much as possible the instruments or special equipment needed for each particular case. The surgeon's preference card should always be consulted. If the need for certain equipment is questionable, it is permissible to ask the surgeon about it *before the patient is anesthetized.*

Danger from the use of certain anesthetic agents such as those that produce conscious sedation (see Chapter 9) is a critical concern of all surgical team members. Patients must be monitored carefully during the use of all types of anesthesia no matter how common the use, or how mild the effects, of the agent used.

Protection From Disease

The practice of *aseptic technique* (see Chapter 8) is the individual responsibility of every team member in surgery. Any break in technique *must be reported immediately even if this causes a delay or if admitting an error is personally embarrassing.* All personnel must follow strict protocol regarding the handling of surgical supplies, tissue specimens, and medical equipment. Because of the widespread occurrence of blood-borne diseases, such as acquired immunodeficiency syndrome (AIDS) and serum hepatitis, negligence in this area can be life threatening. Thus, strict personal hygiene and adherence to prescribed methods of cleanup and decontamination (see Chapter 6) require unfaltering surgical conscience.

Emotional Protection

Protection from psychological insult is the responsibility of everyone in the operating room. The patient must not be allowed to overhear or misinterpret matters discussed that are intended to be confidential or are offensive. Research has indicated that even the unconscious patient may be affected by comments made during surgery, including those that are in poor taste or are inappropriate. Tasteless or vulgar action or speech must never, under any circumstances, be tolerated in the operating room. If the technologist should witness such actions he or she should not become involved but should report it to the operating room supervisor or other appropriate authority. Likewise, idle chatter in hallways or in the surgical suites must be kept to a minimum. Horseplay can be a disturbing sight to a patient about to enter the operating room. The patient must be made to feel that his or her well-being is the primary concern of all those around him or her.

The personal dignity of a patient must be guarded at all times. Unnecessary exposure of the patient should not be allowed. This is particularly true in the preoperative areas and hallways where the patient is exposed to nonhospital personnel or other patients. The surgical patient is generally ill at ease and frightened. Unnecessary embarrassment further assaults the patient emotionally and should be avoided. Never assume that a premedicated patient has lost his or her sense of dignity.

Environmental protection in the form of warmth and comfort is essential in good patient care. The patient must not be forced to lie shivering either on a gurney or on the operating table while he or she awaits surgery. Constant neglect of care and compassion are symptomatic of a poorly organized and non–patient-oriented staff.

Anxiety and fear accompany nearly every patient to the operating room. Even though preoperative medications are effective in controlling anxiety, they cannot replace the warm touch or understanding voice of a staff member. Although it is not always practical to spend extended periods of time talking to the patient (in fact this can adversely affect the action of the preoperative medication), a few words of assurance or comfort demonstrates good surgical conscience—that of a caring person.

SURGICAL ETHICS

Ethical behavior in the operating room is inseparable from surgical conscience. It requires a high level of moral conscience coupled with sound judgment and professional honesty. Numerous practices in surgery are affected by the professional ethics of the employee. Some common areas of concern are discussed here.

The patient has an ethical and legal right to privacy.

His or her condition must *not* be discussed outside the surgery department where relatives, friends, or passersby might overhear. The information contained in the medical record is not a topic for public discussion, debate, or criticism. The patient's condition must never be discussed in any setting where the patient or family members might overhear and misinterpret information. Public areas of the hospital such as hallways, elevators, and cafeterias must never be the site of discussions regarding the patient's medical history or condition. Only designated members of the surgical staff should speak to members of the news media regarding the condition of a public figure who is a surgical patient.

Any action or occurrence in surgery that either causes harm or has the potential to cause harm to the patient is called an *incident.* In addition, any occurrence that prevents the safe or professional conduct of staff members is also an incident. Should an incident occur, one or more of the team members involved personally, or as a witness, should submit a description of the incident *in writing* to a member of the staff designated by the hospital to receive such reports. The purpose of the incident report is to accurately describe the occurrence in the event legal or disciplinary action is subsequently taken. Incident reports must be completed regardless of the implications they carry. It is grossly unethical for any staff member to ignore occurrences that have harmed or could harm the patient or staff members. Although it would be impossible to list all possible incidents that require a report, the following are some that are common.

- Inaccurate sponge, needle, or instrument counts, when the count is not resolved by the close of surgery
- Sponge, needle, or instrument left in the patient
- Gross contamination of the surgical wound
- Any injury to the patient as a result of negligent or inadvertent action by any staff member
- Substance abuse by a staff member either witnessed or suspected
- Theft of medications suspected or witnessed
- Gross misconduct by any staff member during the course of work
- Gross equipment failure that results in patient or staff injury
- Patient fall. Any fall of the patient from the stretcher or operating table must be reported as an incident. Even if the team members save the patient from actually landing on the floor, the incident must be reported. The patient may have suffered injury to joints, ligaments, and tendons.

Admission of an error in the operating room reflects a high degree of professional ethics, especially when the error causes loss of integrity or embarrassment. There must be no motivation greater in admitting an error than the safety of the patient. Two common errors are contamination of the surgical field and inaccurate sponge, needle, or instrument counts.

SITUATIONS THAT UNDERMINE SURGICAL CONSCIENCE AND ETHICS

Poor morale in the operating room may be caused by a number of problems within the department. These may involve the whole staff or merely certain persons. Although most graduates of surgery programs and experienced personnel are anxious to provide the best patient care possible, certain situations can cause a person with a good attitude to become apathetic. Apathy and poor morale are enemies of good patient care, and the cause should be of major concern to all involved.

Peer Apathy

When morale is low in the surgical department, even those who are normally very attentive to detail may feel, "No one else cares, so why should I?" This type of attitude can cause the whole department to lose sight of its primary goal—the treatment of illness and disease and the compassionate care of the patient. Occasionally a new staff member (usually a recent graduate) enters the department hoping to practice sound technique and is shunned or criticized by apathetic staff members. This type of behavior is defensive; the staff may feel threatened by the newcomer. The new employee, now feeling disillusioned and discouraged, allows his or her standards to fall to the level of the group.

Once group apathy has set in it is difficult to remedy. Most professionals feel guilty about sliding standards, which in turn provokes defensive behavior when they are confronted. This snowball effect can be prevented in its early stages by staff meetings and "airing sessions" to help determine the causes of the problem. The sessions will work if the problem is viewed as one that is shared by all rather than by placing the blame on individual staff members.

Stress, Fatigue, and Poor Health

The operating room is an extremely stressful place, and the responsibilities carried by staff members are great. One of the major causes of errors and morale problems in surgery is fatigue. Although the operating room must be run at an efficient level, the workload must never exceed the staff's ability to function safely and professionally. Likewise, a staff member's poor health may greatly influence his or her ability to work under such pressure.

Personal Problems

Any staff member who has overwhelming personal problems should seek counseling to prevent these problems from influencing the care of his or her patients.

The staff member's immediate supervisor can sometimes resolve problems that involve professional issues or staff relations. Clinical preceptors may also offer help in resolving these problems. Many hospitals now have an employee assistance program whose purpose is to counsel and refer personnel who experience personal or professional difficulties. A leave of absence from work may be needed to resolve the problem.

Staff Relations

It is common for surgery personnel to show some preferences as to which surgeons they work with. There are, of course, some surgeons to whom all nursing and technical personnel are pleased to give first-rate assistance and attention to detail. Regardless of the surgeon, however, the professional attitude of the staff must be the same. The quality of patient care should never be dictated by the personality of the surgeon.

Questions for Study and Review

1. What does "surgical conscience" mean to you?
2. What areas of your work are most deeply concerned with surgical conscience?
3. In what area do you need to improve your surgical conscience?
4. What common excuses do you think are given for *not* having good surgical conscience?
5. Discuss ethical responsibility in the operating room.
6. What are some ways in which you can combat apathy in the operating room?
7. In what specific area of your work do you tend to show apathy?

Bibliography

Association of Operating Room Nurses: Recommended Practices for Documentation of Perioperative Nursing Care. Denver, 1991.

Davidhizar R: Honesty: The best policy in nursing practice. Todays OR Nurse, 30–34, January 1992.

Koener M, et al: Communicating in the operating room. AORN J 36(1), 1982.

Ponthieu-Black JF: Hints for dealing with employee stress. AORN J 36(1):57–58, 1982.

Surgery and the Law

Learning Objectives

After reading this chapter you should be able to

- ◆ *Understand* why it is important to know laws that pertain to surgery.
- ◆ *List* the federal regulations that affect surgical technologists.
- ◆ *Define* the nurse and medical practice acts.
- ◆ *Distinguish* between certification and licensure.
- ◆ *Discuss* the two areas that place the surgical technologist at the highest risk for exceeding the scope of practice.
- ◆ *Define* "negligence" and discuss those situations most affected by it.
- ◆ *Define* "defamation."
- ◆ *Discuss* four categories of errors that occur in the operating room.
- ◆ *Respond* appropriately to the four types of errors.
- ◆ *Understand* malpractice insurance.
- ◆ *Know* how to seek a competent attorney.

Key Terms

certification: Formal recognition by a private organization that a person has demonstrated certain skills or has received certain training.

complaint: The legal document that begins a civil lawsuit and designates who is suing whom and why.

damages: Money awarded in a civil lawsuit to compensate the injured party.

defamation: A derogatory statement concerning another person's skill, character, or reputation.

defendant: In a lawsuit, the person or corporation being sued; in a criminal case, the person being prosecuted.

delegate: To assign one's duties or tasks to another person.

deposition: A statement given by a witness, under oath, and transcribed by a court reporter during the pretrial phase of a civil lawsuit.

informed consent: Permission given with full knowledge of the risks involved.

insurance: A contract in which the insurance company agrees to defend the policyholder if he or she is sued for acts covered by the policy and to pay any damages.

liable: Legally responsible.

license: Governmental permission to perform an act or possess property.

malpractice: Negligence committed by a professional.

negligence: The failure to exercise due care. See *tort*.

plaintiff: In a civil lawsuit, the person filing the suit; the injured party.

scope of practice: The limits of professional duties set by law, training, and experience.

slander: Spoken defamation.

subpoena: A court order requiring its recipient to appear and testify at a trial or deposition.

summons: A court-issued document that is received by a person being sued, notifying the person that he or she is a defendant in the lawsuit.

theft: Taking the property of another with the intention of keeping it.

tort: A wrongful act, other than a breach of contract, that can result in a lawsuit for money.

WHY KNOW THE LAW?

Surgical technologists and nurses need to know the law to protect their patients, their hospital, and themselves. Knowledge about safety regulations protects the patient from harm. Knowing and following state and federal laws protects the professional and the hospital from civil lawsuits and protects the professional from criminal penalties.

THE ROLE OF THE ASSOCIATION OF SURGICAL TECHNOLOGISTS

The Association of Surgical Technologists (AST) and its Liaison Council on Certification is a private organization that certifies surgical technologists after they meet specific educational requirements and pass a certifying examination. Certification by AST or any other private organization confers no special legal status to the certificate holder. It is not a substitute for a state license to practice medicine or nursing.

SOURCES OF THE LAW

Federal Regulations

A number of federal regulations apply to health care personnel. Those issued by the Department of Health and Human Services (HHS) prescribe standards for hospitals receiving federal funds under Medicare. The Occupational Safety and Health Administration (OSHA) issues and regulates standards for the prevention of transmission of human immunodeficiency virus (HIV) and hepatitis B virus. The Environmental Protection Agency (EPA) regulates the use of chemicals for disinfection and sterilization. The Food and Drug Administration (FDA) tests and regulates the use of antiseptic agents.

State Law: Medical and Nurse Practice Acts

Under the constitution of the United States, each state has the power to regulate businesses and professions, including the practice of medicine, and the laws differ from state to state. It is the responsibility of each person to become familiar with the laws of the state in which he or she works.

Each state has *medical* and *nurse practice acts*. These acts state that a license is required for a person to practice medicine or nursing. A *license*, as it applies to medicine, is official permission given by a governmental agency to perform specific duties (e.g., surgery) or to possess certain substances (e.g., pharmaceutical products). For example, physicians may diagnose and treat disease, cut and suture tissue, prescribe drugs, and pronounce death. Nurses may administer medications that are prescribed by a physician. These laws, by giving permission to licensed professionals and by defining the profession, *restrict* the activities or scope of practice of those persons that are not licensed. Because surgical technologists are *not* licensed by any state, they must not exceed the scope of their practice and violate the medical or nurse practice acts. To do so is usually a criminal offense that can result in severe penalties.

AREAS OF CRIMINAL LIABILITY

Exceeding the Scope of Practice

Two roles that place the surgical technologist at extreme risk for exceeding the scope of practice are that of first assistant to the surgeon and that of circulating nurse.

Role as First Assistant

Because medical practice acts differ from state to state, a technologist must proceed very cautiously when acting as a first assistant. The surgeon may permit or even require the technologist to perform certain invasive functions such as suturing or incising tissue that are strictly forbidden by that state's medical practice act. *It is the technologist's responsibility, not the surgeon's, to determine whether these acts are legal in the state where he or she works.* When a surgeon asks a technologist to perform invasive functions, he or she delegates (hands over) that task to the technologist. Some states allow the delegation of duties and others specifically forbid it. Unfortunately, the language in some states' medical practice acts is so vague that it is difficult to determine whether delegation is permitted. When in doubt, the technologist should seek the advice of the hospital's legal staff or even a private attorney. If a lawsuit or threat of criminal prosecution should arise, the technologist who has sought legal advice before proceeding with assigned tasks is in a more defensible position than one who proceeded blindly.

Most states permit a properly trained registered nurse to be first assistant. In a 1989 survey of all 50 states and U.S. territories, the Association of Operating Room Nurses found that 42 states and territories permit the registered nurse to be first assistant; in Guam, New Jersey, Ohio, and Oklahoma it is forbidden. The status of the registered nurse first assistant is uncertain in Hawaii, Illinois, Indiana, Rhode Island, and Puerto Rico.

Both the Association of Operating Room Nurses and the Association of Surgical Technologists are lobbying legislatures in those states that forbid first assisting, or in which it is not clearly permitted, to allow the practice for their members. This may result in changes in the law.

Role as Circulating Nurse

Circulating includes duties that are usually restricted to licensed nurses. These duties include the delivery of medications and patient assessment and charting. The federal guidelines that govern hospitals that treat Medicare patients permit surgical technologists and licensed practical nurses to "assist in circulatory duties" under the supervision of a registered nurse who is "immediately available to respond in emergencies." Neither "assisting in circulatory duties" nor "immediately available" is defined in the regulations. Hospital policy varies, and the technologist may have greater responsibility and less immediate supervision in rural hospitals where nursing resources are scarce. The federal regulations do not preempt or overrule state nursing laws. Whether a nurse can delegate duties requiring a license varies from state to state. It is therefore critical that the technologist become familiar with the laws of the state in which he or she works.

Theft

Taking property that is not one's own with the intention of keeping it is theft. Operating room personnel must protect the property of patients and that of the hospital.

Patient Property

Patients occasionally arrive in the operating room with valuables such as wedding rings, watches, or dentures or other prostheses. Care must be taken to protect these items from loss or theft. A record should be made of all property stored for the patient, listing the items and either their place of storage or to whom they were entrusted. This record should appear in the patient's chart.

Hospital Property

Damaged instruments and other hospital property must not be removed from the hospital without the specific consent of the operating room manager or other appropriate authority. Never assume that these items can be taken without permission. Damaged items can often be repaired or may be used in other areas of the hospital. The fact that "everyone does it" is not an appropriate defense against charges of theft.

CIVIL LIABILITY

Criminal acts can result in fines or imprisonment. Civil wrongs (called *torts*) result in lawsuits in which money (called *damages*) is awarded to the injured party. The law divides these civil wrongs into two categories: negligence and intentional torts.

Negligence

Negligence is defined as "the failure to exercise due care, or the care that an ordinary prudent person would exercise under the circumstances." If the violator is a professional, such as a physician, nurse, or surgical technologist, then the standard of care is that of a "reasonable professional with similar training and experience." This definition is necessarily vague, since no law can foresee every circumstance and dictate the correct conduct.

There are many situations in the operating room in which negligence can injure patients or fellow workers. These injuries can result in lawsuits against the individual professional as well as the hospital. The hospital, like any employer, is *liable* for the negligent acts of its employees and can be sued for those acts. It is beyond the scope of this text to discuss every possible situation that might result in liability; only those activities or situations that carry the highest risk of harm are discussed. The reader should refer to specific chapters related to the topics below to fully appreciate and understand the risks associated with each area. The surest way to avoid risk and liability is to develop constant awareness of one's actions and to acquire knowledge about every phase of the job. "Not thinking" is one of the major causes of tragic accidents that occur in the operating room.

Side Rails, Supports, Positioning

It is the responsibility of all operating room personnel to ensure that the patient is protected against falls from stretchers, tables, or beds. The technologist or nurse should be certain that side rails and restraining straps are in place at all times. Similarly, supports used for positioning the patient (see Chapter 10) must be placed and padded correctly to prevent injury. Improper positioning can cause permanent damage to nerves and blood vessels.

Burns

The patient can be burned by faulty grounding of electrocautery equipment or improperly aerated equipment that has been gas sterilized. Lasers can severely damage the eyes of patients and operating room personnel and can cause fires. The use of alcohol-based prep solutions in conjunction with electrosurgery or laser surgery can lead to fire, with tragic results. The improper use or storage of disinfectants can cause burns to patients and personnel. Whenever hyperthermia blankets are in use during surgery, the temperature must be carefully monitored; also, all fittings must be inspected for integrity before use.

Electrical Shock

Faulty grounding of electrical equipment can cause burns or shock or can kill both patients and operating room personnel. All equipment must be properly grounded, and plugs and wiring must be undamaged. In addition, all equipment must be visually inspected *before use*.

Gas Cylinders

Gases stored in steel cylinders are under tremendous pressure. Failure to properly handle the relatively fragile valves, regulators, and fittings can turn a cylinder into an unguided missile propelled by escaping gas. This can cause substantial damage or even kill personnel in the path of the cylinder.

Patient Identification, Side, and Site of Surgery

There is no excuse for performing surgery on the wrong patient or on the wrong side of the patient, yet these mistakes do happen. All patients must be correctly identified at least twice before surgery begins. The patient chart, identification bracelet, and identification card (where applicable) should all agree. The patient should be asked to identify himself or herself and to confirm on which side the operation is to be performed.

Loss of an Item Within the Patient

A large number of lawsuits arising from surgery involve foreign objects left in the patient. The technologist, together with the circulating nurse and surgeon, is responsible for correct sponge, needle, and instrument counts. Except in the most urgent surgery, the technologist and nurse must not allow a busy surgeon (or one who is behind schedule) to bully them out of a proper count. If the count does not agree, the surgeon must be advised immediately. If the surgeon does not follow up by searching for the missing object or ordering a radiograph of the patient, that fact must be fully documented in the incident report.

Medications and Solutions

It is not unusual for the technologist to have several medications or solutions on the instrument table at the same time. Each one must be identified clearly so that the wrong drug or solution is not administered to the patient inadvertently. If there is any doubt about the contents of a particular cup or basin, it should be disposed of and replaced by the circulating nurse. When transmitting medications, both the deliverer and the receiver should state the contents (and dilution, if appropriate) to avoid any possibility of error.

Explosion

Although explosive anesthetic agents are no longer permitted in the operating room, there remains a danger of explosion from other agents and from the presence of in-line oxygen or oxygen stored in tanks. Oxygen supports combustion and creates a substantial fire hazard. If there is any doubt about the integrity of oxygen bottles, valves, or supply lines, it should be reported immediately and the equipment should not be used.

Abandonment of the Patient

Patients, regardless of their level of sedation, should never be left unattended. Responsibility for a patient should be passed specifically from one person to another. Never assume that someone will be along shortly to take care of a patient. Pediatric patients can be particularly curious and may attempt to escape from the stretcher, crib, or operating table. The incompetent or combative patient must be properly secured and attended at all times. The sedated or unconscious patient may be in danger of cardiopulmonary arrest and must be closely watched.

Specimens

The preservation and identification of specimens are crucial. The technologist and nurse should be sure that each specimen is properly identified, preserved, and labeled. Any tissue or item that is removed from the patient is considered a specimen unless specifically stated otherwise by the surgeon. This includes previously implanted prostheses or even debris such as metal or glass fragments. Bullets or other items originating from a weapon may be required for police inspection.

Informed Consent

Many lawsuits charge that the patient did not consent to the surgery or that the surgery went beyond the scope of the written or verbal consent. Although this is primarily the responsibility of the surgeon, the technologist and nurse can help reduce the number of these lawsuits. First, make sure that the chart includes the written authorization for the surgery (informed consent) signed by the patient or the patient's guardian. If the patient is sufficiently alert, the technologist or nurse should ask him or her what surgery is to be performed and, if applicable, on which side. If there is no written authorization or if the patient's oral response differs from that on the written form, the surgeon and operating room manager should be advised immediately. If it appears that the surgeon is about to exceed the limits of authorization ("While we're here let's . . ."), the technologist or nurse should advise the surgeon that there is no consent and should be sure that the records reflect the situation. If the surgeon persists, the technologist or nurse should not dispute the matter further but should document the incident *fully* after surgery.

A minor (a patient younger than the age of 18) may sign his or her own informed consent provided he or she is in one of the following categories:

- Fifteen years old, living apart from parents or guardian, and managing his or her own finances
- On active duty with the United States Armed Forces
- Pregnant
- Married, whether or not the marriage has been terminated by dissolution

An informed consent is not necessary under extreme emergency when the proposed procedure prevents further deterioration of the patient's condition.

Intentional Torts

Negligent acts are accidental; they are not intended by the person. However, operating room personnel can commit intentional acts that are not crimes but that cause harm. Two common examples of intentional torts are defamation and invasion of privacy.

Defamation

Operating room personnel occasionally see surgery that they believe is performed incompetently or know

physicians whose skills they believe are questionable. These opinions should not be shared with anyone outside the operating room unless the health and safety of the patient is in jeopardy. Derogatory statements made about one person to another is *defamation*. If the comment is made in writing, it is called *libel*; if made orally it is called *slander*. In either case the physician can sue unless the charges are proven to be true. This places the technologist and nurse in a sensitive position because the law states that the patient can sue these professionals for *not* reporting a physician who demonstrates a consistent lack of skill or exhibits other dangerous characteristics, such as symptoms of drug abuse or alcoholism.

The best course of action is to report the facts as they were observed in writing, as an incident report, and to the operating room manager, without inserting any opinion. For example, one could state, "This morning Dr. X was shaking and had alcohol on his breath, his speech was slurred, and he kept dropping instruments" rather than "Dr. X was drunk."

Invasions of Privacy and Patient Communication

The patient is entitled to privacy regarding all aspects of his or her illness. Legally, the patient's medical condition is confidential. Physicians are bound to keep all information about the patient's condition in confidence unless the patient gives specific permission to the physician to act differently. The technologist and nurse must honor that obligation and observe the same rules. They must not discuss patients with anyone outside the operating room.

The technologist must not discuss the specifics of the patient's disease, surgery, or prognosis with the patient. This could be construed as practicing medicine without a license and could also lead to problems such as raising false hopes (or fears) or misleading the patient.

ERRORS IN THE OPERATING ROOM

Errors and incidents occur in the operating room despite all precautions. Surgery personnel should be prepared for four types of incidents:

1. Errors made by themselves
2. Errors made by other technologists or nursing personnel
3. Physician error
4. Failure of a mechanical device

Technologist Errors

If a technologist realizes that he or she has made or might have made a mistake, the first thing to do is to admit it. Errors can often be rectified if caught early. There is no excuse for compounding the mistake by concealing it. Make sure that both the mistake and the corrective measures taken are reflected in an incident report.

In case of serious errors, such as an item left within the patient, the technologist should consult with the operating room manager and hospital administration to make sure that the legal department and insurance carriers are promptly notified of a potential claim. The technologist should report any mistakes he or she has made (or might have made) to his or her malpractice insurer.

Errors by Nursing Personnel or Other Technologists

If one technologist believes that an error has been made by a nurse or another technologist, he or she should first bring it to the attention of the person who committed the error. If the error is of a serious nature and is unresolved, it must be reported to the operating room manager, who can then decide whether to take further action.

Physician Errors

Physician error is a delicate problem. If the physician acknowledges the error and takes steps to correct it, the nurse or technologist should probably do nothing. If the physician errs and seems unaware of it, *and the error lies within the competence of the nurse or technologist to recognize,* it must be called to the attention of the physician and documented in an incident report. Examples of such errors are a foreign object's being left in the patient or the surgeon's gross contamination of the surgical wound.

In rare cases of a conspicuously incompetent or impaired physician, the facts should be carefully documented and reported to the operating room manager, as discussed earlier. These instances are unusual and should be discussed only with one's immediate supervisors to avoid defamation.

MECHANICAL FAILURES

The practice of surgery relies on numerous complex machines and instruments whose failure can injure both the patient and the hospital personnel. Regardless of the type of failure, the safety of the patient and others in the operating room suite must be ensured first. Once the situation has been stabilized, the defective equipment should be removed from service and labeled to avoid its use by the next team, who would otherwise be unaware of the problem. Next, the failure should be documented so that those responsible for repair can learn what happened and what service is required.

In the event of injury to a patient or staff member, further steps must be taken. Because a lawsuit could arise from the failure, the evidence should be preserved. Any broken parts should be saved and labeled, and perhaps photographs should be taken of the equipment as it was when the failure occurred. The hospital administration should be alerted through the operating room manager in the event of patient or staff injury so that the legal staff can be sure that everything necessary is done to protect the evidence. No part of the defective equipment should be given to a manufacturer's representative without specific authorization from the hospital administration.

Since 1991, the federal Safe Medical Devices Act has required hospitals to report within 10 days any incident in which a medical device "has or may have caused or contributed to" the death, injury, or serious illness of a patient. The act also requires hospitals to report "significant adverse device experiences," which may include injuries to persons other than patients and major malfunctions whether or not anyone was hurt. Every hospital should have forms and procedures for collecting the information for these reports.

DOCUMENTATION AND INCIDENT REPORTING

Every hospital policy manual prescribes which incidents and accidents are to be documented and what information the record should contain. The technologist and nurse should conform specifically to those standards, but some general rules also apply. Facts are important; opinions are not. Any report should contain only what was seen, done, or heard. Opinions and statements of conclusions not only are inappropriate and unprofessional but also add nothing to the report. "When in doubt, document" is also a good rule. Because it cannot always be determined what will be important following an incident or accident, it is best to note in writing anything and everything that has occurred. If witnesses were present during the incident, their names should be included in the report.

INSURANCE

Insurance is available to cover many risks, most of which should be familiar to the technologist and nurse from daily life. Insurance is also available for risks incurred in this profession and is usually called *errors and omissions* or *malpractice* insurance.

Coverage

Most errors and omissions policies cover the insured (policyholder) for accidents that result in claims made during the policy period, whenever the accident might have happened.

Is Insurance Needed?

Most technologists and nurses are employed by a hospital and covered by that hospital's policy. If this is the case, a separate policy is usually unnecessary. If the technologist or nurse is not employed by a hospital or if the hospital policy does not provide protection, then it is vital to have such coverage. Even if the technologist or nurse is blameless, the cost of hiring a lawyer to defend a lawsuit can be staggering.

What Does Insurance Do?

All errors and omissions policies provide that the insurance company will pay for the lawyer to defend a lawsuit and pay for a monetary award up to the policy limit.

What Does Insurance Cost?

Errors and omissions coverage for the technologist is available through AST at reasonable rates. At the time of this writing it is considerably less than the equivalent coverage on automobiles. Nurses can obtain coverage through their professional organization.

How Much Coverage Should One Have?

For the average technologist, the basic policy (with limits of $1 million per occurrence, up to a total of $3 million per year) should be more than sufficient. If the technologist has a number of valuable assets, additional policy should be purchased. An insurance broker familiar with medical malpractice insurance should be able to assist in the purchase of insurance with limits higher than those available through AST or nursing organizations.

LEGAL REPRESENTATION

The average technologist or nurse may never need a lawyer. Each person should, however, be able to recognize when one is necessary and be able to select one that is competent.

When Is a Lawyer Necessary?

A lawyer is needed when legal papers arrive. If a technologist or nurse is handed or receives any legal document, it should be shown to a lawyer immediately. Almost any lawyer will be able to explain the significance of the document, which usually will be a subpoena or a summons.

Subpoena

A subpoena (Fig. 3–1) is an order to appear as a witness to an incident. If a technologist or nurse is required to testify about an incident at the hospital, he or she should check with the hospital administration before doing so. In some cases the hospital (or its insurance carrier) may provide a lawyer to be present during the testimony.

There are two types of testimony that might have to be given. The most common is called a *deposition*. This is the testimony taken in a lawyer's office or in some other informal location and is given under oath and transcribed by a court reporter. All lawyers involved in the case are allowed to question the witness. The witness may have a lawyer present and will certainly have one if he or she is also involved directly in the lawsuit. The deposition can be read to the jury during trial if the witness is not available, or it can be read while the witness is testifying during the trial to show that the testimony has changed or to refresh the witness's memory.

The second form of testimony is that given in court during a trial. If required to testify at a trial, a technologist or nurse should inform the hospital administration and consider consulting an attorney, depending on the seriousness of the case and the degree of involvement in the suit. Anyone who receives a subpoena should remember that it is a court order requiring his or her presence; to disobey the subpoena can result in criminal penalties.

Summons

The second type of document is a summons (Fig. 3–2). A summons differs from a subpoena in that the summons makes its recipient a *party* to the lawsuit. If a person receives a summons, he or she is being sued. Attached to the summons is usually the *complaint* or *petition* that the lawyer for the injured person has filed with the court to initiate the suit. The person who was injured and is suing is called the *plaintiff*. The person being sued is the *defendant*.

All summonses require action by the recipient within a limited time (usually 20 to 30 days). One should take the papers to a lawyer or an insurance company immediately. Failure to do so could cause the case to be lost without ever having had the chance to defend oneself.

Selection of a Lawyer

If a technologist or nurse is insured, either personally or through the hospital, the insurance company will appoint a lawyer to handle the case. If the insurance company is not involved (such as when the nurse or technologist is not a party to the lawsuit), the best way to choose a lawyer is by referral. Any lawyer in the community can refer a person to another lawyer who specializes in a particular discipline. In most cases, the best lawyer for the nurse or technologist is one who defends medical malpractice cases. Lawyers who represent defendants (such as physicians and hospitals) will generally be more suitable than ones who represent

ATTORNEY OR PARTY WITHOUT ATTORNEY *(Name and Address)*:	TELEPHONE NO.:	FOR COURT USE ONLY

ATTORNEY FOR *(Name)*:

NAME OF COURT:
STREET ADDRESS:
MAILING ADDRESS:
CITY AND ZIP CODE:
BRANCH NAME:

PLAINTIFF/PETITIONER:

DEFENDANT/RESPONDENT:

CIVIL SUBPENA

☐ **Duces Tecum**

CASE NUMBER:

THE PEOPLE OF THE STATE OF CALIFORNIA, TO (NAME):

1. **YOU ARE ORDERED TO APPEAR AS A WITNESS in this action at the date, time, and place shown in the box below UNLESS you make a special agreement with the person named in item 3:**

   a. Date: Time: ☐ Dept.:   ☐ Div.:   ☐ Room:
   b. Address:

2. AND YOU ARE
   a. ☐ ordered to appear in person.
   b. ☐ not required to appear in person if you produce the records described in the accompanying affidavit and a completed declaration of custodian of records in compliance with Evidence Code sections 1560, 1561, 1562, and 1271. (1) Place a copy of the records in an envelope (or other wrapper). Enclose your original declaration with the records. Seal them. (2) Attach a copy of this subpena to the envelope or write on the envelope the case name and number, your name and date, time, and place from item 1 (the box above). (3) Place this first envelope in an outer envelope, seal it, and mail it to the clerk of the court at the address in item 1. (4) Mail a copy of your declaration to the attorney or party shown at the top of this form.
   c. ☐ ordered to appear in person and to produce the records described in the accompanying affidavit. The **personal attendance** of the custodian or other qualified witness and the production of the original records **is required** by this subpena. The procedure authorized by subdivision (b) of section 1560, and sections 1561 and 1562, of the Evidence Code will not be deemed suffficient compliance with this subpena.

3. **IF YOU HAVE ANY QUESTIONS ABOUT THE TIME OR DATE FOR YOU TO APPEAR, OR IF YOU WANT TO BE CERTAIN THAT YOUR PRESENCE IS REQUIRED, CONTACT THE FOLLOWING PERSON BEFORE THE DATE ON WHICH YOU ARE TO APPEAR:**
   a. Name: b. Telephone number:

4. **Witness Fees:** You are entitled to witness fees and mileage actually traveled both ways, as provided by law, if you request them at the time of service. You may request them before your scheduled appearance from the person named in item 3.

DISOBEDIENCE OF THIS SUBPENA MAY BE PUNISHED AS CONTEMPT BY THIS COURT. YOU WILL ALSO BE LIABLE FOR THE SUM OF FIVE HUNDRED DOLLARS AND ALL DAMAGES RESULTING FROM YOUR FAILURE TO OBEY.

Date issued:

. . . .   ▶
(TYPE OR PRINT NAME)   (SIGNATURE OF PERSON ISSUING SUBPENA)

                                        (TITLE)
                (See reverse for proof of service)

Form Adopted by Rule 982   **CIVIL SUBPENA**   Code of Civil Procedure, §§ 1985, 1986, 1987
Judicial Council of California
982(a)(15) [Rev. January 1, 1991]

Figure 3–1. Example of a subpoena. (Courtesy of the Judicial Council of California.)

SUMMONS
(CITACION JUDICIAL)

NOTICE TO DEFENDANT: *(Aviso a Acusado)*

YOU ARE BEING SUED BY PLAINTIFF:
(A Ud. le está demandando)

You have *30 CALENDAR DAYS* after this summons is served on you to file a typewritten response at this court.

A letter or phone call will not protect you; your typewritten response must be in proper legal form if you want the court to hear your case.

If you do not file your response on time, you may lose the case, and your wages, money and property may be taken without further warning from the court.

There are other legal requirements. You may want to call an attorney right away. If you do not know an attorney, you may call an attorney referral service or a legal aid office (listed in the phone book).

Después de que le entreguen esta citación judicial usted tiene un plazo de 30 DIAS CALENDARIOS para presentar una respuesta escrita a máquina en esta corte.

Una carta o una llamada telefónica no le ofrecerá protección; su respuesta escrita a máquina tiene que cumplir con las formalidades legales apropiadas si usted quiere que la corte escuche su caso.

Si usted no presenta su respuesta a tiempo, puede perder el caso, y le pueden quitar su salario, su dinero y otras cosas de su propiedad sin aviso adicional por parte de la corte.

Existen otros requisitos legales. Puede que usted quiera llamar a un abogado inmediatamente. Si no conoce a un abogado, puede llamar a un servicio de referencia de abogados o a una oficina de ayuda legal (vea el directorio telefónico).

The name and address of the court is: *(El nombre y dirección de la corte es)*

CASE NUMBER. *(Número del Caso)*

The name, address, and telephone number of plaintiff's attorney, or plaintiff without an attorney, is:
(El nombre, la dirección y el número de teléfono del abogado del demandante, o del demandante que no tiene abogado, es)

DATE:
(Fecha)

Clerk, by _____, Deputy
(Actuario)   *(Delegado)*

[SEAL]

NOTICE TO THE PERSON SERVED: You are served
1. ☐ as an individual defendant.
2. ☐ as the person sued under the fictitious name of *(specify)*:
3. ☐ on behalf of *(specify)*:

under: ☐ CCP 416.10 (corporation)   ☐ CCP 416.60 (minor)
        ☐ CCP 416.20 (defunct corporation)   ☐ CCP 416.70 (conservatee)
        ☐ CCP 416.40 (association or partnership)   ☐ CCP 416.90 (individual)
        ☐ other:
4. ☐ by personal delivery on *(date)*:

Form Adopted by Rule 982
Judicial Council of California
982(a)(9) [Rev. January 1, 1984]

(See reverse for Proof of Service)
SUMMONS

*CCP 412.20

Figure 3–2. Example of a summons. (Courtesy of the Judicial Council of California.)

plaintiffs (unless a person wishes to file a lawsuit, in which case that person will be a plaintiff). Because lawyers are costly, several may be interviewed before one is selected.

Questions for Study and Review

1. What is the legal status of certification by the Association of Surgical Technologists?

2. What four agencies of the federal government issue regulations pertaining to health care personnel?

3. Define *medical practice acts*.

4. Investigate whether your state allows you to act as first assistant to the surgeon.

5. What should you do if a patient arrives in the operating room and he or she is wearing a watch?

6. Give a legal definition of *negligence*.

7. Give a legal definition of a *tort*.

8. Discuss three hypothetical accidents that might be caused by negligence in the operating room.

Bibliography

Association of Operating Room Nurses: Legislation: 1989–1990 Legislative Committee updates RN first assistant survey. AORN J 51(6):1591–1598, 1990.

California Business & Professions Code §§ 2051, 2052, 2732, 2725, 2725.1

Colorado Revised Statutes § 12-36-106.

Creighton H: Law Every Nurse Should Know, 5th ed. Philadelphia, WB Saunders, 1986.

Illinois Revised Statutes (1981). chap 111.

New York Education Law, § 6521.

Title 21, United States Code, § 360i.

Title 42, Code of Federal Regulations § 482.51(a) (3).

Witkin B: Summary of California Law, 9th ed. Vol 5–6. San Francisco, Bancroft-Whitney Co, 1988.

Organization of the Operating Room: Personnel and Environment

Learning Objectives

After reading this chapter you should be able to

♦ *Define* the roles of those who work in surgery.
♦ *Review* the specific responsibilities of a circulator.
♦ *Determine* which circulating duties are restricted to the registered nurse.
♦ *List* the duties of the scrub technologist.
♦ *Discuss* the duties of the technologist when he or she is neither scrub nor circulating.
♦ *Describe* the protocol for the movement of supplies and personnel in the operating room.
♦ *Describe* the various work areas of the operating room.
♦ *Describe* the equipment found in the operating room suite.

Key Terms

circulator: Surgical team member who does not perform a surgical hand scrub or don sterile attire, and thus does not work within the sterile field.
frozen section: A fine slice of frozen biopsy tissue that is microscopically examined for the presence of disease.
gurney: Stretcher.
JCAHO: Joint Commission on Accreditation of Healthcare Organizations.
nurse anesthetist: Registered nurse who administers anesthesia under the supervision of an anesthesiologist.

PACU: Post-anesthesia care unit.
pathologist: Medical doctor who specializes in the identification of diseased tissue.
unit secretary: Secretary of the operating room.
vector: An intermediate source that transmits bacteria from one surface to another.

Part I ◆ PERSONNEL

The responsibilities and functions of every member of the surgical department are clearly defined in writing in the hospital's *operating room policy or procedure manual.* These policies are written to clarify the job description and to establish the accountability of each employee. They comply with state and federal laws and ensure that the hospital meets the minimum standards set by the Joint Commission of Accreditation of Healthcare Organizations (JCAHO). These policies must be strictly followed because they define the scope of practice for each employee and provide a chain of command necessary to the safe and efficient operation of the department. The number and type of personnel who compose the operating room staff depends on the size of the hospital and the activity of the surgical case load. The organization, titles, ranking, and educational requirements of staff members vary from hospital to hospital.

SURGEON

The operating surgeon's role is often compared to that of a ship's captain. During surgery he or she is the person who ultimately guides the flow and scope of what happens in the surgical suite. The surgeon operates under the prescribed policies of the hospital in which he or she works and is licensed under the medical practice acts in his or her state.

ANESTHESIOLOGIST

The anesthesiologist is a physician who is specially trained to administer anesthetic agents to the surgical patient. He or she is also responsible for the meticulous monitoring and adjustment of the patient's physiologic status during surgery. The anesthesiologist is trained to render immediate care in the event of physiologic crisis. The nurse anesthetist is a highly trained registered nurse who renders the same care as the anesthesiologist but must work under the supervision of an anesthesiologist.

OPERATING ROOM SUPERVISOR

The operating room supervisor is responsible for overseeing all clinical and professional activities in the department. He or she helps to set policies concerning major clinical and professional practices in the operating room. It is also his or her duty to implement and enforce these policies. This position is ideally held by a registered nurse who holds a master's degree in nursing or business administration with at least 3 years operating room and post-anesthesia care unit (PACU) experience. Depending on the hospital, the operating room supervisor is accountable to the director of nurses or the nursing director of the operating room and PACU. The operating room supervisor may represent the department at supervisory meetings by helping to coordinate activities in other departments with those of the operating room. He or she may also develop and supervise educational programs and seminars within the department.

NURSE MANAGER

The nurse manager assists the operating room supervisor in his or her duties. If the supervisor is absent from the department, the head nurse assumes the role of supervisor. He or she may or may not participate in surgery and is responsible to both the supervisor and the director of nurses.

CLINICAL NURSE

The clinical or staff nurse is a highly educated clinical professional. He or she holds a current license in nursing and may also have advanced degrees in a clinical specialty. The staff nurse functions on the surgical team in one of several ways. He or she may act as a circulating nurse, or "circulator," an instrument or scrub nurse, or a surgical first assistant. The clinical nurse performs his or her duties in accordance with the scope and type of education, individual level of clinical experience, and the laws of the state. The staff nurse is accountable to the head nurse, operating room director, or operating room supervisor. All paraprofessional personnel, including operating room technologists, are accountable to the staff nurse. Although exact duties vary from hospital to hospital, the following describes the functions of the staff nurse circulator.

Perioperative Duties of the Staff Nurse Circulator

Preoperative Phase

Patient Arrival in the Operating Room

1. Greets the patient on arrival in surgery and assesses his or her level of consciousness.
2. Verifies with the patient the site and side of the procedure.

3. Reviews the chart and establishes that the surgeon's preoperative orders including preparation of the wound site have been completed.

4. Completes a preoperative care plan that includes assessment, plan implementation, evaluation, and expected outcome of nursing care during the perioperative period. Briefly explains the perioperative phases to the patient.

5. Answers any questions the patient may have about the procedure.

6. Communicates to the surgeon any irregularities noted in the preoperative preparation of the surgical site.

7. Communicates to the surgeon any irregularities noted in the patient's physical, physiologic, or emotional condition.

8. Communicates to the scrub technologist or nurse any conditions that would directly affect his or her preparation for this surgery.

9. Prepares the patient for any sights, smells, or sounds that might be disturbing.

Patient Arrival Within the Surgical Suite

1. Assists in the safe transfer of the patient from the stretcher (gurney) to the operating table.

2. Assists the anesthesiologist or nurse anesthetist with the patient preparation for anesthesia.

3. Directs or participates in the initial sponge, needle, and instrument counts.

4. Applies patient grounding device when applicable.

5. Ensures that the patient is warm and comfortable while awaiting the start of the surgery.

6. Offers emotional support to the patient before and during induction of anesthesia.

Intraoperative Phase

All Cases

1. Assists the anesthesiologist or anesthetist during induction of anesthesia.

2. Assists in the safe positioning of the patient.

3. Maintains an aseptic environment within the surgical suite.

4. Receives nonsterile ends of suction tubing, electrical cords, power cables, electrocautery pencils, and other items that must be connected to nonsterile units.

5. Ties the gowns of scrubbed personnel.

6. Adjusts the surgical lights as needed.

7. Prevents the unnecessary movement of personnel into and out of the surgical suite.

8. Directs and participates in sponge, needle, and instrument counts.

9. Aseptically opens and delivers any additional sterile supplies needed by scrubbed team members.

10. Documents supplies used during surgery.

11. When their presence is required in the suite, notifies support personnel such as the x-ray technician or pathologist.

12. Documents any irregularities or incidents that occur during surgery.

13. Delivers any medications needed to the scrub technologist or nurse.*

14. Obtains blood components or other fluids as needed by the anesthesiologist.*

15. Correctly identifies type and location of any specimens obtained during surgery including tissue, fluids, foreign bodies, or prosthetics. Documents and preserves specimens.

16. Strictly follows procedure for Universal Precautions (described in Chapter 5) during the case.

17. Communicates to PACU any necessary equipment that will be needed based on the patient's physical and physiologic needs.

Local or Regional Anesthetic Cases

1. Assesses the patient's cardiac and pulmonary status. Documents status.*

2. Reports changes in the patient's pulse, respiration, temperature, and blood pressure.*

3. Provides emotional support to the patient during the procedure.

Postoperative Phase

1. Assists the anesthesiologist during the patient's emergence from general anesthesia.

2. Assists the surgical team in the transfer of the patient from the operating table to the gurney.

3. Accompanies the patient and anesthesiologist to PACU.

4. Reports to the family, spouse, or significant other on the patient's condition.

5. Reports the identity and physical status of the patient to the PACU nurse.*

6. Reports the type and site of operative procedure.

7. Reports any impairment resulting from the operative procedure.*

8. Reports the type and site of drains, catheters, and tubing.*

9. Communicates necessary equipment needs based on the physical assessment of the patient.*

Duties of the Scrub or Instrument Nurse

The role of the staff nurse when he or she is functioning as a scrub or instrument nurse is nearly identical to that of the scrub technologist (see later).

Duties of the Registered Nurse First Assistant

In 1984 the Association of Operating Room Nurses (AORN) defined the role of the registered nurse (RN) first assistant:

---

*May be strictly forbidden by the state's nurse practice act, even under the supervision of a registered nurse.

The RN first assistant to the surgeon during a surgical procedure carries out functions that will assist the surgeon in performing a safe operation with optimal results for the patient. The RN first assistant practices perioperative nursing and has acquired the knowledge, skills, and judgment, necessary to assist the surgeon, through organized instruction and supervised practice. The RN first assistant practices under the direct supervision of the surgeon during the first assisting phase of the perioperative role.

The first assistant does not concurrently function as a scrub nurse. Behaviors unique to the RN first assistant may include the following:

- Tissue handling
- Providing exposure using instruments
- Suturing
- Providing homeostasis

The RN first assistant always functions under the direct supervision of the surgeon, and not all states allow the practice of first assistant by a registered nurse.

SURGICAL TECHNOLOGIST

The duties of the surgical technologist are defined by the written policies of the hospital in which he or she works and by his or her level and type of education. The scope of practice is limited by the nursing or medical practice acts for the state in which he or she practices. The technologist, when functioning in a circulating or scrub role, does so under the supervision of the registered nurse. The policies of the JCAHO explicitly state that when the technologist acts as a circulator, a registered nurse must be *immediately available* to respond to emergencies. Because the technologist (or other paraprofessional personnel) may not be trained to evaluate and respond to critical emergencies, *it is inappropriate for a hospital to force the technologist into this role without immediate professional supervision. Likewise, no technologist should endanger the patient's safety by violating these critical standards.*

As Circulator

The role of the surgical technologist as circulator is defined earlier under the heading of Perioperative Duties of the Staff Nurse Circulator. Duties that are followed by an asterisk (*) may be strictly forbidden by the state's nurse practice acts, *even under the supervision of a registered nurse.* Some of these activities involve the choice and distribution of medications or blood components, an area in which the technologist is neither educated nor licensed. Others require the physical or physiologic assessment of the patient, another area of critical care in which the technologist is not licensed.

As Scrub Assistant

The functions discussed below comprise a broad range of activities performed by the technologist. He or she

may perform all or some of these, depending on the needs of the specific operating room and the skills of the technologist. Each of these will be discussed in detail later in the text.

1. Assists in the sterile gowning and gloving of the surgeon and his or her assistant.
2. Is responsible for the maintenance of an orderly surgical field. He or she must keep the instrument table neat so that supplies can be handed quickly and efficiently.
3. Prevents injury to the patient by removing heavy or sharp instruments from the operative site as soon as the surgeon has finished using them.
4. Prevents contamination of the surgical field by the strict practice of aseptic technique.
5. Prevents the possible contamination of team members by blood-borne pathogens by following Universal Precautions standards set by the hospital.
6. Is constantly alert to any intraoperative dangers to the patient.
7. Takes part in sponge, needle, and instrument counts, as needed. All of these items must be accounted for during the procedure. The technologist takes part in counting the items before, during, and after surgery to ensure that they are not left in the wound. The count is done in an orderly way and is performed using accepted technique.
8. Accepts and properly identifies any medications or solutions and does so in a prescribed manner.
9. Properly identifies and preserves specimens received during surgery. The technologist is responsible for maintaining the specimens in a prescribed manner so that the material can be subsequently examined by the pathologist.
10. Anticipates the needs of the surgeon by watching the progress of the surgery and knowing the various steps of the procedure. He or she passes instruments and other supplies in an acceptable manner so that the surgeon does not have to turn away from the wound site to receive them.
11. Assists the surgeon by tissue retraction, suture cutting, fluid evacuation, or sponging the wound when asked to do so.
12. At the end of the procedure, assembles all instruments and supplies and prepares them for decontamination and resterilization and assists in the safe clean-up of the operating suite following Universal Precautions.

As First Assistant

In some hospitals, the surgical technologist may act as first assistant to the surgeon. The duties of the technologist as first assistant vary according to his or her level of education and qualifications and the state in which he or she practices. In this role, the technologist works under the direct supervision of the surgeon and assists in such duties as hemostasis, suturing, and wound dressing.

State sanction of the technologist as first assistant is varied and complex. In some states the practice is forbidden, and in others its legality is ambiguous or uncertain. Chapter 3 includes a more complete discussion of this issue.

Other Functions of the Technologist

When the technologist is neither scrubbed nor circulating he or she has other responsibilities in the department, including the following:

1. Assists in ordering and stocking supplies for the department. The technologist may be responsible for ordering new supplies from the manufacturer or from the materials supply department.
2. Prepares instruments and supplies for sterilization. The technologist takes part in cleaning instruments and supplies and in wrapping them properly for sterilization. He or she is knowledgeable about sterilization techniques and knows which methods of sterilization are best for a given piece of equipment. He or she is responsible for maintenance of equipment and makes sure that it is sent out for repair when necessary.
3. May assist in the safe transportation of patients in and out of the department.
4. May perform the preoperative preparation of the surgical site on the patient's ward.
5. Assists in restocking the operating room suites and removes those items that need resterilization.
6. May assist in the preparation and selection of equipment for scheduled procedures.

LICENSED PRACTICAL OR VOCATIONAL NURSE

The duties and scope of practice of the practical or vocational nurse are virtually the same as those of the surgical technologist. The type and extent of the education of the licensed practical nurse or licensed vocational nurse dictate the role and to what extent that role is fulfilled. As with the surgical technologist, the professional or vocational nurse's role depends on the supervision of a registered nurse.

UNIT SECRETARY

The surgical unit secretary receives scheduling requests from the surgeons or their representatives. He or she must also answer the telephone and relay messages into and out of the surgical department. In the event of emergency he or she must reschedule any cases that have been canceled (or "bumped") and notify all personnel involved in those cases. The unit secretary is under considerable strain to maintain an orderly schedule and to satisfy the scheduling needs of many different surgeons. Consequently the job requires a composed and efficient personality. He or she must be knowledgeable about medical and surgical terminology, have excellent communication skills, and be able to cheerfully but firmly cope with the many demands made during the workday.

SURGICAL ORDERLY/AIDE

The function of the surgical orderly or aide depends on the size of the hospital and the availability of other types of paraprofessional personnel. The orderly participates in many types of patient care services, including the transportation of the patient to and from the surgical department, the preoperative preparation of the wound site, and the transfer of patients on and off the operating table. He or she may also participate in the safe cleanup of the surgical suite after procedures and in the restocking of supplies. He or she assists in the preparation of supplies and instruments for decontamination and sterilization. The job of the orderly is demanding because there are many requests for his or her attention by many members of the surgery department. He or she must be knowledgeable in patient care and Universal Precautions, have a caring attitude toward his or her patients, and be able to switch job assignments very quickly.

RELATED PERSONNEL

The *pathologist* is a medical doctor who specializes in the identification of disease tissue. He or she is available to examine biopsy or resection tissue while surgery is in progress. Fine slices of tissue are made of the biopsy specimen after it has been quickfrozen and are then examined under the microscope. These slices are called *frozen sections*. If malignancy is discovered, the decision to proceed with radical surgery can be made immediately. This prevents the need for a subsequent separate operative procedure to remove the area of malignancy.

X-ray personnel are available to come into the surgical suite and take radiographs during procedures such as operative cholangiography or in orthopedic cases.

Part II ◆ STRUCTURE AND DESIGN OF THE OPERATING ROOM

PHYSICAL LAYOUT

There are many different types of layouts suitable for the modern operating room. Although layouts vary from institution to institution, the goals of all design concepts are patient safety and work efficiency. Because of the constant danger of contamination to the surgical patient, design engineers strive clearly delineate "clean" from "hazardous" or contaminated areas of the surgical department. In this text the term *unrestricted* refers to hazardous areas. The functions of the area or room define whether it is restricted. Unrestricted areas are those that carry a high potential for cross-contamination by disease-carrying organisms. All personnel must un-

derstand which areas are clean, which are contaminated, and which are mixed. The patient receiving area, dressing rooms, lounges, and office are considered unrestricted. The hallways between various rooms in the department, instrument and supply processing area, storage areas, and utility rooms are semi-restricted. The operating suites themselves, scrub sink areas, and sterile supply rooms are all restricted. Full surgical attire, including masks, must be worn in these areas.

A common floor plan used in the modern operating room is one in which the surgical suites are arranged around a central core work area (Fig. 4–1). The administrative offices, lounges, dressing rooms, preoperative areas, and PACU are located in adjoining but separate

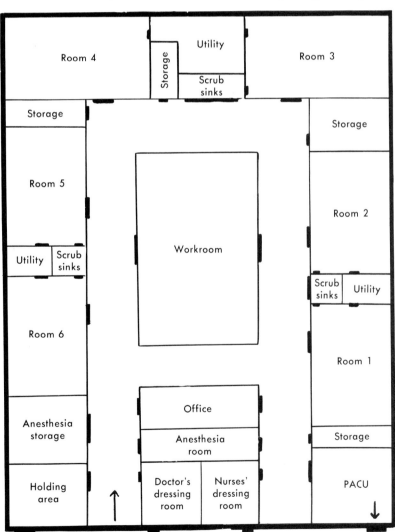

Figure 4–1. Floor plan of the surgery department. Note that the workroom is centrally located. (From Brooks SM: Fundamentals of Operating Room Nursing, 2nd ed. St. Louis, CV Mosby, 1979.)

areas. When traffic and equipment move from one area to the next, a certain protocol must be followed. Hospital protocols may vary slightly, but all follow the same principle: clean areas are restricted to clean traffic, and contaminated areas are restricted to contaminated traffic.

Protocol for the Movement of Supplies and Personnel

1. Persons entering the department from outside should not enter restricted areas unless clothed in surgical attire (discussed fully in Chapter 8).

2. Surgical personnel leaving the department must cover their clothing with appropriate attire such as lab coat and shoe covers. These items must be discarded before entering the surgical department.

3. Doors between clean and hazardous areas must be kept closed at all times.

4. Shipping cartons that contain surgical supplies for the department must be discarded before the supplies are accepted. Only the inner packaging is acceptable in a clean area.

5. Food and drink must be restricted to the lounge areas.

6. If the central supply and instrument processing area is located away from the operating room, a dumbwaiter, elevator, or conveyer system must be used to carry contaminated equipment out of the department. Two separate systems should be in place: one for soiled or contaminated equipment and one for clean equipment or instruments.

7. Clean or sterilized equipment received from outside the department should arrive draped or wrapped with an outside barrier cover that is dust and water resistant. The cover must be discarded before the supplies pass into clean area.

8. Soiled linen and trash must be kept in a restricted area while awaiting transfer out of the department.

9. Patients are commonly transported to surgery on a gurney, not a hospital bed. When it is necessary for the patient to be transported in a bed, such as an orthopedic bed, the bed must not be brought into the clean area of the department before being cleaned with a disinfectant.

DESCRIPTION AND FUNCTION OF AREAS IN THE OPERATING ROOM

Preoperative Area

The preoperative area is where patients are received before surgery. This area provides a quiet atmosphere where patients are not disturbed by traffic into and out of the department. It should be located adjacent to the surgical suite and be supplied with any equipment or medications that might be needed in the event of an emergency, such as suction, a defibrillator, or oxygen. The room must also be equipped with an emergency alarm system. The use of a separate preoperative area provides a safe place for the patient and prevents obstruction of hallways with patient beds and gurneys. In addition, it allows the patient privacy while awaiting surgery. Many patients feel justifiably disturbed when left in the midst of the traffic and noise of department corridors while awaiting surgery. This "cattle car" arrangement can be demoralizing and dangerous to the patient. Patients in the preoperative area must never be left unattended or unguarded. The preoperative room can be used by surgery personnel to complete the preoperative check-in, review the medical chart, and assess the physical and emotional status of the patient. The operative wound site may be prepared here. Intravenous lines and urinary retention catheters may also be inserted in this area.

Dressing (Locker) Rooms

Dressing rooms are used by surgical personnel to change into surgical attire from their street clothes. Each dressing room or locker room should be equipped with shower and toilet facilities. Personnel may obtain their surgical attire before entering the locker room, or scrub suits may be available in closed cabinets within the area. This area may adjoin the lounge area, but personnel should not enter the lounge area unless fully attired in scrub clothing.

Surgical Office

The surgical office is the workplace of the unit secretary or the operating room supervisor and his or her assistant. Guests may be received here at a pass-through window that overlooks the corridor leading into the surgery department. This design prevents personnel in street clothing from entering the office. When the office is directly adjacent to the entry doors of the department, the surgical secretary or supervisor can control the entry of unauthorized personnel into the department and also ensure that those who do enter are properly attired.

Instrument Workroom

The workroom is the area where soiled instruments and equipment are decontaminated, washed, and then wrapped or packaged for resterilization. The area must be subdivided into two separate areas to prevent the contamination of clean supplies by those that are contaminated. Some hospitals employ a system in which the processed, clean unwrapped instruments pass through a washer-sterilizer and then are received on the other side to be wrapped. This system prevents personnel from physically carrying clean instruments through the contaminated area into the clean one. Some hospitals employ a case cart system of cleanup whereby all soiled instruments and supplies are sent directly out of the department to a central processing area in the hospital by way of a dumbwaiter or conveyor system. Clean supplies are then sent back to the department through a separate transportation system. Further discussion of the case cart system can be found in Chapter 6.

Sterile Supply Room

The sterile supply room is a clean area and houses all sterilized and packaged instruments and supplies needed for surgery. Unless a case cart system is in use, surgery personnel assemble items needed for a particular case from the supply located in this room. The supplies must be arranged neatly on shelves whose lowest point is not more than 8 inches from the floor and whose highest point is not less than 18 inches from the ceiling. Supplies here are routinely checked for "outdates" (expiration dates for the sterility of the prepackaged supplies) and for package integrity.

Equipment Room

The equipment room is used to store large apparatus such as the operating microscope, image intensifier, and laser machine. Some hospitals also store their gas anesthesia machines in this area. The equipment stored here should be kept free of dust and cleaned routinely just as in any other area of the operating room. The equipment room is a valuable area because it prevents the storage of such equipment in hallways where it could be a hazard or become damaged.

Housekeeping Supply Room

The housekeeping supply room is an area where supplies used to decontaminate the surgical suites and those used in general operating room cleanup are stored. The area may also contain a hopper where contaminated liquids and fluids are disposed of. The cleanup equipment and supplies stored here must be restricted to use within the operating room to prevent cross-contamination from other areas of the hospital. Large operating rooms may have several cleanup and supply areas.

Anesthesia Supply Room

As the name suggests, the anesthesia supply room is where all equipment needed by the anesthesiologists is stored. Anesthesia machines, hoses, catheters, airway devices, and other equipment are located in this area. This room may also contain a cabinet to house nongaseous anesthetic agents.

Substerile Rooms

Substerile rooms are located between one or more operating suites. These rooms typically contain a refrig-erator for small tissue grafts, medications, and solutions. A blanket warmer and utility sink are usually found here also. The substerile room contains an autoclave for sterilizing unwrapped instruments and equipment. Some also contain a washer-sterilizer.

Scrub Sink Area

Scrub sink areas (Fig. 4–2) are found in various locations close to the operating suites. Caps, masks, antiseptic soap, scrub brushes, and eyeglass defogging agents are located at each scrub station. Protective eyewear for use during management requiring Universal Precautions may also be found in this area. The scrub sink area must be located away from wrapped sterile supplies because of their possible contamination by water droplets and spray from the sinks. Scrub sinks must never, under any circumstances, be used for the cleanup of equipment or instruments.

The Operating Suites

Design and Environmental Control

In this text, the term *operating suite* is used to designate the individual room where surgery is performed. All operating suites are similar in design. They are roomy enough to allow scrubbed personnel to move around nonsterile equipment without contamination. The architectural design is uncluttered and simple so that dust is not trapped in areas that would be difficult to clean. The operating suite, like other areas of the operating room, is designed for maximum patient safety. The floors, ceilings, and other surfaces are smooth, nonporous, and constructed of fireproof materials. The smooth surfaces allow thorough cleaning and prevent

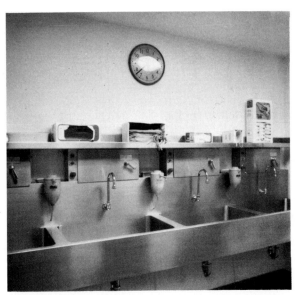

Figure 4–2. Scrub sink area. These sinks are operated by a push button. The water shuts off automatically after the scrub.

the trapping of biologic material that could cause cross-contamination. All surface materials are made to withstand frequent washings and cleaning with strong disinfectants. In older operating rooms where flammable anesthetic gases are used, the floors are conductive. However, there has been a trend away from the use of these agents, and consequently many new operating rooms do not have conductive flooring.

The *ventilation system* in the surgical suite is engineered to prevent the possible contamination of the clean environment by air-borne bacteria. The current requirements call for 20 exchanges of air per hour, 4 of which must be fresh. Clean air exchange depends on the positive pressure of air within the suite. This air is derived directly from the outside to avoid circulating air that might be contaminated by passage through other areas of the hospital. There should be no more than 20 exchanges per hour because the turbulence thus created would cause a great amount of dust and bacteria to be swept about the room. The humidity is also controlled to minimize static electricity and consequent ignition of any flammable solutions or objects used in the operating room. The ideal humidity level to achieve minimal static and also reduce microbial growth is 50% to 55%. The air temperature is maintained at 20°C to 24°C (68°F to 75°F). Scavenging systems that pull anesthetic gases out of the environmental air and shunt them away from the surgical suite have gained favor in recent years. These systems are now in place in modern operating rooms.

Lighting in the operating suite is achieved by the use of main overhead fluorescent lights and by the surgical spotlights themselves. Halogen lamps are used within the surgical spotlights. Halogen lamps have a higher color temperature (measurement of the hue that a light emits) than incandescent light. Hence, the halogen light emits a pale bluish cast that is less fatiguing to the eyes. The bluish cast is an indication of immense energy. The energy is given off in brightness (intensity) rather than heat and is thus safe to use near delicate tissue. The overhead surgical spotlights are mounted on a post that is suspended from the ceiling. Typically, two spotlights are attached to each post, although a third satellite lamp may be added for increased visibility or extension of the lighted field. Track lights are undesirable in the surgical suite since dust and bacteria are trapped in the tracks, which are difficult to keep clean.

In some operating suites, closed-circuit television cameras are mounted within the framework of the surgical lights so that the course of the operation can be viewed by students or auxiliary personnel outside the department.

The *electrical* system in the operating room meets minimum standards set by the National Fire Protection Association (NFPA). All outlets are grounded and explosion proof. In modern operating suites, rigid outlet columns that extend from the ceiling are equipped to receive electrical cords, suction, and compressed air. These prevent the draping of cords across the floor, where they might become a hazard to personnel. A system that ensures that no piece of equipment is grounded through a higher resistance than any other piece of equipment is called an *equal-potential grounding system*. This system, in place in the surgical suite, ensures that the shortest distance to the ground is not through the patient.

Operating Suite Equipment

The *operating table* on which the patient is positioned for surgery is fully adjustable for height, degree of tilt in all directions, orientation in the room, articular breaks, and length. This allows manipulation of the patient in any position while maintaining proper body alignment. The surface is covered with a firm pad that can be removed for cleaning.

Many accessories are available to meet the needs of different types of surgery. *Removable armboards* allow extension of the patient's arms and hands for intravenous lines. The *surgical armboard* is wider and provides a broader surface on which to place the hand and arm for surgery in these areas. *Stirrups*, used in gynecologic and some general surgical procedures, connect to the mid-break of the table, which is flexed downward and away or removed altogether. *Leg holders* may be attached to the sides of the table for access to the knee or for the scrub prep of the leg when it must be held up away from the table surface. A special tabletop *cassette attachment* that accepts x-ray cassettes is added to the table surface for operative procedures that require radiographs.

The *back table* is a large table on which all instruments and supplies except those in immediate use are placed during surgery. Before surgery a sterile linen pack is opened onto the table and sterile supplies are deposited there. After gowning and gloving, the scrub technologist or nurse arranges the supplies in an orderly fashion.

The *Mayo stand* is a tray supported by two legs that is placed immediately adjacent to the operative site. The scrub technologist or nurse places instruments that will be used frequently during a procedure on this stand where they are immediately accessible. The stand is adjustable in height and may also be placed directly over but never in contact with the patient.

The *Gerhardt (overhead) table* is a combination Mayo stand and back table. The overhead table is positioned over but not touching the patient and is used frequently in craniotomy cases, although it may be used for other types of procedures. The large surface of the table provides the scrub technologist or nurse immediate access to numerous instruments and supplies without the use of a back table.

The *kick bucket* is used by surgical team members to discard soiled sponges during surgery. The bucket frame has wheels so that it can be easily moved about the suite.

A gas *anesthesia machine* is kept in each surgical suite. Other accessory equipment such as physiologic monitor, anesthesia supply cart, intravenous standards, and sitting stools are also supplied to each room. The *intercom system* is the primary link between the surgical team and personnel outside the surgery suite. All intercom systems are equipped with an emergency call button that can be activated by foot or knee. This emergency system allows scrub personnel to remain sterile while alerting outside personnel of the emergency. Routine communication is carried out by push button. A call light is also mounted so that incoming calls are identified visually rather than by the sound of a buzzer. The intercom system establishes communication throughout the department. Calls that must be made to outside auxiliary personnel, such as the pathologist or x-ray technician, are usually placed by the surgical secretary or operating room supervisor.

Supply cabinets located in each room are used to store such items as suture material, dressings, intravenous solutions, sponges, and a few commonly used instruments. Supplies should be stacked in wire baskets so that accumulation of dust is minimal. In some operating rooms the cabinets are double sided so that they may be accessed from either the surgical suite or the hallway outside the suite.

Post-Anesthesia Care Unit

The post-anesthesia care unit (PACU) (Fig. 4–3) is located immediately adjacent to the operating room and is supervised by that department's nursing and administrative personnel. Patients are taken to the PACU immediately following surgery so that they can be continuously monitored while emerging from general or light anesthesia. This area of the department is staffed by highly qualified nursing personnel who can quickly assess the patient's cardiac, respiratory, and physiologic status and respond immediately with appropriate assistance. The course of the patient's emergence is meticulously documented and reviewed by the anesthesiologist, as needed. Each recovering patient is assigned to a separate cubicle that is equipped with oxygen, suction, electrical outlets, and extensive monitoring equipment. An emergency cart is centrally located and equipped with a defibrillator, airway maintenance supplies, emergency drugs, and other supplies. The PACU is linked directly with the surgical office and operating room supervisor's office by intercom. Emergency call buttons are located throughout the department.

Surgical Outpatient Department

In recent years there has been a large increase in the number of patients undergoing surgery on an outpatient basis. With the advent of conscious anesthetic agents (described in Chapter 9), more and more patients are choosing recovery at home rather than in the hospital setting. The outpatient rooms are equipped with the same facilities as those described for the surgical suites. Some hospitals use the outpatient facilities for endoscopic procedures such as esophagoscopy and gastroscopy except when extensive x-ray equipment is needed.

Questions for Study and Review

1. Which circulating duties are restricted to the registered nurse?

2. When may a technologist circulate alone?

3. May a technologist distribute a medication to a scrub technologist if a registered nurse is in the room?

4. Discuss the duties of the scrub technologist.

5. Why must the humidity be controlled in the operating room?

6. What is the NFPA?

7. Why are halogen lights used in the operating suite?

8. Why is circulating air in the operating room brought in from outside the hospital?

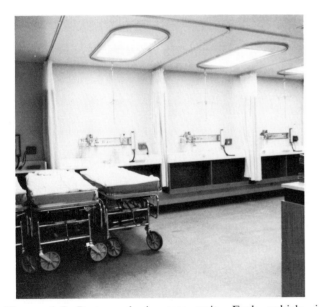

Figure 4–3. Post-anesthesia care unit. Each cubicle is equipped with suction, blood pressure monitor, and separate overhead light.

Bibliography

Association of Operating Room Nurses: Recommended Practices for Traffic Patterns in the Surgical Suite. Denver, 1988.
Groah L: Operating Room Nursing: Perioperative Practice, 2nd ed. Norwalk, CT, Appleton & Lange, 1990.

Microbiology Overview and Acquired Immunodeficiency Syndrome

Learning Objectives

After reading this chapter you should be able to

- ◆ *Understand* bacterial structure and physiology.
- ◆ *Understand* the process of disease transmission.
- ◆ *Discuss* the process of infection.
- ◆ *Discuss* the body's protective mechanisms.
- ◆ *Identify* different wound classifications.
- ◆ *Name* the common pyogenic bacteria.
- ◆ *Understand* the significance of hepatitis B in the health care setting.
- ◆ *Understand* the causes and form of acquired immunodeficiency syndrome (AIDS).
- ◆ *Discuss Universal Precautions.*
- ◆ *Identify* the body fluids through which AIDS may be transmitted.

Key Terms

aerosol effect: The release of minute particles of liquid in the air. Liquid may harbor bacteria, which thus spread through the air droplets.

AIDS: Acquired immunodeficiency syndrome, a fatal disease transmitted by blood and body fluids.

animate surface: Living tissue.

binary fission: Bacterial form of reproduction in which the cell splits to reproduce a copy of itself.

endotoxin: Toxin released when a cell dies and breaks up.

exotoxin: Toxin released from living bacteria.

facultative bacteria: Bacteria that can live with or without the presence of oxygen.

fomite: A substance that is capable of harboring and transmitting disease.

HBV: Hepatitis B virus.

HIV: Human immunodeficiency virus—the cause of AIDS.

host: Organism that provides nutrition for parasites.

inflammatory response: The body's reaction to injury or disease.

morphology: The study of structure and form.

parasites: Organisms that derive nutrients from a living source.

pathogenic: Disease-causing.

personnel protective equipment: Special barrier attire worn to prevent the cross-communication of blood-borne diseases.

phagocytosis: The process by which white blood cells engulf bacteria.

saprophytes: Organisms that feed on dead or decaying material.

spore or **endospore:** Protective reproductive form of the bacterium that contains all the genetic material capable of becoming a living bacterial cell. Some are extremely difficult to destroy.

strict aerobes: Bacteria that cannot survive without oxygen.

strict anaerobes: Bacteria that cannot survive in the presence of oxygen.

suppuration: The accumulation of bacterial cells, dead white blood cells, and cellular fluid.

systemic infection: Infection that has spread from one area to other parts of the body through the bloodstream.

toxigenicity: A bacterium's ability to release toxic substances.

Universal Precautions: Precautionary standards issued by the Occupational Safety and Health Administration (OSHA) and the Centers for Disease Control (CDC) for the containment and isolation of blood and body fluids.

Part I ◆ MICROBIOLOGY OVERVIEW

BACTERIAL STRUCTURE AND PHYSIOLOGY

Bacteria are partially identified by their structure. The study of form and structure is referred to as *morphology*. There are three separate forms or shapes of bacteria: (1) spherical (cocci), (2) rod-shaped (bacilli), and (3) spiral or curved (spiral forms). In addition, each type of bacteria may group together in a particular way, such as in small clusters or in long chains. A detailed discussion of the internal structures of bacteria is beyond the scope of this text. However, knowledge of basic *bacterial physiology* is important in understanding how and why infection occurs and the processes necessary to prevent it.

Environmental Requirements

Bacteria have certain environmental requirements necessary for their growth and reproduction. These include specific temperature ranges, amounts of moisture, the presence or lack of oxygen, specific nutrients, and ranges of pH.

Temperature

Bacteria that cause disease in humans prefer an environment in which the temperature is the same as that of the human body. They multiply rapidly at temperatures ranging from 20°C to 37°C (68°F to 98.6°F). However, certain forms of bacteria can withstand temperatures above the boiling point and below freezing.

Moisture

A moist environment is best suited to the growth and reproduction of bacteria. It is important to note, however, that most bacteria can live in dried pus, sputum, or blood for long periods of time.

Oxygen

The amount of oxygen necessary for bacterial growth gives rise to three major classifications. Those bacteria that require oxygen for survival are called *strict aerobes*. Those that cannot survive in the presence of oxygen are termed *strict anaerobes*. This type of bacteria usually lives in soil, the intestines of mammals, or in other areas where air cannot penetrate. Those bacteria that can live in both aerobic and anaerobic environments are called *facultative* bacteria.

Nutrition

There are two general groups of bacteria, classified according to the source of their nutrition. *Autotrophs* utilize simple carbon dioxide to synthesize nutrients from inorganic substances. *Heterotrophs* require complex organic compounds from which they derive carbon to synthesize nutrients. Since there is a great deal of overlap between these groupings, several systems of classification have been developed. These are based on complex biochemical reactions that are beyond the scope of this text.

Among the heterotrophs are two distinct groups that are of medical significance. These are the *saprophytes* and the *parasites*. Saprophytes are organisms that feed on dead or decaying material, while parasites derive nutrients from a living source (called the *host*). The relationship between the parasite and the host may be beneficial, such as that between the parasitic organisms that dwell in the human intestinal tract and aid in the synthesis of vitamins. Some parasites, however, derive their nutrition at the expense of or to the detriment of the host. These include the pathogenic bacteria, discussed later in this chapter.

pH Requirements

Most bacteria require an environment that is neutral or slightly alkaline. Should the pH change, the bacterial cell's growth and metabolism are greatly decreased or may cease altogether.

Bacterial Reproduction and Spore Formation

Bacteria reproduce by a process called *binary fission*. In binary fission the bacterial cell simply splits apart to reproduce a copy of itself. Some bacteria also produce *endospores* (commonly referred to as *spores*). The spore is a protective reproductive form of the bacterium that contains all the genetic material capable of becoming a living bacterial cell. When conditions for bacterial growth are unfavorable, the spore remains dormant. Its thick coating protects it from temperature extremes or strong chemicals. Because of the existence of spores, we employ very precise, exact, and rigorous methods of sterilization when processing surgical equipment and supplies. By definition, an object is sterile only when it harbors no living microorganisms, *including spores*.

DISEASE TRANSMISSION

Now that we are familiar with the environments favored by bacteria, we can study how bacteria or other microorganisms are transferred from one source to another. There are numerous ways that disease is transmitted, and these should be studied by *all* operating room personnel so that steps can be taken to prevent the spread of infection.

For bacteria to be transmitted from one surface to another they must be carried by an intermediate source. This intermediate source is called a *vector* and may be animate, such as an insect, or inanimate, such as a contaminated instrument. A substance that is capable of harboring and transmitting disease is referred to as a *fomite*. Examples of fomites in the hospital are bed linens, wound dressings, and contaminated surgical instruments. Fomites in our everyday environment include

such objects as money, eating utensils, toys, and clothing.

Common Sources of Transmission

The following are some common sources of transmission. Table 5–1 lists various methods that help to prevent these sources from acting as vectors in the operating room.

Moisture

Bacteria can be attached to droplets of moisture that remain suspended in the air or to droplets that settle on a surface. Moisture from the mouth and respiratory system contains millions of potentially harmful bacteria that are released during talking, coughing, and sneezing. This is called an *aerosol effect*. For this reason talking is kept to a minimum while surgery is being performed. Another process of transmission by moisture is through the hand washing of soiled instruments. Washing instruments by hand can release minute droplets of wash water into the environment, possibly contaminating both the environment and those working in it.

Dust

Because bacteria can live for long periods of time on dried surfaces, dust may serve as a carrier. In addition to what is commonly referred to as dust (minute particles of "dirt"), there are other forms of dust commonly found in the hospital that are potentially dangerous carriers of disease. These include dried sputum, pus, and blood.

Direct Contact

Bacteria can be transferred from one source to another by direct contact. An example of direct contact is the contamination of the surgical wound by a contaminated surgical instrument or through patient contact with contaminated bed linens.

Insects

Insects, particularly silverfish, flies, and roaches, are dangerous carriers of disease and can carry bacteria from surface to surface. Insects are a particular problem in surgery because they can gain entrance to sterile surgical supplies through the package's wrapper. It is for this reason that live plants are not allowed in the surgical department, nor should food be stored in lockers unless it is in insect-proof containers. Shipping cartons should also never be brought into restricted areas of the operating room.

Ingestion

Some bacteria are transmitted in food and water, resulting in what is commonly called food poisoning.

Table 5–1. COMMON PATHOGENS RESULTING IN INFECTIONS

Bacteria*	Normal Flora/Location	Infection	Prevention and/or Control of Infection†
I. Aerobic Bacteria			
A. Gram-positive cocci			
1. *Staphylococcus aureus*	Skin, hair Nasopharynx and oropharynx	Boils (furuncles) Wound infection Pneumonia Urinary tract infection Septicemia	1) Strict aseptic technique 2) Hand washing 3) Isolation of infected persons 4) Disinfection of all discharges
2. *Streptococcus pyogenes*	Nose Nasopharynx	Cellulitis Puerperal fever Wound infections Urinary tract infection	1) Strict aseptic technique around wounds 2) Hand washing 3) Disposal of all discharges 4) Environmental sanitation 5) Adequate ventilation with appropriate air changes
3. *Streptococcus pneumoniae*	Nose Nasopharynx and oropharynx	Lobar pneumonia Conjunctivitis Peritonitis Meningitis	1) Exclusion of infected persons or carriers from the surgical suite 2) Strict adherence to aseptic technique 3) Environmental sanitation 4) Hand washing
B. Gram-negative cocci			
1. *Neisseria gonorrhoeae*	Genitourinary tract Rectum, mouth Eye	Gonorrhea Pelvic inflammatory disease Septicemia Conjunctivitis	1) Environmental sanitation 2) Early diagnosis and treatment including all contacts
2. *Neisseria meningitidis*	Nose Oropharynx	Meningitis Pneumonia	1) Identification of carriers 2) Environmental sanitation 3) Strict adherence to aseptic technique 4) Hand washing
C. Gram-negative bacilli			
1. *Escherichia coli*	Large intestine Perineum	Septicemia Inflammation of the liver and the gallbladder Urinary tract infection Peritonitis	1) Hand washing 2) Strict aseptic technique during bladder catheterization 3) Isolation of bowel contents and instruments during large bowel resection
2. *Pseudomonas aeruginosa*	Intestinal tract Skin Soil	Wound infections Urinary tract infection Burns	1) Use aseptic technique when handling wounds and burns 2) Proper disposal of contaminated materials 3) Environmental sanitation
3. *Salmonella typhosa*	Intestinal tract	Typhoid fever	1) Isolation 2) Disinfection of feces and urine 3) Sanitary control of food, water, and sewage disposal 4) Hand washing
4. *Shigella sonnei*	Intestinal tract	Bacillary dysentery or shigellosis Gastroenteritis Septicemia	Same as for *S. typhosa*
5. *Hemophilus influenzae*	Respiratory tract	Bacterial meningitis Acute airway obstruction	1) Disinfection of respiratory secretions
D. Gram-positive bacillus			
1. *Mycobacterium tuberculosis*	Respiratory tract Urine (occasionally) Lymph nodes	Tuberculosis 　Peritonitis 　Meningitis 　Lungs 　Bone 　Skin 　Lymph nodes 　Intestinal tract 　Fallopian tubes	1) Early diagnosis and treatment 2) Environmental sanitation 3) Disposal of all discharges from respiratory tract 4) Disinfection and sterilization of contaminated equipment 5) Isolation of person with active infection

Table continued on following page

Table 5–1. COMMON PATHOGENS RESULTING IN INFECTIONS *Continued*

Bacteria*	Normal Flora/Location	Infection	Prevention and/or Control of Infection†
II. Microaerophilic Bacteria			
A. Gram-positive cocci			
1. Hemolytic streptococci, α type	Respiratory tract	Abscess in gums or teeth Subacute bacterial endocarditis Meningitis	1) Identification of carriers 2) Adherence to aseptic technique 3) Proper handling of contaminated masks 4) Exclusion of personnel with upper respiratory tract infection from operating room 5) Hand washing
2. Nonhemolytic	Respiratory tract	Endocarditis Urinary tract infection	Same as for hemolytic
III. Anaerobic Bacteria			
A. Gram-positive cocci			
1. *Peptococcus*		Abscess of skin or or respiratory and intestinal tract	1) Strict aseptic technique
2. *Peptostreptococcus*	Vagina (premenopausal)	Abscess of respiratory and intestinal tract Septic abortions	1) Strict aseptic technique
B. Gram-positive bacilli			
1. *Clostridium perfringens* 2. *C. novyi* 3. *C. septicum* 4. *C. histolyticum*	Soil Dust Manure Human feces Vagina	Gas gangrene (rare) Food poisoning (common)	1) Strict aseptic technique 2) Cleansing of all wounds by irrigation with copious amounts of solution to eliminate extraneous material and necrotic tissue
5. *C. tetani*	Soil Dust Feces	Tetanus (lockjaw) Surgical tetanus	1) Tetanus toxoid 2) Tetanus antitoxin 3) Sterilization of all instruments and dressings
C. Gram-negative bacillus			
1. *Bacteroides* species	Nasopharynx Intestinal tract Vagina	Wound infections Rectal, brain abscess Endocarditis Osteomyelitis	1) Strict aseptic technique 2) Environmental sanitation 3) Hand washing 4) Plaster casts should be bivalved or removed outside the operating room.
2. *Fusobacterium* species	Nasopharynx Intestinal tract	Anaerobic infections of brain and respiratory tract Vincent's angina (trench mouth) Cellulitis	1) Strict aseptic technique 2) Good dental hygiene
Nonbacterial Infections			
IV. Fungi			
A. *Candida albicans*	Respiratory tract Gastrointestinal tract Female genital tract	Candidiasis or thrush	1) Avoid disturbance of normal microbial flora
V. Viruses			
A. Hepatitis A virus	Water contaminated by human sewage Shellfish from naturally contaminated sources Blood, urine from infected persons Food prepared or handled by infected persons who practice poor hygiene	Infectious hepatitis	1) Sanitary disposal of sewage 2) Use disposable syringes and needles on infected persons 3) Exercise care in handling syringes, needles, and instruments used on infected persons 4) Sanitary food processing 5) Enforce good hygiene with all food-processing personnel (i.e., hand washing) 6) Gamma globulin immunization within 2 weeks

Table 5–1. COMMON PATHOGENS RESULTING IN INFECTIONS *Continued*

Bacteria*	Normal Flora/Location	Infection	Prevention and/or Control of Infection†
V. Viruses *Continued* B. Hepatitis B virus	Blood Saliva Other body fluids Feces	Serum hepatitis	1) Hand washing 2) Use disposable presterile needles and syringes whenever possible 3) Nondisposable items must be sterilized or disinfected following use 4) Careful disposal of contaminated syringes, needles, knife blades, and suture needles 5) Wear gloves when handling contaminated items 6) Scrub nurse must exercise care not to puncture own skin with needles or knife blades 7) Gamma globulin immunization within 7 days
C. Human immunodeficiency virus	Blood Saliva Semen Cerebrospinal fluid Tears	AIDS	1) Wear gloves when touching blood, saliva or mucous membranes 2) Wear masks and protective eyewear when splashing of blood or saliva is likely 3) Do not recap needles 4) Nondisposable items must be sterilized or disinfected following use 5) Impervious gowns or plastic aprons should be worn during procedures that are likely to generate splashes of blood or other body fluid 6) Carefully dispose of contaminated syringes, needles, knife blades, and suture needles 7) Team members should refrain from all direct patient care when they have exudative lesions or weeping dermatitis 8) Scrub nurse must exercise care not to puncture own skin with needles or knife blades 9) Follow institutional policy after any exposure

*Bacterial infections may be mixed (e.g., aerobic and anerobic microorganisms, gram-positive and gram-negative microorganisms, and synergistic microorganisms).
†Strict handwashing technique is the most important precaution in the prevention and control of infections.
Modified from Groah L: Operating Room Nursing: Perioperative Practice, 2nd ed. Norwalk, CT, Appleton & Lange, 1991.

Some forms of food poisoning are very mild whereas others such as botulism, caused by *Clostridium botulinum,* are deadly.

THE PROCESS OF INFECTION

It is important to know not only how infection is transmitted but also how it is contracted and who is likely to succumb to an infection. There are several factors that determine whether an infection will develop in a person.

Location of Entry

The exact point at which bacteria or other microorganisms gain entry into the body may cause or prevent the onset of infection. For example, the bacterium *Escherichia coli* is normally found in the intestine of healthy persons and causes no harm. If, however, the bacteria are allowed to proliferate in the abdominal cavity, the person is in danger of peritonitis. Bacteria usually gain entry to deep body tissues through breaks in the skin caused by trauma, insect bites, or surgical intervention. Certain areas of the body are more resistant to infection than others. In general, the more vascular an area, the greater its resistance to infection.

In addition, the body has other mechanisms to prevent infection; these will be discussed later in the chapter.

Dose of Organisms

For an infection to develop, there must be sufficient numbers of bacteria (called the *dose*) at the entry site. Gross contamination of the surgical wound, such as that occurring from bowel leakage into the abdomen, is far more likely to lead to an infection than is contamination caused by a puncture hole in one of the operator's gloves.

Condition of the Person

A healthy, young, well-nourished person is more likely to resist infection than one whose condition is compromised in some way. Any patient who is debilitated by disease, advancing age, or stress or is nutritionally imbalanced is more likely to develop an infection. Consequently, the risk of postoperative infection is often great, *and it is important to practice strict asepsis in the operating room.* In addition to the fact that the surgeon exposes the sensitive inner tissues of the body during surgery, the patient has the added disadvantage of physiologic and emotional stress. Many patients are also undergoing surgery because of lengthy or critical illness.

Aggressiveness and Toxigenicity of the Invading Microorganism

In addition to the entry location, dose of microorganisms, and condition of the patient, the aggressiveness and toxigenicity of the microorganism determine whether an infection will develop following its entry into the body.

Some bacteria are more resistant to the body's protective mechanisms than others are. Normal, so-called resident bacteria are harmless when prevented from entering deep body tissues; they do not exhibit aggression. However, if these bacteria (those that normally reside in skin and other areas, such as the mouth and respiratory tract) are transmitted from their normal environment, they may become *aggressive* owing to lack of resistance in their new location and can cause serious illness.

The *toxigenicity* of a bacterium is its ability to release certain toxic substances. Not all bacteria release toxins, but many of the toxins released by the pathogenic bacteria are potentially fatal if allowed to remain unchecked in the body. There are two types of toxins released by certain bacterial cells. *Endotoxins* are components of the bacterial cells and are released when the cell dies and breaks up. *Exotoxins* are released from the living bacteria through the cell membrane. Toxins from each type of bacteria are specific to that type of bacteria, and each may have different effects. One toxin may affect only the liver or heart, while another affects only

certain nervous tissue in the host. This explains the relationship of certain pathogenic microorganisms to the specific diseases they cause.

Inflammatory Response

When pathogenic bacteria penetrate body tissue, or if the body is injured, it responds in a distinctive manner. The process by which the body defends itself against invading pathogens is called an *inflammatory reaction* and occurs at the focal point of the injury or bacterial invasion. The response to infection proceeds in the following way.

First, the blood supply to the injured area increases and the blood vessels dilate at the site. This brings an increased number of white blood cells to the area, causing *redness*. The white blood cells engulf the bacteria by a process called phagocytosis. The blood then begins to flow very slowly at the site. The area may become swollen (edematous) because of fluid formation, which in turn causes pressure on sensory nerves in the area, resulting in *pain*. The increase of the blood supply to the site causes *heat* to be generated there. As the white blood cells continue to engulf the bacterial cells, the accumulation of dead and living bacterial cells, dead white blood cells, and tissue fluids forms a milky substance known as *pus*. This process is called *suppuration*, and any infection that results in the formation of pus is said to be suppurative. If the bacterial growth is not arrested at the site of the injury or invasion, the vessels of the lymphatic system pick up the pathogens and carry them to regional lymph nodes, where more concentrated phagocytosis takes place. If the infection is too overwhelming for the body to fight, the infection may invade the bloodstream and thereby spread to other parts of the body. In this case the infection is said to be *systemic*. Systemic infection is accompanied by fever, malaise, headache, and loss of appetite.

PROTECTIVE MECHANISMS OF THE BODY

The human body has efficient protective mechanisms that prevent the entry of microorganisms, the onset of infection and disease, and the proliferation of pathogens.

Skin

The skin is perhaps the body's greatest protective mechanism. Not only is skin a thick barrier, but its secretions may also prevent the proliferation of bacteria. However, if the skin is broken, as is the case during injury or surgery, microorganisms have a free path through which to enter the body. This is of great significance, not only to the surgical patient but also to all health care personnel. Accidental inoculation of pathogenic microorganisms can occur through contaminated hypodermic needles, scalpel blades, and other sharp objects or by direct contact between the patient's contaminated tissues (including his or her blood) and a small break in the skin of a healthy person. For this reason, surgery personnel should *never handle soiled surgical instruments or equipment with bare hands.* An apparently healthy patient might nonetheless be harboring a disease, such as hepatitis.

Mucous Membranes

The moist mucous membranes of the nose, mouth, throat, and respiratory and genitourinary tracts offer extra protection because of the increased blood supply in these areas. The bloodstream can quickly carry away and destroy invading organisms. In addition, some mucous membranes harbor normal flora that serve a protective function. For example, the lactobacilli of the vaginal mucosa keep it acidic, in a pH range that inhibits the growth of many pathogenic bacteria and yeasts. *Cilia,* tiny hairlike projections on the surface of some mucous membranes, sweep foreign bodies away from inner body cavities.

Tears

Tears help to protect the eyes by constantly washing away debris and microorganisms. Tears also contain a natural bactericidal agent that adds further protection.

Lymphatic System

The fluid-filled vessels of the lymphatic system defend the body by transporting white blood cells, which engulf and destroy bacteria. In addition to the white blood cells, certain tissue cells called *histiocytes* engulf and destroy foreign material, including bacterial cells. Unlike white blood cells, histiocytes are immobile and remain fixed in the body tissues.

Antibody Formation

Some foreign materials, both living and nonliving, stimulate the production of *antibodies.* These are proteins that act in a complex manner to destroy specific foreign organisms, such as bacteria. The foreign substance that initiates the formation of the antibody is called an *antigen.* The production of antibodies can be naturally or artificially induced by inoculating a specific antigen to form an antibody that can fight a specific disease.

SURGICAL WOUND INFECTION

A surgical wound infection is a type of hospital-acquired infection. Postoperative surgical wound infec-

tions can be caused by many different conditions. Of course, there must be a specific microorganism present to initiate the infection, but other conditions influence the outcome of any surgical procedure. These include the following:

1. The age of the patient. Older patients may be more prone to postoperative infection because of poor circulation or other physiologic deficits.
2. Concurrent disease. Patients with preexisting disease may be susceptible to postoperative infection. Patients with diseases of the circulatory system or those that indirectly affect the circulatory system are far more likely to develop a postoperative infection than a healthy person.
3. Nutritional status. Well-nourished persons are able to tolerate surgery better than those whose nutrition has been compromised or is otherwise imbalanced.
4. Length of operative procedure and damage to tissue. Any condition that impairs the circulation of healing tissue predisposes it to infection. Gentle manipulation of tissues during surgery prevents circulatory compromise. Crushing, bruising, or maceration of tissue by retractors or even manually can disrupt normal blood flow and increase the chance of postoperative infection. During lengthy procedures, delicate tissues can dry out; this may further disrupt circulation or even cause sloughing.

Classification of Wounds

The following classification of wounds may determine which are more likely to develop postoperative infection. The least likely to become infected are wounds in category 1. Those most at risk are in category 4.

Category 1: Clean Wound

A clean wound is one in which there was no break in asepsis during surgery. These wounds do not involve the alimentary, respiratory, oropharyngeal, or genitourinary tract. No wound drain is used.

Category 2: Clean Contaminated Wound

This type of wound is one in which the alimentary, oropharyngeal, respiratory, or genitourinary tract has been entered. However, no unusual contamination occurred during surgery. Also included in this category are wounds that require some form of drainage.

Category 3: Heavily Contaminated Wound

These wounds include those in which a major break in aseptic technique occurred during surgery, those in which acute inflammation without pus was encountered, and those in which the surgical incision was made near contaminated skin.

Category 4: Infected or Dirty Wound

This type of wound includes those that have not been freshly incised (old wound) and those in which perforated viscera are encountered. These wounds almost always have bacteria present within them before the surgical procedure begins.

PATHOGENIC MICROORGANISMS

The following section describes some major groups of pathogenic microorganisms and the diseases they cause. The pathogens discussed represent the most common forms and those seen most frequently in the hospital setting. Table 5–1 presents a list of specific organisms and their associated diseases.

Pyogenic Bacterial Infections

Those bacteria that cause infection are termed *pyogenic*. Included in this group are the streptococcal, staphylococcal, meningococcal, pneumococcal, and gonococcal organisms and the coliform (intestinal) bacilli. These organisms typically cause suppuration and tissue destruction and may lead to systemic involvement, resulting in death.

Streptococcal Infections

There are several clinically significant infections caused by the streptococci. The lesions of a streptococcal infection appear as watery, blood-stained abscesses. The streptococci are responsible for such diseases as rheumatic fever, glomerulonephritis, impetigo, bacterial endocarditis, tonsillitis leading to otitis media, and severe postoperative wound infection. Transmission is by direct contact with a contaminated source, by droplet, and by dust particles.

Staphylococcal Infections

There are two common types of staphylococcal bacteria, each carried on the skin. *Staphylococcus albus* is a harmless resident bacterium often found on the hands. However, in the debilitated or weakened carrier the organism may become pathogenic. *S. aureus* is frequently carried in the nasopharynx as well as on the skin. It is responsible for causing such conditions as carbuncles and boils and is the most common cause of postoperative wound infection.

Meningococcal Infections

Meningococci reside normally in the nasopharynx but can produce meningitis (inflammation of the meninges) in persons who are susceptible to the disease. Meningitis, which can be fatal, may reach epidemic proportions when many persons are crowded together in a confined space. It is transmitted through droplet formation from the mouth, nose, and throat or from direct contact with the contaminated source.

Pneumococcal Infections

There are many different types of pneumococci, some of which are found in the throats of healthy persons. Some types of pneumococci are harmless, while others can cause lobar pneumonia of varying degrees of severity. The disease is capable of spreading to other organ systems, where local infection occurs. It is transmitted chiefly through direct contact and through droplet formation from the nose, mouth, and throat of the carrier. The elderly and debilitated are particularly susceptible.

Gonococcal Infections

Gonococcal bacteria cause the disease gonorrhea, which is transmitted through sexual intercourse. The disease presents, in the male, as an acute urethritis accompanied by discharge. In the female, urethritis may present or there may be no symptoms. If left untreated, the disease spreads to the reproductive systems in both the male and female and may result in permanent sterilization in both sexes. In addition to involvement of the genitourinary and reproductive systems, gonorrhea may be transmitted to the conjunctiva by direct contact with bacteria from the hand. When the disease invades the bloodstream, it may cause serious septicemia.

Coliform Bacterial Infections

The coliform bacteria are so named because they normally reside in the intestines of healthy persons, where they cause no harm. If, however, they are released from the bowel, as during rupture or injury of the intestine, severe peritonitis or other localized, suppurative infections may result. Because they are also found normally in the perianal area of the body, they are often responsible for urinary tract infections. Of particular significance is their introduction into the bladder during catheterization or the introduction of endoscopes. Three common coliform bacteria are *Escherichia coli*, *Proteus mirabilis*, and *Pseudomonas aeruginosa*.

Anaerobic Bacterial Infections

As previously noted, the anaerobic bacteria are those that can live only in an oxygen-free environment. Most anaerobic bacteria are spore forming and may normally reside in the intestine of the healthy person. These bacteria are often found in soil, a significant factor for the patient who has suffered injury in the presence of dirt.

Gas Gangrene

Gas gangrene, initiated by the bacillus *Clostridium perfringens*, is the result of a complex process aided by the presence of other clostridial organisms. This relatively rare disease must not be confused with the type of gangrene caused by vascular insufficiency, which results in the necrosis of an organ or limb. (For example, we often refer to a "gangrenous" foot or leg seen in cases of severe atherosclerosis, where major blood vessels are so occluded with plaque that they are unable to transmit blood to the lower limbs.)

In true gas gangrene, the injured tissues of the wound are destroyed by the toxins of the *C. perfringens* bacillus. *C. novyi* bacilli, another type, invade the necrotic tissue and release toxic gases within the tissue, and absorption of these gases leads to death. The disease is transmitted directly from a contaminated substance to an open or penetrating wound.

Tetanus

Tetanus (commonly called "lockjaw") is primarily a disease of the nervous system caused by the bacillus *Clostridium tetani*. The toxins released by this bacillus travel along the peripheral nerve pathways, eventually reaching the central nervous system. Painful muscle spasms, convulsions, and eventual involvement of the respiratory system lead to death from asphyxia. The bacillus is commonly found in soil and in the normal intestinal tract. Transmission is by direct contact of the bacillus with an open or penetrating wound.

Mycobacterial Infection

The mycobacterial infections of importance include tuberculosis and Hansen's disease. Both diseases are rarely encountered, with Hansen's disease found even less frequently than tuberculosis; therefore, only tuberculosis will be discussed.

The bacillus *Mycobacterium tuberculosis* is the cause of the disease tuberculosis. There are two strains of the bacteria, the human strain and the bovine strain. The human strain causes dense nodules or tubercles to form in localized areas of the body, including the liver, spleen, and bone marrow. Lung involvement occurs in all cases and is the main organ affected by the disease. Tuberculosis is spread by inhalation of droplets or dust in the form of dried sputum released by the person with pulmonary tuberculosis.

Spirochetes

Among the spirochetal diseases, those caused by spirochetes, syphilis is the most significant. The cause of syphilis is the spirochete *Treponema pallidum*. The disease is generally spread through sexual intercourse, although the bacteria can gain entrance through other tissues of the body. Initially, the disease produces a small sore, or *chancre*. After a few weeks, the chancre disappears, indicating that the spirochetes have left the location of entry and have infiltrated other areas of the body through the bloodstream. The disease progresses through three subsequent phases and produces a wide range of symptoms. It can be fatal if left untreated.

Viral Hepatitis

Hepatitis is a disease of the liver that is caused by one of three different types of viruses. Hepatitis A and B are significant in the hospital setting.

Hepatitis A Virus

Hepatitis A virus is transmitted by ingestion and by close contact with an infected person. Fecal and oral routes are the common methods of transmission. This virus cannot be cultured, but the diagnosis of hepatitis can be made through a serologic test that shows the presence of hepatitis A virus antibodies. This disease is rarely fatal, and one infection causes permanent immunity to the disease. Its symptoms are most often subclinical. There is no vaccine available for hepatitis A.

Hepatitis B Virus

Hepatitis B virus, or *HBV* as it is commonly called, is a disease of the liver that is both a serious and a significant threat to patients and health care workers, especially those who work in the surgical setting. HBV may lead to permanent liver damage and cancer of the liver. It is *not* 100% detectable in blood donated for transfusion, and there are now over 200 million chronic carriers of the disease worldwide. *This disease is transmitted through blood, blood products, and nearly all other body fluids. Operating room personnel who work in an environment where there is almost constant contact with blood and blood products are at extreme risk.* In addition to contact with blood and blood products, this disease is transmissible through eating utensils, razors, urine, perspiration, and sexual contact. Patients who are at high risk for getting this disease include blood transfusion recipients, drug addicts, both homosexuals and heterosexuals with multiple partners, and infants with carrier mothers. *In the surgical setting, all patients are considered potential carriers of HBV.* To prevent cross-contamination of this disease, certain strict precautions regarding handling of equipment and patient contact have been established. These precautions are called *Universal Precautions* and are discussed later in this chapter and throughout this book where applicable. Health care personnel must understand these precautions and why they must be followed. In addition to following all Universal Precautions, all health care workers including surgical personnel must be vaccinated against HBV.

INFECTION CONTROL IN THE HOSPITAL

Infection control is the responsibility of all who work in the hospital. In surgery, infection control is accomplished with *knowledge* of the processes and causes of infection, *adherence* to certain minimum regulations set by the hospital and the Joint Commission on Accreditation of Health Care Organizations (JCAHO), and the strictest practice of aseptic technique (see Chapter 8).

All hospitals have an infection control committee whose major function is to prevent and control nosocomial infection (infection resulting from hospitalization). The infection control committee, usually headed by a physician, infection control nurse, or nurse epidemiologist, carries out its duties in many ways. Following standards set by the JCAHO, it provides the hospital with an effective program with the following goals:

1. Investigate the *source* of infection. The source may be a person in the hospital, either a patient or an employee, or may be the practices of one or more employees (in surgery, for example, one team member may be the source of postoperative infections because of poor aseptic technique, or a team member may be harboring a specific disease organism that is transmitted to those patients in his or her care).

2. Provide effective isolation of infected patients, when necessary. Infected patients may be placed in an isolation ward or other area away from healthy persons to prevent cross-contamination (contamination from patient to patient, from patient to a vector or carrier, and from patient to employee). Those working in isolation wards follow strict rules of asepsis to prevent such contamination. In surgery, if a patient must undergo a procedure even in the presence of infection, he or she may not go to the post-anesthesia care unit following the procedure but may be cared for by trained personnel in an area where the infection cannot be spread to other postoperative patients.

• •

Part II ♦ ACQUIRED IMMUNODEFICIENCY SYNDROME

CLINICAL SIGNIFICANCE

It has been more than 2 decades since the Centers for Disease Control first reported the increase of certain rare disorders, among them Kaposi's sarcoma, *Pneumocystis carinii* pneumonia, and severe herpes simplex. Shortly thereafter, physicians and other members of the scientific community described a condition in which a patient *acquired* a defect in his or her immune system and that defect led to crippling disease and eventual death. Furthermore, it was quickly noted that the disease was transmitted by distinct modes: sexually by both homosexuals and heterosexuals, through transfusion of infected blood either clinically or through shared needles of intravenous drug users, and through the placenta of an infected mother to her child. The name *acquired immunodeficiency syndrome*, or *AIDS*, was given to this devastating disease, and research as to the cause and cures was begun immediately. We now know the cause of AIDS. *Human immunodeficiency virus (HIV)* attacks the CD4, T4, and B-cell components of the body's immune system and renders it helpless to fight infection and disease. We also know that AIDS transmission requires the direct entry of *blood* or *body fluids* of the infected person into another's bloodstream through a mucous membrane or nonintact skin surface.

There are three distinct strains of HIV, and each causes a clinically different picture. In addition to AIDS, two other syndromes have been identified: AIDS-related complex (ARC) and AIDS dementia complex (ADC). Whether a patient develops one or another of these syndromes depends on what type of cells the HIV organism attacks. None of the forms is curable.

The significance of AIDS and HIV infection in the operating room setting is the extreme burden of exposure that occurs there. Nearly every activity within the surgical environment presents the hazard of contamination with blood or body fluids. Hence, all surgical personnel must follow the standards set by the Occupational Safety and Health Administration (OSHA) regarding blood-borne pathogens. These standards (Universal Precautions) will be emphasized and described repeatedly throughout this text. These discussions may seem redundant. However, there are few topics that deserve more emphasis or, if misunderstood, could cause such harm. The issue at hand is not one of possible disease—it is one of possible death.

UNIVERSAL PRECAUTIONS

Universal Precautions are activities whose goal is to prevent cross-contamination of blood-borne pathogens such as HBV and HIV. These have been developed by OSHA and apply to all health care settings and all personnel in those settings. Wherever the phrase "body fluids" is discussed with regard to Universal Precautions, it refers to those fluids that can transmit the AIDS virus:

- Human blood components (e.g., plasma)
- Products made from human blood
- Semen
- Vaginal secretions
- Tears
- Cerebrospinal, synovial, peritoneal, and amniotic fluids
- Saliva in dental procedures
- Any body fluid visibly contaminated with blood
- All unrecognizable body fluids
- Any unfixed tissue or organ (other than intact skin) from a living or dead human
- Cells or tissue cultures containing HIV or HBV, or blood, organs, or tissues from experimentally infected animals

Surgical Standards

1. Protection with appropriate barriers
   - Hands, and other contaminated skin surfaces, must be washed immediately and thoroughly
     - when contaminated with blood or body fluids.
     - before and after all patient contact.
     - after removal of gloves.
   - Gloves must be worn when there is a high probability that the hands will come in contact with blood, body fluids, mucous membranes, or nonintact skin of patient.
   - A gown must be worn during all invasive operative procedures on patients; an apron must be worn when cleaning bloody instruments or equipment contaminated with blood. Material must provide a moisture barrier (i.e., be fluid resistant) to protect the wearer from splashes.
   - Protective eyewear is to be worn during all invasive procedures that may generate splashes of blood, body fluids, or bone chips and during cleaning of instruments.
   - Masks are to be worn during all invasive procedures.
   - Employees who have exudative lesions or weeping dermatitis should refrain from all direct patient contact and from handling patient care equipment until the condition resolves.
2. Prevention of puncture injuries
   - Needles and sharp instruments must be discarded in puncture-proof containers.
   - Needles are not to be recapped, bent, or broken before disposal or left on beds, stuck into armboards, or disposed of in routine waste containers.
3. Care of specimens
   - Specimens are to be transported in sealed plastic bags or in leak-proof containers with proper labeling.

4. Protection of oral mucosa
   - Ventilation devices for resuscitation should be available to prevent the need for emergency mouth-to-mouth resuscitation.
5. Decontamination
   - Instruments must be thoroughly cleaned before sterilization or high-level disinfection.
   - Surfaces of furniture and floors must be cleaned with detergent-disinfectant. Spills of blood and body fluids should be wiped up immediately.
   - Waste must be properly contained for transport or disposal.

Modified from Welch TC: AIDS: Viewpoints. Point View 28(2):13, 1991, with permission of Ethicon, Inc., Somerville, NJ.

For specific applications of the Universal Precautions, refer to the particular chapter for which the precautions apply. For example, as they apply to aseptic technique during surgery, see Chapter 8.

PERSONAL PROTECTIVE EQUIPMENT

Personal protective equipment is special attire or equipment that health care personnel must wear when working in a high-risk environment. *Any* worker who may come in contact with the fluids listed earlier must wear protective equipment. This equipment includes gloves, mask, eye and face shield, and outerwear that provides an effective barrier against liquids.

Questions for Study and Review

1. What are the environmental requirements of all bacteria?
2. What are spores?
3. Describe a vector. Give an example of one in the operating room.
4. What is the "aerosol effect"?
5. Name the body's protective mechanisms against disease.
6. What is pus?
7. Define *pyogenic*.
8. Give an example of the four classifications of wounds.
9. How is hepatitis B transmitted?
10. *Briefly* discuss the cause of AIDS.
11. How is AIDS transmitted?
12. What are Universal Precautions?
13. Name the body fluids that can carry the AIDS virus.
14. What is the goal of Universal Precautions?

Bibliography

Ackerman V, et al: Microbiology: An Introduction for the Health Sciences. Sydney, Harcourt Brace Jovanovich, 1991.

Altemeier WA, et al: Manual on Control of Infection in Surgical Patients. Philadelphia, JB Lippincott, 1984.

Bell DM, et al: HIV and the Surgical Team. Todays OR Nurse 12(11):24–27, 1990.

Centers for Disease Control: Update: Universial precautions for prevention of transmission of human immunodeficiency virus, hepatitis B virus, and other bloodborne pathogens in the health-care settings. MMWR 37(24):A-1–B-16, 1990.

Occupational Safety and Health Administration, Department of Labor: Occupational exposure to bloodborne pathogens; final rule, 1991. Washington, DC, U.S. Government Printing Office, 1991.

Welch TC: AIDS: View points. Point View 28(2):13, 1991.

Disinfection and Decontamination

Learning Objectives

After reading this chapter you should be able to

◆ *Distinguish between* disinfection and sterilization.
◆ *Distinguish between* antisepsis and disinfection.
◆ *Understand* the classification of patient care equipment.
◆ *Recognize* the hazards associated with the use of chemical disinfectants.
◆ *Be familiar with* different disinfectant agents.
◆ *Understand* what sanitation is and how it is accomplished.
◆ *Be familiar with* the process of instrument decontamination.
◆ *Be familiar with* the postsurgical duties of the scrub assistant.
◆ *Be familiar with* Universal Precautions as they apply to decontamination.
◆ *Understand* what personal protective equipment is.

Key Terms

antisepsis: A process that destroys most pathogenic microorganisms from animate surfaces.
bactericidal: Able to kill bacteria.
bacteriostatic: Capable of inhibiting the growth of bacteria but not of killing them.
cavitation: A process in which air pockets are imploded (burst inward), releasing particles of soil or tissue debris.
cleaning: A process that removes organic or inorganic soil or debris.
contaminated: Refers to any surface, living or nonliving, that is known to harbor microorganisms.
critical items: In medicine, those items that must be sterile before their use on a patient; items that penetrate body tissues or the vascular system.
decontamination: A process of disinfection.

disinfection: A process by which most but not all pathogenic microorganisms are destroyed on inanimate objects.

high-level disinfection: Disinfection process that kills spores.

inanimate: Nonliving.

sanitation: A process that cleans an object.

sporicidal: Able to kill spores.

sterilization: A process by which all types of microorganisms are destroyed.

terminal disinfection: A process in which an area or object is rendered disinfected after contamination has occurred.

ultrasonic cleaner: Equipment that cleans instruments through cavitation.

virucidal: Able to kill viruses.

washer-sterilizer: Equipment that washes and sterilizes instruments following an operative procedure.

Part I ◆ DISINFECTION

DEFINITIONS AND CLARIFICATION

Disinfection is a process by which *most but not all* pathogenic microorganisms on *inanimate objects* are destroyed. This process is clearly distinguished from *sterilization,* which is the destruction of *all* microorganisms on an object. In the operating room, sterilization (discussed in Chapter 7) is used to destroy all microorganisms on all objects that enter the body, such as instruments, catheters, and needles. Quite different from disinfection and sterilization is *antisepsis,* which is a process that destroys most pathogenic microorganisms on *animate (living) surfaces.*

The distinction among these terms is critical. Disinfection is used in the operating room and elsewhere in the hospital to render objects nearly free but not completely free of microorganisms. Patient care objects such as respiratory therapy equipment and patient furniture are examples of objects that are disinfected. *Antiseptics,* used only on living tissue, are used on the skin of the surgical site and for the surgical hand and arm scrub of sterile team members. Antiseptics are discussed in Chapter 11. These do not sterilize the skin but do kill many pathogenic microorganisms.

Several other terms are important to the understanding of disinfection. The suffix *-cidal* means to destroy or kill. Thus, if a product is bactericidal, it destroys bacterial cells. A sporicide destroys bacterial spores, the vegetative form of the bacteria that is very difficult to kill by any means. Generally, if a product is sporicidal, it is highly effective against all types of microbes and is said to achieve a *high level of disinfection.* A virucide is a product that is effective in killing viruses, and a germicide is any agent that kills microorganisms. A tuberculocidal agent is one that kills tubercle bacilli. The suffix *-static* refers to a process of controlling or inhibiting growth. Thus, a bacteriostatic disinfectant is one that inhibits the growth of bacteria on a surface but does not necessarily destroy the bacteria. Once the disinfectant is removed, the bacteria freely proliferate. A hospital-grade disinfectant is one that claims effectiveness against *Salmonella, Staphylococcus aureus,* and *Pseudomonas aeruginosa.* These are all significant microorganisms in the hospital setting.

CLASSIFICATION OF PATIENT CARE EQUIPMENT

The following is a system of classification for items that are commonly disinfected or sterilized in the hospital. Although many of these items are not encountered in the operating room setting, it is important to understand the distinctions made and why they fall into various groupings. These distinctions were developed in the past 2 decades and remain in use today. The categories are based on *the degree of risk of infection* associated with each item. Items in categories II and III are disinfected according to their classification. That is, they are disinfected with a specific process and substance to achieve the needed level of disinfection. *High-level disinfection* is a process that destroys all forms of microorganisms except bacterial spores. *Intermediate-level disinfection* is a process that inactivates *Mycobacterium tuberculosis,* vegetative bacteria, most viruses, and most fungi but may not destroy bacterial spores. *Low-level disinfection* is a process that destroys some virus and fungi and most bacteria. However, this process is not reliable in killing tubercle bacilli or bacterial spores.

Category I: Critical Items

Critical items are those that must be sterile. These objects enter sterile tissue or the vascular system. In most cases, sterilization requires special equipment and critical monitoring. Examples of critical items include

- Surgical instruments
- Cardiac and urinary catheters
- Implants
- Needles

Category II: Semicritical Items

Items in this category come in contact with mucous membranes or skin that is not intact. The items in this category must be completely free of microorganisms except for bacterial spores. This is because mucous membranes are resistant to bacterial spores but have little or no defense against bacteria such as tubercle bacilli and viruses. Semicritical items are disinfected away from patient care areas and require some special equipment for disinfection. This group of items includes

- Respiratory therapy and anesthesia equipment
- Endoscopes

Category III: Noncritical Items

This group of items comes in contact with skin but not mucous membranes. Skin is effective in protecting the inner tissues of the body against bacteria and viral invasion; thus, this category includes items that are commonly found in patient care areas:

- Blood pressure cuffs
- Bed linens
- Bedside tables
- Crutches
- Some food utensils
- Bed frames
- Floors
- Walls

SELECTION AND USE OF DISINFECTANTS

In the operating room and elsewhere in the hospital, the most common disinfection process is with the use of a liquid disinfectant. Disinfectants commonly used in patient care fall into chemical types. These are discussed below and in Table 6–1. The *selection* of a disinfectant is based on the result required. Some disinfectants are effective in destroying a limited number of microorganisms; others are very effective in killing all organisms, including bacterial spores. Some are extremely corrosive, while others are relatively harmless to common materials found in the hospital.

Factors that affect a disinfectant's activity or "cidal" ability include the concentration of the solution, the number of microorganisms present on the object being disinfected, water hardness and pH, temperature of the solution, and presence or absence of organic matter. Most disinfectants have a dilution factor that is critical to their efficacy. Therefore, it is very important to follow mixing instructions *exactly*. Some disinfectants can be extremely harmful to materials such as plastics, rubber, or tile. Mixing errors can be costly in terms of both destruction of equipment and simple economic use of the product. Nearly all disinfectants are considerably weakened in the presence of organic material such as blood, sputum, or tissue residue. Therefore, *cleaning* (removal of organic debris and soil) must occur before a disinfection process. Cleaning is accomplished with detergent, water, and mechanical action and should never be confused with disinfection or sterilization.

Precautions and Hazards

Many disinfectants are *unsafe for use on human tissue, including skin.* This means that personnel must be extremely cautious when handling certain liquid disinfectants. Warnings and instructions for use must be strictly followed. *Do not be misled by the mild odor of some disinfectants.* Many chemicals are preferred for commercial or medical use because they do not give off noxious fumes. *This is not an indication of any lack of toxicity to skin or the respiratory system.* Because of the toxicity of some disinfectants, the following precautions should always be exercised:

1. All disinfectants should be stored in well-ventilated rooms and their containers kept *covered.*

2. The following personal protective attire must be worn when personnel handle a chemical disinfectant:

- Protective eyewear
- Gloves
- Masks
- Full protective body wear such as a jumpsuit, apron, or cover gown

3. Data concerning the safe use of chemical disinfectants are kept by every hospital.

4. Never change the dilution of a liquid chemical unless instructed to do so by an appropriate supervisor.

5. When mixing liquid disinfectants with water, always use a measuring cup designated for that purpose. Do not rely on haphazard technique or guesswork when preparing solutions.

6. Never mix two disinfectants together. This could create toxic fumes or unstable and dangerous compounds.

7. Dispose of liquid chemicals as directed by hospital policy and label instructions. Some chemicals are unsafe for disposal through standard sewage systems.

8. Never use an unlabeled bottle or container. Be aware of what chemical is being used and its specific purpose.

DISINFECTANT CHEMICALS

The following are disinfectants that are commonly used in the hospital environment. These are regulated and registered by the Environmental Protection Agency (EPA).

Alcohol

Alcohol is a commonly used disinfectant that is composed of two components: ethyl alcohol and isopropyl

Table 6–1. COMMONLY USED CHEMICAL DISINFECTANT AGENTS

Agent	Microorganism Destroyed and Time Required (″ = Minutes)	Mechanisms of Action	Practical Use	Usefulness Disinfectant	Usefulness Antiseptic	Precautions
Mercurials	Weak bacteriostat	Oxidation combines with proteins	None	None	Poor	
Phenolic compounds	Bactericidal—10″ Pseudomonacidal—10″ Fungicidal—10″ Tuberculocidal—20″	Surface active—disrupts membrane Inactivates enzymes Denaturation of proteins	Walls, furniture, floors, equipment	Good	Poor	Unpleasant odor, tissue reactions on skin and mucous membrane; personnel must wear gloves when using agent.
Quaternary ammonium compounds ("quats")	Bactericidal—10″ Pseudomonacidal—10″ Fungicidal—10″	Surface active—disrupts cell membrane Inactivation of enzymes Denaturation of proteins	Limited hospital use since these do not destroy gram-negative pathogens and tubercle bacilli	Fair	Fair	Neutralized by soap; active agent is absorbed by gauze and fabrics, thus reducing strength.
Chlorine compounds	Most gram-negative bacteria, *Pseudomonas* Virucidal	Oxidation of enzymes	Spot cleaning of floors and furniture	Good	Fair	Inactive in presence of organic debris, unpleasant odor, corrosive to metal.
Iodine compounds (iodine + detergents = iodophors)	Bactericidal—10″ Pseudomonacidal—10″ Fungicidal—10″ Tuberculocidal—20″ with minimum concentration of 450 ppm of iodine	Oxidation of essential enzymes	Dark-colored floors, furniture, walls	Good	Good	Iodine stains fabrics and tissues; may corrode instruments. Inactivated by organic debris.
Alcohol (usually isopropyl and ethyl alcohol 70%–90% by volume)	Bactericidal—10″ Pseudomonacidal—10″ Fungicidal—10″ Tuberculocidal—15″	Denaturation of proteins	Spot cleaning Damp dusting equipment	Good	Very good	Inactivated by organic debris; becomes ineffective when it evaporates. Dissolves cement mounting on lensed instruments and fogs lenses, blanches floor tile.
Formaldehyde: aqueous formalin 4% or 10%	Bactericidal—5″ Pseudomonacidal—5″ Fungicidal—5″ Tuberculocidal—15″ Virucidal—15″	Coagulation of proteins	Lensed instruments	Fair	None	Irritating fumes, toxic to tissue; rubber and porous material absorb the agent.
Alcohol formalin (8% formaldehyde and 70% isopropyl alcohol)	Tuberculocidal—10″ Virucidal—10″ Sporicidal—12 hours	Coagulation of proteins	Instruments	Good	None	Dissolves cement mounting on lensed instruments; toxic to tissue, irritating fumes.
Glutaraldehyde	Vegetative microorganisms—5″ Tubercle bacilli—10″ Spores—10 hours	Denaturation of proteins	Disinfection of instruments in 10″. Useful for lensed instruments Effective liquid chemosterilizer in 10 hours	Good	None	Unpleasant odor, tissue reaction may occur, instruments must be rinsed well in distilled water.

From Groah L: Operating Room Nursing: Perioperative Practice, 2nd ed. Norwalk, CT, Appleton & Lange, 1991.

alcohol. Both are water soluble (mix easily in water). Alcohol is not sporicidal but is bactericidal, tuberculocidal, and virucidal. It is effective against cytomegalovirus and human immunodeficiency virus. Alcohol's optimum disinfection ability occurs at a 60% to 70% dilution factor. Alcohol must never be used on surgical instruments because it is not sporicidal and is very corrosive to stainless steel. In the hospital, alcohol is most commonly used to disinfect patient thermometers and medication vial stoppers. It is damaging to shellac mounting on lensed instruments and must never be used repeatedly on rubber or plastic tubing since it causes swelling and hardening of these substances.

Alcohol is also frequently used to cleanse patient

injection sites. It greatly reduces the number of bacteria on skin when used as a hand rinse in the absence of water and antiseptic soap. However, toxicity has been reported when it is used on children as a sponging liquid to reduce fever. Alcohol is extremely drying to skin and irritating to mucous membranes.

Because it is *highly flammable and volatile,* alcohol must never be used in the presence of electrocautery or lasers. Alcohol must be stored in a *cool, well-ventilated area.*

Chlorine Compounds

Hypochlorite (sodium hypochlorite) is a broad-spectrum disinfectant that is limited in use because of corrosiveness to metal. However, it is commonly used to clean floors and countertops. The Centers for Disease Control (CDC) has recommended this product for use in spot cleaning of blood spills because it is very fast acting. However, it is deactivated in the presence of organic material, so the area must first be cleaned before application of hypochlorite. It is unstable (decomposes easily) and can be toxic. When hypochlorite solution comes in contact with formaldehyde, *bis*-chloromethyl ether is produced. This chemical is a carcinogen. When hypochlorite is mixed with an acidic solution, toxic chlorine gas is produced.

Formaldehyde

The common form of formaldehyde is formalin, a 37% solution of formaldehyde in water. It is a bactericide, tuberculocide, fungicide, virucide, and sporicide. Its primary use in the hospital is in the preservation of tissue specimens, although it has been used to disinfect renal dialysis equipment. Formaldehyde emits extremely irritating fumes and is toxic to tissue.

Phenolics

Phenol (carbolic acid) is available in detergent form for use in routine hospital cleaning. It is not sporicidal but is tuberculocidal, fungicidal, virucidal, and bactericidal. Because there are not much data relating to the specific effects of phenol on microorganisms, its use is restricted to disinfection of noncritical items. It is extremely important to follow the manufacturer's label instructions for dilution and mixing because phenolic mixtures have been indicated in a number of studies involving toxicity to certain patients. Phenol has a very noxious odor and causes skin lesions and respiratory irritation.

Quaternary Ammonium Compounds

The quaternary ammonium compounds (commonly called "quats") are sensitive to environmental conditions such as hardness of water, soap, and some types of soil, all of which may render them ineffective. Benzalkonium chloride and dimethyl benzyl ammonium chloride have been widely used as disinfectants. Although the quats have traditionally been used on skin, the CDC has recently advised that this practice cease because of the incidence of infection associated with their use as an antiseptic. More recently developed quats such as twin-chain or dialkyl quats are much more effective in hard water than those traditionally used in the hospital. They are reported to be fungicidal and bactericidal but are not sporicidal or tuberculocidal and are not effective against certain types of viruses. In addition, the disinfectant qualities are greatly reduced when they are used in conjunction with an object such as gauze or sponges; the sponge or gauze absorbs the active ingredient in the quat and thus renders the disinfection process ineffectual.

Glutaraldehyde

Glutaraldehyde is a widely used disinfectant that is sporicidal, bactericidal, and virucidal. It is completely safe to used on instruments such as endoscopes, which is its major use in the hospital. It can be used safely on respiratory therapy and anesthesia equipment. However, it is toxic to tissue; therefore, items that have been disinfected or sterilized in glutaraldehyde must be completely rinsed before patient use or handling by personnel. To render glutaraldehyde effective as a sterilizer, the item must soak in solution for 10 hours. It is, however, tuberculocidal in 10 minutes. This disinfectant is weakened considerably by unintentional dilution, such as occurs when instruments are wet when placed in an immersion bath of glutaraldehyde, and by the presence of organic matter. When glutaraldehyde solutions are mixed and kept for repetitive use, the solution must be completely renewed after 2 weeks since it is ineffective after that time. Occupational hazards from glutaraldehyde are most commonly found when the solution is kept in open immersion baths in a poorly ventilated work area. The safe level of glutaraldehyde in the air is under 0.2 ppm. Any amount over that causes irritation to the eyes and nasal passages.

Part II ◆ DECONTAMINATION

DEFINITIONS AND CLARIFICATION

To render the operating room environment, which includes all cleanable surfaces, as disease free as possible, certain regimens are followed on a scheduled basis. The routines are the general responsibility of everyone in the department. In certain settings, the responsibility belongs to specific personnel assigned by the nurse manager, or by the job description given to them by the hospital. At the present time, the emergence of human immunodeficiency virus and other blood-borne pathogens has produced an element of urgency and extreme focus on the practices of sanitation and decontamination. The duties and tasks must never be taken lightly. The devastating results of carelessness in this area testify to its importance.

Disinfection or *sanitation* is the process by which *any* surfaces, materials, and equipment are cleaned with specific substances (disinfectants) that render them safe for their intended use. The term *decontamination* implies that a surface or object was either known or assumed to harbor pathogenic microorganisms and is cleaned and disinfected in a manner that renders it safe for its intended use. Therefore, any item that is soiled with organic matter such as blood, tissue, or any body fluids is considered *contaminated*. The process that renders it safe is decontamination. The disinfection or sanitation process may achieve the same result as decontamination, but an item's status with regard to contamination may or may not be known. *Cleaning* refers to the process by which any type of soil, including organic material, is removed. This is accomplished with detergent, water, and mechanical action. *Cleaning precedes all disinfection processes. The purpose of sanitation and disinfection is to prevent cross-contamination between patients and between patients and personnel.*

DECONTAMINATION OF THE SURGICAL SUITE

Before the Workday

All furniture, surgical lights, and fixed equipment used in the operating suites must be damp dusted with a clean, lint-free cloth and a hospital-grade chemical disinfectant. Environmental dust falls to horizontal surfaces, carrying disease-causing microorganisms with it.

During Surgery

In the past, certain cases were considered "contaminated" or "dirty" depending on the type of surgery and on the disease organisms known to be present during the case. At this time, all cases are considered contaminated and treated accordingly. During surgery it is the duty of the circulator and his or her assistants to ensure that the environment in the surgical suite is kept as disease free as possible. This is accomplished by *confining and containing* all potential contaminants. The following activities describe how this is accomplished. These activities are called Universal Precautions and must be carried out to prevent cross-contamination of blood-borne pathogens.

1. Any blood spills or contamination of other organic material should be *promptly* removed with a hospital-grade disinfectant. The use of household bleach for this purpose is discouraged because of its potential to damage certain equipment and instruments.

2. All articles used and discarded in the course of surgery must be placed in containers that are leak proof. This prevents spilling of contaminated liquid onto other surfaces.

3. Any contaminated or suspect item must be handled in a manner that protects personnel from contamination. Personal protective equipment must be worn by all nonscrubbed personnel. These include gloves, cover gown, face shield or mask, and protective eyewear. It is permissible to use an instrument (called no touch method) to transfer contaminated articles to a waste or other receptacle.

4. Tissue specimens, blood, and all other body fluids must be placed in a leak-proof container for transport out of the department. The outside of any specimen container that is passed off the surgical field to the circulator must be cleaned with a hospital-grade disinfectant.

5. Because paper products are difficult or impossible to decontaminate, all attempts should be made to keep patient charts, laboratory slips, x-ray reports or radiographs, and other paper documentation from contamination.

6. Contaminated sponges must be collected in the kick bucket, in which a plastic bag or liner has been previously placed. Sponges must not be lined up on the floor for counting. Sponges can be counted and immediately placed in plastic bags representing incremental numbers such as 5 or 10 sponges.

7. Instruments that fall off the surgical field must be retrieved by the circulator and placed in a basin or pan containing a noncorrosive hospital-grade disinfectant. In this way organic debris on the instrument is prevented from drying and becoming air-borne. If the instrument is needed to continue surgery it may be cleaned in the substerile room and flash sterilized. During this proce-

dure the circulator must wear gloves and take precautions not to splash or contaminate surfaces in the sub-sterile room.

After Surgery

Following a surgical procedure, duties are shared between the scrub person, who handles equipment and instruments directly related to the performance of the surgery, and the personnel responsible for case cleanup. These can be housekeeping personnel, surgical technologists, or surgical aides. Regardless of the type of personnel participating in the cleanup, all must be attired in personal protective equipment. During this time, the circulator assists the anesthesiologist in emergence (if a general anesthetic has been used) and in transportation of the patient to the post-anesthesia care unit. He or she is also responsible at this time for completing any documentation pertinent to the surgery.

Decontamination of Supplies and Equipment

All contaminated disposable equipment is placed in leak-proof containers that are appropriately labeled. These containers are usually color coded.

All linen used during the case, soiled or not, should be removed from the surgical field with as little activity as possible. This prevents the spread of contaminants that can be spread by lint or other air-borne particles.

All blood and tissue debris is removed from metal instruments. Box lock instruments are then opened fully and placed in a perforated tray. Delicate lightweight instruments should be separated from heavier ones to prevent damage to the lighter ones. Instrument trays can then be placed in plastic bags and transported by other personnel maintaining the upright orientation of the tray to a separate cleaning area. Here they can be processed in one of the following ways:

1. Instruments are processed through a washer-sterilizer.
2. Instruments are autoclaved for 3 minutes at 270°F for 3 minutes or 250°F for 15 to 20 minutes.
3. Instruments are placed in a metal basin to which 2% trisodium phosphate and water have been added and sterilized for 30 minutes at 270°F or 45 minutes at 250°F. If this final process is employed, the fast exhaust cycle should be used.

Decontamination of Surgical Instruments

Surgical instruments represent a significant threat of cross-contamination between the patient and surgical personnel. Therefore, they merit special discussion. The most common method used to decontaminate stainless steel instruments is with the washer-sterilizer. This process not only cleans but also sterilizes instruments. However, before processing through the washer-sterilizer, some hard-to-clean areas of the instruments must be scrubbed to remove bits of tissue and debris. Of special concern are the serrations of hemostatic and other tissue clamps, rasps, and saw blades that contain bits of bone and tissue. Instruments are washed by placing them in a basin with a mild detergent that is neutral or slightly alkaline. Extreme care must be taken to prevent splashing and spraying of contaminated material; when a brush is used to clean the instruments it must be kept below the level of the water. Personal protective attire must be worn during the washing procedure. Following cleansing, instruments may be placed in the washer-sterilizer in mesh trays. All box locks must be opened and hinges extended to their widest adjustment.

The *washer-sterilizer* operates much the same as the steam sterilizer. The washer-sterilizer sends copious amounts of soapy water over the instruments. Steam under pressure and air are then injected into the water, which activates the water significantly. As the water is drained from the chamber, tissue debris and scum are filtered off and steam fills the entire chamber. The temperature is then maintained at 270°F for 3 minutes. Near the completion of the cycle, the steam is released through the exhaust system.

Following processing in the washer-sterilizer, all instruments should be placed in the *ultrasonic cleaner.* This process further removes particles and debris through a process called *cavitation.* During cavitation, high-frequency sound waves are generated through a water bath in which the instruments are placed along with a neutral to slightly alkaline detergent. Cavitation causes tiny air spaces trapped within the debris to explode inwardly (implosion), and this causes their release from the surface of the instrument. Following cavitation, instruments are rinsed thoroughly and dried. Because cavitation is *not* a disinfecting or sterilizing process, all instruments subjected to it must first be processed by the washer-sterilizer. In addition, if the washer-sterilizer has not been used to process instruments before their ultrasonic cleaning, the immersion bath of the ultrasound cleaner must be rinsed and cleaned often, since it contains tissue debris that can culture potentially harmful microorganisms.

All solutions used are suctioned into disposable suction units using disposable tubing. Suction tips may be flushed at this time with *clean* water. The suction tubing can then be disconnected from its wall fixture. However, this must be done by personnel other than the scrub person, who at this time still wears contaminated gloves.

All sharp instruments (e.g., knife blades, needles) are placed in a closable container in a manner that will not injure personnel handling the container next. The disposal of these containers is dictated by hospital policy.

Any items that require gas sterilization must be cleaned with a hospital-grade disinfectant and then transported to the appropriate work area for processing.

When all supplies, instruments, and linens have been contained as described earlier, the scrub assistant then removes his or her gown and gloves and places them in the proper receptacle, thus completing the equipment cleanup. In some hospitals, a case cart system is employed (see later), and at the completion of the cleanup an open cart is covered by drawing its cover over the top of the supplies (handling only the clean edge of the cover) and removing it to the workroom. If a case cart is used, its doors should be secured before transport to the processing area.

Case Cart System

The case cart system is a method of reprocessing all surgical and hospital equipment by personnel in a central processing area outside the surgical department. The cart system may require specific architectural planning to provide a means of transporting contaminated equipment *separately* from sterile-wrapped or decontaminated equipment. A two-dumbwaiter system—one for clean and one for contaminated equipment—is commonly used to transport goods to and from the operating room. The central processing department may be directly underneath or adjacent to the operating room, or it may be located on the same floor but in another area of that floor.

The system utilizes one of several types of stainless steel carts for transportation of goods. Case carts that contain doors are more efficient in preventing contamination of goods than open, unprotected carts. Following a surgical procedure, all contaminated equipment is loaded onto the cart, which is transported directly to central processing, where trained personnel decontaminate, resterilize, assemble, wrap, and store the equipment. All equipment used in a particular surgical procedure is standardized and computerized so that assembly of the case carts is uniform. This requires the communication between personnel in the operating room and the central processing department. In addition to standard case carts, emergency carts are maintained. The goals and advantages of a case cart system are as follows:

1. The risk of cross-contamination and disease is reduced through separate handling and transport of sterile versus contaminated goods.
2. Quality control measures are more efficiently implemented when designated personnel and work areas are centralized.
3. Packaging standards are consistent when processing is centralized.
4. The need for duplicate surgical equipment throughout the hospital is eliminated, thus reducing expense.
5. Duplication of processing equipment by different departments in the hospital is eliminated.
6. When operating room personnel are relieved of decontamination and reprocessing duties, more of their working time can be spent on patient care.

Decontamination of Furniture and Fixed Equipment

Once all equipment, instruments, and supplies have been contained following surgery, the room itself and its furniture and fixed equipment can be cleaned and disinfected.

Disposable suction containers are disconnected from wall units and disposed of in accordance with hospital policy. Regulations about these containers concern their contamination of sanitary sewer systems, and these regulations are formed according to specific state and local ordinances.

All equipment and furniture used during a surgical procedure are thoroughly cleaned with a hospital-grade disinfectant. During the cleaning process, mechanical friction is instrumental in the destruction of microorganisms.

Floors should be cleaned using a wet-vacuum system. This can be a centralized built-in system or a portable wet-vacuum. If neither is available, the following procedure may be used:

1. Two buckets are filled with disinfectant/detergent.
2. Mop heads must be sterilized or a disposable mop head (used once only) used in the operating room suite.
3. Solutions and mop heads are changed for each suite and the buckets cleaned before new solution is mixed.

The pads of the operating table are removed to expose the undersurface of the table. All surfaces of the table and pads are cleaned with particular attention to hinges, pivotal points, and castors. It is necessary to move the table to clean under the supporting post and castors.

Doors and walls are spot cleaned with disinfectant. Additional attention should be paid to supply cabinet doors in the area around the latches or handles.

Linen bags are sealed and removed to the appropriate disposal area.

The surgical spotlights should be cleaned only after they have been allowed to cool, to prevent them from cracking. Some light's manufacturers recommend a specific type of cleaner to prevent buildup of detergent or disinfectant film over the light's surface.

DECONTAMINATION OF OTHER AREAS IN THE OPERATING ROOM

During the Day

Areas around the surgical suite are cleaned according to need during the day. Scrub sink areas need particular attention during the day, particularly because water, a vehicle for bacterial contamination, is frequently splashed on the floors and walls. Scrub areas are frequented by surgeons who may or may not have removed protective shoe covers between cases. Frequently, in the course of a busy schedule, blood and debris can be tracked from one surgical suite to another through pooled water at the scrub sinks.

The halls and doorways of the operating room are frequented by heavy traffic and also need particular attention. Studies have shown that sticky mats placed outside the doorways of the operating room actually transfer bacteria from the mat to the shoes of those entering the department rather than the reverse; thus, their use is discouraged.

Patient stretchers must be cleaned with disinfectant after each use. Linen must be removed and disposed of in the proper receptacle, and both sides of the stretcher pad must be disinfected. Side rails, legs, and castors must also be cleaned.

End of Day Cleanup

At the close of the workday, all operating room suites, scrub sink areas, utility rooms, hallways, furniture, and other equipment must be cleaned in preparation for the following day's activities. This is called *terminal disinfection or cleaning.* Specific areas include

- Surgical lights and slide tracks
- All ceiling-mounted equipment
- All furniture including castors or wheels
- Door and cabinet handles including push plates for automatic doors
- All horizontal surfaces including shelves, counters, work tables, and autoclave cabinet tops
- All floor surfaces in the department. A fresh mop head must be used for each operating room suite.
- Kick buckets and other movable objects in the operating suites
- Scrub sinks
- Soap dispensers. Because soap dispensers have been found to contain significant numbers of microorganisms, these must be completely disassembled and disinfected before refilling.
- Outpatient areas including treatment and holding areas, including all furniture and equipment. The outpatient areas often become "orphaned" because of their location away from the operating room in some hospitals, but their decontamination and sanitation must not be neglected.

Other areas that may be cleaned daily according to operating room policy include

- Locker rooms
- Dictation and conference rooms
- Lounges
- Special equipment storage areas

Weekly Cleanup

According to operating room and hospital policy, the following surfaces and areas are cleaned and disinfected on a weekly basis:

1. Ventilation and air conditioning/heating duct grills must be vacuumed to prevent the release of bacteria-laden dust into the surgical environment.

2. Inside shelves of supply cabinets must be cleaned.

3. In some hospitals, utility and supply carts are steam cleaned.

4. Utility rooms, including those used to store housekeeping supplies, sewer hoppers, and linens, must be cleaned.

Questions for Study and Review

1. What is the difference between *disinfection* and *sterilization*?

2. What is the difference between *disinfection* and *antisepsis*?

3. What is a bactericide?

4. What is the difference between a bacteriostatic agent and a bactericide?

5. Give two examples of patient care equipment for each classification.

6. What does "cidal" mean?

7. Discuss the precautions that should be taken when mixing or using disinfectants.

8. Why can't one dispose of used chemicals in any drain?

9. What disinfectant is used in your operating room to clean the floors and walls? What type of disinfectant is it?

10. Why must hospital equipment be decontaminated?

11. What is meant by *cleaning*?

12. Why must items be cleaned before they are disinfected?

13. How does one handle an instrument that has fallen from the surgical field during surgery?

14. Discuss the duties of the scrub technologist immediately following a surgical case.

15. Why are the scrub sink areas so troublesome to keep clean and decontaminated?

16. Describe the proper decontamination process for surgical instruments.

17. What is cavitation?

18. Describe the case cart system. What are its advantages? What do you think are its disadvantages?

Bibliography

American Hospital Association: OSHA's Final Bloodborne Pathogens Standard: A Special Briefing, Chicago, IL, 1992.

Association of Operating Room Nurses: Good procedures belong in front of case cart setup. AORN J 38(3):389–392, 1983.

Association of Operating Room Nurses: Recommended Practices for Disinfection, Denver, 1992.

Association of Operating Room Nurses: Recommended Practices for Care of Instruments, Scopes, and Powered Surgical Instruments, Denver, 1991.

Association of Operating Room Nurses: Recommended Practices for Sanitation in the Surgical Practice Setting, Denver, 1992.

Centers for Disease Control: Update: Universal precautions for prevention of transmission of human immunodeficiency virus, hepatitis B virus, and other bloodborne pathogens in the health-care settings. MMWR 37(24):1990.

Chlysta M: Case carts and centralized processing: A better way. J Operating Room Res Inst, November-December 1980, pp 14–17, 20–21, 35–37, 40.

Dominick B, American Convertors—Division of American Hospital Supply Corporation: Case Cart Training Program for Central Supply Personnel, Evanston, IL, April 1991.

Occupational Safety and Health Administration, Department of Labor: Occupational exposure to bloodborne pathogens; final rule, 1991. U.S. Government Printing Office, Washington, D.C.

Reichert M: Automatic washer/disinfectors for flexible endoscopes. Infect Control Hosp Epidemiol 12(8):497–499, 1992.

Rutala WA: Disinfection in the O.R. Todays OR Nurse, October 1990, pp 30–36.

Welch TA: Case cart system. AORN J 52(5):993–998, 1990.

Sterilization: Standards and Practice

Learning Objectives

After reading this chapter you should be able to

◆ *Define and understand* sterility.
◆ *Distinguish between* the process of sterilization and other processes that only render objects clean or disinfected.
◆ *Describe* the different methods of sterilization used in the operating room.
◆ *Properly load* the steam sterilizer.
◆ *Understand* and *practice* safety precautions when using any type of sterilizer.
◆ *Determine* which sterilization process is approved for which equipment.
◆ *Understand* the principles of gas sterilization.
◆ *Describe* the environmental concerns associated with the use of the gas sterilizer.
◆ *Prepare* equipment for sterilization.

Key Terms

biological control: A method that determines the presence of pathogenic bacteria on objects subjected to a sterilization process.
cobalt 60 radiation: A method of sterilizing prepackaged equipment; ionizing radiation.
ethylene oxide gas: Highly flammable, toxic gas that is capable of sterilizing an object.
glutaraldehyde: Chemical capable of rendering objects sterile.
gravity displacement sterilizer: Type of sterilizer that removes air by gravity.
high vacuum sterilizer: Type of steam sterilizer that removes air in the chamber by vacuum.
lumen: Hollow tube.
peracetic acid: Chemical capable of rendering objects sterile.
shelf life: The amount of time a wrapped object will remain sterile after it has been subjected to a sterilization process.

steam sterilizer: Sterilizer that exposes objects to high-pressure steam.
sterilization control monitor: Method of determining whether a sterilization process has been completed; does not indicate whether the items subjected to that method are sterile.

Sterility is defined as the absence of any living microorganism, including bacteria, viruses, and spores. An object is either sterile or not sterile. Because the inner tissues of the body are sterile, any equipment or supplies that come in contact with these tissues must also be sterile. Contamination of body tissues with nonsterile items can lead to serious infection or disease. It is therefore critical that all personnel working in surgery or those working with surgical supplies and equipment understand the process of sterilization. One point is of critical importance: *disinfection does not render an item sterile.* The numerous methods used to sterilize equipment are discussed in this chapter.

STEAM STERILIZATION

Steam under pressure is the most common method of sterilization for supplies used in the operating room and elsewhere in the hospital. Steam alone is inadequate for sterilization; however, when steam is pressurized, its temperature rises. It is this moist pressurized heat that causes the destruction of microbes by coagulation and denaturation of the protein within the cells. The relationship between temperature, pressure, and exposure time is instrumental in the destruction of microbes. When steam is contained in a closed compartment and the pressure is increased, the temperature will increase provided the volume of the compartment remains the same. If items are exposed long enough to steam at a specified temperature and pressure, the items will be rendered sterile. The unit used to create this atmosphere of high-temperature pressurized steam is called an *autoclave.*

Types of Steam Sterilizers

Gravity Displacement Sterilizer

The gravity (or "downward") displacement sterilizer (Fig. 7–1) uses the principle that air is heavier than steam. Within the sterilizer there is an inner chamber where goods are loaded and an outer jacket-type chamber that ejects steam forcefully into it. Any air in the inner chamber blocks the passage of pressurized steam to the surface of the goods and thus prevents sterilization. All the air must be removed because every surface of the supplies must be exposed to the pressurized steam to ensure sterilization. Therefore, the sterilizer is constructed in such a way that air is pushed downward by gravity (hence the name "gravity displacement sterilizer"). The air exits the chamber through a tempera-

ture-sensitive valve. As the amount of steam builds up in the chamber, the temperature increases, and when the sterilization temperature is reached, the valve closes. Careful loading of supplies in this type of sterilizer is critical because if the load is too dense or improperly positioned, air may be trapped in pockets. Items in these air pockets will not be sterilized because the steam cannot displace the air, which acts as an insulator.

Prevacuum Sterilizer

The prevacuum sterilizer (Fig. 7–2) does not rely on gravity to remove air from the inner chamber. Instead, the air is pulled out of the chamber, which creates a vacuum in the chamber. Steam is injected into the chamber to replace the air. This type of sterilizer offers greater steam penetration in a shorter time than the gravity displacement sterilizer. When the designated time, pressure, and temperature have been reached and maintained, the steam is removed through a filter and the chamber is reduced to normal (atmospheric) temperature and then cools to a level safe for personnel to handle the sterilized goods. A new alternative method of removing air from items in the sterilizer provides a more effective method of removing air from the chamber during sterilization. The *Joslyn steam sterilization process* removes the air by a process of steam flushes and pressure pulses at *above atmospheric level.* This process is not affected by air leaks that may occur through the valves and around the door seal and thus provides a more reliable method of sterilization.

Flash Sterilizer

The flash sterilizer has traditionally been used in the operating room and in other areas of the hospital to quickly sterilize items that are unwrapped. It has been common practice to flash sterilize any instrument that had become contaminated during surgery. If the instrument was still required to complete the surgery, it was flash sterilized and returned to use. However, this type of sterilizer should now be used only when no other alternative is available. The efficacy of the flash sterilizer is currently being challenged, and it may soon be phased out of use. Because unwrapped goods are normally sterilized in the flash sterilizer, the risk of contamination of the processed items is great. When any item is flash sterilized, its manufacturer's recommendations for time and temperature must be followed. Implants should be flash sterilized only when there is no other possible means to render the implant sterile, and only when a biologic indicator (discussed later) is used during sterilization.

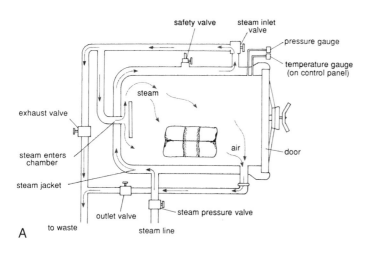

Figure 7–1. *A.* Gravity displacement steam sterilizer. (From Ackerman V, Dunk-Richards G: Microbiology. Philadelphia, WB Saunders/Bailliere Tindall, 1990.) *B.* AMSCO Eagle 3000 steam sterilizer. (Courtesy of AMSCO Healthcare, Pittsburgh, PA.)

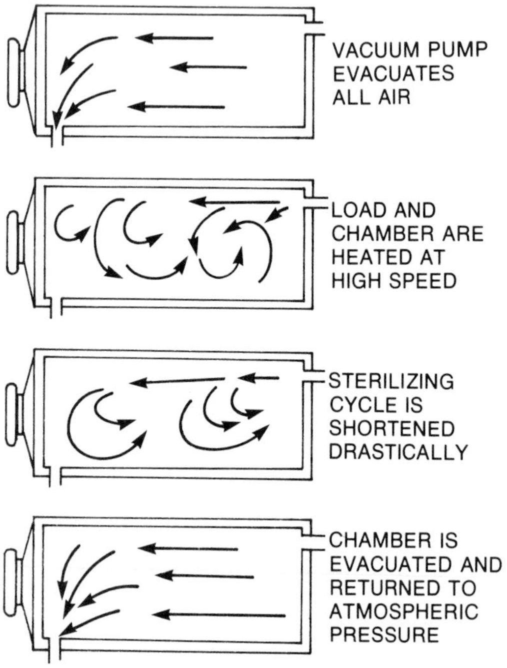

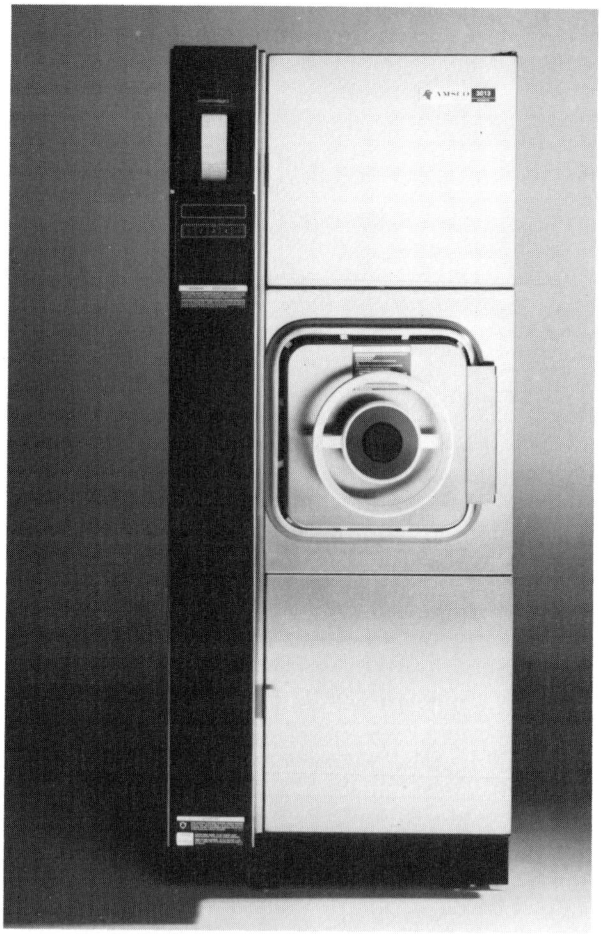

VACUUM PUMP EVACUATES ALL AIR

LOAD AND CHAMBER ARE HEATED AT HIGH SPEED

STERILIZING CYCLE IS SHORTENED DRASTICALLY

CHAMBER IS EVACUATED AND RETURNED TO ATMOSPHERIC PRESSURE

Figure 7–2. Prevacuum steam sterilizer. (From Hofmann RE: Automation of Hospital Sterile Processing. Coral Gables, FL, Ross Hofmann Associates.)

Goods that have been sterilized in a flash sterilizer are removed with sterile handles individually packaged and used by a team member who is not in sterile gown and gloves. The sides of the mesh tray in which the goods were sterilized are grasped with the pickup forceps, and the tray is offered to a scrub assistant for transfer to the surgical field. When the instrument tray is removed from the sterilizer and carried to the surgical team, the technologist's arms and hands must be positioned away from the tray to prevent fallout contamination. A scrub assistant should remove the sterile item from the tray with sterile forceps. The tray should not be left on the sterile field, and *under no circumstances should a scrub assistant leave the sterile field or room to retrieve the item from the sterilizer.*

Loading and Operation

Because steam sterilization depends on direct steam contact with all surfaces of the items, the sterilizer must be loaded so that the steam will penetrate through each pack. This is best done by placing packs on their sides. Packs should touch loosely, and small items should be placed crosswise over each other. An efficient method of loading the sterilizer is shown in Figure 7–3. Heavy packs should be placed at the periphery of the load, where steam enters the chamber. Basins, jars, cups, or other containers should be placed on their sides with the lids slightly ajar so the air can flow out of them and steam can enter. Any item that has a smooth surface on which water can collect and drip during the cooling phase of the sterilization cycle should be placed at the bottom of the load.

Most modern steam sterilizers are controlled by push buttons that are clearly labeled (Fig. 7–4). The operator sets the temperature and time and then initiates the cycle. The sterilizer passes through its phases automatically. Adjacent to the time and temperature panel is a graph that registers the maximum temperature reached during the cycle. This graph must be monitored to ensure that the items in the sterilizer have been adequately exposed to the prescribed amount of heat. The total time necessary to expose goods to pressurized steam and sterilize them depends on the density of the goods and on the temperature within the sterilizer. The minimum temperature–time standards are as follows:

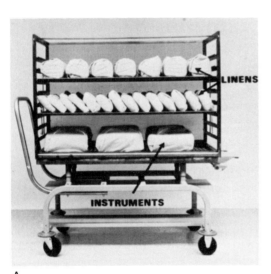

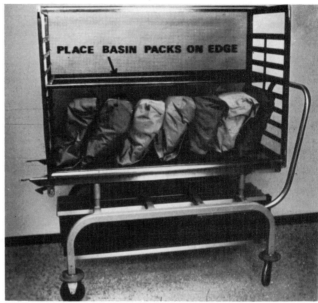

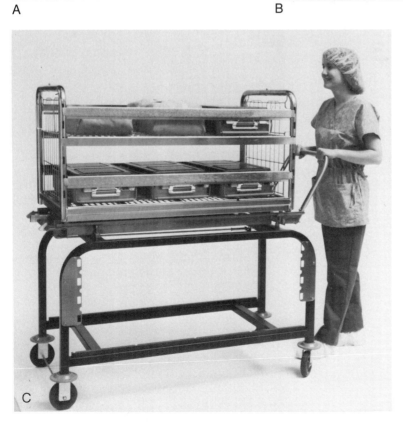

Figure 7–3. *A* and *B*. Proper methods of loading packs in the steam sterilizer. *C*. A loading car with containers and wrapped instrument trays. (Courtesy of AMSCO Healthcare, Pittsburgh, PA.)

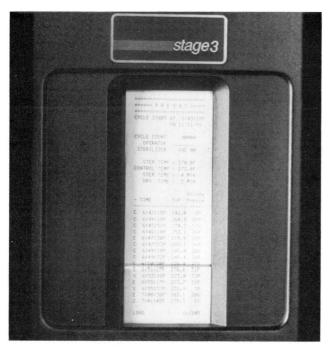

Figure 7–4. Steam sterilizer control panel printout, showing a completed prevacuum cycle. (Courtesy of AMSCO Healthcare, Pittsburgh, PA.)

Table 7–1. EXPOSURE PERIODS FOR STERILIZATION IN GRAVITY DISPLACEMENT STERILIZERS

Article	Minimum Time Required in Minutes	
	250–254°F (121–123°C)	270°F* (132°C)
Brushes, in dispensers, in cans, or individually wrapped	30	15
Dressings, wrapped in paper or muslin	30	15
Glassware, empty, inverted	15	3
Instruments, metal only, any number (unwrapped)†	15	3
Instruments, metal, combined with suture, tubing, or other porous materials (unwrapped)†	20	10
Instruments, metal only, in covered and/or padded tray†	20	10
Instruments, metal, combined with other materials (in covered and/or padded tray)†	30	15
Instruments wrapped in double-thickness muslin†	30	15
Linen, packs (maximum size 12 × 12 × 20 inches and weight 12 pounds)	30	
Needles, individually packaged in glass tubes or paper, lumen moist	30	15
Needles, unwrapped (lumen moist)	15	3
Rubber catheters, drains, tubing, etc. (lumen moist), unwrapped	20	10
Rubber catheters, drains, tubing, etc., individually packaged in muslin or paper (lumen moist)	30	15
Treatment trays, wrapped in muslin or paper	30	
Utensils, unwrapped, on edge	15	3
Utensils, wrapped in muslin or paper, on edge	20	10
Syringes, unassembled, individually packaged in muslin or paper	30	15
Syringes, unassembled, unwrapped	15	3
Sutures, silk, cotton, or nylon wrapped in paper or muslin	30	15

Solutions	Slow Exhaust
75–250 mL	20
500–1000 mL	30
1500–2000 mL	40

*Frequently referred to as "flash sterilizer."
†Maximum weight of each instrument tray is 16 pounds.
From Groah L: Operating Room Nursing: Perioperative Practice, 2nd ed. Norwalk, CT, Appleton & Lange, 1991.

> Gravity displacement cycle: 10 to 25 minutes at 270°F to 275°F (132°C to 135°C) or 15 to 30 minutes at 250°F (121°C)
> Prevacuum cycle: 3 to 4 minutes at 270°F to 275°F

These exposure times and temperatures do not reflect the entire time needed to include all phases of the sterilization process. These minimum standards apply only to the amount of time necessary for the pressurized steam to contact all surfaces of the load. Total exposure time includes the warm-up phase, holding phase (sometimes called the "kill time"), a factor of safety time, and an exhaust phase. Because these times may vary from load to load, depending on the items to be sterilized, the operator should always check the specifications of the item's manufacturer, not the sterilizer's manufacture, for recommended sterilization times and temperatures. Many items, especially heavy instruments and power-driven orthopedic tools, require longer periods of sterilization and cooling. The required exposure time for various equipment is given in Table 7–1.

Precautions and Hazards

In spite of safety features that are built into the steam sterilizer, *accidents occasionally happen.* The operator should be particularly careful when opening or closing the door. It is held in the lock position by a pressure-sensitive valve that prevents the door from being opened when the chamber is under pressure. Because the door has a tremendous amount of inside pressure exerted on it by the steam, the valve is designed to withstand very high temperatures and force from within. If the valve malfunctions for any reason, the operator may be able to open the door while the chamber is partially pressurized with steam. If this happens, he or she will be exposed to a rapid burst of hot steam when the door is cracked open. *Always check the pressure gauge on the control panel before opening the door!* If the pressure has not dropped to atmospheric (0) level at the completion of the sterilization cycle, wait for it to do so. If the pressure remains elevated, do not attempt to open the door. Do not attempt to resolve the malfunction. The malfunction should be reported so that trained personnel can be called for assistance.

Occasionally the operator may fail to close the door all the way. This is usually caused by the misalignment of the spokelike locks that are mounted on the front of the door. When this happens, the chamber receives a constant flow of steam that then escapes from around the edges of the door. The escape of steam may be so great that the operator cannot approach the sterilizer control panel to turn the unit off. Most models have a steam shutoff valve located close to the floor, below the sterilizer. The valve can be turned to the "off" position only if it is approachable without risk of injury. Steam should then be allowed to dissipate from the sterilizer until it is safe to open the door completely. Do not attempt to reach the valve unless the area around it is completely cool and free of steam.

When removing a sterile tray from a flash sterilizer, remember that the walls of the inner chamber are very hot. If the sterilizer has just cycled, be extremely cautious when removing trays or items.

Preparation of Items

Steam sterilization should be used only for items that can withstand high temperatures and pressure. Some items are impenetrable by steam, and these should be sterilized by another method. If unsure about which method to use on a given piece of equipment, the operator should always check with the manufacturer's specifications. Below is a list of items commonly sterilized by steam under pressure. These are listed because of their need for preparation before sterilization. This discussion assumes that equipment has already been thoroughly cleaned and is ready for sterilization (see Chapter 6 for a complete discussion on decontamination and cleaning procedures).

Stainless steel instruments must be open and strung together by means of a hairpin-type loop designed for that purpose. When assembling instrument trays, make sure that any sharp or pointed items are turned down to avoid injury or glove puncture when the pack is opened and sorted at the sterile instrument table. Most operating rooms keep file cards that list the various types of instruments to be included in a certain tray. Make sure that all instruments listed on the card are included in the tray. If an item is missing, locate the item before processing the instrument tray. Do not simply leave it out of the tray. Instrument trays should have a mesh bottom so that steam can circulate up through the tray and adequately cover all surfaces of the instruments (Fig. 7–5). Be sure that no instrument tips are caught in the perforations where they could become damaged. Always place heavy instruments on the bottom of the tray and pack or nest the instruments so that they cannot shift and damage each other during processing. Instruments should be checked periodically for proper function. To do this, first examine the instrument. The shanks of instruments such as hemostats, needle holders, and scissors should be straight. The instrument should be opened and shut several times. Do the ratchets mesh properly? Does the instrument stay shut once it is closed? With time, hemostats and needle holders may spring open unexpectedly. This is annoying and dangerous. To determine whether the

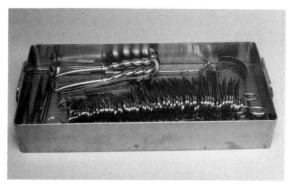

Figure 7–5. Mesh tray used to hold instruments for sterilization.

instrument is "sprung" (will not stay closed), close the jaws and lock the ratchets in place. Rap the edge of the finger rings gently on a firm surface. An instrument that is sprung will pop open. Cutting instruments such as scissors, curettes, and osteotomes should be examined for chips along the cutting edge. Any instrument that is found to be malfunctioning should not be packaged and sterilized. It should be sent out for repair.

Linen must be freshly laundered when it is used as a wrapping material or is the item being wrapped. The minute amount of water trapped between the individual fibers of linen vaporizes and pushes the air out of the fabric when steam sterilized. Fabric that is not freshly laundered contains no water, and thus air trapped within the fibers prevents adequate steam penetration. The largest acceptable linen pack size is $12 \times 12 \times 20$ inches and should have a density of no more than 7.2 pounds per cubic foot based on a weight of 12 pounds.

Basins should be stacked together with a towel or absorbent cloth between each separate basin. This allows steam to penetrate the cloth and wick it to all surfaces of the container. Bowls or cups should be prepared in the same manner.

Items with a lumen should have a small amount of sterile water flushed through them immediately before sterilization. This water vaporizes during sterilization and forces air out of the lumen. Any air that is left in the lumen may prevent sterilization of its inner surface.

Powered surgical instruments (e.g., drills, saws) should be sterilized by prevacuum steam sterilization unless the manufacturer's specifications contradict this. The equipment should always be disassembled before sterilization. Hoses can be coiled loosely during packaging, and all delicate switches and parts should be protected during preparation. Before sterilization, power instruments should be lubricated according to the manufacturer's specifications. Some instruments require that the motor be operated during lubrication to distribute the lubricant through the internal mechanism. Always consult the manufacturer's specifications before choosing a lubricant. Do not run the instrument unless you have been specifically taught how. Excessive force in pounds per square inch (psi) can irreversibly damage the instrument. Finally, before sterilization, all switches and control devices should be in the *safety* position.

Solutions do not require special preparation, but they must not be included in loads when the fast exhaust phase is in effect. If fast exhaust is used, the bottles can boil and burst. Solutions must therefore cycle through slow exhaust.

Items that should not be sterilized by steam include rubber bands or sheeting (steam does not penetrate rubber), wood items (such as tongue depressors), or any item that would obviously be severely damaged by high temperature and pressure such as lensed instruments, those with delicate parts, or those that contain materials that could melt. When in doubt about whether an item can tolerate steam under pressure, *wait, seek assistance,* and *follow instructions.*

ETHYLENE OXIDE (GAS) STERILIZATION

Ethylene oxide is a flammable explosive liquid that when mixed with carbon dioxide or freon becomes a highly efficient and cost-effective method for sterilization. For equipment that cannot withstand the extreme temperature and pressure of the steam sterilizer, ethylene oxide, commonly called "gas sterilization," is an acceptable alternative. The gas sterilizer is illustrated in Figure 7–6. Items such as endoscopes, plastics, power cables, cameras, and many other heat- and pressure-sensitive items are routinely sterilized with ethylene oxide. Ethylene oxide kills microorganisms and their spores by interfering with the metabolic and reproductive processes of the cell. The process is enhanced with both heat and moisture. The chamber of the ethylene oxide sterilizer is maintained at 20% to 40% humidity and at temperatures ranging from 120°F to 140°F (49°C to 60°C). Timing of goods depends on the concentration of ethylene oxide, humidity, temperature, and the density and type of materials to be sterilized. The manufacturer's recommendations for ethylene oxide exposure time must always be followed.

Unlike steam sterilization, items sterilized with ethylene oxide require *aeration* to dissipate any residual gas remaining on the items. *The manufacturer's recommendations for aeration are critical to the safety of the patient and to hospital personnel handling equipment that has been gas sterilized.* Aeration takes place in a special aeration chamber or may be accomplished with room air provided that safety precautions are followed (see later). The aeration time for an object depends on its porosity and size.

The Joslyn Ethylene Oxide Sterilization Process

A new technologic concept in ethylene oxide sterilization has been developed by the Joslyn Sterilizer Corporation, Macedon, New York. The Joslyn system uses three processes. The *preconditioning process* removes air from the inner chamber of the sterilizer by a combination of steam flushes and pressure pulses at below

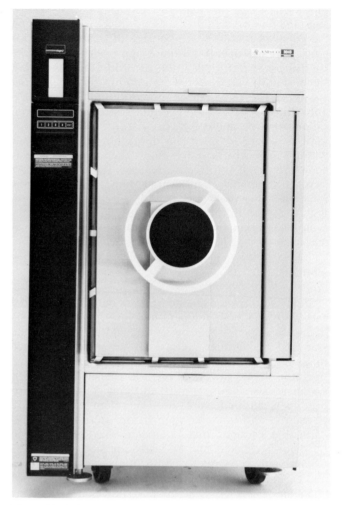

Figure 7–6. Gas sterilizer. (Courtesy of AMSCO Healthcare, Pittsburgh, PA.)

atmospheric pressure. This enhances the penetration of humidity and ethylene oxide gas into the materials in the chamber. In the second process, the *detoxification* phase, the sterilant is removed from both the sterilizing chamber and the materials. This is accomplished through the use of subatmospheric, low-temperature steam, which is delivered in a series of flushing and pulsing sequences. With this process, the sterilized goods are flushed of ethylene oxide residue in a fraction of the time traditionally required. In the third phase of the system, the "patented detoxification process," most of the ethylene oxide gas is captured out of the system, reprocessed, and made available for reuse. This process prevents the release of ethylene oxide into the environment and reduces the overall cost of sterilization.

Preparation of Items for Ethylene Oxide Sterilization

All items to be gas sterilized must be *clean* and *dry.* Any moisture left on equipment will bond with ethylene oxide gas and produce a toxic residue. This residue can cause burns or toxic reaction to those who contact it. Any organic material or soil that is exposed to ethylene oxide may also produce toxic residues; thus, all items must be scrupulously clean. Items are loaded in the sterilizer loosely so that the gas is free to circulate over every surface (Fig. 7–7). Every attempt should be made to load items that have similar aeration requirements. Some items must not be gas sterilized. These include acrylics and some pharmaceutical items. Because ethylene oxide does not penetrate glass, solutions contained within a glass vial or bottle will not be rendered sterile by this method.

Any instruments that have fittings or parts should be disassembled before gas sterilization. This facilitates their exposure to the gas.

A general rule when preparing any equipment for gas sterilization is that loose is better than restricted. For example, rubber sheeting, such as that used in the manufacturing of Esmarch bandages, should always be loosely folded rather than tightly rolled. Any two surfaces that are held tightly together will not receive the gas and hence will not be rendered sterile.

Precautions and Hazards

The environmental and safety hazards associated with ethylene oxide are both numerous and grave. Any employee who encounters this sterilization process should follow all recommended guidelines to prevent injury to himself or herself, to patients, and to others in the hospital environment. Ethylene oxide can cause the following:

- Burns to skin and mucous membranes
- Nausea, vomiting, headache, weakness
- Irritation of the respiratory system

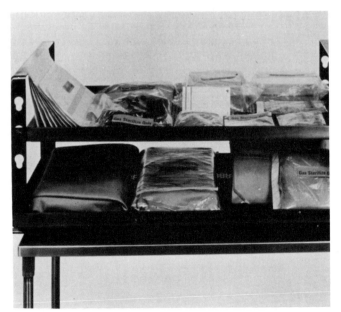

Figure 7–7. Proper method of loading goods in gas sterilizer. (Courtesy of AMSCO Healthcare, Pittsburgh, PA.)

- Destruction of blood cells (when undissipated gas contacts the circulatory system)

To prevent injury due to ethylene oxide exposure, the Occupational Safety and Health Administration (OSHA) has issued recommendations for air sampling in areas that are likely to contain high concentrations of ethylene oxide. The level of ethylene oxide must not exceed 0.5 ppm in any area. Documentation of sampling is made in accordance with federal, state, and local regulations. Other safety precautions include the installation of an exhaust system that vents the gas to the outside of the building through an exhaust vent located above the chamber door. Six to 10 exchanges of fresh air per hour are delivered to the sterilization area.

Items that have been gas sterilized must go through a complete aeration cycle (see earlier). Hazards associated with incomplete aeration are reduced when the following standards are followed:

1. Immediately following the sterilization phase, the door to the sterilizer should be cracked open and left ajar for approximately 15 minutes. This allows a majority of the gas to escape from the chamber.
2. Aeration should take place in a mechanical aerator.
3. The manufacturer's specifications for aeration must be followed exactly. If a mechanical aerator is unavailable, the room in which the sterilized goods are aerated *must be ventilated by negative pressure* to the outside of the building. No other equipment should be stored in this area, and personnel are restricted from entering during the aeration period.
4. Items transported from the sterilizer to the aerator must remain on a transport cart or other appropriate system while being transferred.
5. Protective gloves must be worn when unaerated items are handled.
6. Items must be transported as quickly as possible to the aerator from the sterilizer.
7. The transportation cart should be pulled rather than pushed (to place personnel in back of the air flowing from the unaerated items).

The Future of Ethylene Oxide Sterilization

Because ethylene oxide sterilization requires the use of chlorofluorocarbon 12 (CFC-12) to render it nonflammable and nonignitable, this environmentally unsound form of sterilization may soon be phased out. CFC-12 has been named as one of the chemicals responsible for the destruction of the Earth's ozone. Thus, the Environmental Protection Agency has declared that the United States will cease using CFC-12 by the year 2000. Currently, alternative forms of ozone-compatible CFC and other types of sterilization processes are being investigated and tested. One new method is *plasma sterilization*, which uses reactive ions, electrons, and neutral atomic particles to sterilize items at low temperature. *Vapor phase hydrogen peroxide sterilization* uses gaseous hydrogen peroxide to process instruments quickly and efficiently. This process cannot be used on linen, paper, or liquids. However, it is sporicidal, and stainless steel instruments can be sterilized with this method in 30 minutes. *Ozone sterilization* uses ozone, which is an unstable gas. When microorganisms are exposed to this gas they are destroyed by a process called oxidation. This process requires 30 to 60 minutes. This process cannot be used on some types of metals, rubber, and plastic. However, most materials are unharmed by the gas.

STERILIZATION BY IONIZING RADIATION

Most equipment available prepackaged from the manufacturer has been sterilized by ionizing radiation (cobalt 60). This process is restricted to commercial use because of the expense. Items such as sutures, sponges, and disposable drapes are just a few of the many types of presterilized products available. Also included are anhydrous materials such as powders and petroleum goods. These products have traditionally been sterilized by dry heat in the hospital setting. However, there is a trend away from dry heat sterilization because of its inconvenience and because these substances are now available as single-use items, packaged in one-dose containers to prevent cross-contamination. Items intended for single use, whether they are supplies for use in the surgical field or substances meant for single use, must *never* be resterilized by conventional (steam sterilization, ethylene oxide, or chemical) methods without the manufacturer's express recommendation to do so. The item might change in composition or deteriorate and could become a hazard to the patient or personnel.

WRAPPING GOODS FOR STERILIZATION

All items to be sterilized by pressurized steam or ethylene oxide must be wrapped *in a prescribed manner.* The procedure for wrapping goods is not based on convenience or personal preference. It is based on one principle—*that of enhancing the ease of sterilization and of preserving the sterility of the item.* In achieving these two goals, certain standard methods must be used. These methods have been subjected to challenge and proven to be effective.

Several different materials are available for wrapping items and equipment to be sterilized. All materials have been chosen because they meet certain specifications. Some materials are better for certain processes than others, and these should always be used with the intended process in mind. The wrapper should protect the item from dust, vermin, and penetration. It should resist tearing or delamination (separation of layers). It should be easy to handle to facilitate wrapping and delivery.

Fabric wrappers are made from high-quality cotton muslin (commonly referred to as "linen"). Muslin has sufficient density to protect goods from contamination and yet is porous enough to allow the penetration of steam or gas. The thread count (number of threads per square inch) must be at least 140 to be effective. Two double-thickness muslin wrappers or the equivalent (one double-thickness wrapper of 280-count muslin) are used to wrap items.

Paper and nonwoven fabrics (such as those used in the manufacturing of disposable drapes) are also used. Nonfabric wrappers should be durable and flexible. These wrappers are intended for *one time use only.* Once used during sterilization, they may lose their ability to prevent contamination. Always check with the manufacturer's specifications to determine whether a wrapping material can be used more than once. Nonwoven fabrics must be used in accordance with their thickness. Lightweight fabrics require the same treatment as muslin (i.e., four thicknesses for complete protection). Heavier fabric may be used according to the manufacturer's specifications. These are valuable for wrapping heavy instruments and flat-surfaced items such as basins and trays or heavy linen. When wrapping goods in linen or nonwoven fabric, the most common method is the envelope technique shown in Figure 7–8.

Combination *plastic and paper wrappers* are available in various compositions and styles. The combination wrappers are manufactured on a large roll that resembles a sleeve. The paper and plastic are laminated back to back along their edges. A designated length is cut from the roll, the item is placed within the sleeve, and the ends are heat sealed or taped. When using this type of wrapper, it is critical that as much air as possible be evacuated before sealing. Failure to do this can cause the package to split open during sterilization. When a mechanical heat sealing device is used, the seal should be checked very carefully to ensure that there are no air pockets along the seal.

Manufactured containers are sometimes used to hold equipment for sterilization. These must not be used for flash sterilization but are convenient and safe for both gas and conventional steam sterilization. These containers incorporate disposable filters within the construction of the container, and these must be in place following sterilization to maintain sterility of the items within.

Identification of Packages

No matter what type of packaging or wrapping system is used, each package must be marked with both the current date and the date of expiration (see later). The name of the item must be *clearly* marked and a lot control number also included. The lot control number is used to identify items that have been included in a load that may have yielded a positive biologic or mechanical control test. All packages must identify which type of sterilization—gas or steam—is appropriate.

STERILIZATION AND CONTROL MONITORS

Several methods are used to determine whether the sterilization process used on any given day or on any

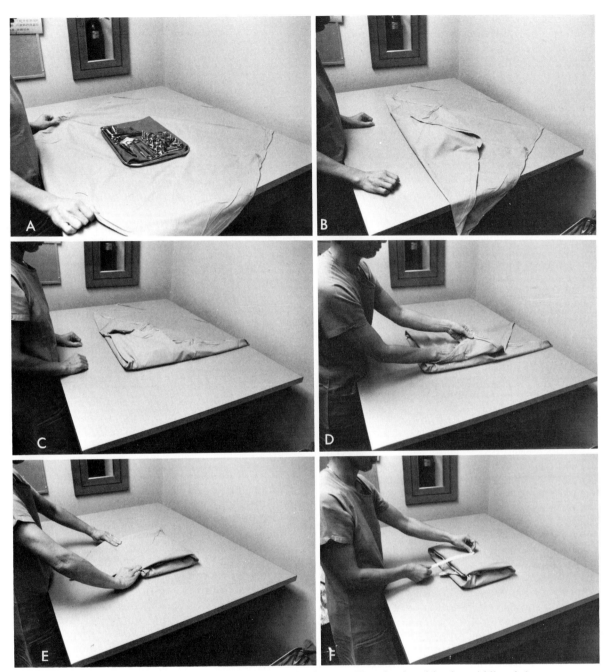

Figure 7–8. Wrapping a package for sterilization. *A.* Tray is placed in the middle of the linen, as shown. *B.* One corner is brought up over the tray and folded back at its edge. *C.* One side corner is brought over the edge. *D.* The second corner is brought over. Note that the excess corner is folded back. *E.* The last corner is brought forward over the tray. *F.* The corner is tucked under the previous layers with a small amount of the corner protruding. Heat-sensitive tape is placed around the edge of the tray.

piece of equipment has been effective. Because contamination of items used in surgery and in other areas of the hospital is critical, monitoring of the sterilization process is exacting and vital. Simply placing an item in a sterilizer and initiating the process does not ensure sterility of the item. Failure to achieve sterility may be caused by mechanical failure of the system used, improper use of the equipment, failure to wrap or load the items properly, or misunderstanding of the concepts involved. The best method for preventing human error is education and attitude. An attitude that is always in favor of the patient provides efficient and positive results. Mechanical failures can be minimized by a complete understanding of the sterilization process and of the equipment used.

Control monitors offer a way to check on the efficiency and efficacy of a sterilization process. A *chemical monitor* is an object that is treated with material that changes its characteristics when sterilized. This may be in the form of special ink that is impregnated into paper strips or tape and placed on the outside of the package, or it may be a substance that is incorporated into a pellet contained in a glass vial. Chemical monitors are available for both steam and ethylene oxide sterilization. The important fact to remember about all chemical indicators is that *they do not indicate sterility—only that certain conditions for sterility have been met.* In other words, the chemical responds to conditions such as extreme heat, pressure, or humidity but does not take into consideration the duration of exposure, which is critical to the sterilization process. A chemical monitor should be placed within and on the outside of all packages to be sterilized, even if it is only one item. To test and monitor the efficiency of the high vacuum sterilizer, a test called the *Bowie-Dick test* is performed daily. In this test, a special package of properly wrapped towels is taped with heat-sensitive chemical monitor tape and stacked to a height of 10 or 11 inches. The package is then placed *by itself* in the sterilization chamber and run for the appropriate time.

Another monitoring method used to evaluate the steam sterilizer is the combined temperature–time graphs that are installed within the control panel of the sterilizer. These graphs provide a permanent written record of all loads that have been processed.

A particular method used to challenge the aerator in the gas sterilization process is to subject a specially designed, highly porous device to sterilization and aeration. This device changes color when impregnated with ethylene oxide but returns to its normal color during complete aeration.

The surest way to determine the sterility of given items is with the use of *biologic controls*. A strain of a highly resistant, nonpathogenic, spore-forming bacteria contained in a glass vial or a strip of paper is placed in the load of goods to be sterilized. For steam sterilization, the dry spores of the bacteria *Bacillus stearothermophilus* are used. The gas sterilization process uses the bacterium *Bacillus subtilis*. The vial or strip is recovered at the end of the sterilization process and cultured. This process is time consuming and the results may not be known for several days, but it is a reliable method of testing the efficacy of a sterilization process. Biologic controls should be administered at least once weekly. If feasible, they should also be used whenever an artificial implant or prosthesis is sterilized and the item withheld from use until the results are known to be negative.

Each package must contain a monitor on both the inside and the outside of the package. Some chemical monitors are available in the form of tape that is placed over the outside of the package.

STORAGE AND HANDLING OF STERILE SUPPLIES

Shelf Life

Shelf life is defined as the length of time a wrapped sterile package remains sterile when in storage. The shelf life of an item or pack is dependent on many conditions. Whether a package remains sterile depends completely on the conditions under which it is stored and on the handling of that package. Any expiration date on any package assumes ideal conditions, which may or may not occur during the life of the package.

The *type and thickness of the packaging material* determines how strong a barrier it provides. Heat-sealed plastic and plastic-paper packages offer the most resistance to contamination. Under ideal conditions these packs will remain sterile for up to 1 year. However, the paper laminate of these packages is somewhat fragile and is subject to tearing or puncturing when the package is handled frequently or if the object within the package is too heavy. The *least resistant* packaging material is nonwoven fabric, which under the best conditions can contain a sterile item for only 30 days. Table 7–2 lists the shelf life for all types of packages under ideal conditions.

Excess handling considerably shortens the shelf life of a package. This is especially true for items that have sharp edges or are pointed. The worst case for excessive handling is when sterile items are stored in deep bins through which personnel must rummage daily to find an instrument or piece of equipment.

Environmental conditions such as temperature, humidity, and air turbulence are important in maintaining ideal shelf life. Excessive temperatures can cause sweating and condensation around packs. Any moisture can wick bacteria from a nonsterile surface through a wrapper and contaminate the contents of the package. Other sources of humidity such as aerosol effect from sinks or cleaning areas may also contaminate wrapped goods. Air turbulence such as that near doorways or halls can sweep bacteria-laden particles over sterile supplies and diminish their shelf life.

The *package closure* also affects shelf life. Heat-sealed packages have a longer shelf life than those that are sealed with tape. Dust covers likewise prevent particulate material from entering the pack. Items that are seldom used can be overwrapped with a plastic dustcover to prevent the need for frequent sterilization.

Commercially prepared and sterilized items may be considered sterile until the expiration date printed on the package.

Table 7–2. SHELF LIFE FOR WRAPPED GOODS

Item	Expiration
Linen (140-thread-count, four thicknesses) (280-thread-count, two thicknesses)	7 weeks
Linen-wrapped items, heat sealed in dust covers after sterilization	9 months
Linen-wrapped items, tape sealed in dust covers after sterilization	3 months
Paper	8 weeks
Plastic–paper combination, heat sealed	1 year
Plastic films, tape sealed	3 months
Plastic films, heat sealed	1 year
Nonwoven fabrics	30 days

From Groah L: Operating Room Nursing: Perioperative Practice, 2nd ed. Norwalk, CT, Appleton & Lange, 1991.

The storage system, whether in the form of open or closed cabinets or open or closed bins, often determines shelf life.

Storage of Sterile Supplies

Ideally, sterile supplies should be stored in an area that prevents their exposure to the adverse conditions listed earlier. They should be stored in areas of restricted traffic, away from ventilation ducts, sprinklers, and heat-producing light. If items are stored in open bins, the bins or drawers should be shallow to prevent excess handling of the items. Closed cabinets are ideal for storage. Mesh or basket containers are preferable over those with a solid surface where dust and bacteria can collect. The area should be cleaned frequently and prevented from exposure to dampness. The temperature and humidity should be controllable. Items should never be stored around scrub sinks, in hallways, or near nonrestricted areas. Packs should be handled as little as possible. They should be inspected for wrapper integrity before they are opened for use. Any suspicious pack should be rewrapped before being resterilized. *Always check the expiration date of an item before offering it for use.*

COLD CHEMICAL STERILIZATION

A number of liquid chemical agents in existence today can sterilize an item immersed in it. However, most of these chemicals are so corrosive and damaging to the equipment being sterilized that they cannot be used for this purpose. Two products that can be safely used for sterilization are a 2% solution of *glutaraldehyde* and *peracetic acid*. (See Chapter 6 for a complete discussion on liquid chemical and disinfectants.) Glutaraldehyde is noncorrosive and provides a safe means for sterilization of delicate lensed instruments such as cystoscopes and bronchoscopes. Most equipment that is safe for immersion in water is safe for immersion in 2% glutaraldehyde. Some items such as fiberoptic endoscopes have a control head that cannot be immersed in liquid. The insertion tube (the part that enters the body), however, is the critical part and can be sterilized with a liquid chemical. Other instruments such as the cystoscope can be completely immersed in solution because the delicate optical portions can be separated. To prepare an item for cold chemical sterilization it must be clean and dry. Any organic matter such as blood or sputum may prevent the liquid from penetrating crevices or joints of the instrument. If the item is wet, the moisture will dilute the sterilizing solution and render it ineffective.

When preparing an endoscope for liquid chemical sterilization, be sure to open all channels and stopcocks. Use a long cleaning brush designed for use with that particular instrument to clean inner channels. Take care that the lens is not scratched and the insertion tube is not allowed to strike a hard surface, because this will cause the glass fibers inside to break. After washing and drying the instrument, place the instrument in a soaking pan containing the liquid chemical. After immersion, the item must be soaked for the full length of time specified by the manufacturer. The immersion time must never be compromised because there is no method for testing the sterility of the item. Alternatively, an automatic washer-disinfector may be used. This equipment is designed to automatically clean and disinfect flexible endoscopes. Problems associated with the use of this type of washer include water quality, the water delivery system, exposure time, temperature, and flow rate. Following sterilization, regardless of the process used, all items must be rinsed *thoroughly* with sterile water and dried with sterile towels. Sterilization of an item in glutaraldehyde requires approximately 10 hours of soaking. Disinfection takes place in approximately 10 minutes. Because it is extremely difficult to thoroughly clean endoscopic accessory instruments such as biopsy brushes, these items are now available as single-use items that are disposable following surgery. Remember that disinfection is not sterilization.

The *Steris System* utilizes a 2% solution of peracetic acid at low temperature (122°F–131°F) for a complete sterilization process. This chemical is used in conjunction with a tabletop unit that provides sterilization within 20 minutes. Fiberoptic endoscopes are routinely sterilized by this method, which provides automatic continuous monitoring of the chemical disinfection as well as a printout of the chemical concentration. Because peracetic acid may be irritating to the eyes, respiratory system, and skin, personal protective equipment should be worn by persons handling the system.

Questions for Study and Review

1. What does *sterilization* mean as it applies to equipment used in surgery?

2. What is the difference between a gravity steam sterilizer and a high vacuum sterilizer?

3. What advantage does the Joslyn system of steam sterilization offer?

4. Why is it important that all air be evacuated from the steam sterilizer?

5. Name the five phases of a steam sterilization cycle.

6. Discuss the proper method of preparing stainless steel instruments for sterilization.

7. Why must linen be freshly laundered before it is used to wrap goods for steam sterilization?

8. What is the largest acceptable linen pack for steam sterilization?

9. What are the symptoms of ethylene oxide poisoning?

10. What is the minimum level of ethylene oxide allowed in the work area environment?

11. Why is CFC-12 being phased out of use in ethylene oxide sterilization?

12. What bacterium is used to monitor a steam-sterilized load?

13. What bacterium is used to monitor a gas-sterilized load?

14. What is the Bowie-Dick test?

15. What is the ideal storage condition for sterilized wrapped goods?

16. What two disinfectants may be used to sterilize fiberoptic instruments?

17. How long does it take to *sterilize* an item with the disinfectants referred to in question 16?

Bibliography

Conviser SA: Hospital sterilization using ethylene oxide: What's next? J Healthcare Materiel Management, July 1989, pp 35–39.

Groah L: Operating Room Nursing: Perioperative Practice, 2nd ed. Norwalk, CT, Appleton & Lange, 1991.

Howard WJ: The controversy of flash sterilization. Todays OR Nurse 13:1, 1991.

Jacobs PT: Plasma sterilization. J Healthcare Materiel Management, July 1989, p 49.

The Joslyn process: A new sterilizer technology. J Healthcare Materiel Management 6(3).

Karlson EL: Ozone sterilization. J Healthcare Materiel Management, July 1989, pp 43–45.

Kem Medical Products Corporation: Emission Control Systems, Sterilant Recovery & Chemical Scrubber Systems, Macedon, NY.

Kem Medical Products Corporation: New Process Technology for Sterilization Systems Using Steam and Ethylene Oxide for Industrial, Hospital and Laboratory Applications, Macedon, NY.

Kem Medical Products Corporation: Joslyn Sterilizer Sterilant Recovery and Emission Control Systems, Macedon, NY.

Rickloff JR et al: Vapor phase hydrogen peroxide sterilization. J Healthcare Materiel Management, July 1989, pp 45–48.

Stoddart GM: Ozone as a sterilizing agent. J Healthcare Materiel Management, July 1989, p 42.

8

Aseptic Techniques and Universal Precautions in the Operating Room

Learning Objectives

After reading this chapter you should be able to

♦ *Describe* aseptic technique.
♦ *Explain* the rules of asepsis.
♦ *Describe* proper surgical attire.
♦ *Discuss* the importance of personal health and hygiene.
♦ *Describe* Universal Precautions as they are practiced during surgery.
♦ *Use* proper technique for hand washing.
♦ *Describe* the techniques used to maintain asepsis in the operating room.
♦ *Practice* aseptic technique properly.

Key Terms

aseptic technique: Methods and practices that prevent cross-contamination in surgery.
closed gloving: Method of donning sterile gloves when a surgical gown is worn.
fallout contamination: Contamination of a sterile surface by particles arising from a source above it.
open gloving: Method of donning sterile surgical gloves when a gown is not worn.
strikethrough contamination: Contamination of a sterile surface by moisture that has originated from a nonsterile surface and penetrated the protective covering of the sterile item.
surgical scrub: Precise method by which all team members who will be working in sterile attire scrub their hands and arms before performing an operation.

WHY ASEPSIS?

The performance of surgery robs the patient of a significant barrier against infection and disease—the skin surface. Whenever the integrity of the skin is disrupted, as it is in surgery, microorganisms have the immediate opportunity to invade inner tissues and to proliferate. To prevent this from occurring in surgery, certain rules and procedures must be followed. These rules are called *aseptic technique.* Aseptic technique is the basis on which nearly every activity is performed in surgery. These rules are not simply guidelines but are the laws of the operating room, and to break them is to subject the patient to infection or disease. In addition to the rules of asepsis, certain practices are followed to ensure that the operating room is as clean and nonpathogenic as possible.

THE RULES OF ASEPTIC TECHNIQUE

1. *Surgical team members in sterile attire keep well within the sterile area.* It is considered poor aseptic technique for scrubbed team members in sterile gown and gloves to leave the sterile field. The *sterile area* is the space that includes the patient, surgical team members, sterile equipment tables, and any other draped sterile equipment. Scrubbed team members must never leave the operating suite during surgery without regowning and regloving. When x-ray procedures are anticipated during a procedure, a lead apron is donned before gowning and gloving so that scrubbed team members do not have to leave the room.

2. *Talking is kept to a minimum during surgery.* Talking releases droplets of moisture laden with harmful bacteria into the air around the sterile field. Although surgical face masks are helpful in eliminating the effect of these bacteria, they are not completely effective. Excessive talking increases the possibility of wound contamination.

3. *Movement is kept to a minimum during surgery.* Team members should move about the operating suite as little as possible. This rule applies to both scrubbed and nonscrubbed personnel. Scrubbed members are restricted to the immediate sterile area. The circulator must not tolerate excessive traffic in and out of the suite during surgery because this may bring dust and bacteria in from outside the operating room. When drapes are handled on the surgical field, they are unfolded and applied gently but deliberately, with as little movement as possible. Any turbulence may move particulate material and bacteria in the air onto the surgical site.

4. *Nonscrubbed personnel do not reach over sterile surfaces.* The circulator must never reach over the back table or Mayo stand to distribute goods on the surgical field. Dust, lint, or other particulate matter containing bacteria may fall on the sterile area. The scrub assistant must set basins and cups to be filled on the edge of the

sterile table. When sterile goods are opened onto a sterile surface, the hand and arm of the nonscrubbed person must be protected by a cuff formed by the inner surface of the sterile wrapper. Alternatively, the scrub assistant may receive the sterile item directly from the nonscrubbed team member.

5. *Scrubbed team members face each other. They face the sterile field at all times.* When scrubbed team members must pass each other or exchange places within the surgical area, they pass back to back. In doing so, they must *never back toward another sterile area such as the back table or Mayo stand.* They may step out a short distance from the sterile area and then pass each other with backs toward each other. Nonscrubbed personnel must never pass between two sterile areas or between scrubbed team members.

6. *Equipment used during a sterile procedure has been sterilized.* Any instruments or equipment that is used during surgery has been processed in a manner that renders it completely free of microorganisms. There must never be any doubt about the sterility of an item that is placed or used within the sterile area.

7. *Scrubbed personnel handle only sterile equipment. Nonscrubbed personnel handle only nonsterile equipment.* "Sterile" personnel are those who have performed the surgical scrub and donned sterile gown and gloves. These team members touch only the operative wound or those items that have been previously sterilized. "Nonsterile" team members touch only those items that have not been sterilized. They pass sterile items in a prescribed manner to avoid contaminating them.

8. *If the sterility of an item is questionable, the item is considered contaminated.* Packages with faded expiration dates, water-stained wrappers, or wrappers that appear defective must be considered contaminated. If there is any question about whether contamination of scrubbed personnel has occurred, it is assumed that it has.

9. *Sterile tables are sterile only at table height.* The surface of the sterile table is the only area of that table that is considered sterile, even if the table has been covered with a sterile drape. Thus, suture ends must not trail over the table edge. Table drapes must not be repositioned once they are put into place, because this would cause a nonsterile area to be brought up to a sterile one.

10. *Gowns are sterile in front from the axillary line to the waist and at the sleeves to 3 inches above the elbow.* The back of a surgical gown should be considered nonsterile even if the gown is a wraparound type. (Contamination of the supposed sterile gown back cannot be observed by the person wearing it.) Hands must be kept within the sterile boundary of the gown. The axillary region is not sterile, and so the arms must never be crossed with the hands positioned into the axillary region.

11. *The edge of any container that holds sterile supplies is not sterile.* Wrapper edges must not be allowed to come into contact with the sterile supplies they hold. When scrubbed personnel receive sterile items from nonscrubbed personnel, they must not touch the edge

of the wrapper with the gloved hand. When sterile solutions such as water or saline are distributed from a bottle, the cap is considered contaminated once the bottle is opened.

12. *Contact with sterile goods is kept to a minimum.* The excessive handling of instruments, drapes, and other supplies invites contamination. Sterile gloves are a thin barrier between sterility and contamination. Equipment should be handled only during preparation or use.

13. *Moisture carries bacteria from a nonsterile surface to a sterile surface.* When water comes in contact with a sterile surface, such as a table drape, it carries bacteria with it. This is called *strikethrough contamination.* It may occur when a hot instrument tray is placed on a sterile linen drape; the condensation of steam moistens the drape and carries bacteria from the nonsterile surface underneath to the sterile surface of the tray. Strikethrough contamination may also occur when sterile supplies are stored near scrub or utility sinks, where splashing may occur.

14. *Some operative areas cannot be sterile. Steps are taken to keep contamination to a minimum.* Operative areas such as the nose, the mouth, and perineal region cannot be made sterile fields. Aseptic technique is observed to prevent contamination of the field by pathogenic bacteria arising from other sources.

SURGICAL ATTIRE

All surgical personnel, and those visiting the operating room who proceed to restricted areas, are required to wear a surgical scrub suit. The scrub suit must be made of static-and flame-resistant, lint-free material. Operating room personnel don a scrub suit at the start of each workday when they enter the department and must change it if it becomes visibly soiled. The scrub suit should consist of pants and top. The sleeves should be short enough to perform a proper hand and arm scrub and also prevent the sleeves from becoming wet during the scrub. The top must be tucked into the waistband of the pants to prevent the front from becoming soaked during the hand and arm scrub and also to prevent it from contaminating sterile equipment and surfaces during surgery. Pants that are closed at the ankle are preferred over loose cuffed pants, because the closure prevents the release of minute skin particles and bacteria (called "fallout"). When pants are donned, they should not be allowed to touch the floor, since dust and bacteria can contaminate them. When personnel leave the department they must cover the scrub suit with a jump suit, cover gown, or lab coat. This covering must be secured in front and not left loosely open—otherwise it is of little use.

Hair is an extremely significant carrier of bacteria. Because of this, surgical caps must be worn at all times and in all areas of the operating room. The cap (or hood) meets the same safety requirements as the scrub suit and should be donned before the scrub suit to prevent the shedding of bacteria from the hair to the suit. All hair surfaces must be covered, including side-

burns. Nondisposable head coverings are permissible only if they are laundered each day by the hospital's laundry facilities. Only materials that prevent the protrusion of hairs from their surface should be allowed.

Shoes worn by surgical personnel should be sturdy, supportive, and closed on all sides. Because personnel spend many hours standing, shoes should be comfortable and well fitted. Sandals or clog-type shoes are hazardous in the operating room because they may slip off or cause a fall if a person must move quickly. Shoes worn in the operating room must be designated for work use only and not worn outside the hospital setting. Shoe covers should be worn anytime surgical personnel leave the department and must be discarded before reentering. Shoe covers should also be worn during procedures in which large amounts of body fluids are likely to be encountered, such as major orthopedic or cystoscopic procedures.

Masks are worn in restricted areas of the operating room. They are constructed of lint-free material and are designed to filter out particulate material from the atmosphere. Breath is a major source of contamination in the operating room. Thus, masks must be fitted so that they do not allow the wearer's breath to escape from the sides. Masks must never be left dangling from around the neck. A fresh mask must be used for each surgical case, and the used mask should be discarded as soon as the wearer is no longer in contact with soiled materials or equipment associated with that case. When the mask is being removed, only the tie strings should be handled. The filtering portion of the mask is laden with harmful bacteria that the wearer can easily transmit if that portion is handled.

Because of the lowered temperatures in the surgical suites, circulating personnel and others in the department may wear a cover gown over the scrub suit. If a cover gown is used, it must comply with the standards of asepsis. It should be closed in front to prevent the contamination of sterile equipment by loose ends or tie strings. A cover gown worn outside the department must never be used in the department.

All forms of surgical attire serve only one purpose— they are a barrier between sources of contamination and the patient or personnel. The standards of asepsis must never yield to individual comfort or fashion trends.

PERSONAL HYGIENE AND HEALTH

Strict personal hygiene is necessary for operating room workers. Daily baths and frequent shampooing aid in the maintenance of a healthy surgical environment. Fingernails must be kept short, since bacteria are easily trapped in the subungual area. Nail polish is strictly forbidden because it serves as a barrier to effective hand cleaning and scrubbing. Excessive make-up should be avoided because minute particles can be shed onto sterile surfaces. Any employee with a respiratory condition, open sores or wounds, moist eczema, or infections of the eyes, nose, or throat must not work in the operating room. These conditions add significantly to the bacterial population of the environment and may contribute to surgical infection of the patient.

UNIVERSAL PRECAUTIONS

The devastating spread of acquired immunodeficiency syndrome and hepatitis B virus of the past decade has resulted in the creation of critically important documents and recommendations for the protection of health care workers and patients. These documents define the health care worker, identify the risks to the worker, and establish practices and recommendations to prevent the transmission of blood-borne diseases. Original regulations for safety were created by the Occupational Safety and Health Administration (OSHA) and by the Centers for Disease Control (CDC). These regulations have come to be known as *Universal Blood and Body Fluid Precautions* or *Universal Precautions*. It is beyond the scope of this text to describe the entire set of regulations for all health care workers, but all surgical personnel must be familiar with those practices that apply specifically to the operating room duties. Because documentation from OSHA and the CDC is meant to serve as a guideline for minimum standards of practice, each hospital's exact protocol may differ slightly. *It is absolutely critical that these standards be respected and followed— not only for the safety of the health care worker but also for the health and safety of his or her patients.*

The basic guidelines for Universal Precautions are as follows:

1. All surgical patients are considered contaminated. In other words, all surgical patients are considered to be carriers of blood-borne pathogens.

2. All personnel must wear gloves when handling blood, body fluids, or contaminated surgical supplies.

Contaminated supplies are those that have touched any body fluids. These supplies include instruments, linen, waste, or any other type of item that is used in patient care or treatment.

3. Gloves must be worn by personnel when they perform or assist in the performance of care that involves touching the patient's mucous membranes or nonintact skin surfaces.

4. During all surgical procedures, with the possible exception of microsurgery, all team personnel must wear protective goggles or a face shield (Fig. 8–1). Ordinary eyeglasses may suffice for protective eye wear as long as the eyeglasses are fitted with side shields that completely protect the eye. Goggles or other protective eye wear must be disinfected following each case.

5. Face masks must be worn during every surgical case and properly disposed of following each case.

6. Whenever it is anticipated that excessive amounts of body fluids will be encountered during a surgical case, all team personnel must wear barrier gowns that prevent the penetration of these fluids to the skin of the team member. If penetration of fluids and soaking of a gown does occur during a procedure, team personnel must shower and change into clean scrub attire immediately following the case. Soiled scrub attire must be discarded into designated linen or waste containers.

7. Any sharp item, including scalpel blades, needles, pointed instruments, or any other item that could penetrate skin, must be handled with *extreme caution* to prevent accidental puncture. Disposable sharp instruments must be discarded into a designated container that is leak and puncture proof. During surgery a sterile container or magnetic board must be used to contain the item and prevent accidental injury. Scalpel blades must never be mounted or removed from the handle by hand. Instead, an instrument must be used for this

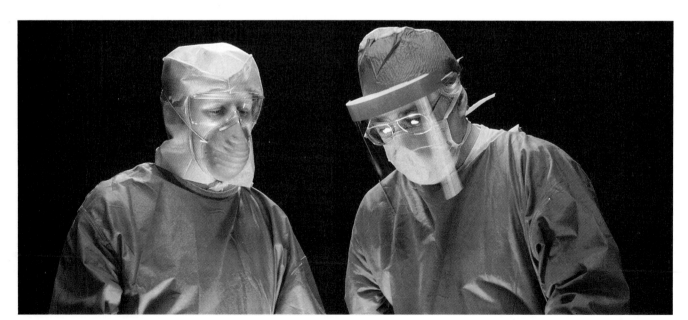

Figure 8–1. Protective goggles (left) and a face shield (right). (Courtesy of ONYX Medical, Greenbrae, CA).

purpose. Likewise, hypodermic needles must never be removed or mounted on a syringe by hand. A needle-locking syringe or one-piece needle-syringe is preferable to a two-piece system. Syringe caps must never be replaced by hand for subsequent reuse. Instead, the syringe must be discarded into a designated container.

8. All personnel must wash their hands thoroughly before and after patient contact, *even if gloves have been worn during the contact.*

9. All personnel must wash their hands thoroughly after contact with body fluids, even if gloves were worn during the contact.

10. When discarding contaminated sponges during surgery, the receiving container must be placed close to the patient and operating team.

11. Soiled linen and waste must be discarded in appropriate containers and not allowed to contact clean uncontaminated areas. Linen hampers must be leak proof.

12. Any tissue, blood, or body fluid specimen, or any specimen that has contacted patient blood or body fluids, must be secured in a leak-proof container. Specimens may be placed in two separate containers. The outside container must be prevented from touching the tissue, specimen, or other body fluids.

13. Personnel responsible for the decontamination of surgical suites following an operative procedure must don protective barrier attire, including gloves, mask, and waterproof apron, when contact with body fluids is anticipated.

14. When blood or body fluids are spilled, an effective disinfectant agent must be poured carefully over the spill before cleanup.

15. When an employee suffers any injury resulting from puncture or interruption of skin by a contaminated object, the injury must be immediately reported and follow-up care begun according to hospital policy.

16. All operating room employees should be vaccinated against hepatitis B virus.

17. Any employee whose exposed skin surface is not intact and is oozing exudate must be excluded from operating room duty until the condition is healed.

ASEPTIC PROCEDURES

Hand Washing

Hand washing, a separate activity from the surgical scrub, should be a routine practice during the course of a workday. Research has shown that hand washing has a dramatic effect on the reduction of disease transmission in the hospital setting. *Hand washing should occur before and after patient contact even if gloves are worn during the contact. Following surgery, all team personnel should wash their hands thoroughly after removing surgical gloves.* Hand washing is essential after removing gloves because the environment under the gloves is ideal to support the growth of bacteria. This means that even though a thorough surgical hand and arm scrub has been completed before donning gloves, some bacteria

that may remain on or in the skin can grow rapidly in the warm, moist environment under the gloves.

Procedure

1. Use an antimicrobial soap, not plain soap.
2. Use 3 to 5 mL of soap per hand wash.
3. For the antimicrobial action to take effect, the soap must be in contact with the skin for at least 10 seconds.
4. When washing hands, pay particular attention to the subungual area. Most of the hand's bacteria are found in this area. Fingernails must always be kept short for this reason.
5. The skin under rings can harbor dangerous amounts and kinds of bacteria. Always remove rings before washing.
6. Health care workers who wash or scrub their hands frequently are subject to cracked or dry skin. Breaks in the surface of the skin, even when very small, can allow the entry of bacteria. Use lotion to prevent this. However, do not use skin lotion immediately before or after hand washing. Lotions can inhibit the residual action of the antimicrobial soap. When lotions are used they must be dispensed in such a way that the user cannot contaminate the lotion remaining in the container.

TECHNIQUES THAT MAINTAIN ASEPSIS

The Scrub

All sterile team members perform the hand and arm scrub before entering the surgical suite. The basic principle of the scrub is to wash the hands very thoroughly and then to wash from a clean area (the hand) to a less clean area (the arm). A systematic approach to the scrub is an efficient way to ensure proper technique.

There are two methods of scrub procedure. One is a numbered stroke method, in which a certain number of brush strokes are designated for each finger, palm, back of hand, and arm. The alternative method is the timed scrub, and each scrub should last for 5 minutes. The procedure for the timed 5-minute scrub consists of the following:

1. Locate scrub brushes, antimicrobial soap, and nail cleaners, which are available at each scrub station.
2. Remove watch and rings.
3. Wash hands and arms with antimicrobial soap.
4. Clean subungual areas with a nail file.
5. Start timing. Scrub each side of each finger, between the fingers, and the back and front of the hand for 2 minutes.
6. Proceed to scrub the arms, keeping the hand higher than the arm at all times. This prevents bacteria-laden soap and water from contaminating the hand.
7. Wash each side of the arm to 3 inches above the elbow for 1 minute.
8. Repeat the process on the other hand and arm, keeping hands above elbows at all times. If at any time

the hand touches anything except the brush, the scrub must be lengthened by 1 minute for the area that has been contaminated.

9. Rinse hands and arms by passing them through the water in one direction only, from finger tips to elbow. Do not move the arm back and forth through the water. Proceed to the operating room suite holding hands above elbows.

The scrub technique is illustrated in Figure 8–2. *Note:* If the hands and arms are *grossly* soiled (dirt is visible), the scrub time should be lengthened. However, vigorous scrubbing that causes the skin to become abraded should be avoided.

Drying

The scrubbed technologist or nurse enters the surgical suite immediately after the hand and arm scrub. The hands are held above the elbows while entering. The procedure for drying the hands is demonstrated and explained in Figure 8–3.

Gowning and Gloving

Gowning Self

The technique for gowning oneself is illustrated and explained in Figure 8–4.

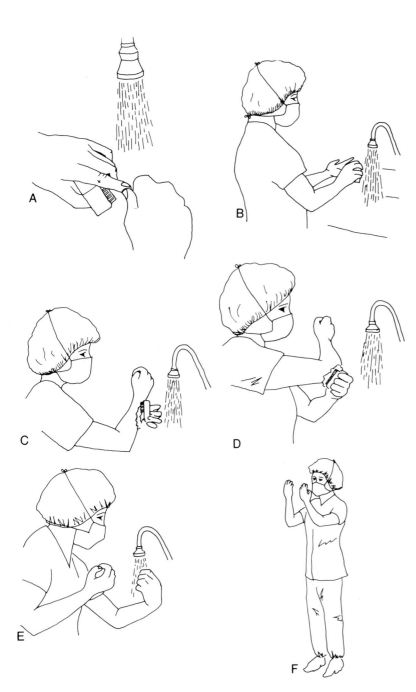

Figure 8–2. Technique for hand and arm scrub.
A. Subungual area is cleaned. Special attention must be given to this area, which is heavily laden with bacteria.
B. The timed scrub begins. Each side of each finger, between the fingers, and the back and front of the hand are scrubbed for 2 minutes apiece.
C. Proceed to scrub the arms, keeping the hands above the elbows at all times.
D. The scrub extends to 3 inches above the elbow (note scrub line). Each side of the arm is scrubbed for 1 minute. Repeat the timed scrub on the other arm.
E. Holding the hands above the elbows, proceed with the rinse. Pass the arm under the water in one direction several times. Do not move the arm back and forth through the water.
F. Proceed to the operating room suite holding the hands well above the elbows.

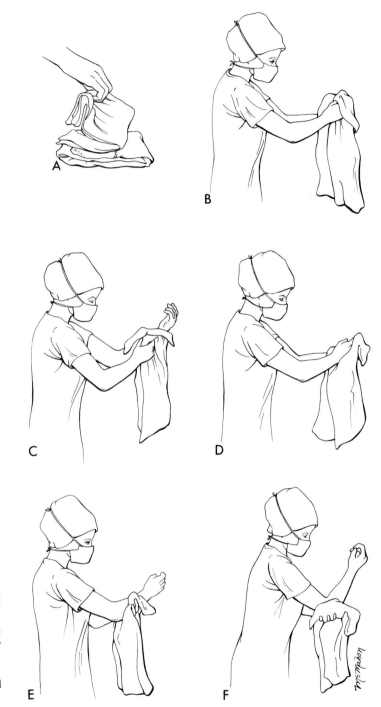

Figure 8–3. Drying the hands and arms.
A. Pick up a sterile towel from the table, being careful not to drip water on the gown beneath it.
B. Fold the towel lengthwise. Use one end of the towel only to dry one hand. Use a blotting motion as you dry.
C. Rotate the arm as you proceed to dry it, working from wrist to elbow. Do not allow the towel to contact the scrub suit.
D. Once the arm is dried, bring the dry hand to the opposite end of the towel and begin drying the other hand.
E. Dry the arm using the blotting rotating motion.
F. Proceed to the elbow. The towel may be discarded in the linen hamper or kick bucket.

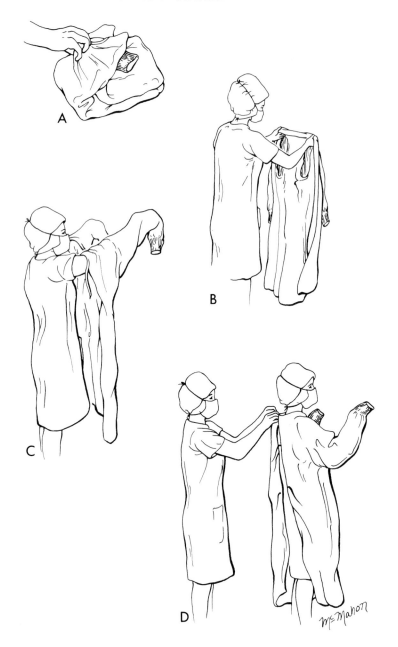

Figure 8–4. Technique for gowning oneself.
A. Grasp the gown firmly and bring it away from the table. It has been folded so that the outside faces away.
B. Holding the gown at the shoulders, allow it to unfold gently. Do not shake the gown.
C. Place hands inside the armholes and guide each arm through the sleeves by raising and spreading the arms. Do not allow hands to slide outside cuff of gown.
D. The circulator will assist by pulling the gown up over the shoulders and tying it.

Gloving Self—Closed Technique

The closed technique for gloving ensures that the hand never comes into contact with the outside of the gown or glove. When gloving is completed, any glove powder may be removed with a moist towel. (Glove powder can cause the postoperative formation of adhesions in the wound.)

By working through the gown sleeve, one glove is picked up from its wrapper. The bare hand must not be allowed to touch the cuff of the gown or the outside surface of the glove. The proper procedure is shown in Figure 8–5.

Gloving Self—Open Technique

The open technique for gloving is used when only the hands need to be covered, such as for catheterization or

the patient scrub preparation. It may also be used during surgery when one glove becomes contaminated and must be changed. However, it is very difficult to achieve complete asepsis using the open technique over a sterile gown. It should *never* be used routinely for gowning and gloving unless it can be performed while preserving complete asepsis. The technique of open gloving is given in Figure 8–6.

Gowning Another Person

The scrubbed technologist or nurse gowns the surgeon after he or she has performed the hand and arm scrub (Fig. 8–7). After handing the surgeon a towel for drying, the technologist or nurse allows the gown to unfold gently, making sure that there is enough room to prevent contamination by nonsterile equipment.

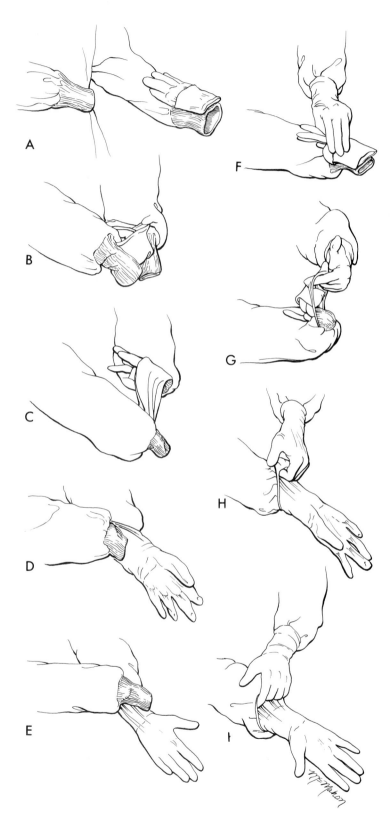

Figure 8–5. Gloving self—closed technique.
A. Lay the glove palm down over the cuff of the gown. The fingers of the glove face toward you.
B and *C.* Working through the gown sleeve, grasp the cuff of the glove and bring it over the open cuff of the sleeve.
D and *E.* Unroll the glove cuff so that it covers the sleeve cuff.
F, G, H, and *I.* Proceed with the opposite hand, using the same technique. Never allow the bare hand to contact the gown cuff edge or outside of glove.

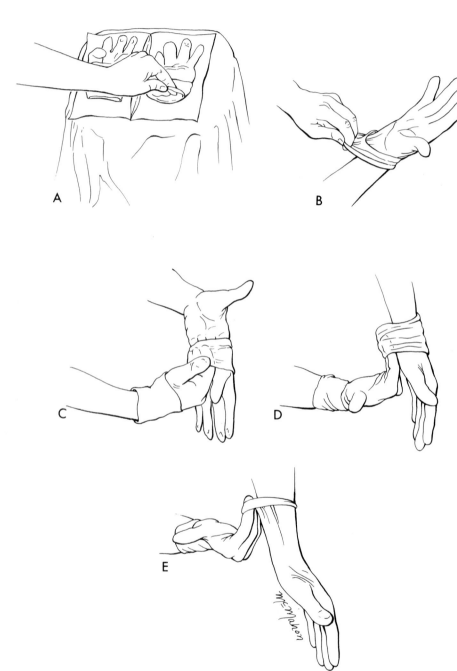

Figure 8–6. Gloving self—open technique.

A. Pick up the glove by its *inside* cuff with one hand. Do not touch the glove wrapper with the bare hand.

B. Slide the glove onto the opposite hand. Leave the cuff down.

C. Using the partially gloved hand, slide the fingers into the outer side of the opposite glove cuff.

D. Slide the hand into the glove and unroll the cuff. Do not touch the bare arm as the cuff is unrolled.

E. With the *gloved* hand, slide the fingers under the *outside* edge of the opposite cuff (not shown) and unroll it gently, using the same technique.

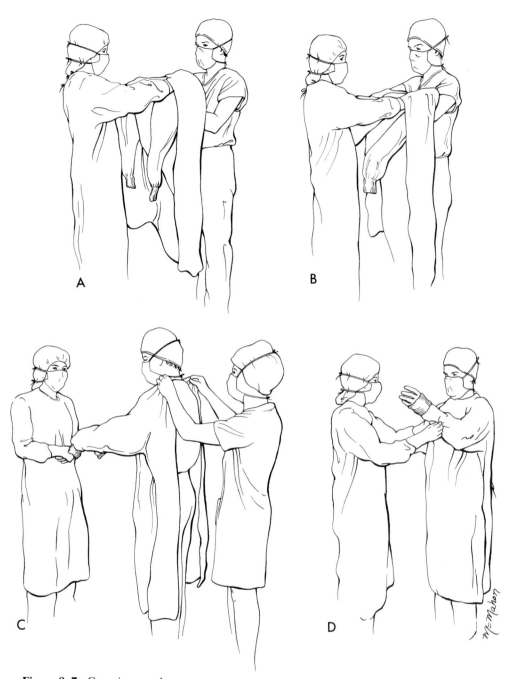

Figure 8–7. Gowning another.
A. Grasp the gown so that the outside faces toward you. Holding the gown at the shoulders, cuff your hands under the gown's shoulders.
B. The surgeon steps forward and places his arms in the sleeves. Slide the gown up to the mid upper arms.
C. The circulator assists in pulling the gown up and tying it.
D. Gently pull the cuffs back over the surgeon's hands. Be careful that your gloved hands do not touch his or her bare hands.

Gloving Another Person

To glove another person the rules of asepsis must be observed. One person's sterile hands should not touch the nonsterile surface of the person being gloved. The proper procedure is shown in Figure 8–8.

Removing Gloves Aseptically

The gloves should be removed so that the bare skin does not come into contact with the outside of the soiled glove. This technique is shown in Figure 8–9.

Distribution of Sterile Goods

Sterile items are packaged to allow personnel to unwrap the item without contaminating it. There are three popular methods of distribution.

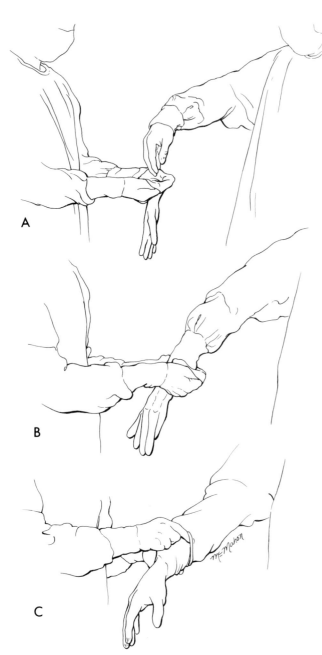

Figure 8–8. Gloving another.
A. Pick up the *right* glove and place the palm away from you. Slide the fingers under the glove cuff and spread them so that a wide opening is created. Keep thumbs under the cuff.
B. The surgeon will thrust his or her hand into the glove. Do not release the glove yet.
C. *Gently* release the cuff (do not let the cuff snap sharply) while unrolling it over the wrist. Proceed with the left glove, using the same technique.

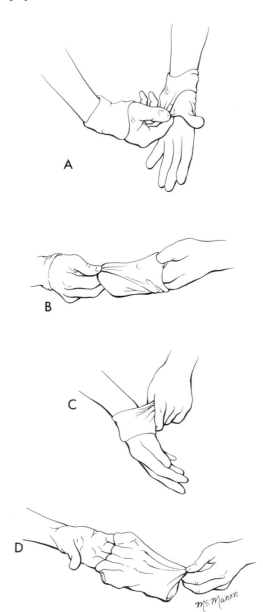

Figure 8–9. Removing gloves aseptically.
A. Grasp the edge of the glove.
B. Unroll the glove over the hand. Discard the glove (not shown).
C. With the *bare* hand, grasp the opposite glove cuff on its inside surface.
D. Remove the glove by inverting it over the hand. Discard the glove (not shown).

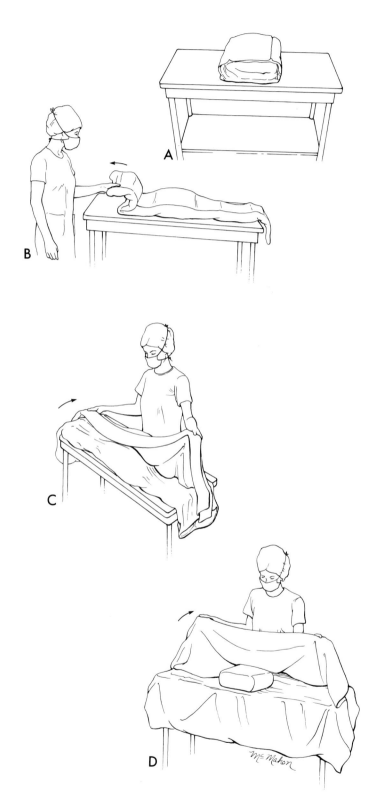

Figure 8–10. Unwrapping a sterile linen pack.
A. The large linen pack is placed in the center of the back table.
B. Layers are always pulled toward the person opening the pack so that the hand and arm do not extend over the sterile area.
C. Handle only the edge of the linen.
D. Follow the same procedure for the final fold.

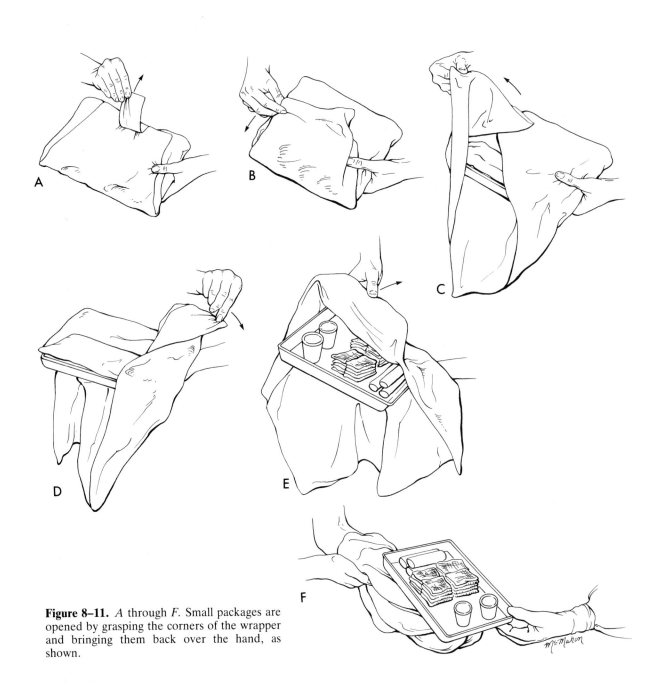

Figure 8–11. *A* through *F.* Small packages are opened by grasping the corners of the wrapper and bringing them back over the hand, as shown.

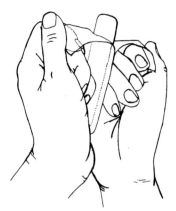

Figure 8–12. A peel-back package. (From Gruendemann BJ, Casterton SB, Hesterly SC, et al: The Surgical Patient, 2nd ed. St. Louis, CV Mosby, 1977.)

1. Large linen packs are placed in the center of the back table and unfolded using the technique demonstrated in Figure 8–10.

2. Small packages, including instrument trays wrapped "envelope style," are held in one hand and the wrapper is removed with the other hand (Fig. 8–11). If

the item or tray is too heavy to be held in the hand, it can be placed on a flat surface and opened there.

3. When supplies are contained in a peel-back wrapper, the package is peeled apart to expose the sterile item (Fig. 8–12).

Solutions such as sterile saline or water are poured into basins. The lip of the solution bottle is protected from contamination by a special cap, whose inside surface is sterile. Solutions must be poured without splashing, with care taken to keep the solution from dripping down the container onto the sterile field (Fig. 8–13). Once a solution bottle has been opened, *its entire contents* must be poured all at once because there is no way to protect the lip from subsequent contamination.

Questions for Study and Review

1. Give one practical example for each of the aseptic rules in this chapter.

2. Why must proper surgical attire be worn in the operating room?

3. When removing a surgical mask, why must only the tie strings be handled?

4. What is the purpose of Universal Precautions?

5. What is the proper procedure for handling and disposing of sharp items during and after surgery?

6. When should hands be washed?

7. What breaks in technique have you observed recently in your clinical rotation?

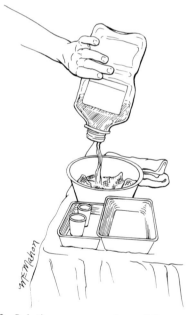

Figure 8–13. Solutions are poured carefully to avoid splashing.

Bibliography

American Hospital Association: OSHA's Final Bloodborne Pathogens Standard: A Special Briefing, Chicago, IL, 1992.

Centers for Disease Control: Update: Universal precautions for prevention of transmission of human immunodefiency virus, hepatitis B virus, and other bloodborne pathogens in the health-care setting. MMWR 37(24):1990.

Jackson M, McPherson DC: Blood exposure and puncture risks for OR personnel. Todays OR Nurse, July 1992, pp 5–10.

Korniewicz DM, Laughon B, Butz A, Larson E: Integrity of vinyl and latex procedure gloves. Nurs Res 38(3):144–146, 1989.

Larson E: Hand washing: It's essential even when you use gloves. Am J Nurs, July 1989, pp 934–939.

Occupational Safety and Health Administration, Department of Labor: Occupational Exposure to Bloodborne Pathogens; Final Rule. Washington, DC, U.S. Government Printing Office, 1991.

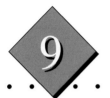

Anesthesia

Learning Objectives

After reading this chapter you should be able to

♦ *Distinguish between* general and conductive or local anesthesia.
♦ *Describe* the phases of general anesthesia.
♦ *Describe* the components of the gas anesthesia machine.
♦ *Define* a semi-closed or open anesthesia system.
♦ *Define* a closed anesthesia system.
♦ *Define* conscious sedation.
♦ *Describe* the characteristics of conscious sedation.
♦ *Be familiar with* common anesthetic agents.
♦ *Distinguish among* the different types of conductive anesthesia.
♦ *Recognize* the adverse affects of local anesthesia.
♦ *Recognize* classifications of anesthetic adjuncts.

Key Terms

caudal anesthetic: An anesthetic agent introduced into the caudal canal to induce a type of epidural anesthesia.

closed anesthesia system: In general anesthesia, the recirculation of anesthetic gases through the gas machine and back to the patient that prevents exposure of personnel to the gases.

emergence: The arousal from general anesthesia after cessation of the anesthetic agent.

endotracheal tube: Tube that is inserted into the patient's trachea for the administration of anesthetic gas.

epidural anesthetic: Type of anesthetic agent that is introduced into the epidural space of the spine.

excitement: The second stage of general anesthesia, in which the patient is sensitive to external stimuli.

general anesthetic: Type of anesthetic agent that causes unconsciousness.

induction: The first stage of general anesthesia, during which the patient's physiologic status is unstable.

infusion pump: Containment and monitoring equipment used when the patient receives intravenous solutions, including anesthetics.

local anesthetic: Type of anesthetic agent that causes loss of sensation or feeling to a localized area.

local infiltration: The anesthetic is injected directly into the operative tissue.

monitored anesthesia care: The patient receives an intravenous sedative anesthetic, which may be given in conjunction with a local anesthetic or by itself.

nerve block: Anesthesia of a large single nerve or nerves.

relaxation: During general anesthesia, the operative phase.

topical anesthetic: A drug used on the surface of tissue such as the eye.

vasoconstrictor: A drug that constricts blood vessels, used in conjunction with local anesthetics.

CLASSIFICATION OF ANESTHESIA

Anesthesia, the absence of sensation or feeling, may be produced systemically or in a specific body area. When the agent given causes unconsciousness, the anesthetic is termed *general*. When loss of feeling is produced in a specific area of the body, the anesthetic is said to be *conductive* or *local*.

The decision to administer a general or local anesthetic is based on many different considerations:

- The physical condition of the patient: existing disease, allergies, medication history, age of the patient, previous history of anesthesia
- The type and scope of the surgery
- The patient's and surgeon's preference
- The mental status of the patient

In addition to these considerations, the American Society of Anesthesiologists has developed a classification system for surgical patients representing five physical status categories. When this system is used, the patient is rated by one of the five categories and an appropriate method of anesthesia is chosen for that particular patient. This system is described in Table 9–1.

Table 9–1. PHYSICAL STATUS CLASSIFICATION OF THE AMERICAN SOCIETY OF ANESTHESIOLOGISTS

Class*	Description
1	No organic, physiologic, biochemical, systemic, or psychiatric disturbances
2	Mild to moderate systemic disturbance; mild, well-controlled diabetes, asthma, hypertension, or obesity
3	Severe systemic disturbance that limits activity; severe organic heart disease, severe diabetes with systemic complications, poorly controlled hypertension
4	Severe systemic disorder that is life threatening; severe angina, advanced renal or hepatic diseases
5	Moribund patient not expected to survive the operation; ruptured abdominal aortic aneurysm with shock, or massive pulmonary embolus with shock

*Emergency operation—The letter E is appended to any of the above five categories to indicate that the contemplated operation is an emergency.

From Goldstein A Jr, Keats AS: The risk of anesthesia. Anesthesiology 33(2):130, 1970.

GENERAL ANESTHESIA

Stages

General anesthetics cause unconsciousness. Depending on the type and amount of agent used, the patient may be slightly or not at all responsive to stimuli. A combination of agents is frequently used to achieve the desired level of muscle relaxation and postoperative analgesia. The period of time occurring immediately after anesthesia begins is called *induction*. When administration of the anesthetic is halted, the patient is in *emergence*. During induction and emergence the patient's physiologic status is unstable. It is the responsibility of the registered nurse circulator to stand beside the anesthesiologist during these phases and assist should an emergency such as cardiac arrest or vomiting occur.

Four dose-related stages of anesthesia have traditionally been described (Table 9–2).

Induction

The first stage begins when the anesthesiologist administers the induction agent. This agent may not be the same as the one that maintains unconsciousness. Sodium pentothal is often used to induce unconsciousness. During induction the patient retains his or her sense of hearing until the last moment before unconsciousness. For this reason it is mandatory that all personnel in the operating suite remain as quiet as possible. The doors to the operating suite should be closed, and all conversation should be halted.

Excitement

During this phase of anesthesia the patient is delirious and sensitive to external stimuli. Involuntary muscle activity and struggling may be seen. The patient is physiologically unstable.

Surgical or Operative Plane

This phase is the level at which surgery may be performed safely. The patient is relaxed, unconscious of

Table 9–2. THE FOUR STAGES OF ANESTHESIA

Stage	Biologic Response	Patient Reaction	Nursing Action
I: Relaxation	Amnesia Analgesia	Feels drowsy and dizzy Exaggerated hearing Decreased sensation of pain May appear inebriated	Close operating room doors Check for proper positioning of safety belt Have suction available and working Keep noise in room to a minimum Provide emotional support for the patient by remaining at his or her side
II: Excitement	Delirium	Irregular breathing Increased muscle tone and involuntary motor activity; may move all extremities May vomit, hold breath or struggle (patient is very susceptible to external stimuli such as a loud noise or being touched)	Avoid stimulating the patient Be available to protect extremities or to restrain the patient Be available to assist anesthesiologist with suctioning
III: Operative or surgical anesthesia	Partial to complete sensory loss Progression to complete intercostal paralysis	Quiet, regular thoracoabdominal breathing Jaw relaxed Auditory and pain sensation lost Moderate to maximum decrease in muscle tone Eyelid reflex is absent	Be available to assist anesthesiologist with intubation Validate with anesthesiologist appropriate time for skin scrub and positioning of patient Check position of patient's feet to ascertain they are not crossed
IV: Danger	Medullary paralysis and respiratory distress	Respiratory muscles paralyzed Pupils fixed and dilated Pulse rapid and thready Respirations cease	Be available to assist in treatment of cardiac or respiratory arrest Provide emergency drug box and defibrillation Document administration of drugs

From Groah L: Operating Room Nursing: Perioperative Practice, 2nd ed. Norwalk, CT, Appleton & Lange, 1991.

pain, and physiologically stable. Breathing is steady and automatic. If this phase is carried to its deepest level, cardiac or respiratory arrest can occur (see Table 9–2).

Danger

This stage begins when the amount of agent causes such severe depression of the central nervous system that the patient is in immediate danger of cardiopulmonary arrest.

Volatile Liquids and Gas

The *anesthesia machine* (Fig. 9–1) is used to administer compressed gas anesthetics, volatile anesthetic liquids that are vaporized within the machine before administration, and oxygen. Gases may originate from tanks mounted on the machine, or they may come from a source elsewhere in the hospital. In the latter case they are piped into the machine from wall or ceiling fixtures. Volatile liquids are poured into the vaporizer, where they are converted and administered in their vaporized form. In the past, the anesthetic gases and vapors traveled from the source directly to the patient through one of several methods (discussed later). The gases were then exhaled either totally or partially into the atmosphere. Fresh gases were added as needed. These systems were called *open* and *semi-closed systems.* However, escaped gases are a serious health hazard to personnel and there is now a trend to scavenge all waste gases to minimize these risks.

A safer, more efficient method of gas anesthetic administration is with the use of a system that collects exhaled gases into a reservoir called a rebreathing bag. The anesthesia machine provides new gases and oxygen,

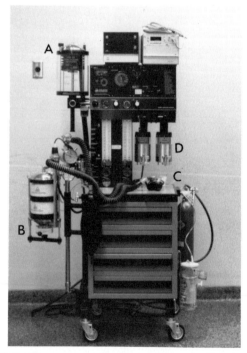

Figure 9–1. The gas anesthesia machine. A, Respirator; B, soda lime canister; C, mask and hoses; D, vaporizers.

filters carbon dioxide out of the expiratory mixture, and monitors the amounts of all three types of gases. This system is called a *closed system* (Fig. 9–2). Modern anesthetic machines are equipped with sophisticated monitoring and alarm systems that prevent the administration of oxygen-poor gas mixtures and alert the anesthesiologist to machine malfunctions.

The route of administration for all gaseous or vaporized anesthetics is by one of two ways. The *endotracheal tube* (Fig. 9–3) is inserted into the trachea following induction, and hoses that carry inhaled and exhaled gas are attached directly to it. Alternatively, a soft rubber face mask may be fitted tightly around the nose and mouth and the hoses attached to it. The commonly used inhalation anesthetics and their relative strengths, effects, and forms are described in Table 9–3.

Intravenous and Intramuscular Injection

Many anesthetic agents are given intravenously or intramuscularly. These agents are often given in conjunction with inhalation anesthetics to enhance their effect or to prevent some undesired effect of the inhalation drug. They may also be given alone or in combination with other intravenous drugs or in conjunction with a local anesthetic to give the desired level of sedation and relaxation. Table 9–3 is a list of commonly used intravenous and intramuscular anesthetic agents.

Monitored anesthesia care, also referred to as conscious sedation, is the administration of an intraoperative intravenous anesthetic with or without a local anesthetic.

When this type of anesthesia is chosen, the anesthesiologist administers the intravenous or intramuscular agents. A local anesthetic may be administered at the same time by the surgeon. The anesthesiologist monitors the patient's physiologic status throughout the procedure.

To be successful, conscious sedation must achieve the following:

- *Alteration of mood.* The patient's anxiety and fear are diminished.
- *Maintenance of consciousness.* The patient must remain conscious and able to cooperate with the surgeon and anesthesiologist during the procedure.
- *Elevation of pain threshold.* The anesthetic agents used must raise the patient's tolerance to pain.
- *Relatively stable vital signs.* The successful use of conscious sedatives does not severely alter the patient's physiologic status. The patient's vital signs are only slightly altered.
- *A desired level of amnesia.* The use of some types of sedatives results in a degree of amnesia that is dose related. This is a desirable effect.

Thus, during conscious sedation, the patient is cooperative, is relaxed, and may occasionally fall asleep. However, the degree of sedation must never be so great as to cause unarousable sleep, depression of the respiratory or circulatory system, or other adverse reactions.

Intravenous liquid agents are administered through a catheter inserted into the patient's vein. An intravenous

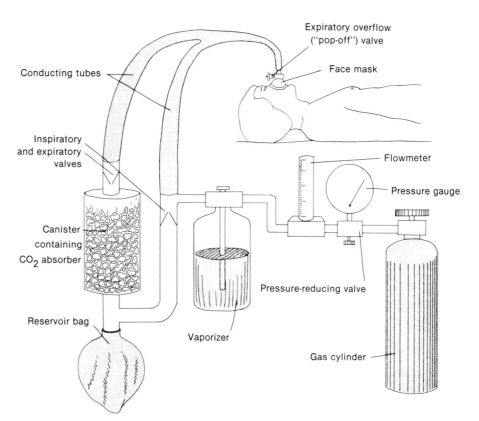

Figure 9–2. Closed gas circuit for the administration of inhalation anesthetics. (From Groah L: Operating Room Nursing: Perioperative Practice, 2nd ed. Norwalk, CT, Appleton & Lange, 1991.)

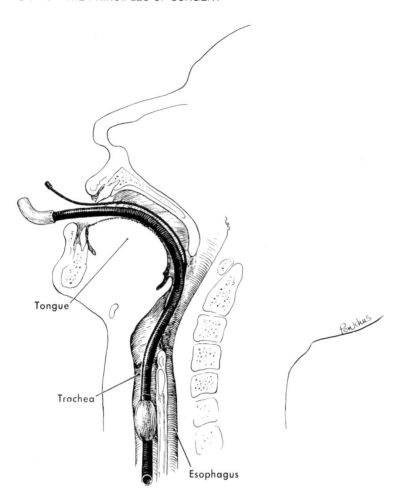

Tongue

Trachea

Esophagus

Figure 9–3. Endotracheal tube in place. (From Gruendemann BJ, Casterton SB, Hesterly SC, et al: The Surgical Patient, 2nd ed. St. Louis, CV Mosby, 1977.)

line also provides a pathway through which other solutions such as saline, electrolytes, blood expanders, and blood can be administered. The *infusion pump* (Fig. 9–4) is frequently used to aid in the administration of these liquids. This system provides outlets for several intravenous lines and continuously monitors the amount and rate of flow for each type of solution installed in the system. A computer module, available for some types of pumps, can be programmed to provide customized administration of solutions.

A combination of *fentanyl citrate* and *droperidol* (*Innovar*) is used to supplement nitrous oxide. It may also be used during local anesthesia as an analgesic.

Propofol (*Diprivan*) is a relatively new anesthetic that

Table 9–3. GENERAL ANESTHETIC AGENTS

Agent	Form	Method	Remarks
Enflurane (Ethrane)	Volatile liquid	Inhalation	Rapid, smooth induction; rapid recovery; moderate relaxation
Fentanyl citrate and droperidol (Innovar)	Stable liquid	IV or IM	Produces amnesia, analgesia; sedative effect; used in conjunction with other agents
Halothane (Fluothane)	Volatile liquid	Inhalation	Slow, smooth induction; potent cardiac depressant; may be toxic to liver
Isoflurane	Volatile liquid	Inhalation	Rapid, smooth induction; rapid recovery; good muscle relaxation; no renal or hepatic damage
Ketamine (Ketalar)	Volatile liquid	IM	Causes dissociative anesthesia, amnesia, analgesia; used in short procedures
Methoxyflurane (Penthrane)	Volatile liquid	Inhalation	Potent; may be toxic to kidney; slow recovery; prolonged analgesia postoperatively
Nitrous oxide	Compressed gas	Inhalation	Weak agent; used with other agents to potentiate their effect, poor muscle relaxation; rapid recovery; very safe
Propofol (Diprivan)	Stable liquid	IV	Rapid induction, extremely rapid recovery; may cause apnea or hypotension
Thiopental sodium (Pentothal)	Stable liquid	IV	Rapid induction; strong respiratory depressant; used almost exclusively for induction

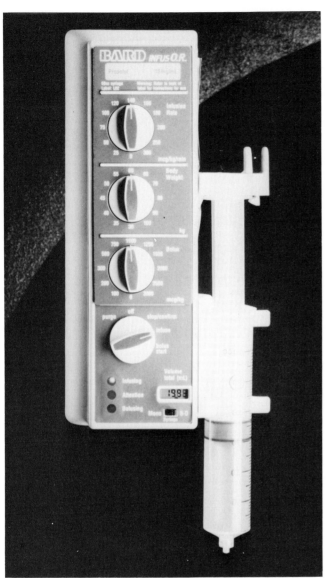

Figure 9–4. Infusion pump for the administration of intravenous medications and anesthetics. (Courtesy of Bard Med-Systems, Murray Hill, NJ.)

produces complete anesthesia in less than 40 seconds and complete orientation after cessation within 8 minutes. Unlike many other anesthetics that may require a rather long recovery time, patients who have had propofol are able to eat, ambulate, and function normally within a very short time. This drug has become extremely useful for outpatient surgery and for procedures that require only a short time to complete.

Thiopental sodium (*Pentothal*) is used almost exclusively for induction because it is very short acting. It is not generally given to sustain deep anesthesia. It is sometimes used in conjunction with nitrous oxide to produce anesthesia for very short procedures. This drug is a powerful respiratory depressant when given in large doses.

Narcotics such as *morphine, meperidine* (*Demerol*) and *fentanyl citrate* are often used in conjunction with inhalation anesthetics to prevent postoperative pain. These drugs may cause respiratory depression postoperatively.

Diazepam (*Valium*) a tranquilizer, is used with other anesthetic agents to potentiate their effects and allow a lower dosage of the primary anesthetic. This drug also produces amnesia postoperatively.

Ketamine is given intramuscularly as a short-acting anesthetic or may be combined with nitrous oxide to potentiate its effect. It is a dissociative drug that produces a trancelike state. Ketamine is often used for diagnostic or other short procedures.

LOCAL OR CONDUCTION ANESTHESIA

The agent used during local anesthesia acts on a single nerve, on a group of nerves, or on superficial nerve endings. During all types of anesthesia, including local infiltration, nerve block, topical, epidural, and spinal, the patient may be given a sedative or other agent to induce conscious sedation, as previously discussed. This increases the patient's comfort during the procedure and also prevents restlessness or excess movement during the surgery.

Local Infiltration

This type of anesthetic is injected directly into the tissues through which the surgeon must incise or manipulate to perform the surgery. Infiltration may be carried to deep tissue provided the surgery is not extensive. It should be noted that high levels of local anesthetic are toxic. Because the administration of local anesthetic takes place as part of the sterile procedure, the technologist should provide a 25-, 26-, or 30-gauge needle and syringe. After the initial injections into the skin have been made, the larger needles can be used because the patient no longer feels the pain of the injection. As the surgeon injects the anesthetic, the technologist and circulator must keep track of how much anesthetic has been used; this must appear on the patient's operative report. Medication is distributed, as needed, to the scrub assistant, who receives it in a glass medicine cup. Metal cups must not be used for this purpose, because they may interact with the drug and alter its composition. When highly vascular areas are injected, *epinephrine* is sometimes added to the anesthetic. Epinephrine is a *vasoconstrictor* (a drug that constricts the blood vessels). It aids in blocking the escape of anesthetic out into the systemic bloodstream and also helps control hemorrhage. Epinephrine is a potent cardiac stimulant, and whenever it is used, the exact amount must be tabulated by the registered nurse circulator. Many local anesthetics are manufactured with epinephrine already added. Anesthetic *with* epinephrine is manufactured in specified strengths, designated on the vial label. If anesthetic both "with" and "without" epinephrine is distributed to the scrub assistant, he or she must be aware at all times during the surgery of which one the surgeon is using so that the *amount and strength* of the drug can be charted.

Nerve Block

This is anesthesia of a large single nerve or nerves, not necessarily at the immediate surgical site. When the agent is injected into and around the nerves, impulses from the area supplied by the nerve are prevented from reaching the brain. Nerve block is commonly used in surgery that is performed on the fingers and toes and may also be used in the treatment of specific neuralgia, such as tic douloureux. For treatment of vascular insufficiency, a block is used to dilate large vessels whose smooth muscle walls are constricted. The nerve that supplies the vessel layers is anesthetized, and the vessel dilates.

Topical Anesthesia

A topical anesthetic is used to numb superficial nerve endings, particularly those of the mucous membranes. The agent may be swabbed, sprayed, or applied in drops, as for eye surgery. Topical agents are useful in preparing the patient for endoscopic procedures such as bronchoscopy or gastroscopy.

Epidural Anesthesia

An epidural anesthetic is introduced into the epidural space of the spine. The agent bathes the nerve roots of the spinal cord, and the area supplied by these nerves is anesthetized. Because the anesthetic is injected outside the spinal canal, there is no direct contact between cerebrospinal fluid and anesthetic.

Caudal Anesthesia

This form of anesthesia is a type of epidural anesthesia that is directed into the caudal canal at the sacrum (Fig. 9–5). It is ideal for obstetrics and procedures on the perineum. Continuous epidural anesthesia is performed when the procedure is lengthy. A plastic catheter is inserted into the epidural space and the agent is given

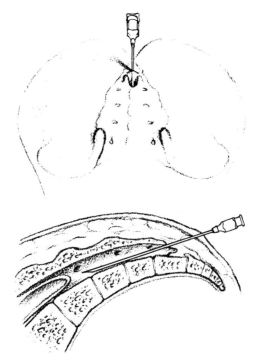

Figure 9–5. Position of the needle for caudal anesthesia. Note that the needle does not enter the spinal canal. (From Nealon TF: Fundamental Skills in Surgery, 3rd ed. Philadelphia, WB Saunders, 1979.)

intermittently, as needed. The catheter remains in place throughout the procedure. This type of anesthesia is also used to control postoperative pain.

Spinal Anesthesia

A spinal anesthetic is introduced into the subarachnoid space at the fourth or fifth lumbar interspace (Fig. 9–6). Here the agent comes into contact with the cerebrospinal fluid and thus travels along the length of the spinal canal. All nerve roots in the path of the agent are anesthetized. The patient is positioned on the tilted operating table so that the head is lower than the feet (Trendelenburg position) for a few moments only, until the desired level of anesthesia is reached. The table is then moved to a slight reverse Trendelenburg position. When the agent is hyperbaric (heavier than cerebrospi-

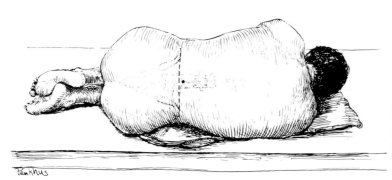

Figure 9–6. Position of the patient for spinal anesthesia. The patient may also sit up with the back arched to widen the vertebral interspaces. (From Gruendemann BJ, Casterton SB, Hesterly SC, et al: The Surgical Patient, 2nd ed. St. Louis, CV Mosby, 1977.)

nal fluid), the level of anesthetic is easily manipulated within the first 5 minutes, after which the agent is fixed in the tissues.

Spinal anesthesia is ideal for surgery of the lower pelvis, such as cesarean section or hernia repair. It is also commonly used for surgery of the lower extremities. Continuous spinal anesthesia, which utilizes the same technique as continuous epidural anesthesia, presents a risk of infection in the spinal canal because of the plastic catheter used. If the puncture site becomes contaminated, the infection could then travel freely in cerebrospinal fluid and thus spread to the brain.

Some commonly used local anesthetics are presented in Table 9–4.

Adverse Reactions

Many patients react adversely to conduction anesthetics, particularly topical agents. Proper monitoring of blood pressure, pulse rate, and heart rhythm is essential. The circulator should monitor the patient continuously every 15 minutes during the procedure. All team members should be aware of the danger signals that accompany an adverse reaction. However, it should be noted that *not all* symptoms occur in *all* patients. These symptoms are often noted during relative overdose, which is by far the most common complication. Relative overdose occurs when the patient receives too much anesthetic too quickly, as when a vein or artery is punctured during the administration of the anesthetic. The anesthetic travels quickly to the brain, and the following features may be observed.

Stimulation

The patient may become very talkative or anxious and exhibit signs of tachycardia (fast heart rate), thready pulse, tremors, or convulsions.

Depression

The patient may appear sleepy and unresponsive. Bradycardia (slow heart rate) may develop, as well as hypotension (decreased blood pressure).

Other Signs

The patient may develop cyanosis or excessive perspiration (diaphoresis), feel cold, and act restless (signs of shock). Fainting, itching, nausea, or sudden headache may also occur.

In treating the reaction, the anesthetic is discontinued immediately and oxygen is administered. Cardiopulmonary resuscitation is initiated, if necessary.

ADJUNCTS TO ANESTHETIC AGENTS

Preoperative Medications

Preoperative medications are given to certain patients according to their specific need before surgery. The current trend is to avoid the use of profound preoperative sedation, which in many cases prolongs the effects of anesthesia and may severely depress the patient's respiratory and circulatory systems.

Anticholinergics. These medications reduce the formation of oral secretions and also block stimuli

Table 9–4. DRUGS USED FOR LOCAL ANESTHETICS

Characteristics	Cocaine	Novocaine (Procaine)	Lidocaine (Xylocaine)	Tetracaine (Pontocaine)	Mepivacaine (Carbocaine)	Bupivacaine (Marcaine)	Chloroprocaine (Nesacaine)
Topical concentration	Eye 1% Other 4%–10%	Ineffective	Eye 0.5% Other 4%	Eye 0.5% Other 1%–2%	Eye 0.5% Other 1%–2%	Not used	Not used
Onset (minutes)	Immediate		3–5	10–20	10–20		
Duration (minutes)	30–60		30–60	60–120	60–120		
Maximum dose	200 mg		200 mg	50 mg	500 mg		
Infiltration concentration	Not used	0.25%–1.0% 2.0, 10%	0.5%–2%	0.05–0.1%	0.5%–2%	0.25%–0.75%	1%, 2%, 3%
Onset (minutes)		5–15	3–5	10–20	5–10	5–10	5–10
Duration of action (minutes), plain		45–60	30–60	90–120	150–240	90–120	30–60
Duration of action (minutes) with epinephrine 1:200,000		60–90	45–90	140–180	240–320	140–180	45–90
Maximum dose, plain		1000 mg or 15 mg/kg	300 mg or 6–8 mg/kg	50–100 mg or 3 mg/kg	500 mg or 6–8 mg/kg	175 mg or 4–6 mg/kg	1000 mg or 15 mg/kg

Adapted from Bridenbaugh LD: Care of the surgical patient under local anesthetics. Gown Gloves 4(2):13, 1979.

from the vagus nerve. Examples: atropine, scopolamine, glycopyrrolate.

Barbiturates. These medications produce sedation. Examples: pentobarbital, secobarbital.

Tranquilizers. These drugs decrease the patient's anxiety and produce sedation. When given intravenously they may sometimes be used during endoscopic procedures. Example: diazepam.

Narcotics. These drugs provide sedation and analgesia. They may cause nausea and vomiting and circulatory and respiratory depression.

Neuromuscular Blocking Agents

Neuromuscular blocking agents are used in conjunction with a general anesthetic to produce profound muscle relaxation. Neuromuscular blocking agents are administered by the anesthesiologist immediately following induction and as needed thereafter during the operative procedure. Even during deep anesthesia the voluntary (striated) muscle may respond to stimulus and thus contract. This phenomenon can interfere with necessary anatomic manipulation that occurs during surgery, especially during abdominal procedures and during intubation (insertion of the endotracheal tube).

Questions for Study and Review

1. What is the difference between general and local anesthesia?

2. What are the phases of general anesthesia?

3. Describe the components of the gas machine.

4. What is a closed anesthesia system?

5. What is conscious sedation?

6. What is the difference between a caudal and a spinal anesthetic?

7. What are some of the adverse effects of a local anesthetic?

8. Why is epinephrine sometimes used during local anesthesia?

9. Why is it important to know how much local anesthetic has been given?

10. What are neuromuscular blocking agents, and why are they used?

Bibliography

Anesthesia equipment profiles. Milestones Anesthesia 1(1):2–3, 1991.

Dripps RD, Eckenhoff JE, Vandam LD: Introduction to Anesthesia: The Principles of Safe Practice, 6th ed. Philadelphia, WB Saunders, 1982.

Malignant hyperthermia. Milestones Anesthesia 2(1) Supplement, 1992.

Martin JT: Positioning in Anesthesia and Surgery. Philadelphia, WB Saunders, 1978.

Osborn I: Case one: Diprivan infusion during magnetic resonance imaging. Milestones Anesthesia 2(1):8–9, 1992.

Sheridan E, Patterson RH, Gustafson EA: Falconer's The Drug, the Nurse, the Patient, 7th ed. Philadelphia, WB Saunders, 1984.

Transporting and Positioning the Surgical Patient

Learning Objectives

After reading this chapter you should be able to

◆ *Transfer* the conscious patient safely from a bed to a stretcher.
◆ *Transport* the patient safely to the operating room or other location in the hospital.
◆ *Describe* the safe positioning of the patient.
◆ *Understand* the need for careful padding and protection during positioning.
◆ *Transfer* the unconscious patient to a stretcher safely.

Key Terms

armboard: Detachable extension on the operating table that accommodates the patient's arms.
dorsal recumbent: Term synonymous with *supine*; position of the patient lying on his or her back.
footboard: Section of the operating table at the foot end that can be removed or angled up or down.
Fowler position: Sitting position.
headboard: Removable section of the operating table at the head end that can be angled up or down.
Kraske position: Operative position used for procedures of the perianal area; also called "jackknife" position or "knee-chest" position. The patient lies in prone position, with the table broken at its midsection so that the head and feet are lower than the midsection.
laminectomy position: Operative position used for spinal surgery; a form of prone position.
prone: A position in which the patient lies face down.

89

reverse Trendelenburg position: Operative position in which the patient lies in supine position, and the operating table is tilted so that the head is higher than the feet.

Sims position: Also called lateral position; position of the patient lying on his or her side.

table breaks: Hinged sections of the operating table that can be folded up or down to create different postures.

Trendelenburg position: Operative position in which the patient lies in supine position with the operating table tilted such that the head is lower than the feet.

The safe transportation and positioning of the patient is a skill that all surgery personnel must develop. The patient must be transported to the operating room before surgery, positioned on the operating table after arrival, and transferred back to the stretcher following surgery. These maneuvers must be accomplished with extreme care.

TRANSPORTATION OF THE CONSCIOUS PATIENT

There are many hazards associated with the transportation of the patient regardless of whether he or she is fully conscious. Patient falls often occur during transfer. Catheters, oxygen tubing, and other medical devices can cause severe tissue trauma if pulled away from the body. Mechanical devices used to adjust and control transport equipment can pinch, bruise, or even cause fractures. Safe transportation requires that personnel are knowledgeable, alert, and gentle. In addition to the safe operation of transport equipment, there remains the hazard of patient care emergencies that may occur during transport.

Transport Vehicles

Transport vehicles are used to convey the patient to various locations in the hospital. The surgical patient is commonly transported to the operating room on a *stretcher* (also called a *gurney*). Stretchers are designed to maximize patient safety and also to accommodate equipment such as oxygen tanks and intravenous solution containers. The safest type of stretcher is one that has the following design features:

- Locking devices on the wheels
- Restraining devices such as safety straps and side rails. Pediatric cribs have side bars that are high enough to prevent the child from falling out of the crib when he or she is standing.
- Adjustable intravenous infusion pole or standard
- Rack for stabilizing an oxygen tank
- Positioning capabilities
- Control levers that are easily accessible by personnel
- Maneuverability
- Sufficient size

- Removable headrests and footboards
- Mattress stabilizing devices
- Easily cleaned surfaces

Transfer to Stretcher

Before moving any conscious patient from his or her bed to the stretcher, the technologist or nurse must *assess* the situation. Does the patient have an indwelling urinary catheter? Is he or she receiving continuous oxygen? Is the patient elderly? Does the patient have obvious physical limitations such as a cast or limb prosthesis? Is the patient alert or sedated? Extra personnel should be available to assist in the transfer if the patient is encumbered by indwelling equipment, is heavily sedated, or is unconscious. *One should never attempt a transfer if unfamiliar with the equipment used to transport the patient.*

To transfer the patient from his or her bed to the stretcher the technologist or nurse should

1. Tell the patient what is about to happen.
2. Free any catheters, intravenous lines, or other tubing that may become entangled in the bed linen during the move.
3. Be certain that all tubing is long enough to accommodate the transfer.
4. Free any bed linen that may become entangled.
5. Align the stretcher with the patient's bed.
6. *Lock all wheels on the stretcher and the bed.*
7. Adjust the height of the stretcher to accommodate the bed height.
8. Position himself or herself on the opposite side of the stretcher to prevent the patient from moving over too far and falling.
9. Ask the patient to move slowly over to the stretcher.
10. Assist the patient during the move.
11. Cover the patient with the stretcher linen.
12. Transfer any patient care devices such as a urinary retention bag or oxygen tank.
13. Check to make sure that all tubing is free and that none is folded or crimped. Intravenous infusion bags or bottles must be positioned away from the patient's head, ideally at his or her feet.
14. Apply safety straps.
15. Raise side rails.

16. Unlock stretcher wheels.

17. Proceed to the destination slowly, pushing the stretcher feet first. Always proceed through doorways, including elevators, positioned at the patient's head and pulling rather than pushing the stretcher.

18. Protect the patient's head at all times.

19. If a patient service elevator is not available and the public elevator must be used, ask occupants to step out to accommodate the patient.

20. On arrival at the destination, notify appropriate personnel. *Do not leave the patient unless other personnel are available to take over the patient's care.*

TRANSFER OF AND POSITIONING THE ANESTHETIZED PATIENT

1. Always *ask* the anesthesiologist's permission before moving the anesthetized patient.

2. *Provide* enough help to move the patient safely.

3. *Pad* all bony prominences and delicate areas where they contact the table. Serious nerve and vascular damage can occur if care is not taken. Note particularly that elbows, knees, toes, and axillary regions are susceptible to damage. The inner surface of the upper arm contains the ulnar nerve, which must never rest on the table or armboard. The brachial plexus, located in the axillary region, must always be protected from strain or pressure.

4. Be *gentle* when manipulating joints. Abducting a limb to an angle greater than 90 degrees may cause injury. The unconscious patient cannot say if he or she is in pain.

5. *Respect* the patient's dignity by avoiding unnecessary exposure of the body.

6. *Align* the neck and spine at all times when positioning the patient. This will prevent injury to the cervical spine and protect the airway.

7. *Protect* the patient's fingers from getting caught in the table break by securing the arm and hand in the draw sheet (Fig. 10–1). Never place the hands under the buttocks.

8. Move *slowly* and *deliberately.* Haste in positioning the patient could cause accident or injury.

9. *Have available* all necessary accessories before anesthesia is induced to save unnecessary anesthesia time and confusion.

10. *Protect* intravenous lines, catheters, and airways from tension.

11. *Teamwork* is important! Move on a count of three when the patient is being lifted. Someone should direct the move.

12. *Use* good body mechanics.

THE OPERATING TABLE

Standard operating tables (Fig. 10–2) may be manipulated in many different ways to achieve the desired position of the patient. The table top is sectioned in several places and may be flexed or extended; the phrase "break the table" refers to the fact that the table is flexed at one or more of these hinged sections. The table may be tilted laterally or horizontally and raised or lowered from its hydraulic base. Sections of the table such as the headboard or footboard may be removed as needed (e.g., in pediatric surgery or when the patient is in stirrups). The technologist and nurse should be familiar with the specific table used in the hospital where he or she works, since the mechanisms vary from manufacturer to manufacturer.

The patient is positioned on the operating table following induction of general anesthesia (when applicable) or just before the administration of local anesthesia. To transfer the conscious patient from a stretcher to the operating table for surgery performed under local anesthesia, the nurse should refer to the guidelines given earlier in the chapter.

POSITIONS

Supine (Dorsal Recumbent)

The supine position (Fig. 10–3) is used for abdominal procedures and for those involving the face and neck, chest, or shoulder. Vascular surgery is also performed with the patient in the supine position. Orthopedic procedures in which there is adequate exposure may also use this position.

Note: The head is in good alignment with the body. The arm rests on the armboard at a 90-degree angle to the body. The arm restraint strap prevents the arm from dropping off the armboard and thereby dislocating. The restraint strap is snug but not tight. The body strap (safety strap) fits above the knees and is snug. A space of about three fingers' breadth is left beneath the strap. The feet lie on the table, *not over the edge,* and they

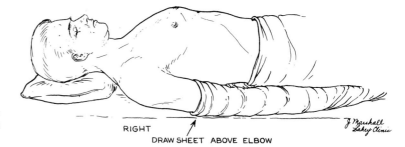

Figure 10–1. Proper position of the draw sheet. (From Ginsberg F: A Manual of Operating Room Technology. Philadelphia, JB Lippincott, 1966.)

RIGHT

DRAW SHEET ABOVE ELBOW

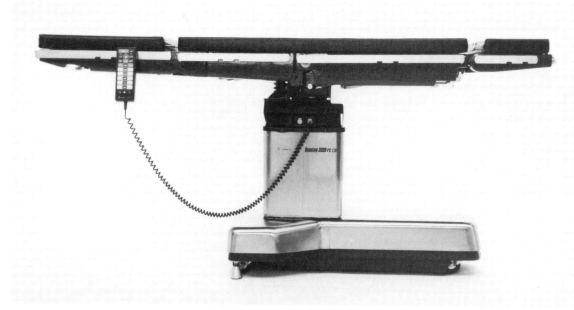

Figure 10–2. Standard operating table. Note control levers at head of table. (Courtesy of AMSCO Healthcare, Pittsburgh, PA.)

are not crossed. Patients often cross their feet while awaiting anesthesia, and care must be taken to uncross them after induction. This will prevent damage to the peroneal nerve, which lies close to the Achilles tendon.

Trendelenburg

The Trendelenburg position (Fig. 10–4) is similar to the supine position except that the table has a horizontal tilt so the patient's head lies lower than the trunk. The table is broken at the lower segment. This position is used primarily for procedures involving the pelvic organs. The goal is to allow the abdominal contents to drop in a cephalic direction (toward the head), thus giving greater exposure to the pelvic contents. This position puts stress on the diaphragm and may restrict breathing. Therefore, the patient does not remain in this position for extended periods of time.

Although some texts recommend an exaggerated Trendelenburg position for treatment of shock, its benefit to the patient is now being questioned.

Note: The armboard, safety strap, and feet are properly placed as described in the supine position. The knees lie over the table break.

Reverse Trendelenburg

Reverse Trendelenburg (Fig. 10–5) is used for surgery of the face and neck. It may also aid in procedures involving the diaphragm and upper abdominal cavity, since it allows the abdominal contents to drop in a caudal direction (toward the feet). Because of this tilt, a footboard is attached to prevent the patient from sliding downward.

Note: Safety straps are in the proper position. The

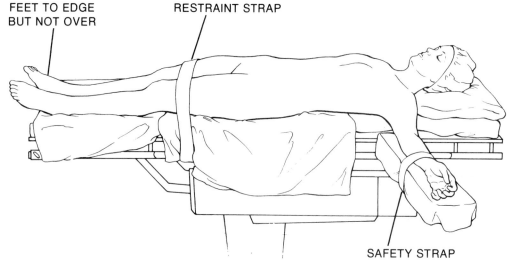

FEET TO EDGE
BUT NOT OVER

RESTRAINT STRAP

SAFETY STRAP

Figure 10–3. Supine position.

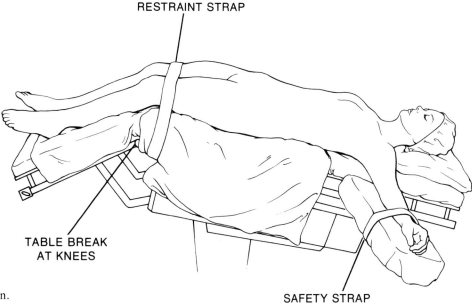

Figure 10–4. Trendelenburg position.

footboard is well padded with a small pillow or soft folded blanket.

Kraske (Jackknife)

The Kraske position (Fig. 10–6) is a modification of the prone position (lying on the abdomen). It is used in rectal and coccygeal surgery. The angle of the table break may be moderate or severe, depending on the needs of the surgeon. The armboards lie forward toward the head of the table so that the elbows may be bent comfortably.

Note: Arm restraints are in the proper position. The elbows rest on the armboard rather than on the edge or hanging off. The down ear is protected by a soft pillow. The break in the table occurs at the hips. The safety

strap lies above the knees. The hips and thighs are cushioned with large pillows. For the male patient in any of the prone positions, it is essential that the genitalia are well cushioned and resting in a natural position. The knees are lifted from the surface of the table by placing a large pillow under the legs. The toes do not rest on the table but are raised by the pillow. The feet do not extend over the end of the table.

Laminectomy

This position (Fig. 10–7) is used for procedures of the spine, particularly thoracic and lumbar laminectomy. The position may utilize a laminectomy brace, which lifts the trunk up off the table. The brace is constructed so that a hollow space between two lateral rests allows

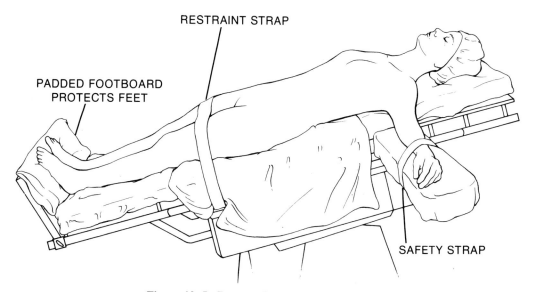

Figure 10–5. Reverse Trendelenburg position.

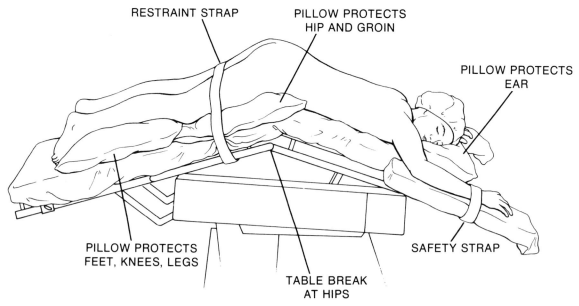

Figure 10–6. Kraske position.

for maximum chest expansion and adequate respiration. The brace is padded with towels for cushioning. Anesthesia is induced on the stretcher with the patient in the supine position before he or she is placed on the operating table. Following induction of anesthesia, and with the anesthesiologist's permission, the patient is gently rolled over from the stretcher to the table and up onto the brace. This maneuver should always be performed by at least six persons. It is essential that the limbs be protected from torsion and that the head be kept in strict alignment with the trunk during the move. Hands must be protected from the weight of the body falling on them during the rolling maneuver.

Note: The arm restraints are correctly placed. The elbow is comfortably bent and padded to prevent ulnar nerve injury. Rolled towels are placed in the axillary regions to protect the nerve plexuses and to aid in respiration. The brace is padded and flexed to the proper height. The safety strap lies above the knees. The knees, lower legs, and feet are well padded with pillows. A footboard extension keeps the patient in good alignment. The feet never rest directly on the footboard but lie on the padding.

Prone With Headrest

This position (Fig. 10–8) is used for craniotomy when the surgeon requests that the patient lie face downward. The headrest shown is horseshoe shaped. The patient is

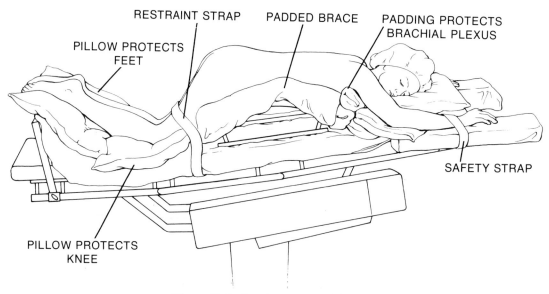

Figure 10–7. Laminectomy position.

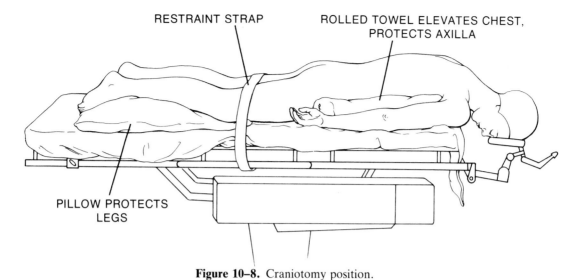

RESTRAINT STRAP

ROLLED TOWEL ELEVATES CHEST, PROTECTS AXILLA

PILLOW PROTECTS LEGS

Figure 10–8. Craniotomy position.

positioned in the routine prone position and the head extends over the edge of the table, with the forehead resting on the padded horseshoe.

Note: The head is in good alignment with the body. The arms are held to the side by the draw sheet. Pressure on the ulnar nerve is avoided. The safety strap lies above the knees. The lower legs and feet are supported by soft pillows.

Lithotomy

This position (Fig. 10–9) is used for vaginal, perineal, and rectal surgery. It utilizes a pair of stirrups that suspend the slightly flexed legs from soft canvas straps.

The straps pass around the instep and over the top of the heel. This position requires two persons to raise the legs. The legs are raised simultaneously with a slight external rotation of the hips. It is essential that the legs be raised slowly, since a rapid change in blood pressure and shock might occur if the change in posture is made too rapidly. The knees must not be allowed to "flop" laterally; this could result in their dislocation. When returning the patient to the supine position, the same precautions are observed.

Note: The armboard lies at an angle no greater than 90 degrees. The opposite arm should lie across the chest. The arm strap is in proper position. The legs and thighs do not come into contact with the metal stirrup bar. The stirrup straps are padded with soft towels to prevent

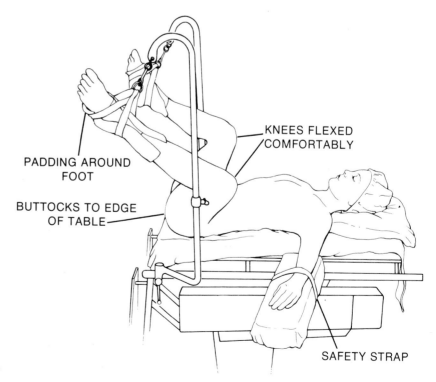

KNEES FLEXED COMFORTABLY

PADDING AROUND FOOT

BUTTOCKS TO EDGE OF TABLE

SAFETY STRAP

Figure 10–9. Lithotomy position.

damage to the peroneal nerve. The knees are only slightly flexed so as not to depress respiratory function. The legs should never hang straight—this puts severe stress on the knees. The buttocks are brought down about 1 inch over the end of the table.

Fowler (Sitting)

The Fowler position (Fig. 10–10) is used when the patient is undergoing surgery of the posterior cervical spine, posterior craniotomy, or procedures of the face and mouth. The sitting position is maintained during general anesthesia by a head support with sterile tongs that penetrate the skull and hold the head in a stable position. When the position is used for procedures other than those of the posterior spine or craniotomy, tongs are not used and the patient's head rests on a padded headrest. The arms are crossed loosely over the abdomen and taped or rest on a pillow on the patient's lap. A footboard helps to steady and maintain the position.

Note: The neck is in straight alignment. The knee strap rests above the knees. The footboard is well padded. The table breaks occur at the knees and hips. The knees are supported by a pillow. As adjustments are made in the table from supine to sitting, the knee strap must be watched for tightness and adjusted as required.

Sims (Lateral)

The Sims or lateral position (Fig. 10–11) is used for surgery of the kidney, ureters, and lung. This is perhaps the most difficult position to attain safely. The patient rests on his or her side with the arms extended on double armboards. The lower leg is flexed. The flank is elevated at the table break and may be given additional support by a mechanical lifter, which is built into the table, or by sandbags that are placed just superior to the iliac crest. There are many potential risks involved with this position, and strict attention to the following guidelines is essential.

Note: The head rests comfortably on a small pillow. The double armboard lies at an angle no greater than 90 degrees. The arm is rotated to prevent table contact with the ulnar nerve. The axillary area of the downside arm is padded with a rolled towel to protect the brachial plexus. The sandbags or kidney rest placed at the waist are well padded. The first table break occurs at the waist. A 4-inch strip of adhesive tape is attached from one side of the table to the other, passing over and securing the iliac crest. This will prevent the patient from falling from his or her side. The safety strap is placed above the knees. The lower leg is flexed and is separated from the upper leg by a large pillow that extends well into the groin. The upper foot may be kept off the table by an additional pillow.

The Orthopedic Table

The orthopedic or fracture table allows the patient to be positioned for hip nailings and other orthopedic procedures. A common hip nailing position is shown in Figure 10–12. The patient rests with the injured leg

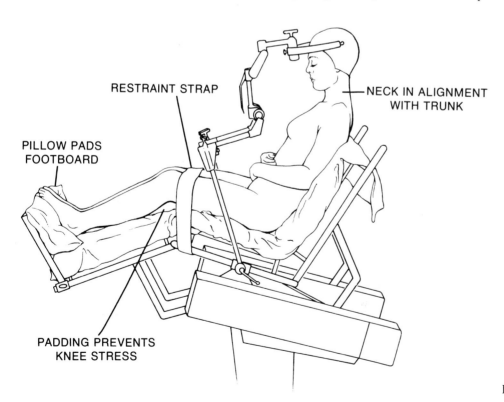

RESTRAINT STRAP

NECK IN ALIGNMENT WITH TRUNK

PILLOW PADS FOOTBOARD

PADDING PREVENTS KNEE STRESS

Figure 10–10. Fowler position.

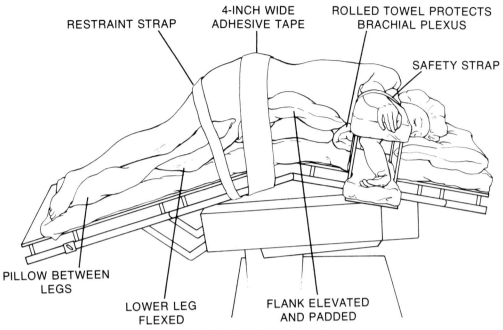

RESTRAINT STRAP 4-INCH WIDE ADHESIVE TAPE ROLLED TOWEL PROTECTS BRACHIAL PLEXUS

SAFETY STRAP

PILLOW BETWEEN LEGS

LOWER LEG FLEXED FLANK ELEVATED AND PADDED

Figure 10–11. Sims (lateral) position.

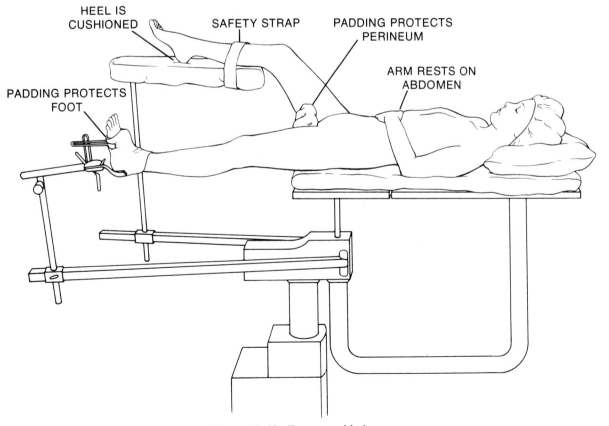

HEEL IS CUSHIONED SAFETY STRAP PADDING PROTECTS PERINEUM

ARM RESTS ON ABDOMEN

PADDING PROTECTS FOOT

Figure 10–12. Fracture table in use.

restrained in a bootlike device. The leg may be rotated, pulled into traction, or released, as the surgery requires. The unaffected leg rests on an elevated leg holder. Radiographs may be taken during the procedure because the unaffected leg is well out of the field of the radiograph. A center post is placed at the perineum and is well padded for protection. Fracture tables vary widely from manufacturer to manufacturer, and the technologist should become well acquainted with the operating mechanisms of the table with which he or she works. Figure 10–12 shows a generalized composite of several fracture tables.

Note: The affected leg is held by a traction device that is well padded to protect the foot. The center post is wrapped with soft towels or abdominal pads. The unaffected leg rests comfortably on the leg support and is well cushioned. If the existing cushion on the legrest puts pressure on the heel, a pillow must be placed under the lower leg to lift it from the legrest. A restraint strap secures the unaffected leg. The arm rests lightly over the abdomen or may rest on an armboard in the manner previously described.

Infant Positions

An infant may be positioned as described earlier, but smaller rolled towels and supports are used. Often the infant is held in the supine position for induction of anesthesia by soft wrist and ankle restraints. These restraints are commercially prepared or can be made by passing soft roller-type gauze around the wrists and ankles and then tying them loosely to the table frame.

Questions for Study and Review

1. Name six design features on a safe type of stretcher.

2. What are some steps involved in patient transfer from the bed to a stretcher that one is likely to forget if tired, in a hurry, or distracted?

3. Why must one enter an elevator pulling the stretcher from the head rather than pushing it from behind?

4. Name two nerves that are in danger of severe injury when safe positioning techniques are not used.

5. Name two surgical procedures that require the following procedures:
   a. Supine
   b. Reverse Trendelenburg
   c. Kraske
   d. Lateral
   e. Fowler
   f. Dorsal recumbent

6. How are infant positions maintained on the operating table?

Bibliography

Association of Operating Room Nurses: Recommended Practices for Safe Care Through Identification of Potential Hazards in the Surgical Environment, Denver, 1991.
Dellasega C, et al: Perioperative nursing care for the elderly surgical patient. Todays OR Nurse 13(6):12–17, 1991.
Dripps RD, Eckenhoff JE, Vandam LD: Introduction to Anesthesia: The Principles of Safe Practice, 6th ed. Philadelphia, WB Saunders, 1982.
Martin JT: Positioning in Anesthesia and Surgery. Philadelphia, WB Saunders, 1978.

Preparation of the Surgical Site

Learning Objectives

After reading this chapter you should be able to

◆ *Define* resident and transient flora.
◆ *Demonstrate* the proper techniques used in removing hair from the surgical site.
◆ *Demonstrate* the proper technique used in the patient skin preparation.
◆ *List* the commonly used antiseptics.
◆ *Know* the different types of commonly used drapes.
◆ *Demonstrate* the proper techniques used in draping.

Key Terms

antiseptic: A chemical agent used on tissue that kills most, but not all, bacteria.
antiseptic solution: Antiseptic mixed with water.
débridement: A process of removing dead skin, debris, or foreign bodies from a wound.
resident flora: Bacteria that inhabit normal skin.
seeding: The breaking away and implantation of cancer cells from the original tumor to a new site.
surgical drape: Sterile cloth or nonwoven material placed around the surgical site to create a sterile field.
tincture: Any agent that is mixed with alcohol.
transient flora: Bacteria that have been acquired from a contaminated source and inhabit skin.

Part I ◆ SKIN PREPARATION

RESIDENT AND TRANSIENT FLORA

Skin harbors two types of microorganisms. *Resident flora* is the name given to bacteria that normally reside on the skin either in the dermis or the epidermis. These bacteria cause no harm unless drawn into the body through a break in the skin. An example of this type of bacteria is *Staphylococcus epidermidis*. Another group of bacteria found on the skin, called *transient flora,* are those that have been acquired from a contaminated source. Transient flora include any type of bacteria that can live on skin, including those that are pathogenic and deadly. To help rid the skin of these two types of bacteria, the incisional site and its periphery are specially prepared before surgery.

PREPARATION ON THE UNIT

The preparation of the incisional site begins before the patient enters the operating room for surgery. All patients are required to bathe (and shampoo, if required by the surgeon). Special attention is given to the operative site during this preoperative bathing.

HAIR REMOVAL

For many years, one of the standard procedures for presurgical skin preparation was a complete dry shave of the incisional site, including a wide margin around it. However, studies have shown that shaving is associated with rashes and exudative lesions, bacterial growth, and an increase in postoperative infection. Therefore, a more clinically sound approach toward skin preparation is for shaving to be omitted from the presurgical prep unless the surgeon specifically requests it.

Because loose hair in the incisional site can carry bacteria into the wound, some surgeons may request hair removal. This can be done either with a *chemical depilatory* or with *electric clippers*. When a depilatory is used, all manufacturer's instructions concerning proper use of the depilatory should be used. All patients must have a patch test before depilatory use to determine any allergic reaction to the chemical. Because chemical depilatories are somewhat messy to use and require pretesting, some surgeons request that the surgical site be shaved with electric clippers. The clippers leave the hairs very short and the skin is not abraded or irritated by the process. *Clipper heads and blades must be sterilized between use on patients, or a disposable clipper head must be used.* When nondisposable clippers are

used, the handpiece should be disinfected after each use. *Do not immerse the handpiece in solution as this would ruin the motor.*

If the surgeon requests that the incisional site be shaved with a razor, the following guidelines should be observed:

1. *Only trained personnel should perform a shave prep.*
2. The shave should occur no more than 2 hours before surgery. This time frame ensures that bacterial growth due to loss of skin integrity is kept to a minimum.
3. The skin must be thoroughly wet and lathered before shaving. Wet hair yields to the cutting edge of the razor more easily than dry hair and helps prevent skin abrasions.
4. The area of the shave is dictated by the surgeon's orders. If these orders are not written in the patient chart, the shave should extend well into areas beyond the actual incisional site. Skin prep boundaries are shown in Figure 11–1.
5. Shave the hair in the direction of growth, not against it.
6. Do not hurry because injury could result.
7. While shaving, pull the skin taut *away from the direction of the shaving, not toward the razor's path.*
8. When the shave is complete, rinse and dry the shaved area gently. Do not rub the skin vigorously as this can further abrade the area.
9. Only disposable razors or those with removable heads that can be sterilized should be used.

Guidelines for All Methods of Hair Removal

1. Always explain to the patient exactly what is going to be done.
2. Assemble needed supplies *before* beginning the shave.
3. Gloves should be donned before beginning the shave.
4. Make sure that the lighting is sufficient before beginning the procedure.
5. Proceed with the shaving in a professional and reassuring manner. Talk with the patient while performing the shave as this helps to reduce anxiety or embarrassment.
6. Never expose the patient unnecessarily. Provide a secluded environment for the patient by closing the bedside curtain.
7. Never shave the eyebrows or cut the eyelashes

100

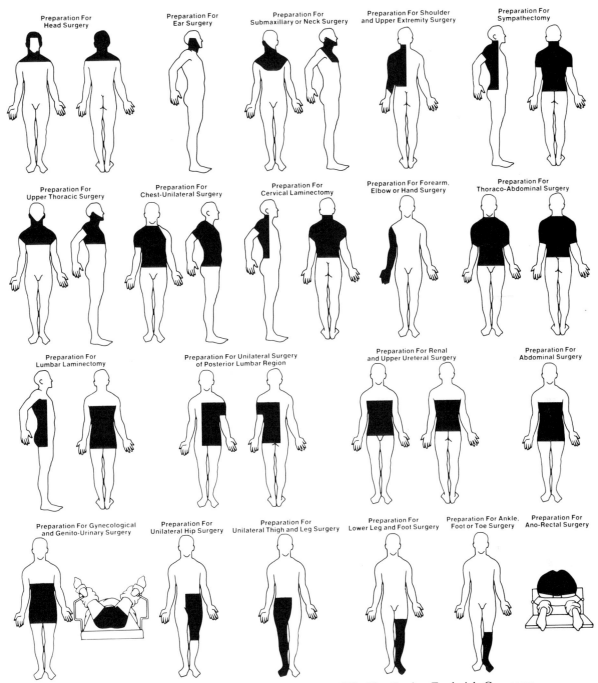

Figure 11–1. Skin prep boundaries. (Copyright © 1971, The Purdue Frederick Company, Norwalk, CT.)

unless specific orders to do so appear in the patient's chart.

8. Scalp hair should never be removed unless specific orders to do so appear in the patient's chart. If the scalp is completely shaved, do not discard the hair. This is the patient's property and should be retained.

9. Always report and document any lesions that were created by the shave prep. If moles, warts, or other irregularities occur within the prep area, carefully avoid them during the shave.

10. Wash hands following the shave prep.

SURGICAL SKIN PREP

Following hair removal, when applicable, the next step in preparing the incisional site is the surgical skin prep. This is a methodical cleansing of the incisional site with an antiseptic-detergent mixture. Following this cleansing, the area is painted with an *antiseptic solution* (antiseptic mixed with water) or *tincture* (antiseptic mixed with alcohol). Disposable prep trays that contain sponges, soap, towels, drapes, and other needed supplies are available and commonly used. The scrub prep takes place after the anesthetized patient has been positioned, just before draping. For patients receiving anesthetic, the anesthetic may be given before or after the skin prep.

ANTISEPTICS

The purpose of the skin prep is to render the incision site and surrounding area as free from microorganisms as possible. To accomplish this, an antiseptic soap approved by the Food and Drug Administration (FDA) must be used. The selection of the antiseptic is based on the germicidal activity of the product, its residual protection, its toxicity, and any known allergies the patient may have to a particular product.

Povidone-iodine (Betadine) is the most commonly used prep solution. This product is a combination of polyvinylpyrrolidone and iodine. It is relatively nonirritating, is nontoxic, and is nonstaining. When used as a skin cleanser, it is batericidal, virucidal, and mycobactericidal but may not kill spores or fungi because their contact with the antiseptic may not be prolonged enough. The "cidal" effect of this product may last up to 8 hours.

Hexachlorophene is used occasionally as a scrub prep solution; however, its use is declining since the FDA issued a warning concerning its neurotoxicity. It is slow acting, and single use of this antiseptic results in a rebound growth of microorganisms. Its only useful recommendation is that it provides long-lasting bactericidal effects. However, because it requires repeated use in order to be effective and because this specific use is contraindicated, its use is limited.

Alcohol is seldom if ever used alone as a surgical scrub or prep agent. However, when mixed with other antiseptics such as iodine, the resulting tincture forms a valuable degreasing antimicrobial agent. Alcohol is an excellent bactericide and is effective against most gram-positive and gram-negative microorganisms. It is also effective against tubercle bacilli. Its main disadvantage is its drying effect on tissue and its potential toxicity. Alcohol and tinctures are highly flammable. Therefore, *when tinctures are used as a surgical scrub the area must be completely dried before the use of electrocautery or laser surgery.*

Chlorhexidine gluconate is a broad-spectrum antiseptic, effective against both gram-positive and gram-negative bacteria. It is only minimally effective against tubercle bacilli but has good residual bactericidal activity for up to 4 hours. However, it is pH dependent and may be neutralized in hard tap water.

Procedure for Surgical Skin Prep

The scrub prep is usually performed by the circulator. However, the surgeon may occasionally wish to perform this prep. All supplies used in the scrub prep must be sterile. These include towels, antiseptic soap, gauze sponges, cotton-tipped applicators, and gloves. Depend-

ing on the area to be prepped, additional items such as cotton balls, nail picks, or a scrub brush may also be needed. The prep is done as follows:

1. Expose the operative site and adjust the overhead lights so that the entire prep area is well lighted.
2. Don sterile gloves.
3. Place sterile towels at the periphery of the scrub area. Make sure that the scrub area is wide enough to include any possible wound drain sites. When the abdomen is being prepped, the edge of the towels can be tucked between the patient and the operating table. Make a cuff in the towel and place your hands within the cuff to do this.
4. Starting at the exact location where the incision will be made, begin washing in a circular motion. Use a "no touch" technique. (Do not touch the patient's skin with a gloved hand. Touch the skin with the soapy sponge only, which may be grasped with sponge forceps.) Keep moving toward the periphery of the scrub area (Fig. 11–2). When prepping the abdomen, use cotton-tipped applicators to remove any dead skin (detritus) from the umbilicus. Do this before beginning the prep.
5. Scrub outward from the incision site and discard used prep sponges and begin again with fresh ones. *Do not return to an area already washed with the same sponge.*
6. Continue this process, using clean sponges for 5 minutes (operating room policy may dictate the length of the scrub).
7. Dry the prep area using the same technique with dry sponges. The site may also be dried by laying a towel over the area and blotting up the antiseptic soap. Do not shift the towel when doing this. Remove the towel by grasping the edge farthest away and "peeling" it back.
8. Antiseptic paint is usually applied immediately after the scrub. Use the same technique as described

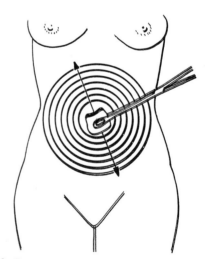

Figure 11–2. Proper direction for prepping. Prepping begins at the incisional site and is carried to the periphery with circular motions. (Reproduced by permission of Ethicon, Inc., Somerville, NJ.)

earlier. Apply antiseptic paint in a circular pattern and never return to an area that has already been painted.

Special Skin Prep Procedures

Ostomy. When the abdomen is being prepped and an ostomy is present, a soapy sponge can be placed over the ostomy before beginning the prep. After the scrub prep, but before the application of antiseptic paint, the ostomy can be cleansed. Care must be taken not to drip any solutions away from the ostomy and onto the area already prepped. The ostomy prep should be confined to that area only. After this is done, the antiseptic paint can be applied, saving the ostomy site until last. Any sponges that have come in contact with the ostomy should not be allowed to touch any other area of the prep.

Limb. When a patient's leg or arm is prepped, the extremity must be prepped around its circumference and along its full length. To accomplish this, the limb must be held in the air, away from the operating table. A second person may be needed to hold the limb for the person performing the prep, or a leg may be suspended on a legrest (accessory to the operating table.) An arm can be suspended from a similar device. *Extreme caution must be exercised so that the limb does not become dislodged from its suspended position. Serious injury can occur if the limb falls away from the operating table.*

Vagina. To prep the vagina, the nurse begins a few centimeters from the vulva and extends the prep outward to include the thighs and lower abdomen. Mounted sponges are used for the vaginal vault. The vulva and anus are cleansed by starting at the top of the vulva and passing the soapy sponge downward. The sponge is discarded after it passes the anus. This is repeated several times, always starting with a new sponge (Fig. 11–3).

Anus. The anal area is prepped as would be done for an ostomy. The prep is begun a short distance away from the anus and continued outward to include the buttocks and upper thighs. The anus is cleansed last, and no sponges should touch the skin area around it.

Biopsy Area with Possible Radical Surgery. When an area such as a breast is being prepped for biopsy and the possibility for a more radical procedure is scheduled or anticipated, the biopsy area should be prepped very *gently*. This is done to prevent malignant cells from *seeding* (breaking loose from the biopsy area and spreading to the lymphatic system or other tissue).

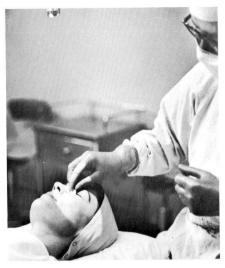

Figure 11–4. Surgeon preparing the face for surgery. (Reproduced by permission of Ethicon, Inc., Somerville, NJ.)

Eye. The eye and surrounding area are prepped with soft cotton balls (Fig. 11–4). The eye is irrigated and rinsed with a bulb syringe, starting from the inner canthus and working toward the outer canthus. A small cotton plug should be placed in the external ear canal of the affected side to prevent prep solutions from draining into it.

Ear. The folds of the outer ear are cleansed with cotton-tipped applicators. The surrounding area is cleansed in routine fashion. Prep solutions must not be allow to drain into the ear canal. A small cotton plug may be placed at the external ear canal opening to prevent this.

Face. The face is prepped by working from the center outward. The nurse should return to the incisional site using clean sponges and prep this area last. The hairline represents a contaminated area, and sponges must not be brought back onto the skin once they have touched that area. Likewise, the mouth and nose must be prepped separately.

Débridement. *Débridement* is the removal of foreign material such as devitalized or necrotic tissue, dirt, gravel, glass, or metal flakes from a wound. This procedure often precedes orthopedic procedures following traumatic injury or may be performed on burn patients. It is often performed in conjunction with the surgical prep that is carried out by the surgeon. In addition to prepping solutions and equipment, the following items should be available:

- Copious amounts of warm sterile saline
- Suction apparatus with two separate suction units and tips
- Thumb forceps (smooth and toothed)
- Cotton-tipped applicators
- Extra sterile towels and impermeable prepping drapes
- Fine tissue forceps
- Scalpel
- Basins or trough drapes to collect saline runoff

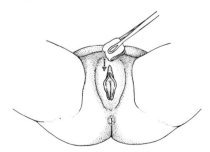

Figure 11–3. Vaginal prep. (Reproduced by permission of Ethicon, Inc., Somerville, NJ.)

- Small basins or cups to collect foreign material (saved as specimens)
- Lavage instrument as needed (uses gentle hydropressure to express foreign matter from superficial tissues)
- Bulb syringe

To perform the débridement, the surgeon uses saline to bathe and irrigate the wound. The technologist or nurse may be required to operate the suction apparatus. The wound is then cleansed of all foreign material, which should be retained as a specimen. The surgeon may use dissecting instruments to scrape or cut away necrotic tissue or remove small bits of dirt and other debris. If further surgery is required, the wound is then prepped in routine manner according to its location.

Points to Remember

1. *Never allow* prep solutions to pool under the patient. These solutions may cause irritation or burns.

Likewise, never allow the solutions to seep under a tourniquet (see Chapter 13).

2. *Never use* x-ray detectable surgical sponges to perform the prep. Their presence in the room may interfere with the operative sponge count.

3. *Use warm solutions.* These solutions prevent the loss of body heat.

4. *Never use* alcohol-based solutions (tinctures) on or around mucous membranes or the eye or on pediatric patients. Alcohol desiccates these delicate tissues and may cause burns.

5. *Use a scrub brush* to scrub the patient's hands or feet if they are visibly soiled. Laying a coat of prep solution over the dirt does not produce adequate asepsis.

6. *Do not rush the prep.* Although the surgeons may be present and waiting during the latter stages of the prep, it is the technologist's responsibility to complete a thorough prep. It is normal to feel rushed, but an insufficient scrub prep can result in serious postoperative infection.

• •

Part II ◆ DRAPING

Drapes may be made of linen (muslin) or paper (nonwoven). A controversy exists over which material is best as a protective barrier against contamination and moisture and which is the most cost effective, although current research strongly supports the use of nonwoven materials. Linen requires laundering, folding, and sterilization by the hospital. It also spreads lint, which can act as a carrier for air-borne bacteria. Since linen is not waterproof, it presents a danger of strikethrough contamination. However, linen is supple and thus falls nicely into folds. Paper drapes are commercially prepared for one-time use. They are waterproof, disposable, and convenient. The paper, however, is somewhat stiff and is therefore more likely to become contaminated in the process of draping.

Because individual hospitals and surgeons use different routines for which drapes to use and where to use them, the technologist should be familiar with the types of drapes available and how to use each one, rather than learning a set of draping procedures that may become obsolete with a change of surgeon or hospital.

BASIC PRINCIPLES

1. Provide a wide cuff for the hand. This prevents contamination of the hand by the nonsterile surface being draped.

2. Drapes are nearly always unfolded at the field to avoid moving them around. Most drapes are fan-folded to allow easy unfolding on the surface to be draped.

3. Once placed, drapes should not be moved. To move a drape after it is placed causes bacteria from unprepped surfaces to contaminate the prepped incisional site. The placement of a sheet over the incisional area and the cuff that protects the hand are shown in Figure 11–5.

4. When linen drapes are used, provide adequate barriers against moisture and contamination. There should be a minimum of four thicknesses around the operative site and two thicknesses elsewhere.

DRAPING MATERIALS AND THEIR APPLICATION

Towels

Towels are usually a basic item in every draping routine. Four towels are placed around the immediate surgical site; this is called "squaring off" the site. Four towel clips secure the towels. These clips may penetrate the skin and towels together or simply join the towels (Fig. 11–6). Some surgeons prefer to sew the drapes to the skin. Once a towel clip has been placed, it is

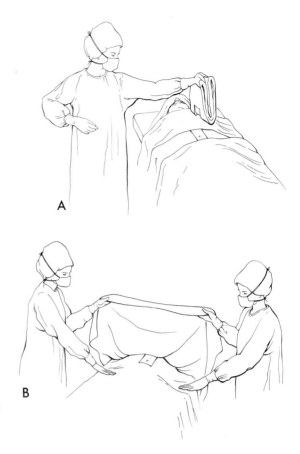

Figure 11–5. *A.* The fenestration is placed directly over the wound site. *B.* The drape is unfolded with the gloved hand protected under a wide cuff.

considered contaminated and must not be returned to the sterile field.

Plain Sheet

This is also called a minor sheet, top sheet, or bottom sheet. It is a large rectangular sheet that may be placed directly above or below the incisional area. It is used in various ways in the draping routine, according to its size.

Plastic Drape

This is a commercially prepared item. Its function is to provide a sterile barrier over the skin at the incisional

site. The sheet is made of thin plastic that is adherent on one side. Some surgeons believe that this type of barrier causes a greater proliferation of bacteria because it increases the perspiration and warmth of the skin it covers. Two or three persons are needed to place the drape. Two persons (usually the surgeon and his or her assistant) hold the drape taut while a third pulls the paper from the adhesive side. The sheet is then lowered onto the patient and smoothed down (Fig. 11–7).

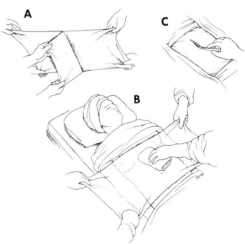

Figure 11–7. *A* through *C.* Application of the plastic drape. (From Rhodes MJ, Gruendemann BJ, Ballinger WF: Alexander's Care of the Patient in Surgery, 6th ed. St. Louis, CV Mosby, 1978.)

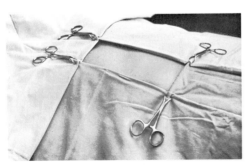

Figure 11–6. Four towels secured with towel clips mark the boundary of the wound site. (From Nealon TF: Fundamental Skills in Surgery, 3rd ed. Philadelphia, WB Saunders, 1979.)

Tube Stockinette

This is a socklike drape made from stretch muslin that is used in limb surgery. The stockinette is prerolled so that it can be unrolled over the limb. The technique for applying the stockinette is shown in Figure 11–8. Note that the person who is doing the draping is careful to avoid touching the patient's skin as the stockinette is unrolled (Fig. 11–8*B*).

Head Drape

This drape is used for procedures about the face other than the eyes, such as tonsillectomy or nose surgery. It is usually composed of two towels or small sheets. The technologist or nurse slides them under the patient's head and then proceeds to wrap the head turban style with the top towel. The draping technique is shown in Figure 11–9. Note that the towel clip is placed well away from the eyes (Fig. 11–9*F*).

Procedure Drapes

A *procedure drape* is the topmost sheet in a draping routine. There are different kinds of procedure sheets designed to fit the needs of a particular surgical position or type of surgery. The sheet has a fenestration (hole) or other access to the incisional site. The fenestration is usually considerably larger than the incision and is reinforced with an extra layer of material surrounding it. The sheet extends the full length of the patient and table and in some cases covers the armboards. Its sides fall well over the table edge but should not touch the floor. The sheet is folded so that the exposed fenestration may be placed directly over the incisional site (see Fig. 11–5). In this way it may be placed and unfolded on the patient without being moved about. The following are basic types of procedure drapes.

Laparotomy Drape

The laparotomy drape (Fig. 11–10) is used for abdominal procedures, laminectomy, and other procedures in which a single, large, rectangular fenestration is required. The fenestration, which lies nearly centered on the drape, may be transverse or longitudinal.

Split Sheet

The split sheet (Fig. 11–11) is used for draping limbs. The body of the sheet, the portion that is not divided, drapes the patient's body, while the "tails" or divided sections are draped out toward the limb and are tucked under it. This drape may also accompany the head drape to provide a sterile surface during facial surgery. In this case the tails are sometimes tucked under the head.

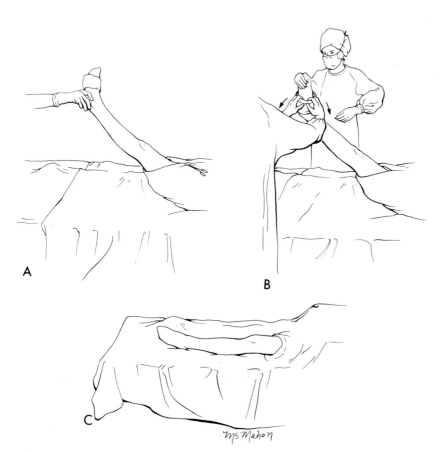

Figure 11–8. *A* through *C.* Application of tube stockinette.

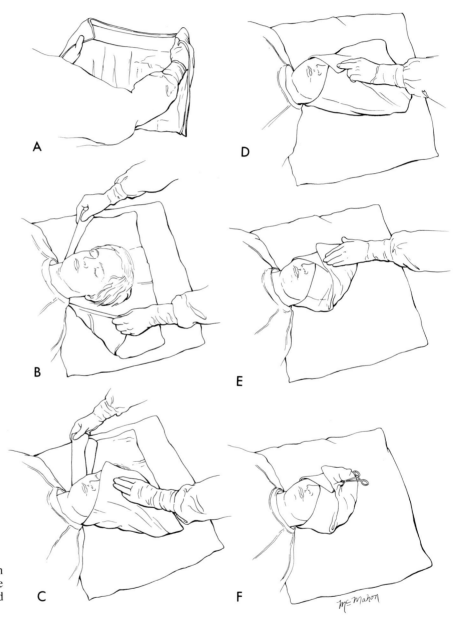

A

B

C

D

E

F

Figure 11–9. *A* through *F.* Application of the head drape. The corners of the towel must be handled carefully to avoid contamination.

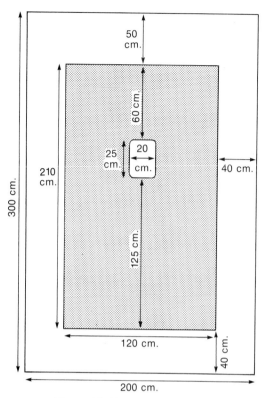

Figure 11–10. Laparotomy drape.

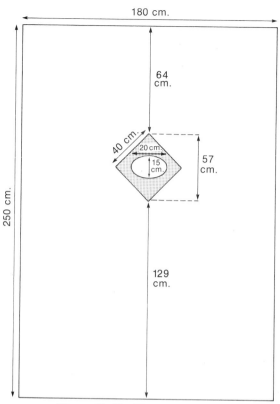

Figure 11–12. Thyroid sheet.

Thyroid Sheet

The thyroid sheet (Fig. 11–12) has a small transverse fenestration located very near the top of the drape. It is used for procedures on the thyroid and associated structures.

Perineal Sheet

The perineal sheet (Fig. 11–13) is used for procedures performed in the lithotomy position (see Fig. 11–9). The sheet has a small low fenestration. Because the

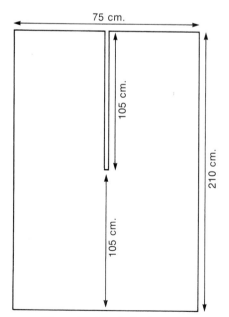

Figure 11–11. Split sheet.

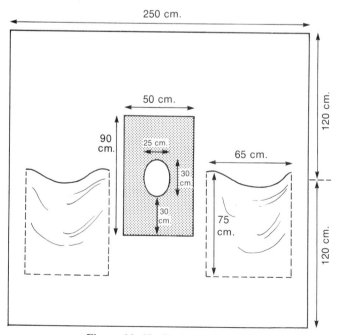

Figure 11–13. Perineal sheet.

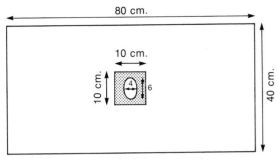

Figure 11–14. Ear or eye drape.

stirrups must also be covered, the sheet may have extending pockets for this purpose. Alternatively, special leggings are used to cover the stirrups fully. These are large pillowcase drapes that fit over each stirrup and extend up into the groin area. Leggings are placed first and then the perineal sheet.

Ear or Eye Drape

This small drape (Fig. 11–14) has a tiny oval fenestration near the center of the drape to allow access to the ear or eye. When the patient is draped for these types of procedures, an additional body sheet is used to cover the patient and operating table.

Craniotomy Sheet

The craniotomy sheet (Fig. 11–15) has an oval fenestration near the top of the drape to allow access to the skull. The sheet may be large enough to cover not only the patient but also the overhead instrument table that many hospitals use during craniotomy procedures. Thus, in covering both the patient and the table with the same drape, a continuous sterile field is created (Fig. 11–16).

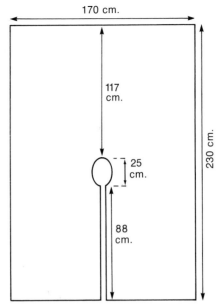

Figure 11–15. Craniotomy sheet.

Draping Rules

1. Handle drapes as little as possible.
2. Never fan or shake drapes. Draping involves slow, deliberate, careful movements. If draping is hurried or if excess movement occurs during the procedure, dust and lint can be released into the immediate environment and act as a vehicle for air-borne bacteria.
3. If a drape becomes contaminated or has a hole in it, discard the drape.
4. When draping for a procedure during which large amounts of fluids are anticipated, a special trough drape, specifically designed to confine the liquids, should be used.

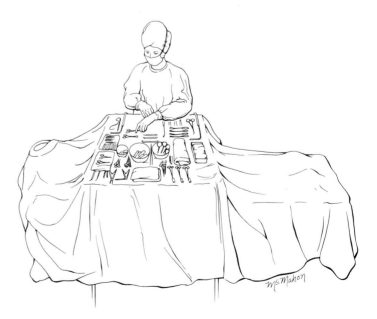

Figure 11–16. Continuous craniotomy drape.

5. Never allow the gloved hands to come into contact with the patient's prepped skin during the draping process. Remember that the gloved hand is sterile, the patient's skin is not.

6. Whenever draping, always provide a cuff for the gloved hand, as this will prevent it from touching nonsterile surfaces during the draping process.

7. Never allow a drape to extend outside the sterile area unless it is to remain there. The drape must not be adjusted once it is placed. If it is placed incorrectly, it must be discarded and another drape used.

8. Do not allow drapes to touch the floor. They can act as a wick and bring bacteria up into the sterile field.

9. Plan ahead when draping. Have drapes ready before the procedure begins. Stack drapes in order of application. The efficient organization of draping materials will save time and prevent confusion.

Questions for Study and Review

1. Define resident and transient flora.

2. Why is a patient's skin prepped before surgery?

3. What methods are commonly used to remove hair from the surgical site?

4. Why is the patient's scalp hair saved if it is removed before surgery?

5. Why is hexachlorophene not commonly used as an antiseptic?

6. What is the most common type of antiseptic used in the operating room?

7. Describe the proper technique of prepping an ostomy? Why is a special technique used?

8. Why are towel clips considered contaminated once they have been placed into the drapes?

9. Why is warm water used when prepping the patient?

Bibliography

Edel M: Impaired skin integrity. Todays OR Nurse 12:7, 1991.
Association of Operating Room Nurses: Proposed recommended practices for aseptic barrier materials for surgical drapes. AORN J 35(5):1982.
Kovach T: Nip it in the bud: Controlling wound infection with preoperative shaving. Todays OR Nurse 12:9, 1990.

Wound Closure

Learning Objectives

After reading this chapter you should be able to

- ◆ *Discuss* the United States Pharmacopeia and its regulation of suture material.
- ◆ *Discuss* suture sizes and what they mean.
- ◆ *Discuss* suture packaging.
- ◆ *Describe* the two main categories of suture materials.
- ◆ *Describe* silk and cotton suture.
- ◆ *Describe* nonabsorbable synthetic materials.
- ◆ *Discuss and demonstrate* the proper handling and preparation of suture materials.
- ◆ *Describe and recognize* different types of surgical needles.
- ◆ *Recognize* the parts of a surgical needle.
- ◆ *Discuss* the advantages of eyeless or atraumatic needles.
- ◆ *Demonstrate* the proper technique for threading and passing suture needles.
- ◆ *Discuss* nonsuture products.
- ◆ *Recognize* and properly *load and unload* cartridges of surgical stapling instruments.
- ◆ *Understand* wound healing.
- ◆ *Describe* the functions of dressings and wound drains.

Key Terms

absorbable suture: Any suture that is digested by body tissue.

anastomosis: The surgical formation of a passageway between two spaces, hollow organs, or lumens.

approximate: To bring body parts or tissue together by sutures or other means.

atraumatic: Refers to a suture-needle combination that has no needle eye. The suture is swaged into the end of the needle shaft.

bleeder: A severed blood vessel.

bolsters: Tubing through which retention sutures are threaded to prevent them from cutting into the patient's skin.

Brown and Sharp (B & S) gauge: Sizing standard used to measure steel sutures.

capillary action: Refers to the absorption of liquids along the length of a suture.

chromic salts: Chemicals used to treat surgical gut suture so that it resists digestion by body tissues.

dehiscence: The splitting apart of a surgical wound postoperatively.

free tie: A term used by the surgeon when he or she requests a length of suture for ligation.

full length: Refers to the length of a suture strand. Full length is 54 or 60 inches.

hold: Indicates that the surgeon wishes to place a small clamp on the end of the suture rather than cut it.

inert: Refers to certain types of suture material, indicating that it causes little or no tissue reaction.

ligate: To tie a length of suture around a vessel or duct and secure it with knots.

memory: A suture's ability to "remember" its configuration during packaging (i.e., coiled or twisted).

monofilament suture: Suture composed of a single, nonfibrous strand of material.

multifilament suture: Suture composed of many fine strands of fiber that are twisted or braided together.

nonabsorbable suture: Suture that is never digested by tissue but becomes encapsulated by it.

precut: Lengths of suture material that are cut to a standard length by the manufacturer.

pursestring: A technique of suturing. A continuous strand is passed in and out around the circumference of a hollow structure and then is pulled tight like a drawstring.

reel: A continuous strand of suture mounted on a spool; used for ligation of many blood vessels in rapid succession.

retention suture: Heavy nonabsorbable suture placed behind the skin sutures and underneath all tissue layers to give added strength to the closure.

running suture: A method of suturing that uses one continuous suture that is passed over and under the tissue edges.

stick tie: Name given to suture ligature—a suture-needle combination that is passed through a vessel or duct before ligation to prevent it from slipping off the edge of the structure.

swage: Area of an atraumatic needle that holds the suture.

tensile strength: The amount of stress a suture will withstand before breaking.

USP: United States Pharmacopeia, the agency that regulates and issues standards of quality for medical products such as suture materials.

Suture materials are used to sew tissue edges together while healing takes place and to *ligate* (tie off) blood vessels or ducts during surgery. There are numerous types of suture materials available. The choice of which type of suture material is used on a particular tissue is based on the individual characteristics of the material, the location and type of the tissue, the age and condition of the patient, and the surgeon's expertise and experience.

During surgery, it is the duty of the scrub technologist or nurse to properly prepare suture materials until the surgeon needs them and to pass the material to him or her in an acceptable manner. Suture products are extremely expensive and, in many cases, delicate. The goal of proper suture handling is to maintain the suture material's inherent strength and integrity and to promote economical use of the materials. In addition to suture, a number of nonsuture products are available that can be used for tissue approximation, and these are discussed later in this chapter.

THE UNITED STATES PHARMACOPEIA

The United States Pharmacopeia (USP) began, historically, as an organization whose physician members set minimum standards for medical products and substances. These standards were adopted by the federal government and are now included in the regulations of the federal Food and Drug Administration (FDA). All substances, including suture products that bear the USP label, must meet minimum standards. Included in the standards for suture materials are those for size, *tensile strength* (the amount of stress that a strand of suture can withstand before breaking), and sterility. Additional standards for packaging, dyes used in the suture, and integrity of needle–suture attachment are also included.

SUTURE SIZE

The *diameter* of a suture strand determines its size. The greater the diameter of the suture, the larger its designated size. Beginning with size 5, the largest suture size available, sizes decrease to 0. As multiples of zeros are indicated in the size, the suture begins to get even smaller in diameter. For example, size 2-0 ("2,0") is smaller than size 0. The smallest diameter suture available is 11-0, which is so fine that it floats in air. Naturally, these very delicate sutures must be handled with extreme care. Very fine sutures are used in microsurgery, and the heaviest sutures can be used to *approximate* (bring together) bone tissue. USP suture sizes are standard in the industry. An additional method called the *Brown and Sharp (B & S) gauge* is used to indicate the size of steel sutures. Stainless steel sizes (called *gauges*) have a different numbering system than other types of suture. The numbers begin at 18 gauge (the thickest gauge) and end with size 38/40 (the most delicate or smallest gauge). Note that as the number of the gauge decreases, the size increases. The B & S gauges and their corresponding sizes are listed in Table 12–1.

The length of suture materials, as they come directly from their package, are standardized. Strands are either *precut* to 17, 18, or 24 inches or are available as *full lengths*. A full length of suture is 54 or 60 inches long. Suture reels contain a continuous length of suture and are used when the procedure requires a rapid succession of ligatures.

SUTURE PACKAGING

Suture manufacturers have developed numerous methods of packaging sutures that facilitate their delivery from the package and also maintain the sterility and integrity of the suture. All sutures are double wrapped in peel-apart envelopes (Fig. 12–1). The inner envelope is sterile both inside and outside. One face of the outer envelope is a transparent film that allows easy inspection of the data printed on the inner package. These data include the type, size, length, needle type and size (when applicable), date of manufacturing, and expiration date of the suture. Inner packages are color coded, according to the type of suture, for quick selection. Each manu-

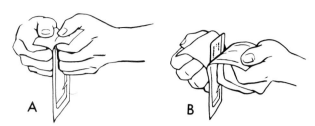

Figure 12–1. To open suture packet, grasp the wrapper edges *(A)* and peel apart *(B)*. (Reproduced by permission of Ethicon, Inc., Somerville, NJ.)

facturer uses its own color coding system. Individual suture packets are boxed with 12 to 36 packets in each box.

TYPES OF SUTURE AND THEIR PREPARATION

Suture materials are classified into two distinct categories: *absorbable* and *nonabsorbable*. The surgeon chooses a category of suture and then the type of suture within that category depending on the type of tissue, its location in the body, the strength of the tissue, and the general condition of the patient.

Absorbable Suture

Absorbable suture is digested by the tissue in which it is placed. The length of time it remains intact depends on the type of tissue, the size and type of absorbable suture, whether the wound is infected, and the general physical condition and the age of the patient.

Nonsynthetic

Surgical gut (formerly called catgut) is manufactured from the intestines of beef and sheep and is made of *collagen*. Because of advances in the manufacturing of synthetic absorbable sutures, surgical gut is rarely used. It is available in two forms: plain and chromicized. Surgical gut is used on tissues that heal rapidly. *Chromicized gut* (treated with chromic salts) resists absorption for a longer period than plain gut. Chromic gut has been used widely in gynecologic as well as genitourinary surgery. Both types of gut are absorbed rapidly in the presence of infection, and their use is contraindicated in wounds that are known to be contaminated and in debilitated patients. Under these circumstances, the use of surgical gut may lead to wound dehiscence (splitting open).

Surgical gut is prepared for use by first being dipped (not soaked) in saline solution. This softens the strands so that they can be straightened into pliable lengths. Surgical gut can be straightened by grasping the strand at each end and pulling gently. One should be careful not to jerk the strands because this weakens them. Handling gut should be avoided as much as possible

Table 12–1. STAINLESS STEEL SIZING

B & S Gauge	#40	#35	#32	#30	#28	#26	#25	#24	#23	#22	#20
USP Size	6-0	5-0	4-0	3-0	2-0	0	1	2	3	4	5

because continued contact with the gloved hand causes fraying of the suture.

Synthetic

Synthetic absorbable suture is made from synthetic polymers and has replaced the use of surgical gut almost entirely. Its advantages over surgical gut are that it causes less tissue reaction, is easier to handle, and has greater tensile strength. In addition, it can be used in the presence of infection and its absorption rate is unaffected by enzymes found in the gastrointestinal tract. Two types of synthetic absorbable sutures have been used for many years: *polyglycolic acid suture* (*Dexon*) and *polyglactin 910* (*Vicryl*). Dexon suture is a synthetic polymer of glycolic acid. Vicryl is a copolymer of lactide and glycolide. Two monofilament absorbable sutures that have been developed are Maxon and *PDS*. These sutures pass through tissue with less "drag" than the two braided synthetic sutures Dexon and Vicryl and may be more resistant to bacterial *wicking* (a process in which bacteria are drawn into the wound along the length of the suture strand).

Nonabsorbable Suture

Nonabsorbable suture is that which the body encapsulates (builds fibrous tissue around) but does not digest. There are a number of types of nonabsorbable suture with which the technologist must be familiar.

Nonsynthetic

Silk suture is manufactured from the degummed threads of silkworm larvae and has been dyed black. It is available as a *multifilament* (single strands braided or twisted together) material. It is easy to handle and is both supple and strong. To resist tissue drag and flaking, it is coated with Teflon or a similar coating. Although silk is not as strong as the synthetic nonabsorbable sutures, it is stronger than cotton, which is the other natural fiber used in the manufacturing of sutures. Silk sutures are often used in eye tissue, gastrointestinal tissue, and blood vessels. They are contraindicated for use in the urinary tract or in the presence of infection. *Virgin silk* suture material is sometimes used in ophthalmic surgery. It has been bleached but not degummed and is available in white or black.

Surgical cotton suture is manufactured from the fibers of the cotton plant. It is a multifilament suture that is supple and easy to use but has not replaced silk suture because of its inferior strength and tendency to flake. Cotton suture can be strengthened by dipping it in saline before use. Its application is similar to that of silk suture. It may also be used for fascia closure and for closing the serosal layer of the gastrointestinal tract. It is not used in contaminated wounds.

Synthetic

Polyester suture or *Dacron* is the strongest of all sutures except for surgical steel. This type of suture produces very little tissue reaction and is used in areas of the body where healing is very slow and the long-term strength and integrity of the suture is extremely important. Dacron is frequently used during the implantation of heart valves and during vascular procedures for *anastomosis* (the suturing together of two hollow structures) of blood vessels.

Polybutester suture or *Novafil* is a monofilament synthetic suture that can be used in all types of soft tissue approximation, except neural or microsurgical procedures.

Polypropylene suture is a monofilament suture that is manufactured from polymerized propylene. This suture is extremely smooth and is used commonly in skin closure and for cardiovascular and microsurgery. It is available in blue or white and has high tensile strength. Polypropylene is coiled during packaging and has a *memory* (springs back to its original shape) when removed from the package. It must be handled carefully to avoid contaminating the ends because they may spring out of control if caught on the gloved hand or surgical drapes.

Nylon suture is manufactured from coal and is available as a monofilament or multifilamented material. Nylon is very inert (nonreactive in tissue, therefore causing little or no inflammation), but it is not used in areas where long-term approximation is important. It has high tensile strength and resists *capillary action* (wicking of fluids along the length of the suture). Monofilament nylon is very smooth and passes easily through the delicate tissues of the eye or blood vessels. The major disadvantage of nylon is its elasticity and stiffness, which necessitate the laying of many knots. These knots tend to untie if placed incorrectly. Nylon suture material is available in a number of colors, including black, green, blue, and clear (for skin approximation in plastic surgery procedures).

Two types of *metal sutures* are available: *stainless steel* and *silver*. Stainless steel is the strongest of all suture materials. It is also the most inert. It is manufactured in the form of monofilament or multifilament strands. It kinks easily and has a "sawing" effect on tissue. Because of its springiness, it is easily contaminated at the field. The sharp ends of the strands can easily puncture a glove, causing contamination and injury to the person handling it. Steel is used primarily in orthopedic surgery to approximate bone fragments or in tendon repair where tissue reaction would cause scarring and malfunction of the tendon as it passes through its sheath. It can also be used on the abdominal fascia when great strength is needed or in the presence of infection. When preparing and using steel sutures, the technologist or surgeon should always cut it with wire scissors. Suture scissors, when used to cut steel, develop nicks and cuts along the cutting edge. Cutting steel sutures may also displace the cutting edges, which renders the scissors useless for delicate suture materials.

Monofilament silver sutures are used primarily to close wounds that have undergone dehiscence. These sutures are softer and easier to handle than steel sutures but must be used with the same precautions.

PREPARING AND HANDLING SUTURE MATERIALS

It is the surgeon, not the scrub assistant, who selects the type and size of suture to be used during a particular case. Therefore, the technologist should always consult the *surgeon's preference card* before surgery to have the correct sutures available on the sterile tables. Because suture material is costly it must not be wasted or handled carelessly. Only a minimum amount should be distributed at the beginning of surgery; more can be easily added as the case proceeds. Strands of suture material can be protected between the layers of a fan-folded towel during surgery. The ends should protrude slightly so that they can be picked up easily. Suture material should never be clamped with a surgical instrument such as a hemostat because this damages the suture. One exception to this is when the surgeon uses a strand of suture to identify or retract an anatomic structure. He or she may sometimes place a clamp on the end of the suture that is used for this purpose.

SURGICAL NEEDLES

Surgical needles are precision-made from high-carbon steel. The combination of metals used in the manufacturing process renders them strong and inert. Needles are available in a number of types according to their shape or curvature, point style, and *eye* (area where suture is threaded or attached). Needles may be disposable (indicated for single use only) or reusable. Most needles used in surgery are disposable.

Needle Shape

The needle shape or curvature may vary according to its use. In general, the deeper the tissue is in the surgical wound, the more acute the curve should be. The curved needle allows the surgeon to dip beneath the surface of the tissue and retrieve the point as it emerges. There are five different angles of curvature available (Fig. 12–2). The ⅝ curvature needle has the greatest amount of

Table 12–2. TRADITIONAL NEEDLE TYPES

Name	Description
Ferguson ("Fergie")	Half-circle; delicate taper shaft
Keith	Straight; medium weight; cutting point
Mayo	Half-circle; heavy; taper shaft and point
Milner	Straight; delicate; taper shaft and point
Surgeon's regular (Martin)	Half-circle; medium weight; cutting point, taper shaft
Trocar	Half-circle; heavy; spear-shaped point, taper shaft

curvature. In descending order of curve are needles with ½, ⅜, and ¼ curve. The straight needle has no curvature and is used primarily on skin. All curved needles are grasped with a *needle holder*. The straight needle is grasped between the fingers just as a normal sewing needle is. Because of the large variety of disposable needles available from suture manufacturers today, many needles are designated by their catalogue number (e.g., P-3 or P-4). These numbers will become more familiar as the products are selected and used. There are, however, traditional names that are still occasionally used to describe a type of needle, and these are given in Table 12–2.

Needle Shafts and Points

Because tissues vary in their elasticity and strength, needles must have different types of points (Fig. 12–3). A *cutting needle* is one that is honed to form cutting edges on three sides. A conventional cutting needle has one cutting edge on the *inside of the needle* curve and one on each side. The *reverse cutting needle* has a cutting edge on the *outside of the needle* curve and one on each side. The cutting needle actually incises the tissue as it passes through it. The *spatula needle* is a type of cutting needle that is flattened on both sides of the needle curve. This type of needle is used in ophthalmic surgery.

Tapered needles have no cutting edge and are used on delicate tissue. This type of needle has a sharp point but does not cut the tissue through which it passes. The *blunt needle* is smooth shafted and has a blunt point. This type of needle is restricted to use on the liver or kidney, in which tissues are soft and spongy and offer no resistance to the needle.

Needle Eyes

The eye of the needle is the point of attachment for the suture. There are several types of needle eyes, and the surgeon's selection depends on the type of tissue to be sutured and on the rapidity with which he or she needs them. Common needle eyes are illustrated in Figure 12–4.

The *conventional* needle eye is rounded, rectangular, or square. The *French-* or *spring-eye* needle has two eyes. This type of needle is used on very delicate tissue, such as gastrointestinal serosa. Only fine sutures are

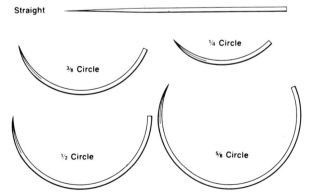

Figure 12–2. Common needle shapes. (Reprinted from Perspectives on Sutures, Courtesy of Davis & Geck, Wayne, NJ.)

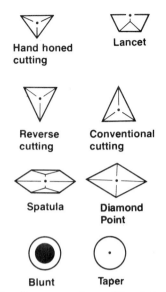

Figure 12–3. Needle cross sections. (Reprinted from Perspectives on Sutures, Courtesy of Davis & Geck, Wayne, NJ.)

used in conjunction with a French-eye needle because large sutures damage the needle's eyes. The proper method of threading a French-eye needle is discussed later in the chapter.

Atraumatic or Eyeless Needles

Because the eye of conventional needles carries a double strand of suture, the hole in which the needle passes is widened by the extra bulk at the eye. An alternative suture–needle combination, the *atraumatic* needle, prevents this trauma. The atraumatic needle is one in which the suture material is inserted by the manufacturer into the shaft of the needle where the eye would normally be. This is called a *swage*, and atraumatic needle and suture combinations are often called *swaged needles*. The diameter or size of the suture is very close to the diameter of the needle shaft so there is little additional tearing of tissue as the suture is drawn through. Atraumatic sutures are available in virtually every size, suture, and needle type. The process of swaging suture is very precise. Thus, this type of suture and needle combination is very costly. However, the advantages of minimum trauma and speed of application far outweigh the relative cost. Atraumatic sutures are

available in *single-arm* (one needle per suture) and *double-arm* (one needle attached to each end of the suture) configurations. Double-arm sutures are used during approximation of a lumen when a continuous suture is needed around the circumference of the vessel. The *suture release needle* (Fig. 12–5) is a type of atraumatic needle that detaches from its suture when pulled sharply. These are commonly used during gastrointestinal anastomosis or fascia closure.

Atraumatic sutures are packaged with many sutures in each packet. This means that there are many needles used and returned in rapid succession. For this reason, they should *always* be used in conjunction with a magnetic needle board or rack to prevent loss of a needle in the surgical wound. When an atraumatic needle is mounted on the needle holder, the jaws should be clamped well away from the swage, which can be easily damaged and cause the suture to be lost from the needle. Different types of shafts and points available on atraumatic sutures are shown in Figure 12–6.

Threading an Eyed Needle

The circulator usually distributes eyed needles to the scrub technologist two at a time. Because the technologist must thread the needle just before use, the process of suturing requires that the surgeon place one suture while the technologist is preparing the next. The surgeon then returns the needle, in its needle holder, ready for the next suture to be threaded. This sequence is one of the skills required of the scrub technologist or nurse and one in which speed and accuracy are developed *with time and practice*. Every scrub assistant must go through this learning process. The proper method of threading the conventional needle is to mount the needle on the

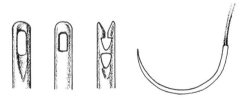

Figure 12–4. Needle eyes. *Left to right:* elliptical, square, French-eye, atraumatic. (From Nealon TF: Fundamental Skills in Surgery, 3rd ed. Philadelphia, WB Saunders, 1979.)

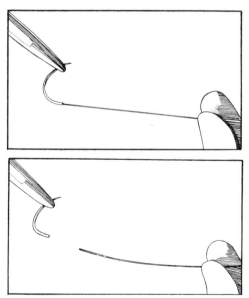

Figure 12–5. Suture release needle head. To release the suture from the needle head, align and pull sharply. (Reproduced by permission of Ethicon, Inc., Somerville, NJ.)

Taper Point Needle — used primarily on soft, easily penetrated tissue, such as peritoneum, intestine, or the heart. This needle is usually preferred where the smallest possible hole in the tissue and minimum tissue damage are desired. The body of the taper point needle is flattened and ribbed to improve its stability in the needleholder.

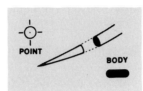

TAPERCUT * **Needle**—specially designed for use on tough tissue where a cutting point is needed and a narrow-bodied needle is desirable. It has a sharp, reverse cutting tip at the point, with the remainder of the needle blending into a taper cross section. All three edges of the tip are sharpened to provide uniform cutting action.

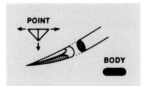

Conventional Cutting Needle — has two opposing cutting edges with a third edge on the inside curvature of the needle. The conventional cutting needle changes in cross-section shape from a triangular cutting tip to a flattened body.

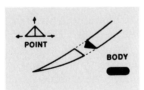

Reverse Cutting Needle — used to cut through tough, difficult to penetrate tissues such as fascia and skin. It has two opposing cutting edges, with the third cutting edge on the outer curvature of the needle. The reverse cutting needle is made with the triangular shape extending from the point to the swage area, with only the edges near the tip being sharpened.

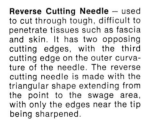

Precision Point Needle — specially designed for the plastic surgeon for use in delicate plastic or cosmetic surgery, and used widely for emergency repair of facial injuries and suturing on children. The Precision Point needle, honed several times, assures smooth passage through tissue, better placement of sutures, and minute needle path that heals quickly.

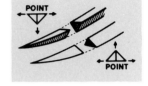

MICRO-POINT * **Reverse Cutting Needle** — an extremely smooth, sharp reverse cutting edge needle for use in ophthalmic surgery. Each needle must be individually honed to extreme sharpness and inspected under high power magnification. This delicate "instrument" has made it possible for ophthalmic surgeons to suture the extremely tough tissues of the eye with optimum precision and ease.

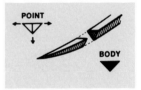

SABRELOC * **Needle**—sharp, flat type, "side-cutting" needle, designed to split through the layers of scleral or corneal tissue, and travel within the plane between them with virtually no resistance. This unique needle is flat on top and bottom; therefore it eliminates undesirable cutting out as a reverse cutting needle would.

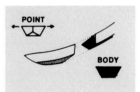

MICRO-POINT Spatula Needle — designed for anterior segment ophthalmic surgery and specially honed for exceptional sharpness. The needle is thin and flat in profile for ease in penetration.

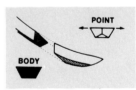

Blunt Point Needle — a taper needle with a rounded blunt point that will not *cut* through tissue. It is used in blunt dissection and in the suturing of friable tissues, such as liver and kidney. It is also used as a swaged ligature carrier on the ligature for incompetent cervix.

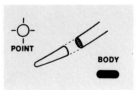

Figure 12–6. Types of swaged needles. *, Registered trademark. (Reproduced by permission of Ethicon, Inc., Somerville, NJ.)

needle holder about one third the distance from the eye. The suture length is passed from the *inside curve of the needle to the outside curve* (Fig. 12–7*A* and *B*). The suture is pulled through the eye of the needle about 2 or 3 inches, and the two strands are twisted once. This will secure the strands so that they are not pulled through the eye of the needle during delivery. An alternative method of securing the suture is to lay both strands between the jaws of the needle holder being

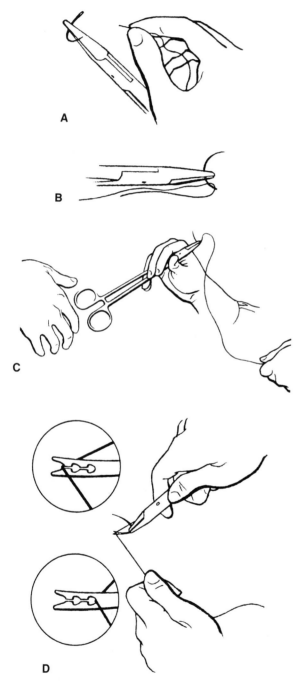

Figure 12–7. How to mount and pass the needle holder correctly. *A.* Suture is passed through the needle eye. *B.* The short end is pulled one third the length of the suture. *C.* The needle holder is passed with the point up. *D.* Threading the French eye needle. (Reproduced by permission of Ethicon, Inc., Somerville, NJ.)

careful not to clamp the suture in the jaws, because this would weaken it.

The method used to thread a French-eye needle is slightly different than that used for a conventional needle. The top eye of the needle is split. Instead of threading the end of the suture through either eye, the needle is placed in the needle holder and one end of the suture is grasped about 3 inches from its end along with the needle holder in one hand. With the other hand, the long end of the suture strand is picked up and drawn down over the split in the top eye and then the bottom eye. The suture will click into place and is ready for use. This technique is shown in Figure 12–7*D*.

Passing the Needle Holder

When the needle holder is passed, it must be oriented so that the surgeon does not have to reposition it for use. To pass the instrument in the proper position, the technologist must first visualize the proper position employed in suturing, that is, with the outside curve of the needle aiming downward and the point aiming upward, in the direction of the surgeon's chin. If the technologist is standing opposite the surgeon, the needle holder should be oriented in mirror image of this position. When passing the needle holder, the long end of the suture should not come in contact with the surgeon's palm as he or she grasps the instrument (Fig. 12–7*C*).

METHODS OF SUTURING

There are two basic methods of suturing and various ways to use the two techniques. The suture is either a *running* or an *interrupted suture*. A running suture uses one continuous strand of suture that is drawn alternately between two edges of tissue. Interrupted sutures are individually placed, knotted, and cut. The continuous suture can be placed rapidly, but if the suture breaks during the healing process, the wound could open along the entire length of the incision. Thus, running sutures are usually used only in areas of minimal stress. Interrupted sutures are more reliable in areas that are under strain because the stress is distributed among all the individual sutures. Some common suturing techniques are shown in Figure 12–8.

Retention sutures (Fig. 12–9) are used in areas where great strength is required, such as in some abdominal incisions. They are used in conjunction with routine abdominal suture layers to add support to the closure. Heavy suture material, usually size 2 or 3 nylon or steel, is placed through the skin and carried down to the fascia or peritoneum on one side of the wound. The suture is then brought up through the layers of the opposite side where it emerges through the skin. After the individual layers of the abdomen are closed, the two ends of the retention suture are threaded through *Bolsters* or *bumpers* (short lengths of rubber or Silastic tubing). The suture ends are then tied together. The bolsters distribute the pressure and prevent the heavy retention sutures from cutting into the patient's skin.

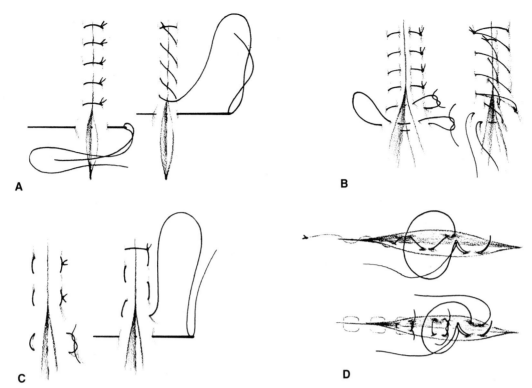

Figure 12–8. Common surgical suturing techniques. *A.* Interrupted and running. *B.* Vertical mattress. *C.* Horizontal mattress. *D.* Subcuticular (buried). (From Nealon TF: Fundamental Skills in Surgery, 3rd ed. Philadelphia, WB Saunders, 1979.)

A *pursestring suture* is used to approximate the open end of a *lumen* (hollow tubular structure) such as a hernia sac or appendiceal stump. The suture is threaded in and out of the edges of the lumen and drawn together like a pursestring (Fig. 12–10).

A *suture ligature* or *"stick tie"* (Fig. 12–11) is used to ligate large blood vessels or ducts. This is a suture-needle combination that is first passed through both sides of the vessel and then tied securely around the vessel. The suture ligature prevents the tie from slipping off the end of the vessel.

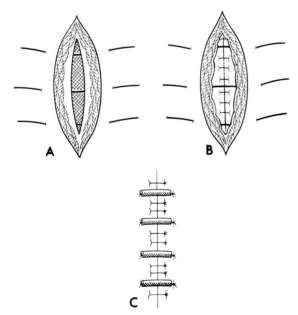

Figure 12–9. *A.* Retention sutures placed through all layers of tissue. *B.* Retention sutures placed in fascia. *C.* Bolsters are used to protect the skin. (Reprinted from Perspectives on Sutures, Courtesy of Davis & Geck, Wayne, NJ.)

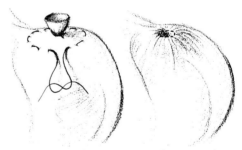

Figure 12–10. Pursestring suture, used commonly on the appendix, as shown here. (From Nealon TF: Fundamental Skills in Surgery, 3rd ed. Philadelphia, WB Saunders, 1979.)

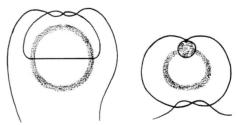

Figure 12–11. Suture ligature. (From Nealon TF: Fundamental Skills in Surgery, 3rd ed. Philadelphia, WB Saunders, 1979.)

SKIN TAPES AND CLIPS

Sterile Tapes

Sterile adhesive tapes are sometimes used to approximate the skin incision. These reinforced surgical tapes are adhesive on one side and are available in various sizes ranging from ⅛ to 4 inches in width. They are used on areas of the body where stress and body moisture are minimal.

Skin Clips

Skin clips (Fig. 12–12) are occasionally used to approximate skin incisions. These are heavy metal clips that are secured with a *clip applier*. Because of the postoperative discomfort they cause and because more technologically advanced methods are available, skin clips are seldom used.

SURGICAL STAPLING INSTRUMENTS

Surgical stapling instruments have advanced the field of wound closure tremendously in the past decade. This family of wound closure products includes vessel ligation and wound approximation instruments as well as those that both divide and approximate or anastomose tissue. The instruments are available in single-use or reusable form. Each type of instrument carries a cartridge that contains a prescribed number and size of staples that fire individually or together in single, double, triple, or quadruple lines. Each type of instrument has specific applications. The advantages of these instruments are listed below:

1. Tissue handling is greatly minimized, thus reducing trauma by manipulation and exposure.

2. The suture lines are strong and dependable.
3. Surgical staples are nonreactive in tissue.
4. Staples are noncrushing, thereby preventing tissue necrosis due to compromised blood and nutrient supply to the tissue edges.

The technologist must become familiar with the proper handling of these instruments and with the loading of staple cartridges. Much aggravation can be prevented during surgery if the instruments are studied carefully before they are needed. There are several manufacturers of surgical stapling instruments, and *all* are reliable. The instruments discussed in this text are available through the United States Surgical Corporation (Norwalk, CT), and the name of each instrument applies to this company only. These instruments have been chosen for discussion because of their widespread use.

Premium Surgiclip

The Premium Surgiclip (Fig. 12–13) is a disposable clip applier used to occlude vessels and other tubular structures and for vagotomy, sympathectomy, and radiographic markings. It consists of an applier shaft with attached handles and an integral cartridge containing 15 or 20 titanium clips (Fig. 12–14). The clip applier jaw is placed around a vessel or other tubular structure. As the handles of the applier are brought together, the clip is closed, occluding the vessel or structure. As the handles are released, a new clip is automatically loaded into the clip applier jaw. Figure 12–15 is a schematic view of the instrument.

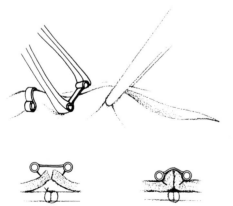

Figure 12–12. Application of wound clips. (From Nealon TF: Fundamental Skills in Surgery, 3rd ed. Philadelphia, WB Saunders, 1979.)

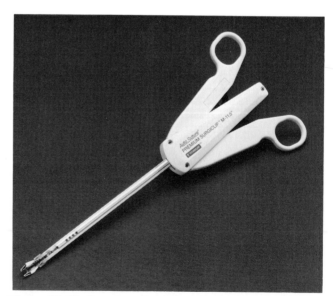

Figure 12–13. Premium Surgiclip clip applier. (Courtesy of United States Surgical Corporation, Norwalk, CT.)

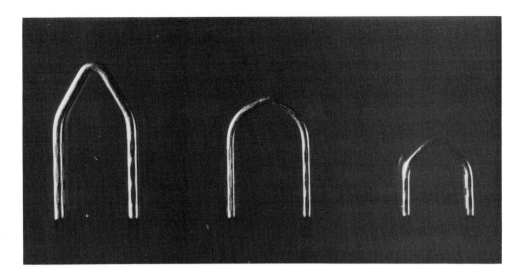

Figure 12–14. Titanium clips used in Premium Surgiclip. (Courtesy of United States Surgical Corporation, Norwalk, CT.)

Powered Disposable LDS Stapler

The powered Disposable LDS stapler (Fig. 12–16) is used in abdominal, gynecologic, and thoracic surgery for ligating and dividing blood vessels and other tubular structures. The instrument places two stainless steel staples to ligate the tissue within the cartridge jaw, and the knife divides the tissue between the two closed staples. The instrument is activated by squeezing the instrument handle. Figure 12–17 is a schematic view of this instrument.

Premium Multifire TA Disposable Surgical Stapler

The Premium Multifire TA Disposable Surgical Stapler (Fig. 12–18) has application in many types of surgical procedures for resection and transection. This instrument places a double or triple staggered row of titanium staples, depending on the model used. The instrument is activated by squeezing the handle. The size of the staple is determined by the selection of the

V, the 3.5, or the 4.8 staple size. Figure 12–19 is a schematic view of the instrument. A description of removing one loading unit and reloading another is provided in Figures 12–20 and 12–21.

Auto Suture TA 90 B and TA 90 BN Stapling Instruments

The Auto Suture TA 90 (Fig. 12–22) and TA 90 BN are used only in bariatric surgery (that dealing with obesity, i.e., stomach stapling procedures). These instruments are nondisposable but use disposable loading units that place four equidistant staggered rows of stainless steel staples. The instrument is activated by squeezing the handle. The notch in the instrument head of the

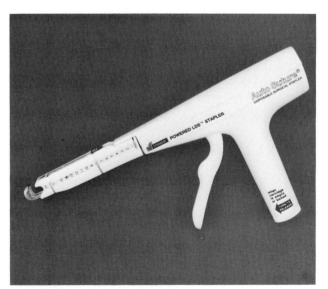

Figure 12–16. Powered Disposable LDS Stapler. (Courtesy of United States Surgical Corporation, Norwalk, CT.)

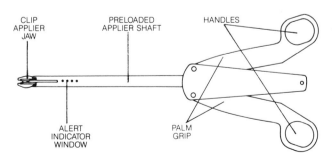

Figure 12–15. Schematic view of Premium Surgiclip. (Courtesy of United States Surgical Corporation, Norwalk, CT.)

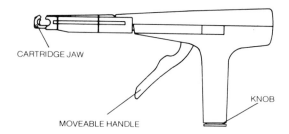

CARTRIDGE JAW

MOVEABLE HANDLE

KNOB

Figure 12–17. Schematic view of Powered Disposable LDS Stapler. (Courtesy of United States Surgical Corporation, Norwalk, CT.)

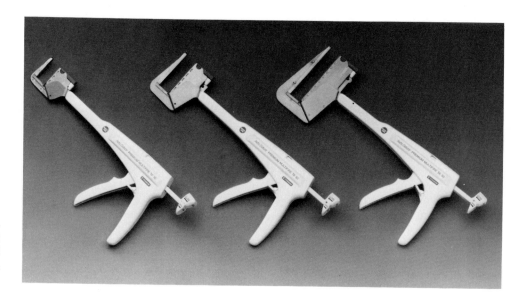

Figure 12–18. Premium Multifire TA Disposable Surgical Stapler. (Courtesy of United States Surgical Corporation, Norwalk, CT.)

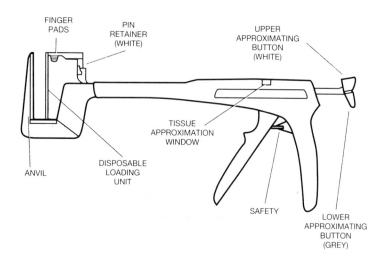

FINGER PADS

PIN RETAINER (WHITE)

UPPER APPROXIMATING BUTTON (WHITE)

TISSUE APPROXIMATION WINDOW

ANVIL

DISPOSABLE LOADING UNIT

SAFETY

LOWER APPROXIMATING BUTTON (GREY)

Figure 12–19. Schematic view of Premium Multifire TA Disposable Surgical Stapler. (Courtesy of United States Surgical Corporation, Norwalk, CT.)

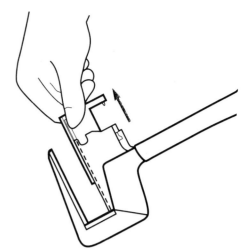

Figure 12–20. Removing loading unit of Premium Multifire TA Disposable Surgical Stapler. Make certain that the safety is in the locked position. To remove the disposable loading unit, grasp the disposable loading unit by the finger pads at the top of the cartridge and pull straight up from the jaws. (Courtesy of United States Surgical Corporation, Norwalk, CT.)

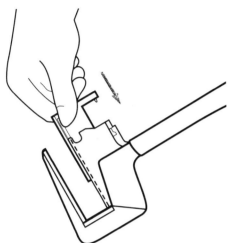

Figure 12–21. To reload the instrument, grasp the unused disposable loading unit by the finger pads, with the staple holes facing the instrument anvil. Insert the disposable loading unit into the metal cartridge housing and push firmly downward until the disposable loading unit clicks into position. *Note:* The instrument jaws will not close if no cartridge has been loaded into the jaws, if the cartridge is not fully loaded into the jaws, or if a fired cartridge remains in the jaws. (Courtesy of United States Surgical Corporation, Norwalk, CT.)

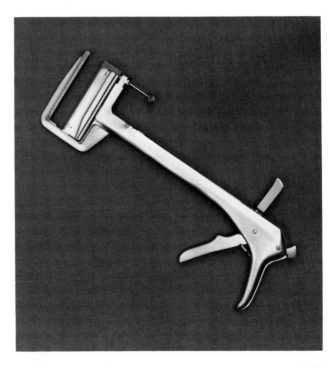

Figure 12–22. Auto Suture TA 90. (Courtesy of United States Surgical Corporation, Norwalk, CT.)

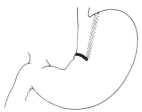

Figure 12–23. Staple results with the Auto Suture TA 90 BN surgical stapling instrument. (Courtesy of United States Surgical Corporation, Norwalk, CT.)

TA 90 BN stapling instrument creates a channel 1 cm wide on activation of the disposable loading unit (Fig. 12–23). The correct method for removing and replacing the loading unit is shown in Figure 12–24.

Auto Suture TA Premium 55 Surgical Stapling Instrument

This instrument (Fig. 12–25) is used in abdominal and thoracic surgery for resection and transection. With the use of a disposable loading unit, the TA Premium 55 places a double row of titanium sutures. When used in conjunction with the Premium Polysorb 55 loading unit (Fig. 12–26), it places a double staggered row of Lactomer absorbable copolymer staples. The size of the staple is determined by selection of the loading unit. The proper loading technique for the titanium loading

cartridge is shown in Figure 12–27, and insertion and removal of the Polysorb 55 disposable loading unit is shown in Figure 12–28.

Multifire GIA 60 or 80 Disposable Surgical Stapler

The Multifire GIA 60 or 80 disposable surgical stapler (Fig. 12–29) and Multifire GIA 60 or 80 disposable loading units have application in abdominal, gynecologic, pediatric, and thoracic surgery for resection, transection, and creation of anastomoses. This instrument places two double-staggered rows of titanium staples and simultaneously divides the tissue between the two double rows. A schematic view of this instrument is shown in Figure 12–30. Unloading and reloading the cartridges is described in Figure 12–31.

Auto Suture GIA 50 Premium Surgical Stapler

The Auto Suture GIA 50 Premium surgical stapler (Fig. 12–32) is a nondisposable instrument that is used in abdominal, gynecologic, pediatric, and thoracic surgery for resection, transection, and creation of anastomoses. The Auto Suture GIA 50 disposable loading unit is used in surgical procedures that require placement of four parallel staple lines. It places two double-staggered rows of stainless steel staples and simultaneously divides

Text continued on page 129

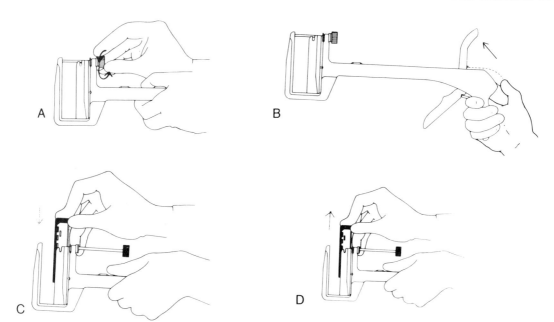

Figure 12–24. Correct method for removing and replacing the loading unit. *A.* Unscrew the retaining pin by turning the knurled knob counterclockwise. *B.* Open the instrument by pushing up on the release lever. Before insertion of the disposable loading unit, always make sure the safety is in the locked position. Failure to do so may result in staples prefiring. *C.* Pull back the retaining pin. (It will lock in place.) Slide the disposable loading unit into the instrument jaw such that the alignment post is within the alignment post slot in the instrument. Failure to do so may cause the cartridge to seat improperly and may result in staple malformation. *D.* Slide cartridge out of the instrument by pulling up on finger pads. (Courtesy of United States Surgical Corporation, Norwalk, CT.)

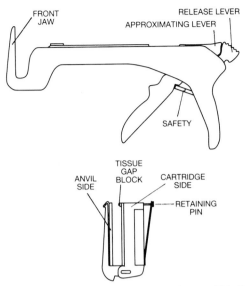

Figure 12–25. Schematic view of Auto Suture TA Premium 55 Surgical Stapling Instrument. (Courtesy of United States Surgical Corporation, Norwalk, CT.)

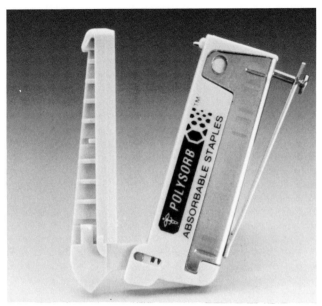

Figure 12–26. Premium Polysorb 55 loading unit. (Courtesy of United States Surgical Corporation, Norwalk, CT.)

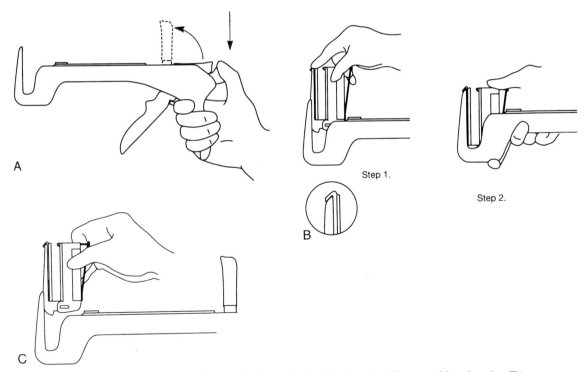

Figure 12–27. Proper loading technique of the titanium loading cartridge for the TA Premium 55. *A.* Open the instrument by pushing the release lever down. Before inserting the disposable loading unit, always make certain the safety is in the locked position. *B. Step 1:* Insert the disposable loading unit into the instrument jaws, taking care to hook the tip of the disposable loading unit anvil side over the top of the front jaw. *Step 2:* Push the loading unit down until firmly seated. *C.* Remove the disposable loading unit by grasping the cartridge side and lifting up. Discard. Never reuse disposable parts. (Courtesy of United States Surgical Corporation, Norwalk, CT.)

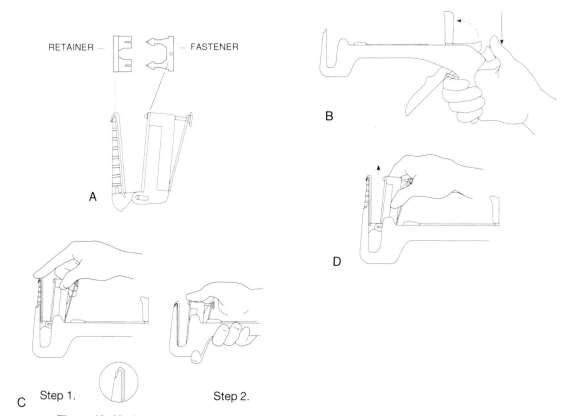

Figure 12–28. Insertion and removal of the Polysorb 55 disposable loading unit. *A.* Each Auto Suture Premium Polysorb 55 disposable loading unit contains 19 staples. Each staple is composed of a fastener, which is loaded into the cartridge portion of the disposable loading unit, and a retainer, which is loaded into the retainer portion of the disposable loading unit. *B.* Open the instrument by pushing the release lever down. Before inserting the disposable loading unit, always make certain the safety is in the locked position. *C.* *Step 1:* Insert the disposable loading unit into the instrument jaws, taking care to hook the tip of the disposable loading unit retainer side over the top of the front jaw. *Step 2:* Push the loading unit down until firmly seated. *D.* Remove the disposable loading unit by grasping the cartridge side and lifting up. Discard. Never reuse disposable parts. (Courtesy of United States Surgical Corporation, Norwalk, CT.)

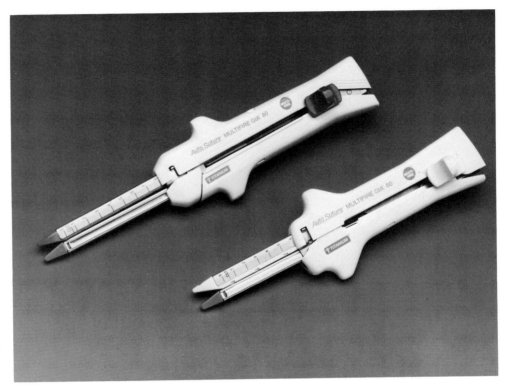

Figure 12–29. Multifire GIA 60 and 80. (Courtesy of United States Surgical Corporation, Norwalk, CT.)

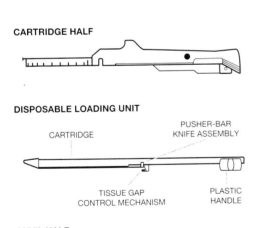

CARTRIDGE HALF

DISPOSABLE LOADING UNIT

CARTRIDGE

PUSHER-BAR
KNIFE ASSEMBLY

TISSUE GAP
CONTROL MECHANISM

PLASTIC
HANDLE

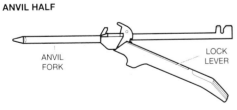

ANVIL HALF

ANVIL
FORK

LOCK
LEVER

Figure 12–30. Schematic view of the Auto Suture Multifire GIA 80 Disposable Surgical Stapler. *Note:* Each disposable loading unit contains a fresh pusher-bar knife assembly and tissue gap control mechanism. (Courtesy of United States Surgical Corporation, Norwalk, CT.)

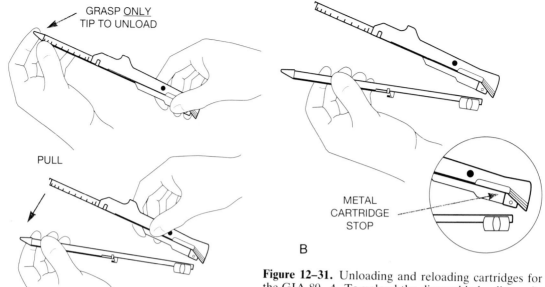

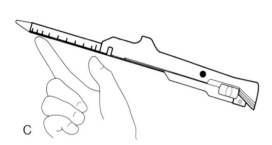

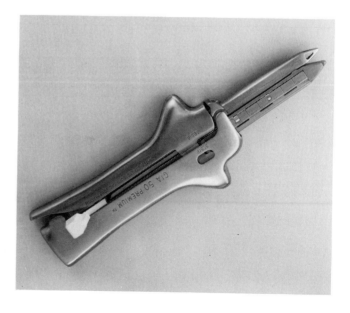

Figure 12–31. Unloading and reloading cartridges for the GIA 80. *A.* To unload the disposable loading unit, grasp the cartridge half with one hand and *the tip* of the disposable loading unit with the other hand. Then pull the disposable loading unit out of the instrument. *B.* To *reload* the cartridge half, insert a Multifire GIA 80 disposable loading unit into the rear of instrument, seating the bottom portion of the cartridge against the metal cartridge stop. *C.* The bottom and top portions of the disposable loading unit should be pressed firmly into place. *Note:* The Multifire GIA 80 can be reloaded only up to seven times for a total of eight applications; otherwise staples may not form correctly. Further applications could compromise the integrity of the staple line, which may result in leakage or disruption of the surgical wound. (Courtesy of United States Surgical Corporation, Norwalk, CT.)

Figure 12–32. Auto Suture GIA 50 Premium Surgical Stapler. (Courtesy of United States Surgical Corporation, Norwalk, CT.)

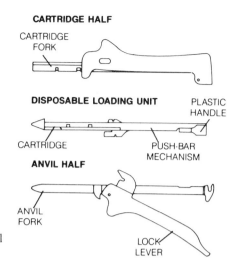

Figure 12–33. Schematic view of the GIA 50. (Courtesy of United States Surgical Corporation, Norwalk, CT.)

the tissue between the two double rows. Figure 12–33 is a schematic view of the GIA 50. Loading instructions are shown in Figure 12–34, and disassembly for cleaning is illustrated in Figure 12–35.

Roticulator 30 and 30-V3 Disposable Surgical Stapler

The Roticulator 30 and 30-V3 disposable surgical staplers (Fig. 12–36) are used in many different types of surgical procedures for resection and transection. The Roticulator 30 places a double staggered row of stainless steel staples, and the 30-V3 model places a triple-staggered row of staples. The size of the staples is determined by the selection of the 3.5, 4.8, or vascular staple size. A schematic view of the instrument is presented in Figure 12–37.

Auto Suture Premium CEEA

The Auto Suture Premium CEEA disposable surgical stapler (Fig. 12–38) is used in general, thoracic, and bariatric surgery for creation of end-to-end, end-to-side, and side-to-side anastomoses. The instrument places a circular, double-staggered row of titanium staples. Immediately after staple formation, a knife blade in the

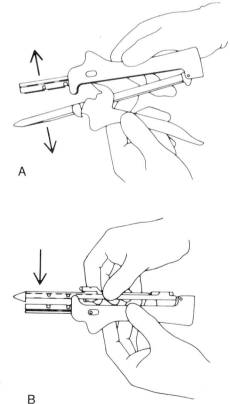

Figure 12–34. *A.* To load the GIA 50, peel open the loading unit package. Prepare instrument for loading by moving the lock lever to the side and separating the instrument in two: an anvil half and a cartridge half. *B.* Insert cartridge into cartridge fork of instrument with open grooves of cartridge facing up. Place the location tabs of the cartridge into the location slots of the cartridge fork. Press down and make certain the front ridge of the cartridge snaps firmly into place. *Note:* Anvil fork is one-piece construction and anvil is not removable. (Courtesy of United States Surgical Corporation, Norwalk, CT.)

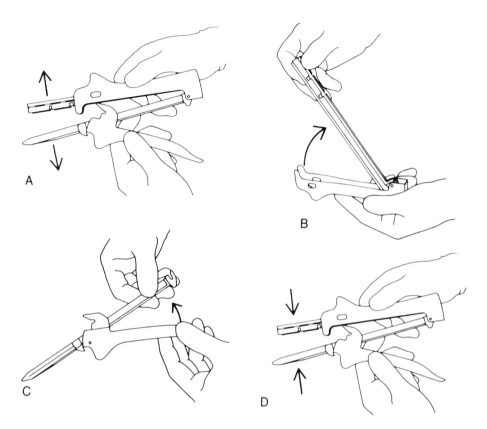

Figure 12–35. Process for cleaning GIA 50. *A.* The GIA 50 is designed to eliminate the need for disassembly and assembly. After each use, the instrument should be opened for cleaning using the following steps. Separate the cartridge and anvil halves. *Do not attempt to disassemble the instrument any further. B.* Grasp the cartridge half and separate the cartridge fork from the hinge site, exposing the open channel for cleaning. *C.* Grasp the anvil half and separate the anvil fork from the hinge site, exposing the open channel for cleaning. Clean with instrument cleaner like any other stainless steel instrument. *D.* Close the instrument by first pushing the cartridge and anvil forks back into the instrument halves. Then join the instrument by holding the lock lever open and engaging the rear hinge assembly. Connect the front of the instrument, and close the lock lever. The audible click will signify that the instrument is properly closed. (Courtesy of United States Surgical Corporation, Norwalk, CT.)

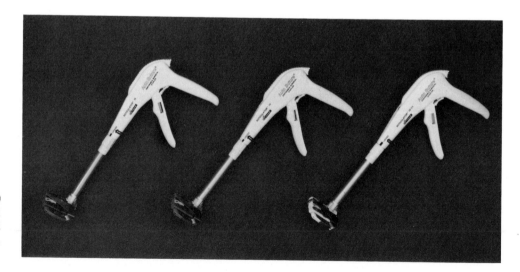

Figure 12–36. Roticulator 30 and 30-V3 Disposable Surgical Staplers. (Courtesy of United States Surgical Corporation, Norwalk, CT.)

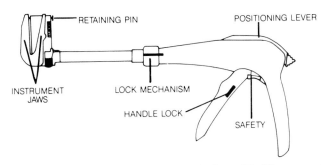

Figure 12–37. Schematic view of Roticulator 30. (Courtesy of United States Surgical Corporation, Norwalk, CT.)

instrument resects the excess tissue, thus creating a circular anastomosis. The instrument is activated by squeezing the handles firmly as far as they will go. The Low Profile Anvil for use with the CEEA is used in procedures in which the anvil normally supplied with the CEEA is too tall for comfortable use. Once the Low Profile Anvil is attached to the center shaft it is permanently affixed to the center shaft and cannot be removed. A schematic view of the instrument is shown in Figure 12–39.

Auto Suture Purstring

The Auto Suture Purstring (Fig. 12–40) is a disposable automatic pursestring instrument. It is used in intestinal, colorectal, and esophageal surgery to place temporary pursestring closures. It places a circumferential strand of 2-0 monofilament nylon held in place by stainless steel staples. The stainless steel staples are attached to the structure or organ where a pursestring closure is desired. A schematic view of the instrument is presented in Figure 12–41.

Auto Suture Multifire Premium Disposable Skin Stapler

This instrument (Fig. 12–42) is used for skin closure in abdominal, gynecologic, orthopedic, and thoracic surgery. It may also be used to close incisions in vein stripping, thyroidectomy, and mastectomy procedures; for closure of scalp incisions; for skin grafts; and in plastic and reconstructive surgery. The instrument places one staple each time the instrument handles are activated. A schematic view of the instrument is shown in Figure 12–43, and proper loading and unloading of the staple cartridges is shown in Figure 12–44.

WOUND DRESSINGS

Dressings are applied to the operative site at the close of surgery to produce one or more of the following effects:

- Absorb or draw away fluids that may drain from the wound during healing.
- Protect the wound from contamination until the wound edges are sealed.

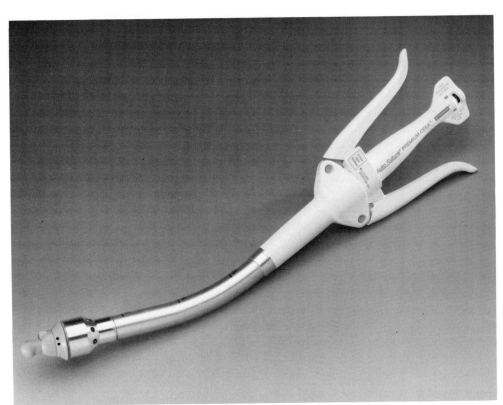

Figure 12–38. Auto Suture Premium CEEA disposable surgical stapler. (Courtesy of United States Surgical Corporation, Norwalk, CT.)

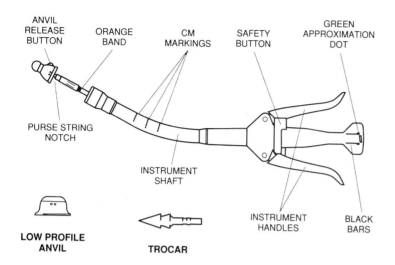

LOW PROFILE ANVIL

TROCAR

Figure 12–39. Schematic view of Auto Suture Premium CEEA. (Courtesy of United States Surgical Corporation, Norwalk, CT.)

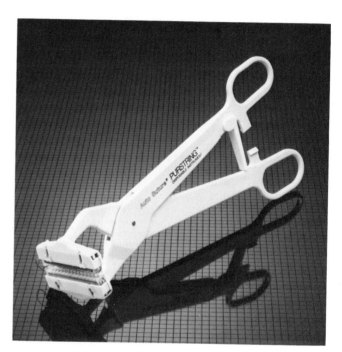

Figure 12–40. Auto Suture Purstring. (Courtesy of United States Surgical Corporation, Norwalk, CT.)

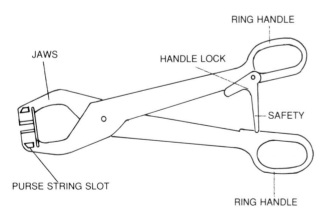

Figure 12–41. Schematic view of Auto Suture Purstring. (Courtesy of United States Surgical Corporation, Norwalk, CT.)

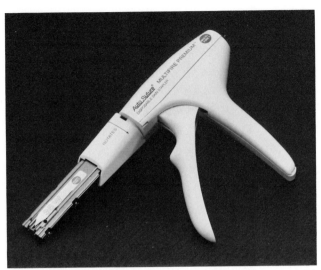

Figure 12–42. Auto Suture Multifire Premium disposable skin stapler. (Courtesy of United States Surgical Corporation, Norwalk, CT.)

- Provide a more aesthetic appearance to the wound than exposed sutures would.
- Provide pressure on the wound to help maintain hemostasis postoperatively.
- Provide support to the wound site.

Not all surgical dressings perform all of these functions. The surgeon chooses the type of dressing to be used based on the following considerations:

- Location of the wound
- Type of surgery performed
- Amount of drainage anticipated
- Postoperative care available to the patient
- Type of tissue encountered during surgery

Simple wound dressings consist of a single layer of polyurethane. These are left in place for approximately 24 hours and provide a moist environment that is beneficial in hastening the primary stages of wound healing. In addition, they help decrease postoperative pain and inflammation.

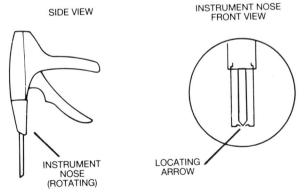

Figure 12–43. Schematic view of Auto Suture Multifire Premium disposable skin stapler. (Courtesy of United States Surgical Corporation, Norwalk, CT.)

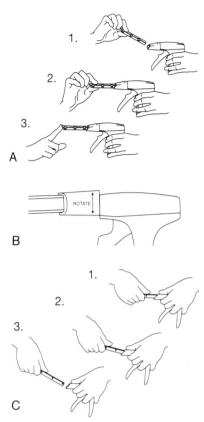

Figure 12–44. Proper loading and unloading of Auto Suture Multifire Premium skin stapler. *A. Loading:* Remove the cartridge from the sterile package. Hold the cartridge with locating arrow away from the instrument nose. Align the metal portion of the cartridge with the slot in the instrument nose. Insert the cartridge firmly into the nose of the instrument until there is an audible click. The instrument is now ready for use. *B.* The nose of the instrument with the cartridge can be rotated for ease of access to any closure. *C. Unloading:* To unload the disposable loading unit: firmly hold the nose as well as the handles of the instrument; grasp the tip of the loading unit; and lift and pull the unit away from the instrument. *Note:* The Multifire Premium disposable skin stapler should not be reloaded more than two times during a *single* surgical procedure. If the instrument is reloaded more than two times, the staples may not form properly. Improperly formed staples may compromise the integrity of the staple line, which may result in leakage or disruption of the surgical wound. (Courtesy of United States Surgical Corporation, Norwalk, CT.)

A three-layered dressing is used when drainage is anticipated or encouraged. This type of dressing is usually left in place longer than 48 hours. When *occlusive* dressings are used, the wound is protected from exposure to air and water.

A pressure dressing is used to occlude *dead space* (areas or pockets where there is no tissue) where fluids may build up and increase the risk of infection or inhibit healing. This type of dressing also helps promote hemostasis within the wound by pressing on small blood vessels. Pressure dressings are composed of layers of fluffed cotton gauze, processed spun cotton, elastic tapes, foam rubber, or a combination of these materials.

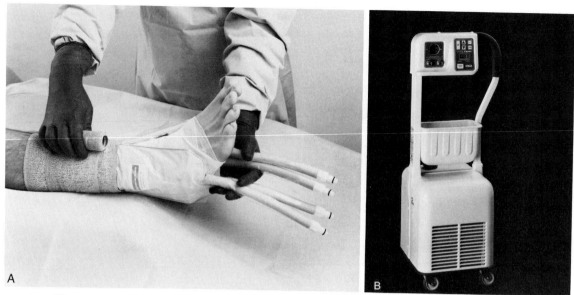

Figure 12–45. Cooltemp localized cold therapy pad. *A.* The pad is applied as part of a dressing routine to deliver constant cold therapy to the operative site. Pads are available in a variety of shapes and sizes to conform to the wound area. Connecting hoses are fully insulated to offer optimum efficiency. *B.* Control unit. (Courtesy of Cincinnati Sub-Zero Products, Inc., Cincinnati, OH.)

Whenever a wound requires external stability, such as after orthopedic surgery, casting materials are placed over, above, and below the wound site. Casting materials are available in several types of materials and weights depending on their application.

Whenever a wound requires postoperative thermal therapy, a hydrothermal pad through which cool water is circulated may be applied under the dressing. This type of dressing is used in orthopedic surgery to reduce postoperative inflammation and pain (Fig. 12–45).

WOUND DRAINS

Because the presence of serum and blood in the operative wound can delay healing, drains are used where the accumulation of these fluids is anticipated. A simple wound drain is the *Penrose* drain (Fig. 12–46). This type of gravity drain may be sutured in place to prevent it from dislodging. The *Hemovac* drain (Fig. 12–47) is used frequently after some orthopedic procedures. It is a self-contained vacuum system that draws fluids away from the wound as they form.

MECHANISMS OF WOUND HEALING

The human body is extremely efficient in its ability to recover from trauma. The patient's surgical wound actually starts healing as soon as the surgeon makes the skin incision.

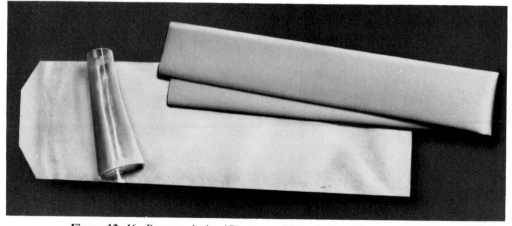

Figure 12–46. Penrose drain. (Courtesy of Davol, Inc., Cranston, RI.)

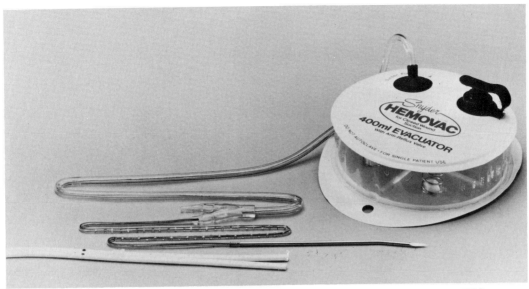

Figure 12–47. Hemovac drain and accessories. (Courtesy of Zimmer, Inc., Warsaw, IN.)

Substrate Phase

The first stage in wound repair is referred to as the substrate phase, which usually lasts from 1 to 4 days. Initially the tissue responds to trauma by a brief period of *vasoconstriction*. Small blood vessels constrict and then dilate. This mechanism brings increased blood supply to the area of injury and also brings with it plasma protein and other agents that defend the injured tissue. This inflammatory stage is followed by one of *hemostasis*. Small blood vessels contract in an attempt to control hemorrhage. Blood platelets begin to fill the lumens of the capillaries and arterioles and act as tiny "plugs." After a complex series of chemical reactions at the site of injury, the body releases a substance called *fibrin* to the wounded tissue, and clotting begins. The fibrin forms into networks that collect red blood cells, platelets, and white blood cells.

About 14 hours after trauma, cellular changes appear at the wound site. Special white blood cells release substances into the tissue that help clean the wound of tissue debris, unneeded cellular components, and bacteria.

Proliferative Phase

This second phase in wound healing lasts from 5 to 20 days. It is during this phase that actual repair of tissue takes place. New cells form and, in some areas of the body, the wound contracts. Wound contraction occurs when a large wound closes without scarring or forming permanent fibrous tissue (cicatrization). Wound contraction takes place on the back, buttocks, and posterior neck.

Remodeling Phase

This last stage of wound repair occurs from the 21st day on. It is during this phase that the wound regains the original strength that existed before trauma.

Through a complex series of cellular activities, *collagen*, a fibrous protein substance that gives the wound its strength, is formed.

WOUND HEALING CATEGORIES

Wounds are classified by the way in which they are repaired and heal. The clean surgical wound that is sutured closed and heals with minimal scarring and without incident does so by *first intention*. If the wound is not closed, such as in the presence of infection, it heals by a process of *granulation* (healing from the bottom up) and is said to heal by *second intention*. When the wound fails to heal by first intention, as when an infection develops at the wound site and the sutures break down, the wound is left open for a period of time until the infection is resolved. The wound is then reclosed. This is called a *secondary suture*. If the wound is known to be infected at the time of surgery and is left open to be sutured at a later date, the closure is referred to as a *delayed primary closure*.

Questions for Study and Review

1. What is the USP?
2. What standards for suture material does the USP establish?
3. How is suture material packaged?
4. What are the two main categories of suture products?
5. Describe the preparation of cotton suture.
6. How should surgical gut be handled and prepared?
7. Name two types of suture needles and describe them.
8. What is a spatula needle used for?
9. What is the difference between a French-eye needle and a conventional needle?
10. What are skin clips?

11. Surgical stapling instruments have many advantages over conventional suture products. What are they?

12. What do you think are the disadvantages of surgical stapling instruments?

13. What are the phases of wound healing?

14. What are the functions of wound dressings?

Bibliography

Ethicon, Inc.: Cardiovascular Surgery: Materials and Methods. Somerville, NJ, Ethicon, Inc.

Groah L: Operating Room Nursing: Perioperative Practice, 2nd ed. Norwalk, CT, Appleton & Lange, 1991.

United States Surgical Corporation: Stapling Techniques in General Surgery. Norwalk, CT, United States Surgical Corporation, 1988.

Hemostasis

Learning Objectives

After reading this chapter you should be able to

- ◆ *Understand* the process of hemostasis.
- ◆ *Understand* the safe use of electrosurgery.
- ◆ *Describe* the components used during electrosurgery.
- ◆ *Differentiate between* a monopolar and a bipolar electrosurgical unit.
- ◆ *Demonstrate* the safe principles and practices of the patient grounding pad, grounding cable, and power unit.
- ◆ *Describe* the different types of sponges used in surgery.
- ◆ *Demonstrate* the proper method for taking a sponge count.
- ◆ *Recognize* the consequences of losing a sponge within the surgical wound.
- ◆ *Understand* how a pneumatic tourniquet operates.
- ◆ *Discuss* different types of pharmaceutical hemostatic agents.
- ◆ *Discuss* hypothermia.
- ◆ *Describe* induced hypotension.
- ◆ *Describe* types of autotransfusion.

Key Terms

autotranfusion: Transfusion using the patient's own blood.

bipolar: Refers to a type of electrosurgical unit in which the electrical current is localized at the tip of the electrocautery probe and does not pass through the patient.

blunt dissection: The separation of tissues or tissue planes with an instrument that has no cutting ability.

bone wax: Medical-grade beeswax used on bone tissue to control bleeding.

dissector: A tiny sponge mounted on a clamp and used to perform blunt dissection.

Esmarch bandage: Rolled rubber bandage that is wrapped around the limb to force blood away from the surgical site before the application of a tourniquet.

four by four (4 × 4): Type of surgical sponge, consisting of loosely woven gauze squares.

Gelfoam: Medical-grade gelatin that is used to control capillary bleeding.
grounding cable: During electrosurgery, the cable connecting the control unit to the inactive electrode.
grounding pad: Gel-covered pad that grounds the patient during electrosurgery; inactive electrode.
hemostasis: The control of hemorrhage during surgery.
intentional hypotension: During surgery, the lowering of the patient's blood pressure to control hemorrhage.
intentional hypothermia: During surgery, the lowering of the patient's core temperature to control bleeding.
laparotomy tape: Also called a "lap tape." The largest surgical sponge available, used during major surgery.
ligation clips: Sometimes referred to as "silver clips." Small V-shaped clips that are applied around blood vessels or ducts in place of a ligature.
microfibrillar collagen hemostat: Substance derived from collagen and used as a hemostatic agent.
monopolar: Refers to a type of electrosurgical unit in which the electrical current passes through the patient and back to the control unit.
oxidized cellulose: Medical-grade cellulose manufactured into mesh squares and used as a hemostatic agent.
patty: A type of sponge used during neurosurgery.
sponge stick: A folded four by four mounted on a sponge clamp.
topical thrombin: Drug used in conjunction with gelatin sponges to halt capillary bleeding.
tourniquet: A device that prevents the flow of blood to the surgical wound.

Hemostasis is the control of hemorrhage. Surgery as it is performed today would be impossible without the many methods used to achieve hemostasis. In addition to controlling vital fluids, hemostasis also allows the surgeon a clear view of the surgical anatomy. The methods used to achieve hemostasis are based on the location of the surgical wound, the type of tissues encountered, and the depth of the surgical wound itself.

ELECTROSURGERY

Electrosurgery, or electrocautery, as a means of achieving hemostasis has been used routinely since the 1920s. Since that time new technology has added variations on electrocautery to the surgeon's armamentarium.

Four separate items are needed to perform monopolar electrosurgery. These are the *power unit* (Fig. 13–1), the *active electrode*, the patient *grounding pad* or *inactive electrode,* and the *grounding cable.* Two types of electrical current are generated by the power unit. One type coagulates tissue, and the other incises it. When either type of current is needed, the surgeon selects the tissue with the tip of the active electrode and activates the power unit either by a foot pedal or by a switch located on the active electrode handle. (Some electrosurgical units are "automatic" and activate when the pencil comes into contact with tissue; however, this type of unit is considered by many to be hazardous because inadvertent tissue damage can occur.)

On a *monopolar* unit, when the electrosurgical unit is activated, electrical current is transmitted to the patient at the tip of the active electrode. As the current travels through the tissue, it seeks a path back to the power unit. The patient grounding pad (inactive electrode) and cable provide this path, thus completing the electrical

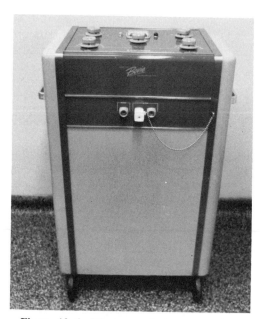

Figure 13–1. Electrosurgical power unit.

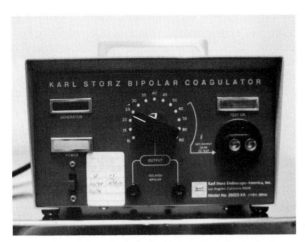

Figure 13–2. Bipolar electrosurgical power unit.

circuit. A grounding pad is therefore necessary when the monopolar unit is used.

When a *bipolar* unit (Fig. 13–2) is used, both the inactive and active electrodes are located at the tip of the instrument. The electrical circuit is completed between the two tips of the instrument, and therefore a grounding pad is not needed.

Safe Use of the Electrocautery Components

Certain safety precautions are critical when electrosurgery is used. Specific precautions concerning the various components of the electrosurgical unit are discussed below:

Whenever ignitable skin prep solutions are used on the surgical site, make sure the sites are completely dried before using the electrosurgical unit. There have been documented cases in which the patient, drapes, and surrounding areas have ignited and caused the death of the patient because of wet, flammable prep solutions (such as alcohol).

Be completely familiar with proper grounding techniques, proper attachment of cables, and dangers inherent in the use of the equipment BEFORE YOU USE IT.

Do not use electrosurgery on a patient who requires an external demand pacemaker. These types of pacemakers are susceptible to electrical interference. The distance between the active electrode and the patient grounding pad should be as wide as possible to prevent injury to a patient who has an implanted pacemaker. The electrosurgical cords must be placed at their full distance from the pacemaker's leads. During any electrosurgical case when a pacemaker is in use, a defibrillator must be located in the room. The patient's cardiac status is continually monitored during the procedure.

Grounding Pad

By far, the greatest risk to the patient during the use of electrocautery is the improper use of the patient grounding pad. The grounding pad is available in several forms. A nondisposable pad consisting of a metal plate with the grounding cable permanently attached is used infrequently. When this type of plate is used, it must be inspected for cracks, pitting, or grooves. The point of attachment to the grounding cable must be intact with no evidence of breakage or fraying. This type of plate must be coated with a layer of conductive gel designated specifically for use with electrosurgical grounding pads. The gel must be spread evenly and in sufficient amounts to prevent drying out during surgery. If the gel is not distributed completely over the surface of the plate, severe burns can occur at the site of application. This type of grounding is similar to a disposable pad composed of a thick foil plate. The disposable plate also requires the use of conductive gel. The most common type of patient grounding pad is a disposable foil plate embedded in a foam pad that is pre-gelled. When this type of pad is used, the connecting adapter for the grounding cable has not been stressed because of prior use and the amount of gel has been measured and applied by the manufacturer. The pads have an adhesive coating that holds the pad securely in place during use.

When applying and using the patient grounding pad the following standards must be strictly followed:

Always place the pad in an area of sufficient "fleshiness." Avoid placing the pad over any bony prominence or areas where the flesh is thin and fragile. This may cause uneven dispersal of electricity and consequent burns. During abdominal surgery the pad is often placed over the patient's thigh on the lateral side midway between the hip and knee. When the patient is in lithotomy position, the pad can be placed at the waist or thigh. The pad should be placed as close to the operative site as possible, but the fleshiness of the area under the pad is more important than its proximity to the wound site.

When a reusable pad is used, spread the electrolyte gel thickly and evenly over the entire surface of the pad. If the procedure is lengthy, the pad should be checked periodically to make sure that the electrolyte gel has not dried out.

Never slide the pad underneath the patient when applying it. When the pad is placed or replaced, the patient should be rolled over, lifted, or turned before the pad is positioned. This prevents materials from being dragged in between the patient's skin and the pad and also ensures that the pad is placed in the correct position and that all surfaces of the pad are in contact with the skin.

If there is excess body hair at the desired pad site, the hair should be removed before applying the pad. Hair can act as an insulator between the patient and the grounding pad.

After surgery, when the pad is removed, inspect the pad site carefully for signs of skin lesions, irritation, or other injury. Document and report any suspicious skin lesion.

Grounding Cable

The grounding cable carries electricity away from the patient grounding pad to the power unit. The cable is coated with clear plastic or vinyl so that the wires inside can be inspected. The following guidelines will prevent patient and personnel injury:

Always check the grounding cable BEFORE USE to make sure that it is fully intact. If there are any signs of broken wires, indentations, or other indications that there is a break in the continuity of the individual wires, the cable must not be used. Never use a cable that has been taped or otherwise "field repaired."

Always make sure that the connection between the cable and the grounding pad is secure. Most connections at the pad are snap-type fixtures that fit tightly and securely. If the connecting snap does not fit to the pad with an audible click, check the integrity of the connection.

Make sure that the connection between the pad and the cable is clean and dry. Cable connections may become soiled or covered with electrolyte gel from a previous case. Always make sure that the connection is unimpeded by this or any other type of soil.

Always attach the grounding cable to the pad before the patient has been draped. This ensures that the cable is attached properly and securely. It is difficult to achieve this while working under a tent of drapes.

Never release the cable from the power unit by pulling on the cable—grasp the plug to release it. Repeated stress on the cable causes the individual wires to weaken and break down.

Power Unit

The power unit supplies all needed electricity to the active electrode and completes the return circuit through the grounding pad and cable. The modern power unit contains a transformer that converts electricity from one voltage level to another and also *isolates the electrical output.* This means that the wall current is prevented from reaching the patient (hence the term *isolated output*). Older power units do not have this important safety feature, and the risk of serious injury is great when they are used. The numerical settings on all types of power units are controlled by the registered nurse circulator during surgery. This unit is a powerful source of electricity, and standards for its safe use must be followed.

Never store liquids such as irrigation solutions or medications on top of the power unit. Fluids and electricity do not mix! The unit should never be used as a table top where fluids might spill inside and cause an electrical short circuit. This could ruin the unit.

The power unit must be in the OFF position and settings placed at 0 BEFORE the grounding cable is connected to it. This prevents the surgeon from inadvertently activating more power than he or she needs. Always wait for the surgeon to dictate what setting he or she needs before turning on the unit.

Be alert to possible malfunctions in the unit. If the surgeon calls for increasingly greater and greater power, the power unit may be defective. Exchange the power unit for another one, check the patient grounding pad and cable for integrity, and make sure that conductive irrigation solutions such as saline have not pooled between the grounding pad and the patient's skin.

SPONGES

Surgical sponges (Fig. 13–3) are used in many different ways to achieve hemostasis. Their primary function is to blot or absorb blood and other body fluids in the surgical wound. Other uses are discussed here.

Sponges, because of their compactibility and pliability when wet, can become lodged in the surgical wound and are difficult to differentiate from tissue. Therefore, all surgical sponges are sewn or impregnated with a radiopaque (x-ray visible) material that can easily identify their location in the surgical wound should the need arise.

Types of Sponges

Four by fours (4×4s) are made of loosely woven gauze that when manufactured and folded measure 4

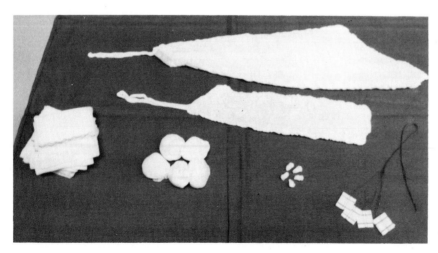

Figure 13–3. Surgical sponges. *Top.* Laparotomy sponge. *Bottom left to right.* Gauze 4×4 inch pads, large dissector, small dissector, and neurosurgical sponges.

inches by 4 inches. This type of sponge is used in superficial surgery when the wound is shallow. It must always be mounted on a clamp for use in deep incisions such as the abdominal or thoracic cavity. To mount a 4 × 4 sponge, the assistant folds it in equal thirds in one direction and then in half in the other direction. The folded sponge is placed on the end of a sponge clamp with the smooth folded portion pointing upwards, away from the body of the clamp. This arrangement is called a "sponge stick" or "sponge on a stick." Sponge sticks are used to blot small bleeding vessels deep within the wound. Open 4 × 4 sponges are often used for blunt dissection (manual separation of tissue planes) in gynecologic surgery such as anterior and posterior repair.

Laparotomy tapes (also called "lap tapes" or "lap sponges") are used whenever the abdominal or thoracic cavity is opened, for major orthopedic surgery, and during any other surgical procedure when large blood vessels are encountered. These are the largest sponges used in surgery. They measure approximately 12 × 12 inches and are manufactured with a cotton fabric loop at one corner. In addition to their use as a blotter and to absorb fluids, abdominal sponges are used to wall off anatomic structures such as the intestines or other abdominal organs that are not the focus of an abdominal procedure. They can serve as padding underneath the blades of large retractors and help prevent bruising and maceration of the wound edges during extended periods of retraction. Abdominal sponges are most often used moistened with sterile saline and wrung dry to increase their absorption of blood and fluids. Some hospitals employ the use of laparotomy rings, which are heavy metal rings that attach to the corner loop. When the sponge is in use deep within the wound, the loop and ring can be draped out and over the edge of the incision to help prevent a sponge from being left in the wound during closure.

A *dissector* is a small compressed cotton wad that is overwrapped with heavy gauze. These sponges vary in size from ½ inch up to 1½ inches and are called a wide assortment of names that resemble their size, such as "peanut," "cherry," or simply "pusher" (as in tissue pusher). Dissectors are *always* mounted on a clamp. The type of clamp used varies with the depth of the incision and the size of the sponge. Most commonly used are Péan or Mayo clamps. This type of sponge is used for blunt dissection and also for blotting and fluid absorption within the wound.

Cotton balls that are specially manufactured to resist shredding and have a small string attached are often used in neurosurgical cases, especially around fragile brain and spinal cord tissue. These sponges may be dipped in warm saline before use to help achieve hemostasis. They are used primarily for absorption of blood and other fluids.

Patties (sometimes called "neuro" sponges) are compressed squares of rayon or cotton with a string attached at one end used in neurosurgical cases involving the brain or spinal cord. They may first be dipped in *thrombin* to achieve hemostasis when direct pressure or other techniques cannot be used.

Sponge Count

Safeguards to prevent sponge loss in the wound include certain rules regarding the use of sponges. These rules are almost universally accepted and should be followed exactly. Infraction of the rules threatens the patient with postoperative infection or disease that can result if a sponge is left inside the surgical wound.

1. The general rule about whether a sponge count is taken at all is that *if a sponge can be lost within the surgical wound, then the complete procedure for the sponge count is followed.*

2. *Sponge counts are the dual responsibility of the scrub assistant and the registered nurse circulator.* Both parties are legally responsible for a correct sponge count.

3. As sponges are used during a procedure, they are dropped into the kick bucket. During the sponge count, the circulator retrieves the sponges using a sponge clamp or gloves and places them in a plastic bag as they are counted. Counts are done audibly.

4. Sponges are counted before the first incision is made. All sponges distributed to the scrub assistant must be counted before the skin incision and whenever sponges are added to the sterile field. This is called the *first count*, and it serves as the baseline for subsequent counts.

5. Most hospitals supply sponges in precounted sets of 5 or 10. If, during the initial count or any subsequent distribution of sponges when the new package of sponges is counted, the package contains more or fewer sponges than indicated on the label, the *entire* package is passed back to the circulator and removed from the room.

6. During all counts, each sponge is separated from the others and counted individually.

7. Counts must be taken in an orderly fashion and not rushed.

8. If laparotomy sponges have been used to wall off the abdominal viscera, the scrub assistant should keep a mental note of how many sponges have been placed in the abdomen.

9. Once the initial count is taken, the next count occurs before a body cavity such as the peritoneum is closed. If any hollow organ such as the bladder has been incised, a count is taken before its closure. After the peritoneal count and each subsequent count, the circulator informs the surgeon the status of the count (whether it is correct or incorrect).

10. In most hospitals, the next count occurs before the fascia layer of an abdominal incision is closed. In other types of surgery, the next count occurs before the closure of any body plane where a sponge could lodge.

11. The final count is taken before the skin incision is closed.

12. If at any time during the course of an operation, one scrub assistant is replaced by another, such as during a shift change, *all* sponges must be counted before the first person leaves the surgical field and the second one takes over. The replacement scrub assistant should be present during the count to verify that this count is

correct. The patient's operative record must reflect the change in personnel and that the sponge count was signed off by the person leaving the case.

Loss of a Sponge

If at any time during a surgical procedure, a count does not coincide with the number of sponges previously counted, certain procedures are followed. The count is repeated to verify the loss. The circulator and scrub assistant search for the sponge individually. Sponges, especially 4 × 4s, are sometimes caught between the folds of the drapes. If at this time the sponge cannot be located, the surgeon is notified of the loss. He or she may then initiate a more thorough search within and around the surgical wound. If the sponge cannot be found, a radiograph may be taken to locate the missing sponge. *The loss of any sponge, whether or not it is finally located, is cause for an incident report* (see Chapter 2). The consequences of a lost sponge are serious. If a sponge is inadvertently left in the surgical wound, the body will respond as it would to any foreign body. Increased inflammation within the wound site, suppuration, fever, and infection are possible consequences. In a debilitated or older patient, this increased burden following surgery can be very serious.

TOURNIQUET

The use of a pneumatic tourniquet on a limb during orthopedic and neurosurgical cases provides a bloodless field and preserves the patient's blood and fluid balance. *Tourniquets should be applied by licensed personnel only.* The nonsterile tourniquet is composed of an inner bladder covered with an outer layer of synthetic material (Fig. 13–4). The tourniquet is connected to an oxygen source and regulator (Fig. 13–5). Before placing the tourniquet on the thigh or upper arm, several layers of compressed rolled cotton are wrapped around the limb where the tourniquet cuff will be placed. There should be no wrinkles in the skin, cotton wrap, or tourniquet

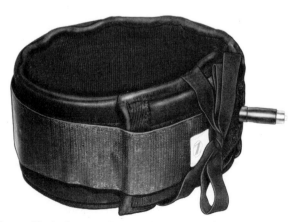

Figure 13–4. Pneumatic tourniquet cuff. (Courtesy of Zimmer, Inc., Warsaw, IN.)

because when the tourniquet is inflated these wrinkles could injure the skin or superficial nerves and blood vessels. Following the skin prep, the surgeon wraps the limb with a sterile roll of sheet rubber called an *Esmarch bandage.* The limb is wrapped tightly beginning at the point on the limb farthest away from the tourniquet and advancing toward the tourniquet in the proximal direction. This maneuver compresses the blood vessels of the limb and pushes most or all of the blood out and away from it. The tourniquet is then inflated and the time noted by the circulator. There is no established safe amount of time that the tourniquet can remain inflated. However, most surgeons believe that 1 to 1½ hours is the maximum duration that they may operate with the tourniquet inflated. This depends on many factors, such as the age and physical condition of the patient, size of the limb, and existing vascular disease. The circulator must inform the surgeon how long the tourniquet has been inflated every 30 minutes. The total duration of time that the tourniquet is inflated is called the *tourniquet time,* and this must be documented in the patient's operative report.

PHARMACEUTICAL HEMOSTATIC AGENTS

Topical thrombin (Thrombostat) is derived from bovine blood components and causes immediate coagulation of small blood vessels. This product is most often used in conjunction with absorbable gelatin sponge. The sponges are dipped in thrombin and then placed over a capillary bed to control oozing.

Absorbable gelatin sponge (Gelfoam) is composed of medical-grade gelatin that has been processed to a dry, spongy, compressible consistency. Gelfoam is manufactured in small thin sheets that can be cut with scissors at the surgical site. The surgeon generally dictates what size patch he or she requires within the wound. These are cut and soaked in topical thrombin by the scrub assistant and placed over the bleeding tissue by the surgeon. Gelfoam is left in the wound, where it is eventually absorbed by the body.

Oxidized cellulose (Oxycel, Hemo-Pak, Surgicel) is cellulose, a vegetable material manufactured in the form of mesh squares. These squares are cut into sections and placed over bleeding capillary beds to control oozing. As the cellulose absorbs blood, it swells and causes clotting at the site. It may be left in the body in most areas except near the spinal cord, optic nerve, and associated structures. Oxidized cellulose becomes tacky when it contacts a wet surface. Therefore, in preparing this product, the scrub assistant should handle it with dry, smooth tissue forceps.

Microfibrillar collagen hemostat (MCH, Avitene) is derived from bovine collagen and is applied in its dry form to the bleeding site, where it is eventually absorbed by the body. It is supplied as a dry powder. When applied to bleeding tissue it causes coagulation. This product is sensitive to moisture and must be handled with dry tissue forceps.

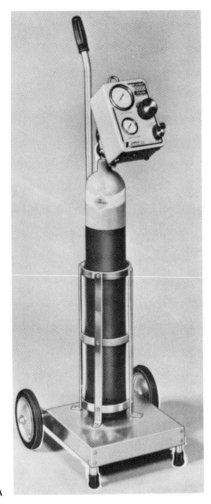

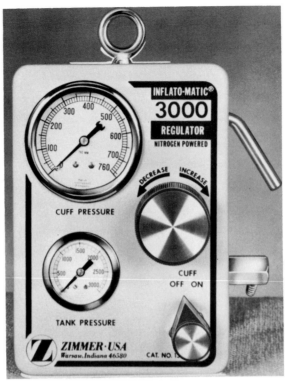

B

A

Figure 13–5. *A.* Oxygen tank and regulator for inflation of pneumatic tourniquet and cuff. *B.* Close-up of regulator. Note that both tank and cuff pressure are regulated. (Courtesy of Zimmer, Inc., Warsaw, IN.)

Bone wax is processed beeswax that is used topically on bone to control oozing from its surface. It is packaged as a thin bar that the scrub technologist must separate into small wads, which are then placed on the edge of a small basin, cup, or flat instrument and offered to the surgeon for use.

LIGATION CLIPS

Ligation clips are tiny V-shaped clips made of stainless steel, titanium, platinum, or absorbable material. These clips are commercially supplied by several companies and are applied across a bleeding vessel and crimped in place. Ligation clips have taken the place of suture ligatures in deep surgery when access is very difficult. The clips are loaded in a long clamp especially designed for this use. Disposable and nondisposable systems are available. A complete discussion of surgical clips is provided in Chapter 12.

HEMOSTATIC CLAMPS

The hemostatic clamp is the most common hemostatic aid used in surgery. Clamps are available in a wide variety of shapes, jaw pressures, sizes, and materials. A complete display of hemostatic clamps is presented in Chapter 15.

SUTURE LIGATURES

Modern suture materials offer the surgeon a wide choice of type, size, and strength. Ligatures are an efficient method for controlling bleeding during surgery. Suture ligatures are discussed in detail in Chapter 12.

HYPOTHERMIA

Intentional hypothermia is the intentional cooling of the patient's body during surgery by internal and external means. This lowers the body's metabolism, and the need for oxygen is decreased; hence the blood flow is slowed. External cooling is achieved by placing the patient on a hypothermia blanket (Fig. 13–6), which is connected to a control unit, or by packing the body with ice. Internal cooling is accomplished by the heat-exchange mechanism of the heart-lung machine. Irrigation of the body with cold fluids also accomplishes hypothermia. When hypothermia is used as a method of hemo-

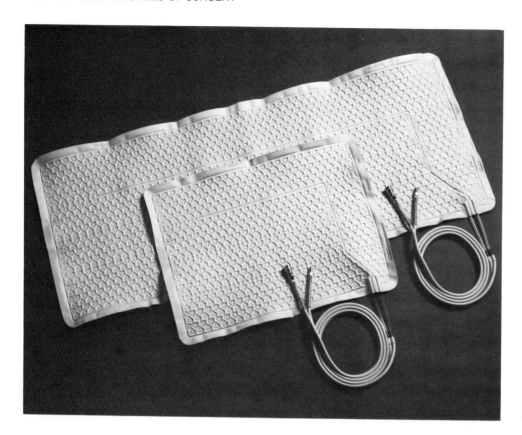

Figure 13–6. Hypothermia blankets. (Courtesy of Cincinnati Sub-Zero Products, Inc., Cincinnati, OH.)

stasis, the patient must be carefully monitored for signs of injury caused by the use of a thermal blanket, such as metabolic acidosis, impaired renal and hepatic functions, cardiac arrhythmia, and other physiologic imbalances. Because of the extreme risks associated with the use of the thermal blanket, only licensed personnel should supervise its use.

HYPOTENSION

Intentional hypotension is the intentional lowering of the patient's blood pressure during surgery to maintain hemostasis. This physiologic state is maintained by the anesthesiologist. There are certain risks associated with induced hypotension, including anuria (absence of urine formation) and coronary thrombosis.

AUTOTRANSFUSION

Autotransfusion or autologous blood transfusion is a procedure by which the patient receives a transfusion of his or her own blood. This procedure has become common in the past decade because of the fear of transmission of acquired immunodeficiency syndrome through untested blood, although only blood from donors known to be negative for the human immunodeficiency virus is routinely transfused. However, increased interest in autotransfusion has caused the development of important autotransfusion equipment that is now commonly used in the operating room. There are four methods of autotransfusion:

1. *Transfusion of the patient's blood* that has been previously donated before surgery and is stored in anticipation of the scheduled procedure can be done. This prevents the need for blood donated by another person.

2. *Hemoconcentration* is dilution of the patient's own blood and is used in open-heart surgery. The blood is diluted preoperatively with special solutions called crystalloids or colloids, which expand the total volume to accommodate the heart-lung bypass circuit. After the procedure, the patient's blood is processed to return it to normal concentration.

3. *Postoperative blood salvage* is a process by which blood is harvested from the surgical wound after its closure. A drainage tube is inserted into the wound and connected to a cell washer apparatus. The blood is then anticoagulated, and the apparatus is transferred with the patient to the post-anesthesia care unit or intensive care unit where the drainage tube is connected to the wall suction outlet. After collection, the blood is transfused to the patient in the normal manner.

4. *Intraoperative blood salvage* is a process that includes collection, concentration, and washing of blood that is lost during surgery. The blood salvage equipment used in this process is a combination centrifuge and cell washer. One type of apparatus used for this purpose is the Cell Saver 4, which is manufactured by the Haemonetics Corporation (Braintree, MA) (Fig. 13–7). During surgery, blood and tissue debris are aspirated

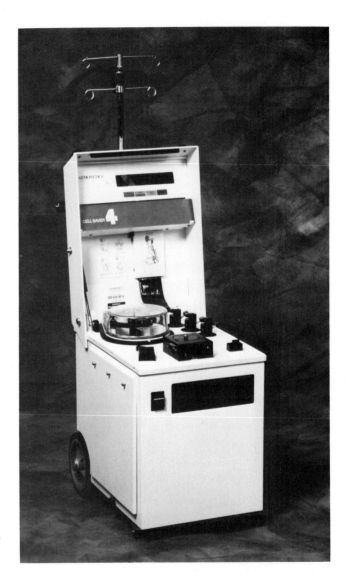

Figure 13–7. Cell Saver 4 Blood Recovery System. (Courtesy of Haemonetics Corporation, Braintree, MA.)

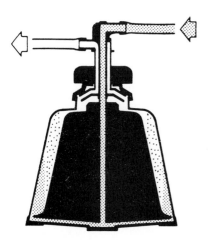

1. BLOOD IS PUMPED IN. SEPARATION BEGINS.

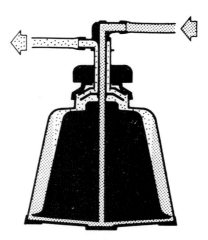

2. THE SUPERNATANT WASTES OVER-FLOW. RBCs STAY IN THE BOWL.

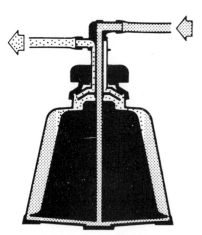

3. AS OVERFLOW CONTINUES, THE HEMATOCRIT IN THE BOWL INCREASES TO 50%-60%.

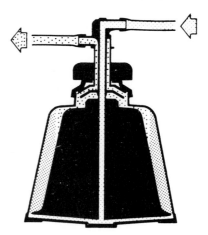

4. NORMAL SALINE CIRCULATES THROUGH THE RED CELL LAYER AND DISPLACES THE WASTE PLASMA.

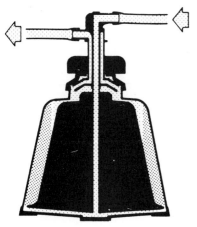

5. THE OVERFLOW RUNS CLEAR. FREE HEMOGLOBIN AND ANTICOAGULANT ARE IN THE WASTE BAG.

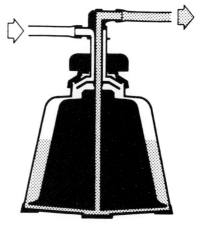

6. THE BOWL STOPS. WASHED, PACKED RBCs ARE PUMPED TO THE REINFUSION BAG.

Figure 13–8. Schematic illustration of blood salvaging process using the Cell Saver 4 Blood Recovery System. (Courtesy of Haemonetics Corporation, Braintree, MA.)

from the surgical wound in the normal fashion using a special aspiration and anticoagulation assembly that is attached to a suction tip. The blood mixture is then pumped into a reservoir bowl and filtered. The supernatant wastes (unwanted tissue and fluid debris) overflow from the reservoir, and the red blood cells remain in the bowl, raising the hematocrit in the reservoir to around 50%. The red blood cells are then washed with normal saline solution, and this removes any unwanted cell or plasma components that remain in the bowl. The centrifuge then removes any plasma, white blood cells, and platelets or other components from the mixture, leaving approximately 50% of the red blood cells originally salvaged. The remaining red blood cell–saline mixture is pumped into a blood bag and can be transfused in the normal fashion. A schematic illustration of the entire process is shown in Figure 13–8.

Questions for Study and Review

1. What does *hemostasis* mean?
2. What are the components used during monopolar electrosurgery?
3. Why are "automatic" active electrodes dangerous?
4. What is "grounding"?
5. Discuss *all* the precautions necessary when applying a patient grounding pad.
6. Why is it important for the grounding pad to have a uniform, thick coating of conductive gel?
7. Why should the power settings on the electrosurgical power unit be off when the grounding cable is attached to it?
8. What is the name given to dissecting sponges used in your clinical rotation?
9. What are "laparotomy rings"?
10. When is a sponge count necessary?
11. Who may take a sponge count?
12. How many sponge counts are necessary during a laparotomy?
13. Why is the sponge count so important?
14. Under what circumstances is a sponge count omitted?
15. Discuss the *form* of the following hemostatics:
    a. Thrombostat
    b. Gelfoam
    c. Oxycel or Surgical
    d. Avitene
16. What is *hypothermia*?
17. What is *hypotension*?
18. What is *autotransfusion*?
19. Name four methods of autotransfusion.

Bibliography

Flynn JC: Perioperative Autotransfusion: Avoiding donated risks. Todays OR Nurse 12:7, 1990.

Groah L: Operating Room Nursing: Perioperative Practice, 2nd ed. Norwalk, CT, Appleton & Lange, 1991.

Haemonetics Corporation: Cell Saver 4 Autologous Blood Recovery System, Owner's Operating and Maintenance Manual. Braintree, MA, Haemonetics Corporation, 1986.

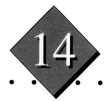

Surgical Pharmacology

Learning Objectives

After reading this chapter, you should be able to

♦ *Convert* from the metric to the apothecaries' systems, and vice versa.
♦ *Perform* basic arithmetical calculations.
♦ *Receive* medications from the registered nurse properly.
♦ *Discuss* the basic types of medications commonly used in surgery.
♦ *List* the names of some medications commonly used in surgery.

Key Terms

antibiotic: A drug that inhibits the growth of, or kills, microorganisms in living tissue.
anticoagulant: A drug that prolongs blood clotting time.
contrast medium: A radiopaque dye (not penetrated by x rays) that is introduced into body cavities to outline their inside surfaces.
corticosteroid: One of a group of complex drugs that have many beneficial uses. In surgery these drugs are used to reduce inflammation.
diuretic: A drug that draws fluid away from tissue.
dye: Any agent that stains tissues.
hemostatic agent: A drug that promotes blood coagulation.
oxytocic: A drug that causes uterine contractions.

WEIGHTS AND MEASURES

Although the surgical technologist does not administer medications to the patient, he or she is occasionally called on to mix solutions such as antiseptics, disinfectants, and contrast media. In other instances the registered nurse circulator may distribute several types of medicines to the technologist, who is then required to mix them in the proper proportions. One example would

be when certain antibiotics are distributed for use as irrigants within the wound. When the technologist receives any medication from the nurse, he or she should be able to identify the drug and to determine the exact amount received. This may require conversion from one system of measurement to another. Because of this, every technologist should be able to perform simple arithmetic calculations and conversions.

In pharmacology the metric system is the most com-

148

Table 14–1. EQUIVALENT WEIGHT AND MEASURES

Apothecaries' Table of Weights

Apothecaries'		Approximate Metric Equivalent	
60 grains	= 1 dram (dr. ʒ)	60 to 65 milligrams (mg)	= 1 grain
8 drams	= 1 ounce (oz. ℥)	4 grams	= 1 dram
12 ounces	= 1 pound (lb)*	30 to 32 grams	= 1 ounce
		370 to 375 grams	= 1 pound
		0.37 to 0.375 kilograms	= 1 pound

Metric System of Weights

Metric		Approximate Apothecaries' Equivalent
1000 micrograms (μg)	= 1 milligram (mg)	gr. 1/60 = 1 mg
1000 milligrams	= 1 gram (g)	gr. 15–16 = 1 g
1000 grams	= 1 kilogram (kg)	2.2 lb. (avoir.) = 1 kg

Apothecaries' Table of Volume

Apothecaries'		Approximate Metric Equivalent
1 minim (m)		= 0.06 mL
60 minims	= 1 fluid dram (fdr)	4 mL = 1 fdr (fl dr)
8 fluid drams	= 1 fluid ounce (foz)	30 mL = 1 foz (fl oz)
16 fluid ounces	= 1 pint (pt. or O)	500 mL = 1 pint
		or 0.5 L
2 pints	= 1 quart (qt)	1000 mL = 1 quart
		or 1 L
4 quarts	= 1 gallon (gal or C)	4000 mL = 1 gallon
		or 4 L

Metric Table of Volume

Metric		Approximate Apothecaries' Equivalent
1000 milliliters (mL)†	= 1 liter (L)	15 minims = 1 mL
1000 liters	= 1 kiloliter (kL)	1 quart = 1 liter or 1000 mL

*Note that in the avoirdupois table there are 16 ounces in 1 lb. in the Troy table there are 12 ounces in 1 lb as with the apothecaries' system.

†One cubic centimeter (cc) is often used in place of 1 milliliter (mL). A milliliter of water occupies approximately 1 cc of space.

From Sheridan E, et al: Falconer's The Drug, The Nurse, The Patient, 7th ed. Philadelphia, WB Saunders, 1984.

monly used system of measurement, but the apothecaries', or English, system is also used. The liter (L) measures volume, the gram (g) measures mass, and the meter (m) measures length. The metric system employs multiple units of 10. The following prefixes are used to denote amounts:

milli means one thousandth; 1 milliliter = 1/1000 liter
centi means one hundredth; 1 centimeter = 1/100 meter.
kilo means one thousand; 1 kilogram = 1000 grams.

The cubic centimeter (cc) is often used to measure liquid amounts. One cubic centimeter is equal to 1 milliliter (mL). Table 14–1 lists approximate equivalents between the two systems of measurement.

REVIEW OF ARITHMETIC

Fractions

A *fraction* defines a number by specifying the *division* necessary to create that number. For example, the fraction ¾ is the number that results by dividing the top number (the numerator), 3, by the bottom number (the denominator), 4. When the numerator is smaller than the denominator, the number is less than 1; if the numerator is larger than the denominator, the number is greater than 1. When the numerator and denominator are the same, the number is 1.

Addition and Subtraction

To add or subtract two fractions, they must have the same denominator. Thus, to compute 1/3 + 1/3 simply add the numerators; the answer is 2/3. To add or subtract fractions that have *different* denominators requires an extra step and the understanding of the concept of *equivalent fractions*. If both the numerator and denominator of a fraction are multiplied (or divided) by the same number, the resulting fraction is equal to the original one. Thus, if both the numerator and denominator of the fraction 1/3 are multiplied by 2, the resulting fraction is 2/6. The fraction 2/6 is exactly equal to the fraction 1/3. Therefore, to add or subtract fractions of different denominators, all that is necessary is to choose an equivalent fraction of each that has the same denominator. The denominator selected should be the *lowest common denominator* (LCD), that is, the lowest number that can be divided by the two denominators you need to add or subtract.

Examples

Addition

$$\frac{1}{2} + \frac{1}{3} \ (\text{LCD} = 6)$$

$$\frac{(1 \times 3)}{(2 \times 3)} = \frac{3}{6} ; \frac{(1 \times 2)}{(3 \times 2)} = \frac{2}{6}$$

$$\frac{3}{6} + \frac{2}{6} = \frac{5}{6}$$

$$\frac{3}{4} + \frac{1}{5} \ (LCD = 20)$$

$$\frac{3}{4} \times 5 = \frac{15}{20} ; \frac{1}{5} \times 4 = \frac{4}{20}$$

$$\frac{15}{20} + \frac{4}{20} = \frac{19}{20}$$

Subtraction

$$\frac{7}{8} - \frac{3}{16} \ (LCD = 16)$$

$$\frac{(7 \times 2)}{(8 \times 2)} = \frac{14}{16} ; \frac{(3 \times 1)}{(16 \times 1)} = \frac{3}{16}$$

$$\frac{14}{16} - \frac{3}{16} = \frac{11}{16}$$

$$\frac{4}{7} - \frac{1}{9} \ (LCD = 63)$$

$$\frac{(4 \times 9)}{(7 \times 9)} = \frac{36}{63} ; \frac{(1 \times 7)}{(9 \times 7)} = \frac{7}{63}$$

$$\frac{36}{63} - \frac{7}{63} = \frac{29}{63}$$

Multiplication and Division

To multiply, simply multiply the numerators of the two fractions, and then multiply the denominators. Thus,

$$\frac{2}{3} \times \frac{5}{8} = \frac{2 \times 5}{3 \times 8} = \frac{10}{24}$$

Any fraction may be *reduced* (simplified) by dividing both the numerator and denominator by the same number.

$$\frac{10}{24} \div 2 = \frac{(10 \div 2)}{(24 \div 2)} = \frac{5}{12}$$

The members 5 and 12 cannot be divided evenly by any number, so ⁵⁄₁₂ is a fully reduced fraction.

To divide fractions, first write the division as a big fraction. Thus,

$$\frac{2}{3} \div \frac{5}{6} = \frac{\frac{2}{3}}{\frac{5}{6}}$$

Then multiply both the top and bottom by the denominator of the lower fraction.

Thus,

$$\frac{\frac{2}{3}}{\frac{5}{6}} = \frac{\frac{2}{3} \times 6}{\frac{5}{6} \times 6} = \frac{\frac{12}{3}}{\frac{30}{6}} = \frac{4}{5}$$

Another method is to invert the divisor and multiply. For example,

$$\frac{2}{3} \div \frac{5}{6} = \frac{2}{3} \times \frac{6}{5} = \frac{12}{15} = \frac{4}{5}$$

Examples

Multiplication

$$\frac{1}{13} \times \frac{2}{3} = \frac{1 \times 2}{13 \times 3} = \frac{2}{39}$$

$$\frac{3}{7} \times \frac{4}{5} = \frac{3 \times 4}{7 \times 5} = \frac{12}{35}$$

Division

$$\frac{1}{3} \div \frac{5}{8} = \frac{1}{3} \times \frac{8}{5} = \frac{8}{15}$$

$$\frac{1}{4} \div \frac{1}{16} = \frac{1}{4} \times \frac{16}{1} = \frac{16}{4} = 4$$

Decimals

The number system we use is the decimal system, which is based on powers (multiples) of 10. Each position to the left or right of the decimal point is a higher or lower power of 10.

Fraction to Decimal Conversion

To convert from a fraction, such as ⅘, to a decimal, just divide the numerator by the denominator (4 ÷ 5 = 0.8). Some fractions do not result in simple decimal numbers. For example, ⅓ is .33333 . . . , and so on forever. For most purposes it is sufficient to round off after three figures. To round off, raise the last digit by 1 if it is 5 or more. Thus, .333333 . . . is .333 but .66666 . . . is .667.

Percentages

A percentage is a fraction expressed as parts of 100. To convert a fraction to a percentage, convert to a decimal and multiply by 100. Thus,

$$\frac{4}{5} = 0.8 \times 100 = 80\%$$

Ratio

A ratio is similar to a fraction. A ratio of 1 to 2 (written 1:2) means that there is 1 unit for every 2 units out of each 3 units (1 + 2) of whatever is being described. To convert a ratio to a fraction, add both terms to make the denominator, and use the first term as the numerator. In the above example,

$$1:2 = \frac{1}{3}$$

Proportions

A proportion is an expression of equality between two fractions. For example, it can be written 1:3 = 2.6. This is the same as ¼ = ⅜. The most common use of proportions is for dilutions. Dilution is usually expressed as a percentage—for example, a 1% solution. A common problem is how much of a chemical to add to a given quantity of liquid. The unknown amount is written as x. For example, to make a 1% solution using 500 mL of water, how much chemical is needed? Written as a proportion, it is

$$\frac{x}{500} \text{ mL} = \frac{1}{100}$$

To solve, multiply the numerator of the first term (x) by the denominator of the second (100) and vice versa (500 × 1). In this case $100\,x = 500$ mL × 1. Multiplying a number times 1 gives the same number, so $100\,x = 500$ mL. To solve for x, divide both sides by 100. Thus,

$$x = \frac{500}{100} \text{ or } 5 \text{ mL}$$

Adding 5 mL of the chemical will produce 505 mL of a 1% solution.

Sample Problems

1. To prepare 30 cc of 50% Hypaque solution, how much 100% Hypaque and how much sterile saline solution are required?
2. To prepare a 1-liter solution of alcohol in water in a ratio of 1:70, how much alcohol is required?
3. To prepare a single solution in which the ratio of bacitracin to neomycin is 1:3 and the ratio of the bacitracin/neomycin mixture to sterile saline solution is 1:1, how much bacitracin, neomycin, and sterile saline solution do you need to make a total of 100 cc of solution?
4. To prepare 30 cc of 0.5% Xylocaine, how much sterile saline solution and how much 1% Xylocaine are required?
5. To prepare a 100-cc solution of Hypaque 1:3, how much 50% Hypaque solution and how much sterile solution should you use?

ACCEPTING MEDICATIONS IN SURGERY

The following rules apply to the surgical technologist, but the general principles should apply in a wide variety of situations, since precise administration of medicines is crucial. Only a registered nurse or physician can legally distribute medications to a surgical technologist, and there is a prescribed manner in which this is done. Because the technologist acts as the intermediate distributor between the nurse and patient, the interaction between the nurse and technologist is very important. The nurse must distribute the drug in a manner that allows the technologist to see the name and understand the amount of drug being received. Once the drug has left the nurse's hands and is distributed to the technologist, it is his or her full responsibility to pass the right medication in the amount specified by the surgeon onto the field of surgery.

Liquid medications are received onto the sterile instrument table in a small cup (commonly called a "medicine glass"). The medication may be poured directly from its vial into these containers, or it may be drawn up into a syringe by the nurse and injected into the sterile container. In both instances, the procedure for accepting medications is the same.

Procedure

1. The technologist makes a medicine glass available to receive the medication.
2. The nurse *shows* the vial to the technologist so that he or she can read both the *name, amount* and, where applicable, the *percentage* (strength) of the drug.
3. The technologist recites *aloud* to the nurse the information described in step 2. For example, "1% Xylocaine, with epinephrine, one to two hundred thousandths, 50 cc."
4. The nurse distributes the drug to the technologist.
5. The nurse shows the vial to the technologist a *second time*. The technologist notes mentally the name and amount of the drug he or she has just received.

In summary, the technologist sees, recites, accepts, and sees again the type and amount of medication received. This routine for accepting medication is sometimes dangerously ignored when a commonly used medication is distributed (e.g., a local anesthetic). The nurse and technologist must not allow supposed familiarity with bottle size and label color to interfere with the proper acceptance of medication. Poor technique and disregard for accepted procedure may cause injury to the patient.

Precautions in Handling Medications

1. Always use accepted procedures when receiving any drug.
2. Never accept a medication from a vial that is cracked or chipped. This might indicate the presence of bacteria or glass chips in the solution.
3. Mark solutions on the instrument table with some kind of marker, such as a particular kind of clamp. Some hospitals use floating glass markers that are imprinted with the names of commonly used solutions. If these are in use, make certain that they are not inadvertently poured into the surgical wound with the irrigation solution in which they lie. There have been cases in which the surgeon, on preparing to close the wound, has found a marker stamped "normal saline" lying inside the wound.
4. Keep a mental note of how much irrigation solution is used within the wound so that blood loss can be accurately determined.

5. Never accept a medication that appears discolored or is otherwise suspicious.

6. If you are uncertain (have forgotten) which basins contain which medications or solutions on the instrument table, *discard* them all and request that new solutions be distributed.

7. Do not accept a medication whose vial or bottle you have not read. Occasionally, in a very rushed procedure, a nurse may distribute a medication onto the instrument table without the scrub person's knowledge and may then inform the scrub person that such and such a drug is in this or that basin. (Or, perhaps, the technologist may be unwilling to turn his or her attention to the nurse.) *This is unacceptable technique.* It is the *dual* responsibility of the circulator and the scrub technologist or nurse to make certain that the correct drug, correct amount, and correct strength are distributed. Likewise, during a *change* or *shift* when one scrub person replaces another at the field, new solutions and medications should be distributed.

8. Many drugs become "outdated" with time, and their composition and effect may be altered. All medications stored in the surgery pharmacy must be periodically checked for "outdates"; these are then discarded or returned to the hospital pharmacy.

MEDICATIONS USED IN SURGERY

Medications used in surgery include those that are injectable, those used topically (on the surface of tissue), irrigating solutions such as antibiotics used to "rinse" the wound, and those introduced into hollow organs or ducts for diagnostic purposes. Also included are those solutions used as blood replacements, blood expanders, and those that keep a continuous intravenous drip patent (open). Table 14–2 lists types and specific names of drugs and their uses.

Specialty medications such as those used in ophthalmic or cardiac surgery are discussed in the chapters with which they are associated.

Anticoagulants

An anticoagulant is a drug that prolongs blood clotting time. In surgery, anticoagulants are used during cardiovascular procedures. When used as irrigating solutions in the wound, they prevent clots from forming around vessels that are the focus of the operation. During surgery they are given intravenously to prevent thrombosis (an obstructing blood clot within the circulatory system). Heparin sodium is most commonly used for this purpose.

Hemostatics

A hemostatic is an agent that promotes blood coagulation. In surgery such agents are used to control bleeding in instances where the usual routine for achieving hemostasis (e.g., clamping, ligating) is impossible or impractical. For example, bleeding arising from tissue that tends to ooze, such as the liver or spleen, can be controlled with the application of a topical hemostatic. Topical hemostatics are available as liquids, powders, or various solids, which differ in composition and form (see Table 14–2).

Oxytocics

An oxytocic is a drug that acts on the uterus to cause its contraction and constriction. In surgery, an oxytocic is given following cesarean section and therapeutic abortion. Given intravenously, these agents cause rhythmic uterine contractions that expel any blood clots or remnants of the placenta that, if left in the uterus, might cause postoperative hemorrhage. In obstetrics, oxytocics are given to induce labor. A commonly used oxytocic is oxytocin (Pitocin).

Corticosteroids

The corticosteroids are a broad group of medications that have many uses, both surgical and nonsurgical. Corticosteroids reduce tissue inflammation. When used during surgery, they help reduce inflammatory reactions in certain tissues that cannot bear the trauma of surgery. For example, in ophthalmic procedures corticosteroids are applied topically to reduce postoperative swelling. In plastic surgery for patients who tend to form keloids (excessive scar tissue), corticosteroids are injected into and around the incision. Two corticosteroids commonly used in surgery are dexamethasone sodium phosphate (Decadron) and polymyxin B–bacitracin–neomycin–hydrocortisone (Cortisporin).

Antibiotics

Antibiotics are medications that either kill or inhibit the growth of microorganisms in the body. They are available in injectable, topical, or oral forms. There are many different types of antibiotics that act on specific organisms. Some are effective for a large range of microorganisms and are termed *broad-spectrum* antibiotics. Others may be specific for only a few types of pathogens and are called *narrow-spectrum* antibiotics. Used during surgery, antibiotics arrest active infection or, in some cases, when used prophylactically, prevent the onset of infection. During the surgical procedure, the surgeon may request that an antibiotic be given intravenously or that the surgical wound be irrigated with antibiotic solution. When suturing of the skin is complete, antibiotic ointments are sometimes applied to the suture line. Antibiotic-impregnated gauze is sometimes used to pack certain body cavities, such as the nose. Names and actions of antibiotics used frequently during surgery are listed in Table 14–2.

Table 14–2. COMMON SURGICAL MEDICATIONS

Generic Name (Trade Names)	Uses	Action
Anticoagulants		
Bishydroxycoumarin (Dicumarol, Dicoumarin) Phenprocoumon (Liquamar)	Prolong the clotting time of blood; treatment of thrombophlebitis, pulmonary embolism, certain cardiac conditions, or any disorder in which there is excessive or undesirable clotting	Prevent the production of prothrombin in the liver. They are often given with heparin to secure both immediate and delayed action.
Warfarin sodium (Coumadin) Heparin sodium (Hepathrom, Lipo-Hepin, Liquaemin)	Prolong the clotting time of blood; treatment of thrombophlebitis and pulmonary embolism; used as an irrigant in cardiovascular surgery to prevent the formation of clots within the wound	Not fully understood, but believed to inhibit conversion of prothrombin to thrombin. It does not dissolve the clots but does prevent the extension of old clots and the formation of new ones.
Coagulants (Hemostatics)		
Absorbable gelatin sponge (Gelfoam)	Local hemostatic agent	Gives a good surface for and aids in clot formation
Oxidized cellulose (Oxycel)	Local hemostatic agent	As above
Microfibrillar collagen hemostat (Avitene)	Adjunct to hemostasis when control of bleeding by ligature or conventional procedures is ineffective or impractical	Absorbable topical hemostatic agent of purified bovine collagen; must be applied directly to the source of bleeding in its *dry state*
Protamine sulfate	Counteracts the effects of heparin	Protamine by itself is an anticoagulant and will cause an increase in clotting time. When mixed with heparin the drugs are attracted to each other and form a stable salt that counteracts the effects of heparin.
Thrombin	Topical hemostatic agent, usually used in combination with an absorbable gelatin sponge (Gelfoam)	Induces clotting on bleeding surfaces where conventional methods of hemostasis are contraindicated, such as on friable or delicate tissue
Oxytocics		
Oxytocic injection (Pitocin, Syntocinon)	Drug of choice to induce and maintain labor; given postpartum to prevent or control hemorrhage	Acts only on the uterus
Sparteine sulfate (Tocosamine)	Induces labor; treatment of uterine inertia	Acts only on the uterus
Corticosteroids		
Betamethasone (Celestone)	Treatment of many inflammatory diseases and conditions	Most of the cortisones are used for their anti-inflammatory properties, both systemic and local.
Betamethasone sodium phosphate (Celestone phosphate)	As above	As above
Dexamethasone (Decadron, Dexameth, Hexadrol)	As above	As above
Antibiotics		
Potassium penicillin G (Cryspen 400, K-Pen)	Treatment of infections caused by α-hemolytic and β-hemolytic streptococci, pneumococci, gonococci, meningococci, and various strains of staphylococci	Bacteriostatic and bactericidal; blocks the synthesis of the bacterial wall and is therefore most effective on cells in their rapid growth phase
Cefazolin sodium (Ancet, Kefzol)	Treatment of respiratory, genitourinary, skin, soft tissue, bone, and blood infections caused by various organisms	As above
Polymyxin B sulfate (Aerosporin)	Effective mainly against gram-negative organisms	Bacteriostatic and bactericidal
Bacitracin	Effective against gram-positive organisms, *Neisseria,* and some spirochetes	Bacteriostatic and bactericidal
Cephalothin sodium (Keflin)	Treatment of respiratory, genitourinary, skin, soft tissue, bone, and blood infections caused by many gram-positive and gram-negative organisms	Blocks cell wall synthesis
Cephapirin sodium (Cefadyl)	Same as cefazolin	Same as cefazolin
Streptomycin sulfate (Streptoduocin)	Most effective against gram-negative organisms	Effective against gram-negative organisms
Gentamicin C sulfate (Garamycin)	Treatment of various bacterial diseases, infections of the eye, and infections of the central nervous system, urinary tract, respiratory tract, and gastrointestinal tract	Bactericidal
Kanamycin A sulfate (Kantrex)	Treatment of tuberculosis and other infections	Bactericidal
Neomycin (Mycifradin)	For preoperative intestinal disinfection and treatment of infections that do not respond to less toxic drugs	
Chloramphenicol (Chloromycetin)	Effective against many organisms, especially gram-negative ones	Bacteriostatic and bactericidal

Table continued on following page

Table 14–2. COMMON SURGICAL MEDICATIONS *Continued*

Generic Name (Trade Names)	Uses	Action
Contrast Media		
Meglumine diatrizoate (Cardiografin)	Radiography of the heart and major blood vessels	When injected, shows as white on radiograph
Iodipamide (Cholografin)	Radiography of the biliary system	As above
Diatrizoate meglumine (Cystografin)	Radiography of the urinary tract	As above
Diatrizoate sodium (Hypaque sodium, Renografin)	Radiography of the biliary tract, kidney, and other internal structures	As above
Dyes		
Methylrosaniline chloride (gentian, aniline, or crystal violet)	Used in colored "marking pens" to draw incisional lines; also has fungicidal effects when used as a topical solution or ointment	Stains the skin
Methylene blue (Hexalol, Urised)	Stains the skin for marking purposes and also for urinary diagnostic procedures.	Turns the skin blue when used topically and turns the urine a greenish color when used systemically
Diuretics		
Mannitol	Helps to measure glomerular filtration and to draw tissue fluids into the urinary system	Mannitol is neither absorbed nor secreted by the kidney tubule. Thus the amount excreted gives an accurate estimation of glomerular filtration.
Analgesics		
Opium (composed of morphine, codeine, papavarine, and thebaine)	Relieves mild to moderate pain	Produces mood elevation, euphoria, and relief of fear and apprehension; gastrointestinal motility is decreased.
"Concentrated opium" (Pantopon)	As above	As above
Morphine sulfate	Relieves moderate to severe pain	As above
Fentanyl citrate (Sublimaze)	Narcotic analgesic	Causes analgesia and sedation
Meperidine hydrochloride (Demerol, Dolosal)	Widely used as an analgesic for moderate to severe pain	Produces analgesia and sedation but does not cause constipation or pupillary constriction, as does morphine; may produce temporary euphoria
Pentazocine (Talwin)	Supposedly nonaddicting narcotic-type analgesic for use in moderate to severe pain	Produces analgesia, which usually occurs within 15 to 20 minutes after injection
Propoxyphene (Darvon, Dolene)	Nonnarcotic analgesic used to relieve all mild to moderate pain	Similar to codeine; has little effect on the gastrointestinal tract
Emergency Drugs		
Aminophylline (Aminocardol, Ammophyllin, Cardophyllin)	Indicated for relief of bronchial asthma, pulmonary emphysema, and acute pulmonary edema	Relaxes smooth muscle, notably bronchial muscle, stimulates the central nervous system, and stimulates cardiac muscle to increase output
Doxapram hydrochloride (Dopram)	Increases depth and rate of respiration in such conditions as asphyxia post anesthesia	Direct stimulant to the respiratory center in the medulla
Digitoxin	Mainly indicated to treat cardiac decompensation and to control the ventricular rate with atrial fibrillation	Stimulates the vagus nerve, thus increasing the strength of the heartbeat while decreasing its rate; reduces high blood pressure
Metaraminol (Aramine)	Mainly indicated for postsurgical or other pathologically induced hypotension	Has a powerful and prolonged vasopressor action
Epinephrine (Adrenalin, Epifrin)	Treatment of shock and cardiac and respiratory failure	Raises the blood pressure; increases the force of heartbeat
Norepinephrine bitartrate (Levophed)	Acute hypotension	A potent vasoconstrictor that raises blood pressure markedly with increased cardiac output
Lidocaine (Xylocaine)	Treatment of cardiac arrhythmias; used intravenously	Exerts antiarrhythmic effect by increasing the electrical stimulation threshold of the ventricles during diastole
Atropine methylnitrate (Harvatrate)	Increases heart and respiratory rates	Acts as an antagonist to the effects of acetylcholine at the peripheral neuroeffector sites
Sodium bicarbonate	Treatment of metabolic acidosis, especially during cardiac arrest; used intravenously	Raises pH of blood
Blood Substitutes		
Dextran (Gentran)	Substitute for blood plasma; especially valuable in the control of shock resulting from hemorrhage	These preparations maintain blood volume until nature can replenish it or plasma can be secured.

Table 14–2. COMMON SURGICAL MEDICATIONS *Continued*

Generic Name (Trade Names)	Uses	Action
Albumin, normal human serum	Generally used the same as for whole blood	These contain all blood factors except cells; thus, they do not produce any additional oxygen-carrying ability.
Plasma protein fraction (Plasmanate)	Combats hypoproteinemia	Maintains blood volume; enhances coagulation
Saline Solutions		
Sodium chloride solution, 0.9% (normal saline solution)	Restores blood volume in hemorrhage and blood pressure in shock; compensates for fluid loss from burns, dehydration, and many similar conditions. Also used as a means of giving needed intravenous medications	Electrolyte solutions are given to maintain balance. The type used depends on the needs of the patient.
Lactated Ringer's solution	As above	As above
Potassium chloride in dextrose	As above	As above
Dextrose solution	Same as for saline solutions but with added nutrients	Dextrose is prepared in isotonic sodium chloride and also in distilled water for use as patient's condition indicates to provide an easily metabolized source of calories.
Blood		
Citrated whole human blood	Replaces blood; also used in the treatment of shock, burns, and certain diseases	If blood is compatible, action is the same as that of patient's blood.
Packed human blood cells	As above	As above

Data from Sheridan E, et al: Falconer's The Drug, The Nurse, The Patient, 7th ed. Philadelphia, WB Saunders, 1984.

Contrast Media

A contrast medium is a radiopaque dye that is injected into an organ, vessel, or duct to identify its inner form. In cardiovascular surgery, contrast media are injected into the bloodstream and radiographs are taken so that strictures or obstructions can be viewed. In biliary surgery, operative cholangiography (injection of contrast media into the bile ducts) can determine the presence of stones, which appear as dark spots against the white background of the contrast medium. Likewise, strictures of the bile ducts can be discovered. When ingested, contrast media are used to determine the shape and structure of the inner surfaces of the gastrointestinal system. The presence of diverticuli, strictures, or tumors are then determined on radiographs.

Diuretics

A diuretic is a drug that draws fluid away from tissue and releases it into the urinary system. This type of drug is given frequently during neurosurgical procedures involving the brain to prevent postoperative and intraoperative swelling of the brain tissues. Mannitol is a frequently used diuretic.

Dyes

Colored dyes are solutions that stain tissue. Before plastic surgery, marking pens that contain dye are used to mark the skin. Lines made with the pen indicate where incisions will be made. In urologic procedures, colored dyes are used for diagnostic purposes. After injection into the bloodstream, the dye is excreted with the urine. The path of the urine can then be directly visualized during procedures involving the ureters and bladder. Two commonly used dyes are methylene blue and indigo carmine.

Central Nervous System Agents

Central nervous system agents are those that affect the body's response to stimuli, coordination of activity, and level of consciousness. This category includes stimulants, depressants, anticonvulsants, and anesthetics. Surgical use of these agents is chiefly limited to anesthetics (discussed in Chapter 9) and depressants (analgesics). Analgesics vary according to their strength and action. They are normally used in the postoperative period to relieve pain. Specific analgesics and their actions are listed in Table 14–2.

Emergency Drugs

Emergency drugs are a part of every operating room pharmacy. An emergency in surgery involves any life-threatening change in the physical status of the patient. Among the most common emergencies are cardiopulmonary arrest, shock, and anaphylaxis. Most operating rooms are equipped with a special cart ("crash cart") that contains the drugs necessary to treat these emergencies. Among them are cardiac stimulants, respiratory stimulants, vasoconstrictors, agents that strengthen the heart's contractions, and those that neutralize the blood's pH. Specific medications are listed in Table 14–2.

Intravenous Solutions and Blood Expanders

Every patient receiving a general anesthetic has a continuous intravenous drip of saline or a mixture of saline or other fluids and electrolytes. The intravenous drip allows the anesthesiologist to administer other drugs or anesthetic agents directly into the bloodstream and keeps the vein open in case of emergency when the patient must receive medication immediately. Blood and blood substitutes are given when the patient has suffered significant blood loss or a drop in blood pressure before or during surgery. These include plasma, dextran, plasma protein fraction, whole blood, and packed blood cells. Table 14–2 has a complete list of intravenous solutions and blood expanders.

Questions for Study and Review

1. Who may distribute medications to the surgical technologist? Why?

2. What is the proper method for accepting a medication?

3. Why is it important to follow a standard for accepting medications?

4. Explain briefly the use of three different categories of drugs.

5. How do you mark solutions in your hospital?

Answers to Sample Problems

1. Answer: 15 cc of each.

$$\frac{x}{30} = \frac{1}{2}$$
$$2x = 30$$
$$x = \frac{30}{2}$$
$$x = 15$$

2. Answer: 14.08 mL

$$\frac{x}{1000} = \frac{1}{71}$$
$$1000 = 71x$$
$$\frac{1000}{71} = x$$
$$14.08 = x$$

3. Answer: Bacitracin 12.5 cc, neomycin 37.5 cc, saline 50 cc. First solve for the amount of saline solution:

$$\frac{x}{100} = \frac{1}{2}$$
$$2x = 100$$
$$x = \frac{100}{2}$$
$$x = 50 \text{ cc}$$

Now you know the remainder must be bacitracin and neomycin, so if you solve for the bacitracin the remainder is the neomycin.

$$\frac{x}{50} = \frac{1}{4}$$
$$4x = 50$$
$$x = \frac{50}{4}$$
$$x = 12.5 \text{ cc}$$

Now subtract the bacitracin from 50 cc to get the neomycin: 50 − 12.5 = 37.5 cc.

4. Answer: 15 cc of each.
0.5% is one half of 1%, so the solution is 15 cc of each.

5. Answer: 50 cc of each.
Hypaque 1:3 is 25% (1/4), so 50% divided by 2 is 25%; thus, 50 cc each.

Bibliography

Asperheim MK: Pharmacology: An Introductory Text, 5th ed. Philadelphia, WB Saunders, 1981.

Physician's Desk Reference, Oradell, NJ: Medical Economics Co., 1992.

Sheridan E, Patterson RH, Gustafson EA: Falconer's The Drug, The Nurse, The Patient, 7th ed. Philadelphia, WB Saunders, 1982.

Thur M: OR/pharmacy drug quality assurance. AORN J 23(4):1976.

Surgical Instruments

Learning Objectives

After reading this chapter you should be able to

◆ *Identify* the components of a surgical instrument.
◆ *Recognize* the different types of instruments by category.
◆ *Care* for instruments by category.
◆ *Use* effective memorization skills in learning the names of surgical instruments.

Key Terms

box lock: The ratchet closure mechanism of many surgical instruments.
clamp: Instrument that is designed to hold tissue, objects (such as surgical needles), or fabric (such as a towel clamp).
cutting instrument: Any instrument with a sharp edge.
dilators: Graduated, rodlike instruments used to enlarge the diameter of a channel or duct.
jaws: The working end of a surgical instrument.
points: The tips of a surgical instrument.
probe: An instrument placed within a lumen to determine its length and direction.
shank: The area of a surgical instrument between the box lock and the finger ring.

Stainless steel instruments are the surgeon's tools. The quality, condition, and type of instruments can affect the outcome of a surgical procedure. These instruments represent a substantial investment and must be cared for in a prescribed manner. A pictorial glossary of the most commonly used surgical instruments is presented in this chapter. The instruments are grouped according to type or application. Some specialty instruments, such as those used in laparoscopic surgery, are discussed within the appropriate chapter describing spe-

cific procedures. The pictorial review gives the proper name of the instrument as well as slang or nicknames when these exist.

PARTS OF AN INSTRUMENT

As shown in Figure 15–1, an instrument has identifiable parts. The *points* of the instrument are its tips. These should approximate tightly when the instrument

157

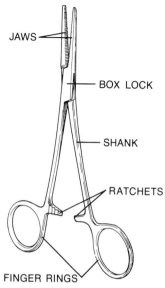

JAWS

BOX LOCK

SHANK

RATCHETS

FINGER RINGS

Figure 15–1. Parts of a clamp.

is closed. (An exception to this rule occurs in some vascular and intestinal clamps that compress tissue only partially.) The *jaws* of the instrument hold tissue securely. Most are serrated, and some have a carbide insert that is replaceable. In needle holders the carbide insert allows great gripping strength and prevents the needle from slipping out of the instrument. The pin that holds the box lock together should be flush against the instrument. The *shank* is the area between the box lock and the finger ring. The *ratchets* of the box lock interlock to keep the instrument locked shut when the instrument is closed. These should mesh together smoothly. See Chapter 7 for a description of how to test an instrument for its integrity and working ability.

TYPES OF INSTRUMENTS

As an aid in memorizing instrument names, it is helpful to know the basic categories of instruments. They are classified according to their function, and most fall into one of four groups. Examples of surgical instruments, including those used in general surgery and in specific procedures and in specific regions of the body, are presented in Figures 15–2 through 15–50.

Cutting and Dissecting

This group includes scissors, scalpels, osteotomes (used for cutting bone), curettes, chisels, biopsy punches, saws, drills, and needles. Any instrument that has a sharp surface, either a blade or a point, can be considered to be a cutting or dissecting tool. Figure 15–

2 illustrates scalpel handles and blades. The most commonly used surgical scissors are illustrated in Figure 15–3.

Grasping and Clamping

A clamp is an instrument that clasps tissue between its jaws. Clamps are available for use on nearly every type of body tissue, from delicate eye muscle to heavy bone. The most common clamps are the hemostatic clamps, designed to grasp blood vessels. Most clamps follow a "finger ring" design and have identifiable parts. The clamp and its parts are shown in Figure 15–1. Grasping instruments are used to retract and manipulate structures. Included in this category are needle holders and tenaculi, used to grasp tissue for dissection or manipulation. Also included are thumb forceps, illustrated in Figure 15–4.

Retracting

Retracting instruments are those that hold tissue or organs away from the area where the surgeon is working. Retractors, like clamping instruments, are available for use in all parts of the body. They may be very shallow, as for skin retraction, or very deep, as for the retraction of abdominal contents. A retractor that is held in the hand, such as a Richardson retractor (see Fig. 15–5), is called a *hand-held retractor*. One that remains extended by mechanical means, such as the Balfour retractor (see Fig. 15–5), is called a *self-retaining retractor*.

Probing and Dilating

Probing instruments are used to enter a lumen that occurs naturally, such as the common bile duct, or one that occurs in a pathologic condition, such as a fistula. Dilators are used to increase the diameter of a lumen, such as the urethra or esophagus.

CARE OF INSTRUMENTS

Instruments can last for many years with proper handling and maintenance. Careless handling of the surgeon's tools results in frustration for the surgeon and great financial loss to the surgery department. The skills of the surgeon are hampered if he or she is forced to work with inferior equipment—scissors that are dull, clamps that will not stay closed over bleeding vessels, needle holders that pop open to release the needle into the wound, or forceps whose teeth do not mesh together properly. It is the technologist's and nurse's responsibility to participate in the maintenance of the instruments. The following guidelines will help increase the life span of instruments and ensure their proper function.

Text continued on page 209

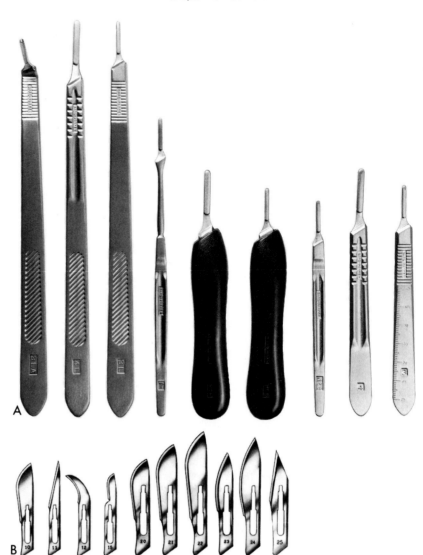

Figure 15–2. Pictorial review of surgical instruments. *A.* Scalpel handles. *B.* Scalpel blades. (Courtesy of Becton-Dickinson & Company, Rochelle Park, NJ.)

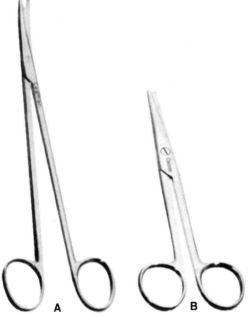

Figure 15–3. General surgery instruments: scissors. *A.* Metzenbaum. *B.* Mayo, straight or curved. (Courtesy of Codman & Shurtleff, Inc., Randolph, MA.)

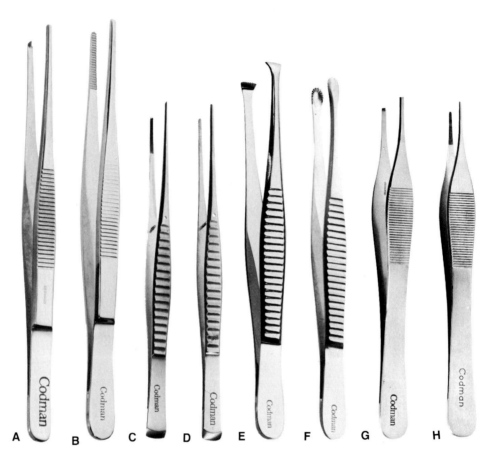

Figure 15–4. General surgery instruments: thumb forceps. *A.* Toothed. *B.* Plain. *C.* Cushing, toothed. *D.* Cushing, plain. *E.* Martin. *F.* Russian. *G.* Adson, toothed. *H.* Adson, plain. (Courtesy of Codman & Shurtleff, Inc., Randolph, MA.)

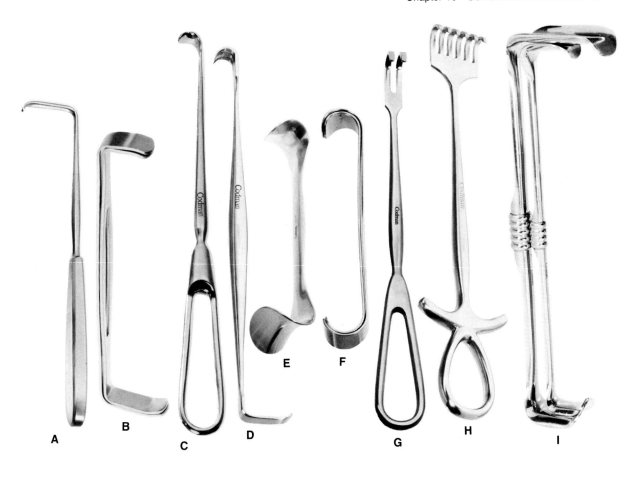

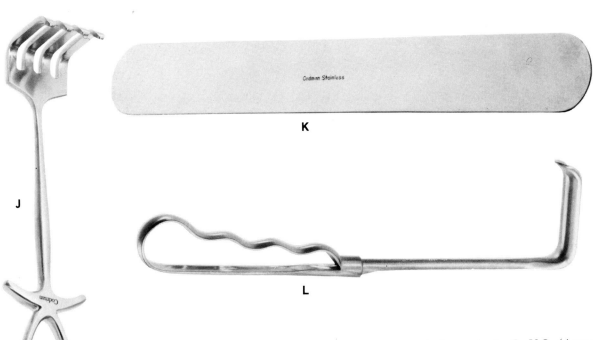

Figure 15–5. General surgery instruments: retractors. *A.* Langenbeck. *B.* U.S. (Army-Navy, USA). *C.* Vein. *D.* Senn (cat's paw). *E.* Goulet. *F.* Parker. *G.* Small rake. *H.* Volkmann, large rake. *I.* Richardson (Rich). *J.* Israel. *K.* Crile, malleable (ribbon). *L.* Richardson appendectomy.

Illustration continued on following page

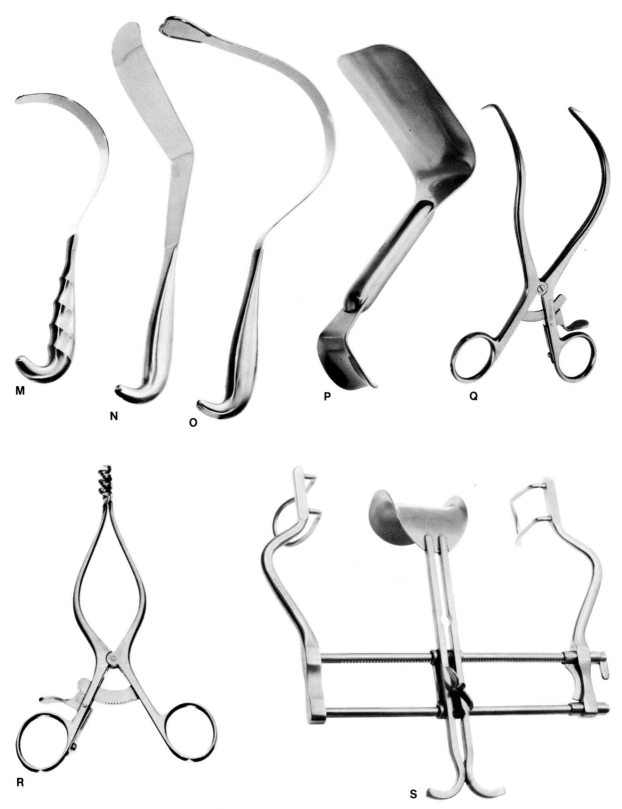

Figure 15–5 *Continued.* *M.* Deaver. *N.* Murphy. *O.* Harrington (sweetheart). *P.* Weinberg (Joe's hoe). *Q.* Gelpi. *R.* Weitlaner. *S.* Balfour, abdominal, with bladder blade. (Courtesy of Codman & Shurtleff, Inc., Randolph, MA.)

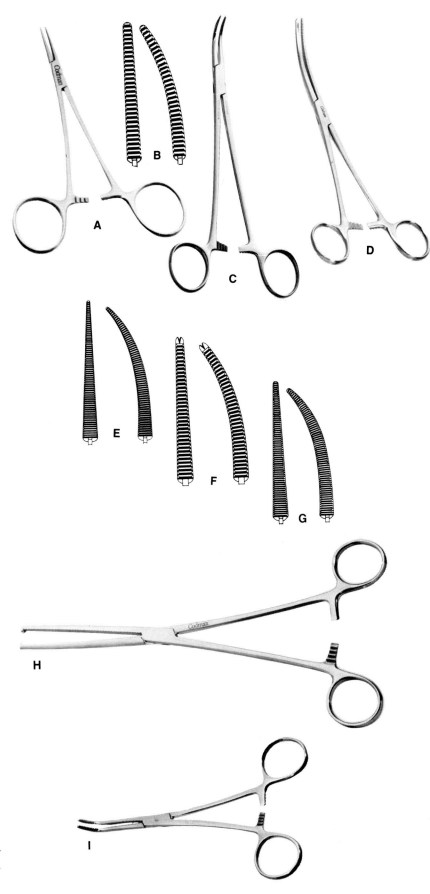

Figure 15–6. General surgery instruments: hemostatic clamps. *A.* Mosquito. *B.* Péan. *C.* Schnidt (tonsil). *D.* Mayo. *E.* Kelly. *F.* Kocher. *G.* Crile. *H.* Ochsner. *I.* Mixter (right angle). (Courtesy of Codman & Shurtleff, Inc., Randolph, MA.)

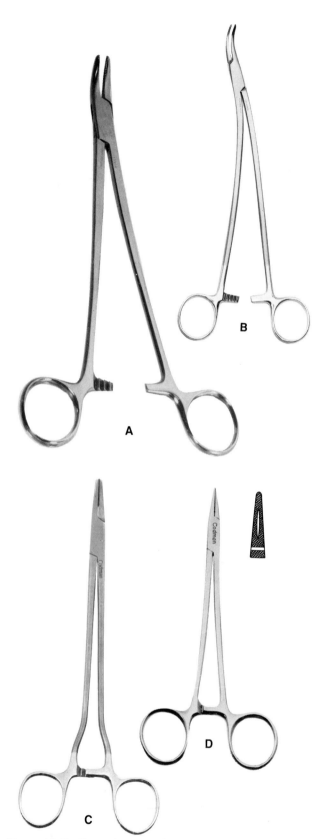

Figure 15–7. General surgery instruments: needle holders. *A.* Heaney. *B.* Stratte. *C.* Rogers. *D.* Crile-Wood. (Courtesy of Codman & Shurtleff, Inc., Randolph, MA.)

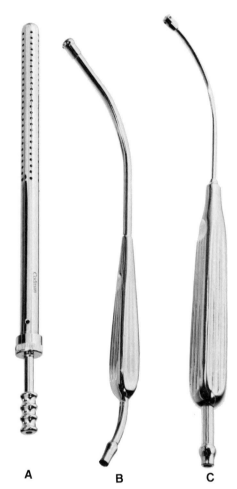

Figure 15–8. General surgery instruments: suction tips. *A.* Poole, abdominal. *B.* Yankauer, tonsil. *C.* Andrews. (Courtesy of Codman & Shurtleff, Inc., Randolph, MA.)

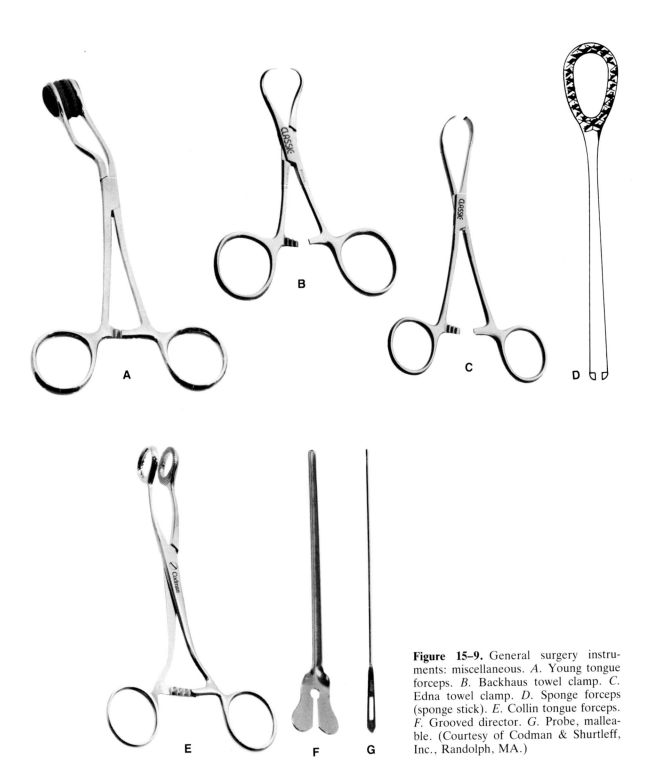

Figure 15–9. General surgery instruments: miscellaneous. *A.* Young tongue forceps. *B.* Backhaus towel clamp. *C.* Edna towel clamp. *D.* Sponge forceps (sponge stick). *E.* Collin tongue forceps. *F.* Grooved director. *G.* Probe, malleable. (Courtesy of Codman & Shurtleff, Inc., Randolph, MA.)

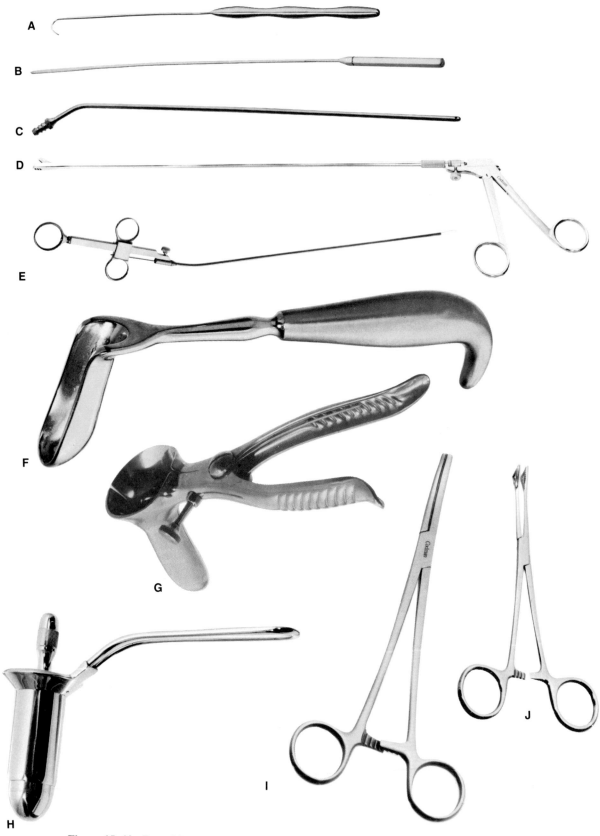

Figure 15–10. Rectal instruments. *A.* Crypt hook. *B.* Fistula probe. *C.* Buie rectal suction tip. *D.* Biopsy forceps. *E.* Rectal snare. *F.* Sawyer rectal speculum. *G.* Pratt rectal speculum. *H.* Proctoscope (anoscope). *I.* Buie pile clamp. *J.* Pennington clamp. (Courtesy of Codman & Shurtleff, Inc., Randolph, MA.)

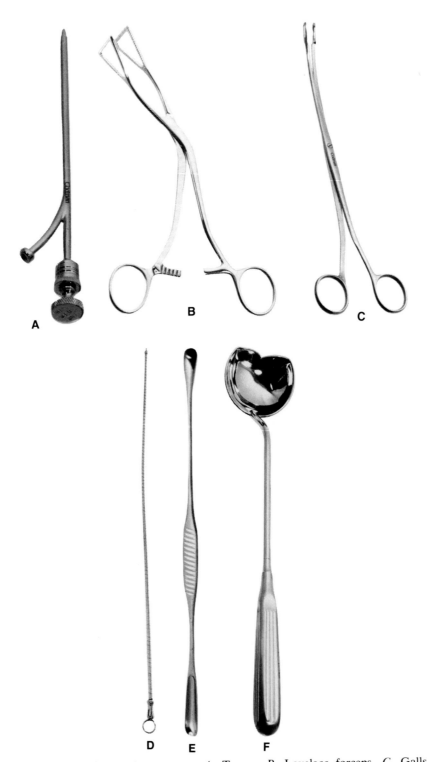

Figure 15–11. Gallbladder instruments. *A.* Trocar. *B.* Lovelace forceps. *C.* Gallstone forceps. *D.* Gallstone probe. *E.* Gallstone scoop. *F.* Moore gallstone scoop.

Illustration continued on following page

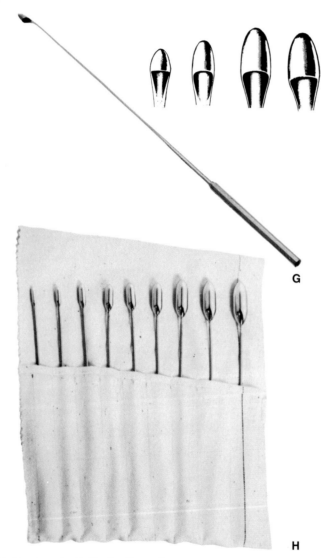

Figure 15–11 *Continued.* *G.* Desjardins gallstone scoop. *H.* Bakes common duct dilators. (Courtesy of Codman & Shurtleff, Inc., Randolph, MA.)

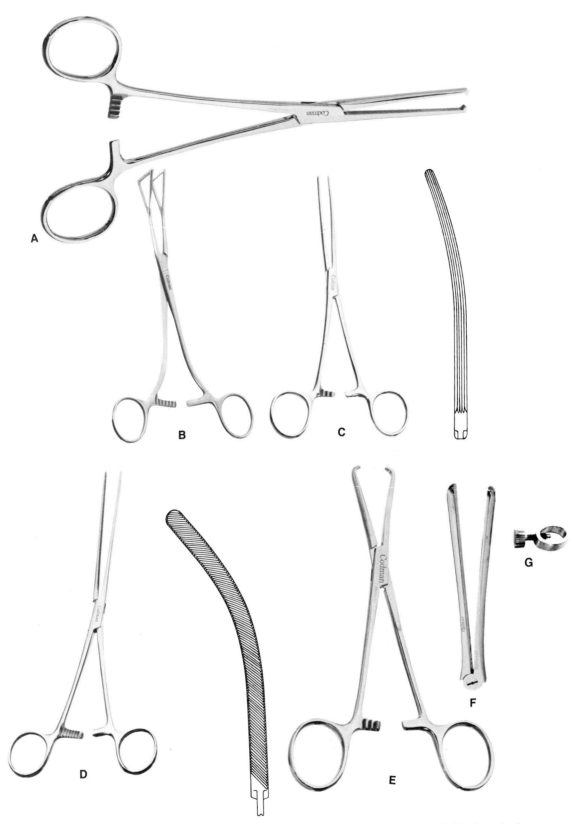

Figure 15–12. Gastrointestinal instruments. *A.* Allen-Kocher clamp. *B.* Collin intestinal forceps. *C.* Bainbridge intestinal clamp. *D.* Doyen intestinal clamp. *E.* Stone clamp applier. *F.* Stone clamp. *G.* Stone locking device.

Illustration continued on following page

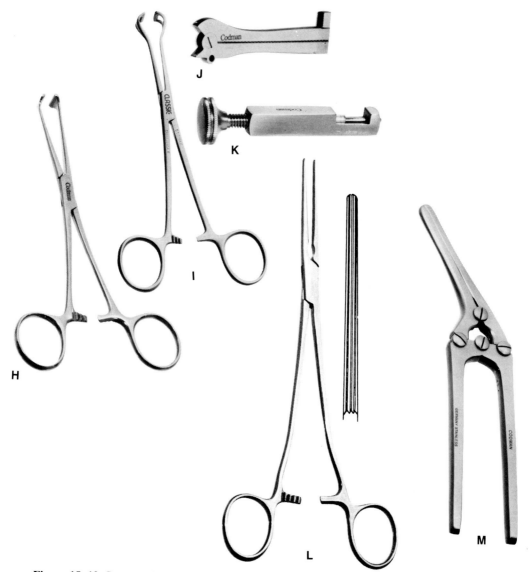

Figure 15–12 *Continued.* *H.* Allis clamp. *I.* Babcock forceps. *J.* DeMartel-Wolfson clamp. *K.* DeMartel-Wolfson clamp holder. *L.* Dennis clamp. *M.* Payr gastrointestinal clamp. (Courtesy of Codman & Shurtleff, Inc., Randolph, MA.)

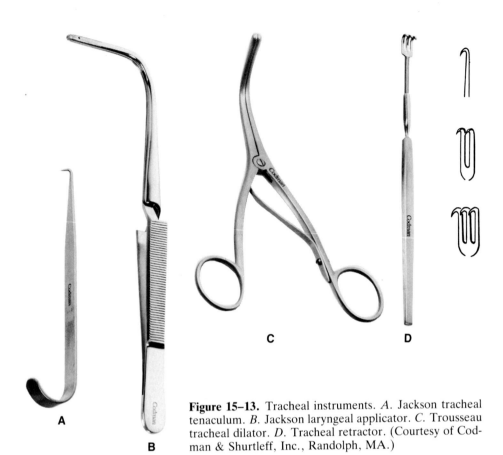

Figure 15–13. Tracheal instruments. *A.* Jackson tracheal tenaculum. *B.* Jackson laryngeal applicator. *C.* Trousseau tracheal dilator. *D.* Tracheal retractor. (Courtesy of Codman & Shurtleff, Inc., Randolph, MA.)

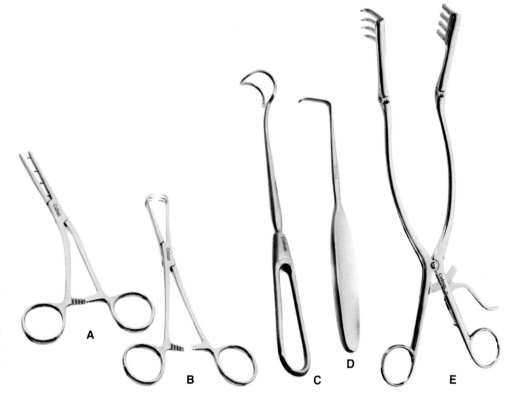

Figure 15–14. Thyroid instruments. *A.* Mastin muscle clamp. *B.* Lahey thyroid tenaculum. *C.* Green thyroid retractor. *D.* Lahey thyroid retractor. *E.* Beckman retractor. (Courtesy of Codman & Shurtleff, Inc., Randolph, MA.)

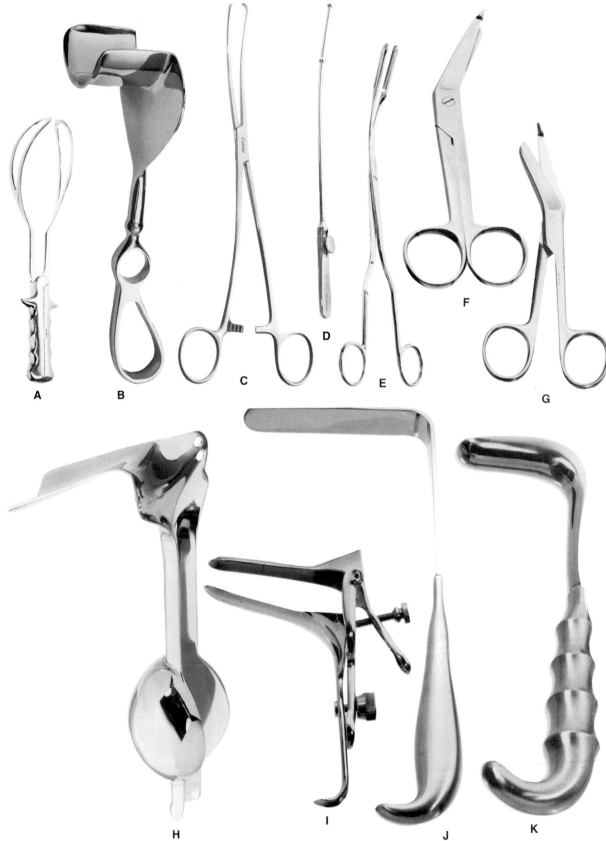

Figure 15–15. Obstetric and gynecologic instruments. *A.* Simpson obstetric forceps. *B.* DeLee retractor. *C.* Iowa membrane puncture forceps. *D.* Wilson amniotic trocar. *E.* Hirst placenta forceps. *F.* Lister bandage scissors. *G.* Episiotomy scissors. *H.* Auvard weighted speculum. *I.* Graves vaginal speculum. *J.* Heaney retractor (lateral retractor). *K.* Sims vaginal retractor.

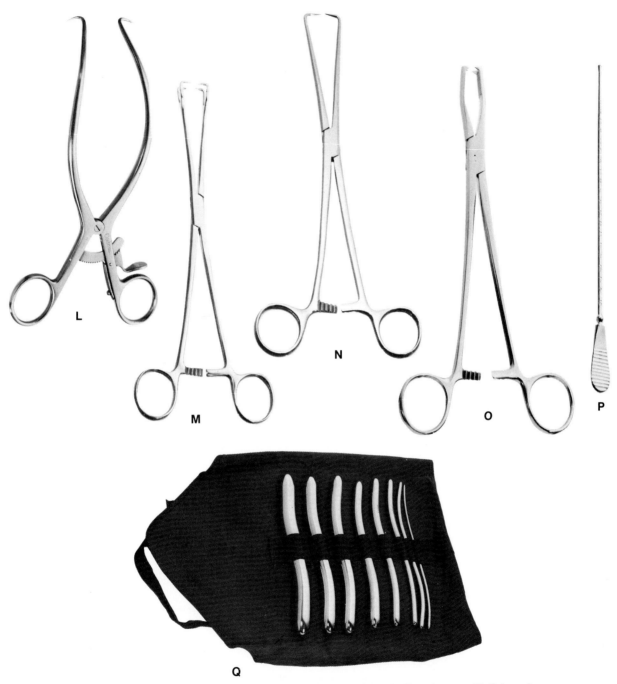

Figure 15–15 *Continued.* *L.* Gelpi retractor. *M.* Schroeder vulsellum forceps. *N.* Schroeder tenaculum. *O.* Jacobs tenaculum. *P.* Uterine sound. *Q.* Hegar uterine dilators.

Illustration continued on following page

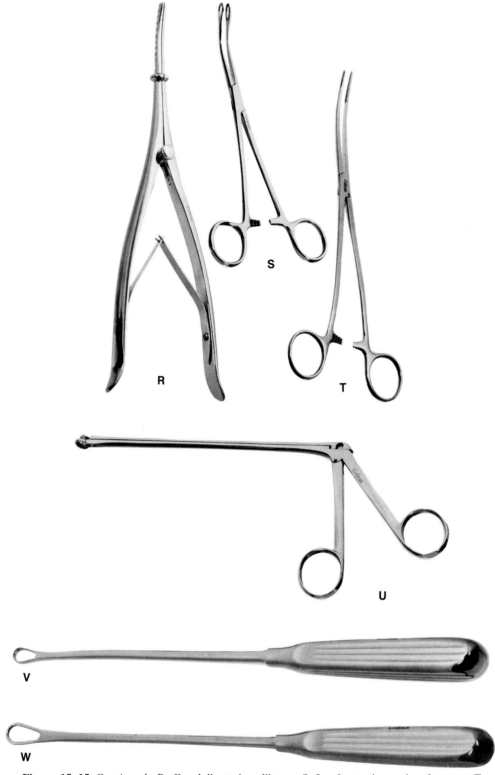

Figure 15–15 *Continued. R.* Goodell uterine dilator. *S.* Laufe uterine polyp forceps. *T.* Bozeman uterine-dressing forceps. *U.* Wittner uterine biopsy forceps. *V.* Uterine curette, sharp. *W.* Uterine curette, smooth. (Courtesy of Codman & Shurtleff, Inc., Randolph, MA.)

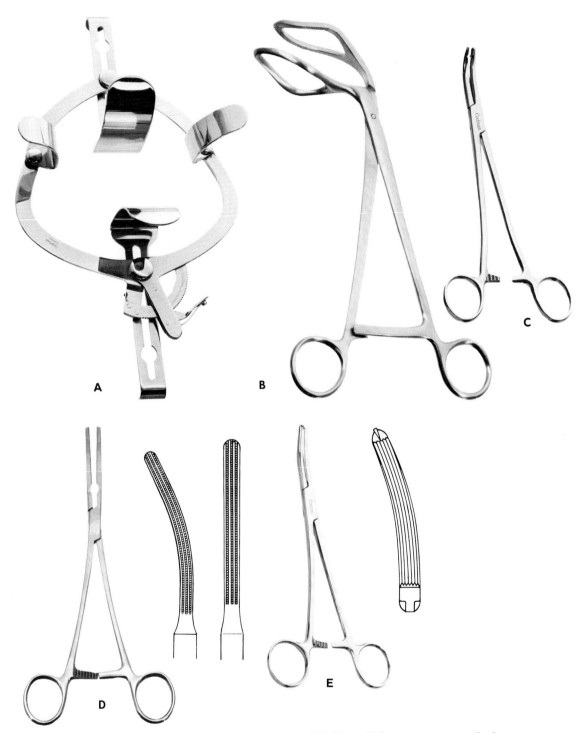

Figure 15–16. Hysterectomy instruments. *A.* O'Sullivan-O'Connor retractor. *B.* Somers uterine elevator (lemon squeezer). *C.* Heaney forceps. *D.* Masterson hysterectomy forceps. *E.* Long hysterectomy forceps. (Courtesy of Codman & Shurtleff, Inc., Randolph, MA.)

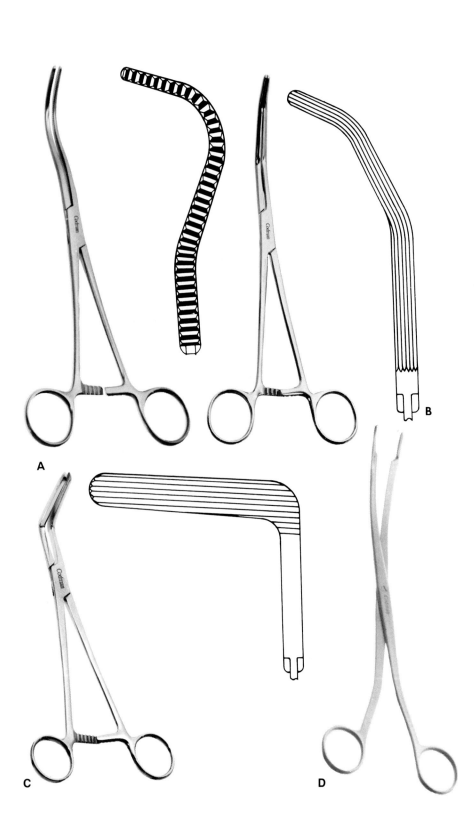

A

B

C

D

Figure 15–17. Genitourinary instruments. *A.* Mayo kidney clamp. *B.* Herrick kidney clamp. *C.* Wertheim-Cullen pedicle clamp. *D.* Randall kidney stone forceps.

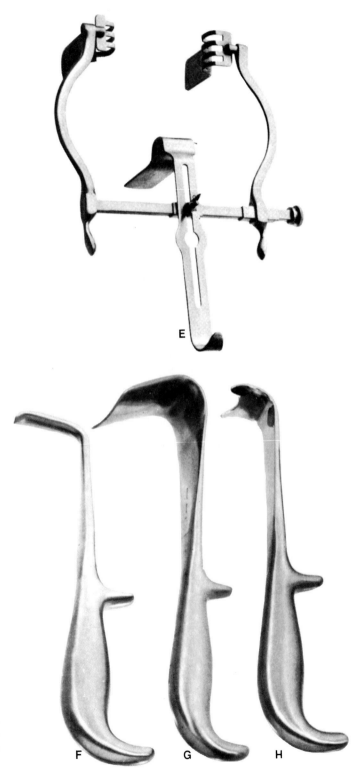

Figure 15–17 *Continued. E.* Judd-Masson bladder retractor. *F.* Young prostatic retractor, lateral. *G.* Young prostatic retractor, anterior. *H.* Young prostatic retractor, bifurcated.

Illustration continued on following page

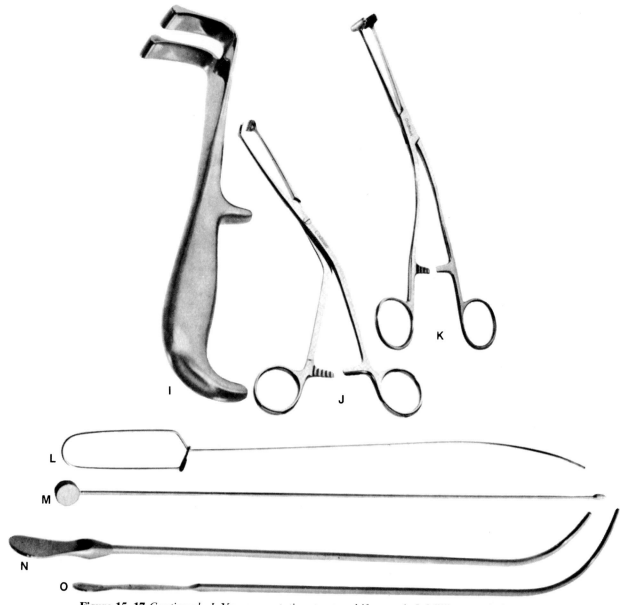

Figure 15–17 *Continued. I.* Young prostatic retractor, bifurcated. *J.* Millin capsule forceps. *K.* Millin T-shaped forceps. *L.* Catheter guide. *M.* Otis bougie à boule. *N.* Otis urethral sound. *O.* Van Buren urethral sound. (Courtesy of Codman & Shurtleff, Inc., Randolph, MA.)

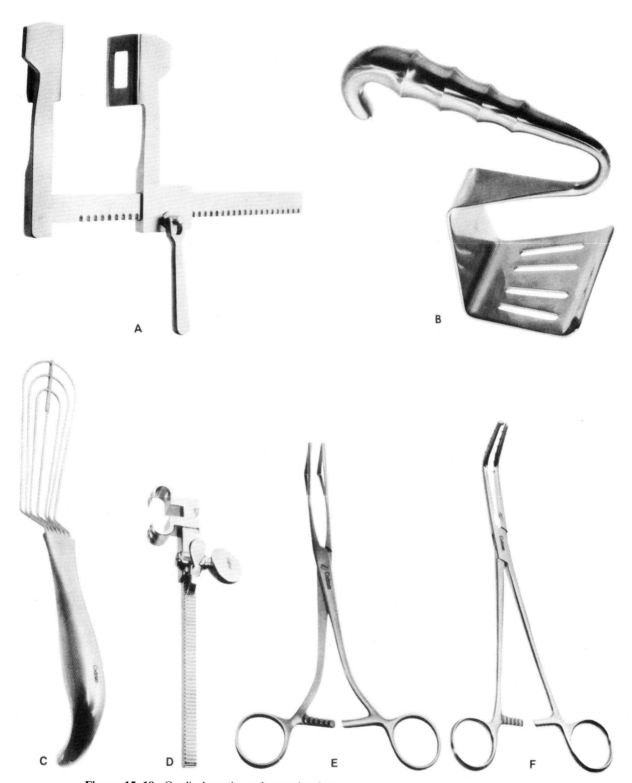

Figure 15–18. Cardiothoracic and vascular instruments: thoracic instruments. *A.* Finochietto retractor. *B.* Davidson scapular retractor. *C.* Allison lung retractor. *D.* Bailey rib contractor. *E.* Duval lung forceps. *F.* Sarot bronchus clamp.

Illustration continued on following page

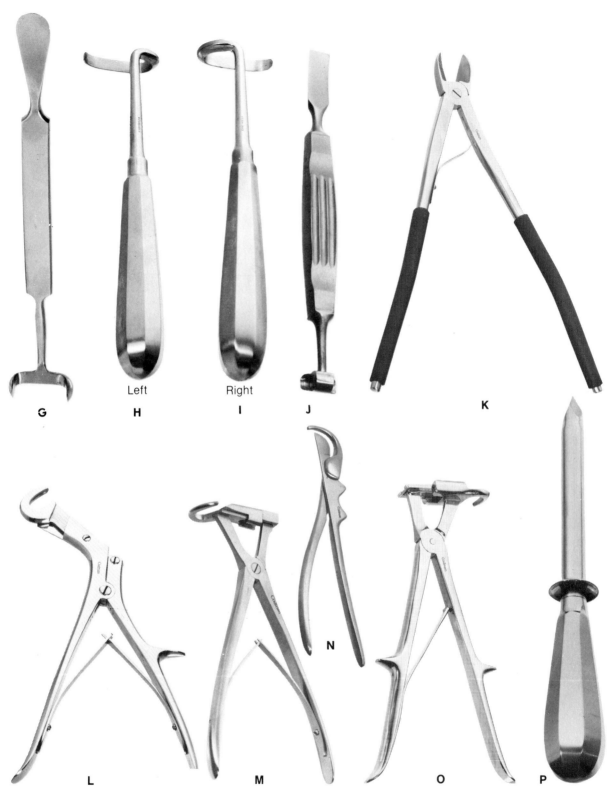

Figure 15–18 *Continued.* *G.* Matson rib stripper. *H.* Doyen rib raspatory, left. *I.* Doyen rib raspatory, right. *J.* Alexander rib stripper. *K.* Bethune rib shears. *L.* Stille-Giertz rib shears. *M.* Shoemaker rib shears. *N.* Gluck rib shears. *O.* Sauerbruch rib shears. *P.* Empyema trocar. (Courtesy of Codman & Shurtleff, Inc., Randolph, MA.)

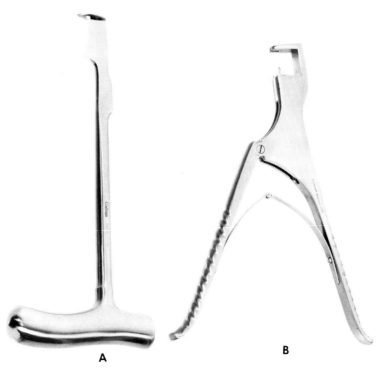

A

B

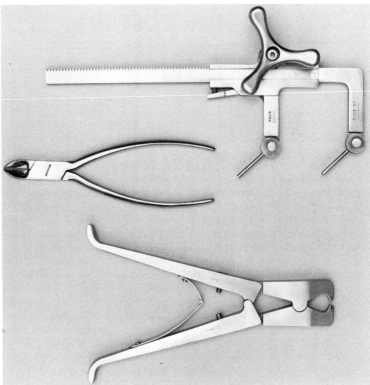

Figure 15–19. Cardiothoracic and vascular instruments: sternal instruments. *A.* Lebsche sternal knife. *B.* Sweet sternal punch. *C.* Pilling Wolvek sternal approximator. (*A* and *B*, courtesy of Codman & Shurtleff, Inc., Randolph, MA; *C*, courtesy of Narco Pilling.)

C

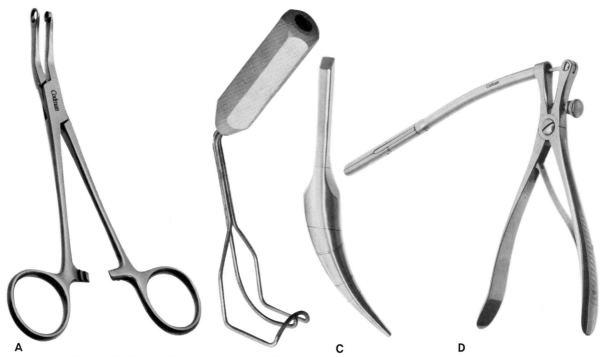

Figure 15–20. Cardiothoracic and vascular instruments: atrial instruments. *A.* Karp aortic punch. *B.* Cooley atrial retractor. *C.* Myocardial dilator. *D.* Tubbs mitral valve dilator. (Courtesy of Codman & Shurtleff, Inc., Randolph, MA.)

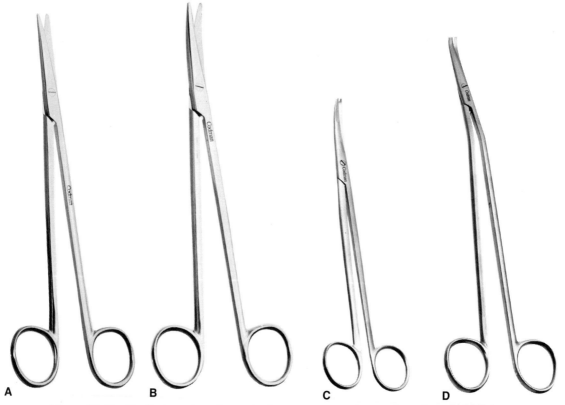

Figure 15–21. Cardiothoracic and vascular instruments: cardiovascular scissors. *A.* Nelson scissors, curved. *B.* Nelson scissors, straight. *C.* Diethrich valve scissors. *D.* Litwak mitral valve scissors. (Courtesy of Codman & Shurtleff, Inc., Randolph, MA.)

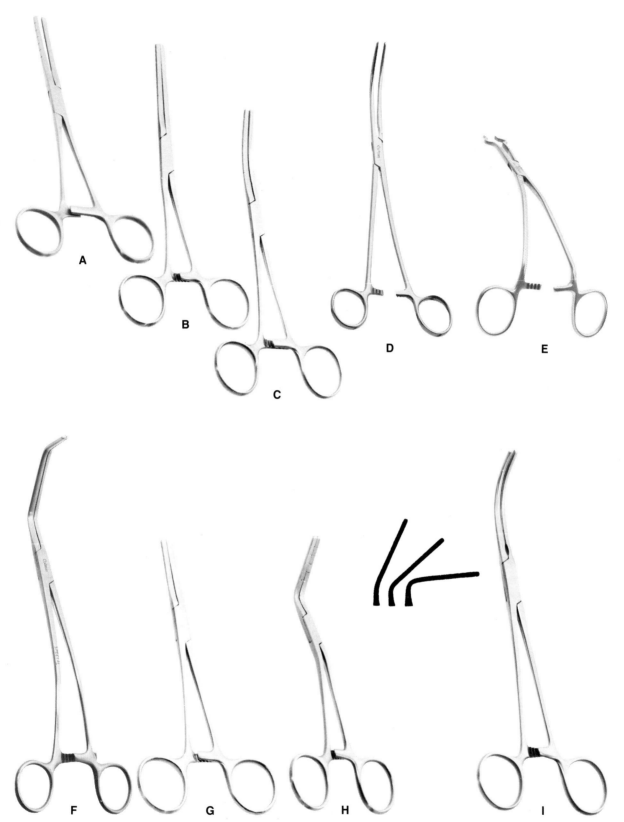

Figure 15–22. Cardiothoracic and vascular instruments: cardiovascular clamps. *A* through *C.* Cooley coarctation clamps. *D.* Crafoord coarctation clamp. *E.* Cooley vena cava clamp. *F.* DeBakey tangential occlusion clamp. *G.* Cooley patent ductus clamp. *H.* Cooley multipurpose clamp. *I.* Glover curved clamp.

Illustration continued on following page

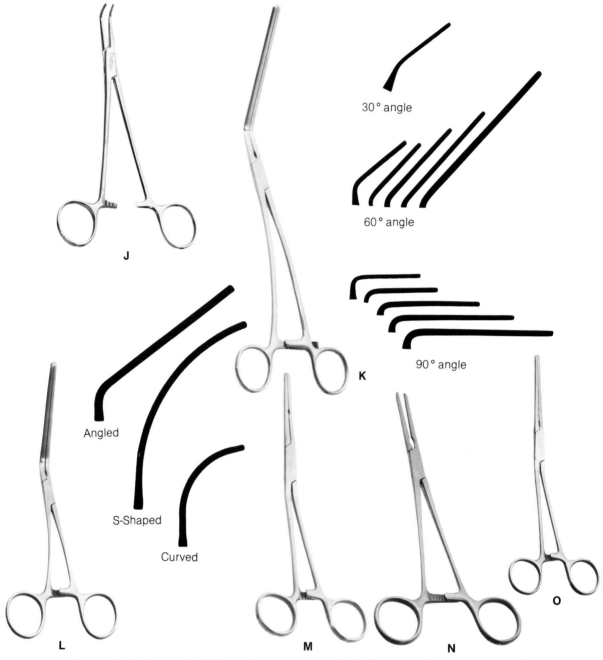

Figure 15–22 *Continued.* *J.* Rumel thoracic forceps. *K.* DeBakey multipurpose clamps. *L.* DeBakey peripheral vascular clamps. *M.* Glover patent ductus clamp. *N.* DeBakey patent ductus clamp. *O.* Glover coarctation clamp.

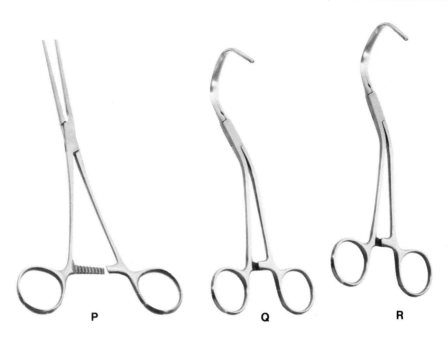

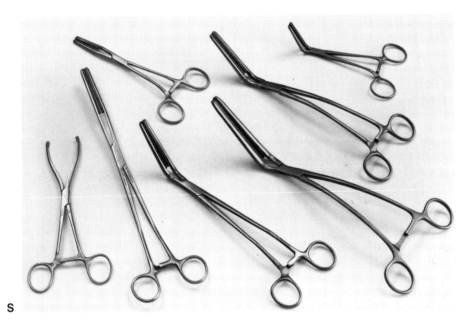

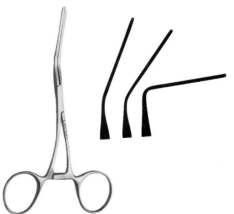

Figure 15–22 *Continued. P.* DeBakey coarctation clamp. *Q.* Kay aorta clamp. *R.* Lambert-Kay aorta clamp. *S.* Fogarty Hydrogrip clamps. *T.* Castaneda multipurpose clamp.

Illustration continued on following page

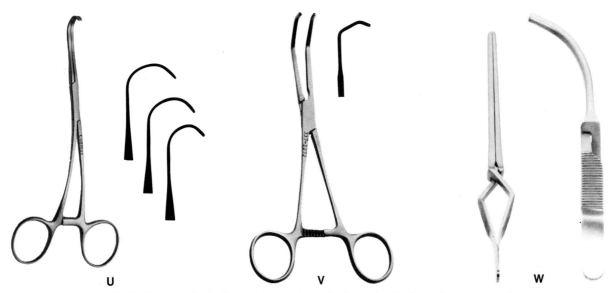

Figure 15–22 *Continued. U.* Castaneda anastomosis clamp. *V.* Beck miniature aorta clamp. *W.* DeBakey bulldog clamps. (*A–R, T–W,* courtesy of Codman & Shurtleff, Inc., Randolph, MA; *S,* courtesy of Edwards Laboratories.)

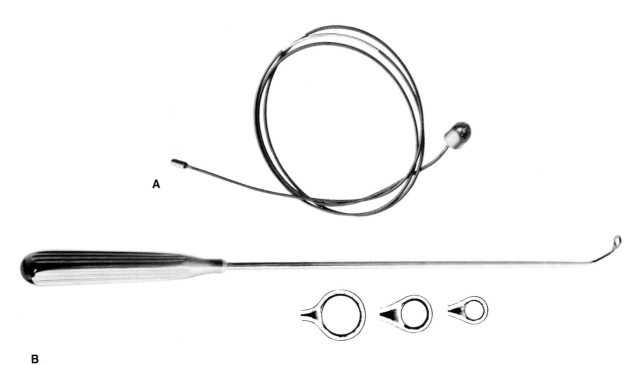

Figure 15–23. Cardiothoracic and vascular instruments. *A.* Internal vein stripper. *B.* External vein stripper. (Courtesy of Codman & Shurtleff, Inc., Randolph, MA.)

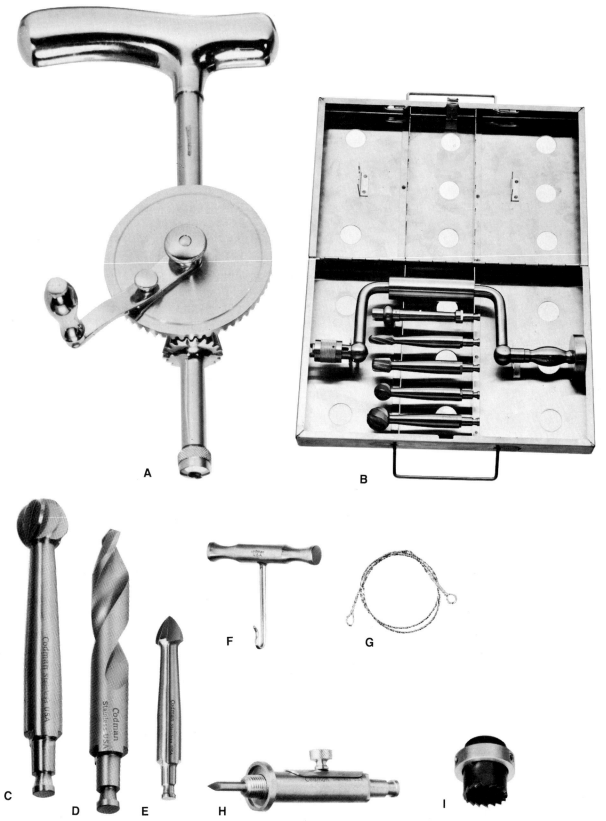

Figure 15–24. Neurosurgical instruments: bone cutters. *A.* Stille cranial drill. *B.* Hudson brace with burs. *C.* McKenzie enlarging bur. *D.* McKenzie perforator drill. *E.* Adson perforating bur. *F.* Gigli-saw handle. *G.* Gigli-saw blade. *H.* Skull trephine handle. *I.* Skull trephine. (Courtesy of Codman & Shurtleff, Inc., Randolph, MA.)

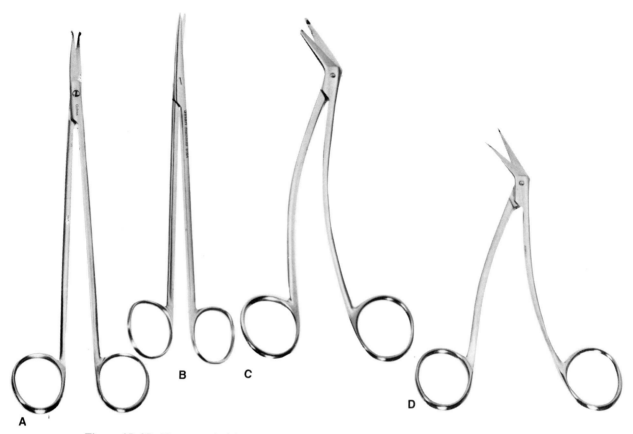

Figure 15–25. Neurosurgical instruments: scissors. *A.* Strully neurologic scissors. *B.* Malis neurologic scissors. *C.* Frazier dural scissors. *D.* Taylor dural scissors. (Courtesy of Codman & Shurtleff, Inc., Randolph, MA.)

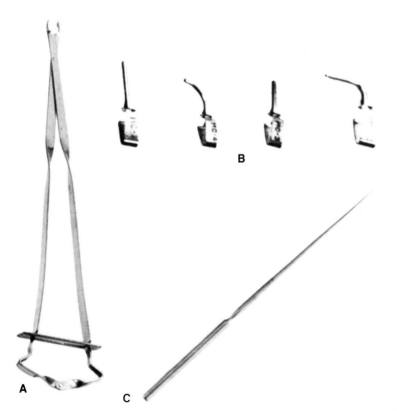

Figure 15–26. Neurosurgical instruments. *A.* Mayfield aneurysm clip applier. *B.* McFadden aneurysm clips. *C.* Adson aneurysm needle. (Courtesy of Codman & Shurtleff, Inc., Randolph, MA.)

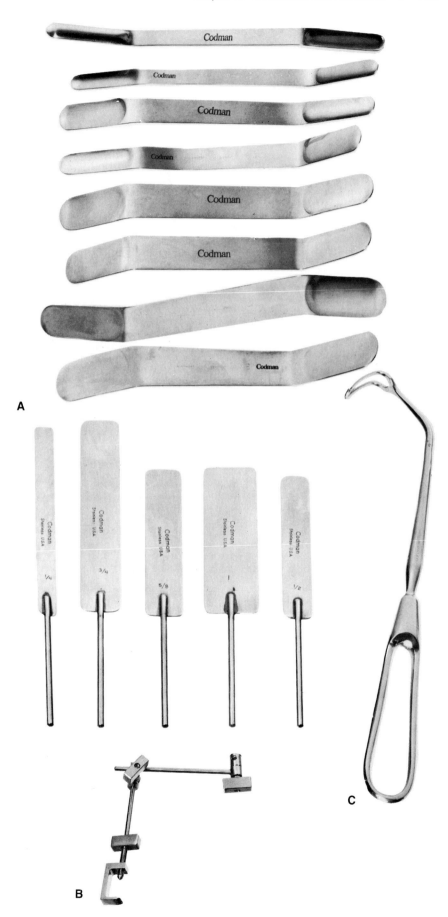

Figure 15–27. Neurosurgical instruments. *A.* Brain spatulas, spoons. *B.* Enker self-retaining brain retractor with malleable blades. *C.* Cushing retractor. (Courtesy of Codman & Shurtleff, Inc., Randolph, MA.)

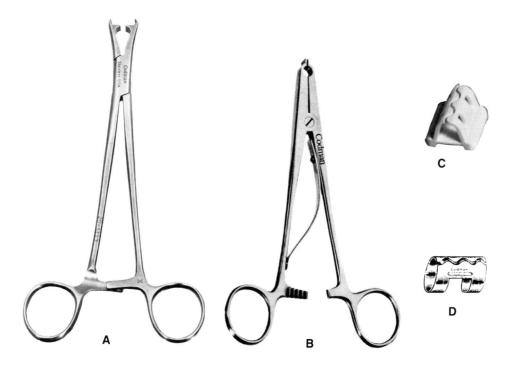

Figure 15–28. Neurosurgical instruments: scalp clips. *A.* LeRoy scalp clip-applying forceps. *B.* Raney scalp clip-applying forceps. *C.* LeRoy disposable scalp clip. *D.* Raney stainless steel scalp clip. (Courtesy of Codman & Shurtleff, Inc., Randolph, MA.)

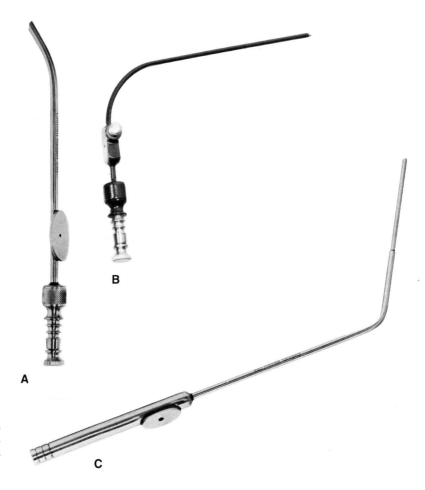

Figure 15–29. Neurosurgical instruments: suction. *A.* Adson suction tube. *B.* Frazier suction tube. *C.* Sachs suction tube. (Courtesy of Codman & Shurtleff, Inc., Randolph, MA.)

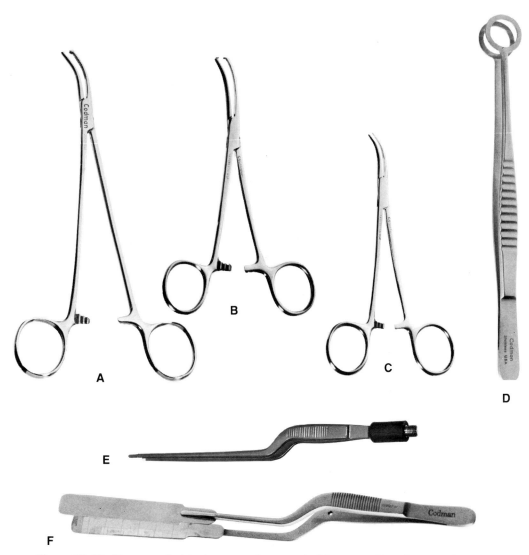

Figure 15–30. Neurosurgical instruments: forceps. *A.* Ligamenta flava forceps. *B.* Dandy scalp forceps. *C.* Hoen scalp forceps. *D.* Johnson brain tumor forceps. *E.* Davis monopolar bayonet forceps. *F.* Scoville brain spatula forceps. (Courtesy of Codman & Shurtleff, Inc., Randolph, MA.)

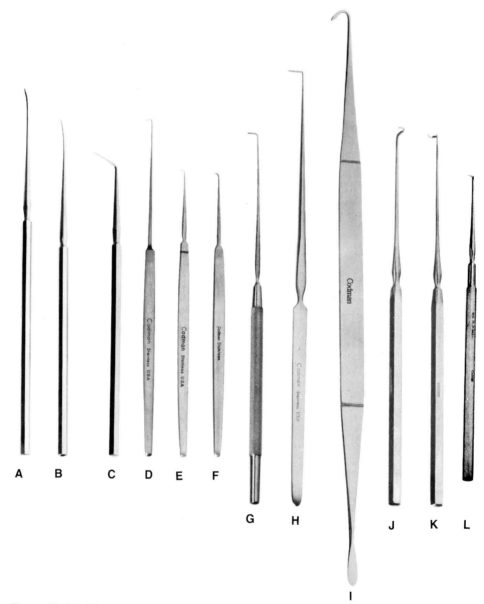

Figure 15–31. Neurosurgical instruments: nerve hooks, separators, and knives. *A.* Sachs nerve separator–spatula. *B.* Davis nerve separator. *C.* Frazier dural separator. *D.* Cloward dural hook. *E.* Cushing dural hook. *F.* Cushing dural hook knife. *G.* Adson dissecting hook. *H.* Hoen nerve hook. *I.* Smithwick nerve hook. *J.* Selverstone cordotomy hook, right. *K.* Selverstone cordotomy hook, left. *L.* Frazier cordotomy knife. (Courtesy of Codman & Shurtleff, Inc., Randolph, MA.)

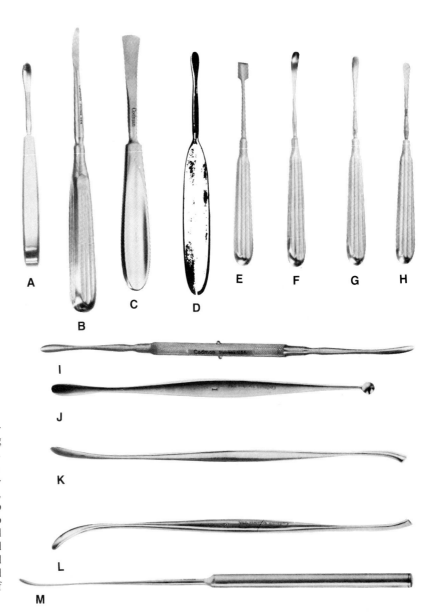

Figure 15–32. Neurosurgical instruments: periosteal and soft tissue elevators. *A.* Cushing elevator (joker). *B.* Cushing elevator, sharp. *C.* Cushing elevator, wide, square edge. *D.* Cushing elevator, small, blunt. *E.* Adson elevator, chisel edge. *F.* Adson elevator, curved, blunt edge. *G.* Cushing elevator, semisharp edge. *H.* Cushing elevator, straight, semisharp edge. *I.* Staphylorrhaphy elevator. *J.* Penfield elevator No. 1 (No. 1 Penfield). *K.* Penfield elevator No. 2 (No. 2 Penfield). *L.* Penfield elevator No. 3 (No. 3 Penfield). *M.* Penfield elevator No. 4 (No. 4 Penfield). (Courtesy of Codman & Shurtleff, Inc., Randolph, MA.)

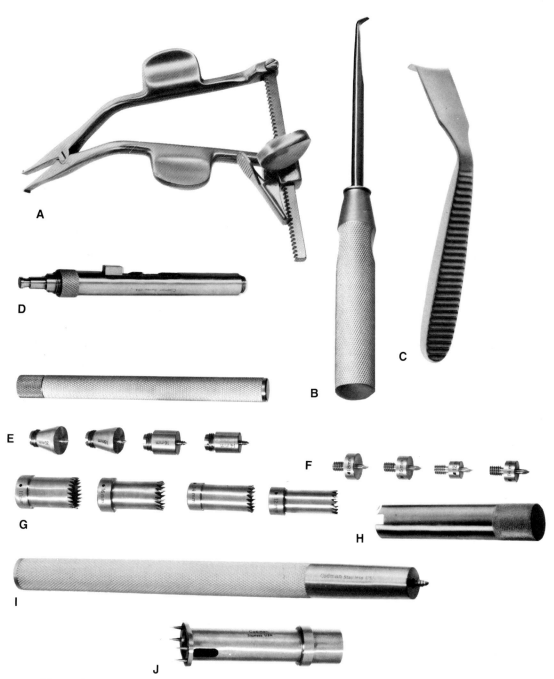

Figure 15–33. Neurosurgical instruments: Cloward laminectomy and fusion instruments. *A.* Vertebral spreader. *B.* Osteophyte elevator. *C.* Blade retractor. *D.* Dowel cutter shaft. *E.* Dowel handle and ejector set. *F.* Dowel cutter center pins. *G.* Dowel cutters. *H.* Dowel ejector. *I.* Bone graft holder and impactor. *J.* Cervical drill guards with bone relief. (Courtesy of Codman & Shurtleff, Inc., Randolph, MA.)

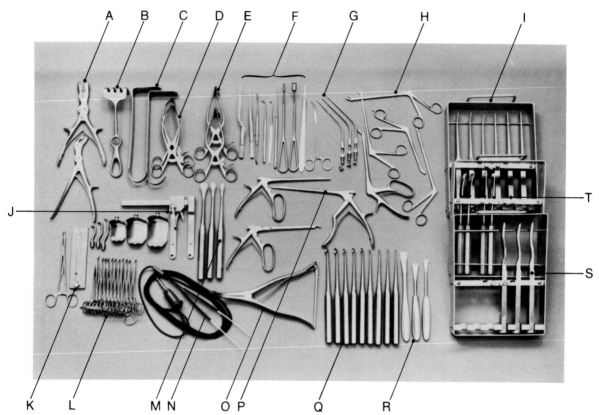

Figure 15–34. Neurosurgical instruments: complete laminectomy set. *A.* Stille rongeurs. *B.* Israel retractor (large rake). *C.* Hibbs retractors. *D.* Gelpi retractors. *E.* Weitlaner retractors. *F.* Fine tissue forceps, delicate retractors, long scalpel, ligamenta flava forceps. *G.* Frazier suction tubes. *H.* Pituitary rongeurs, assorted sizes. *I.* Osteotomes. *J.* Large self-retaining retractor, assorted blades. *K.* Ligation clips. *L.* Hemostats. *M.* Heavy periosteal elevators. *N.* Bipolar coagulation forceps, insulated. *O.* Vertebral spreader. *P.* Kerrison rongeurs. *Q.* Curettes, assorted sizes. *R.* Small periosteal elevators. *S.* Gouges, assorted sizes. *T.* Chisels, assorted sizes. (Courtesy of Zimmer, Inc., Warsaw, IN.)

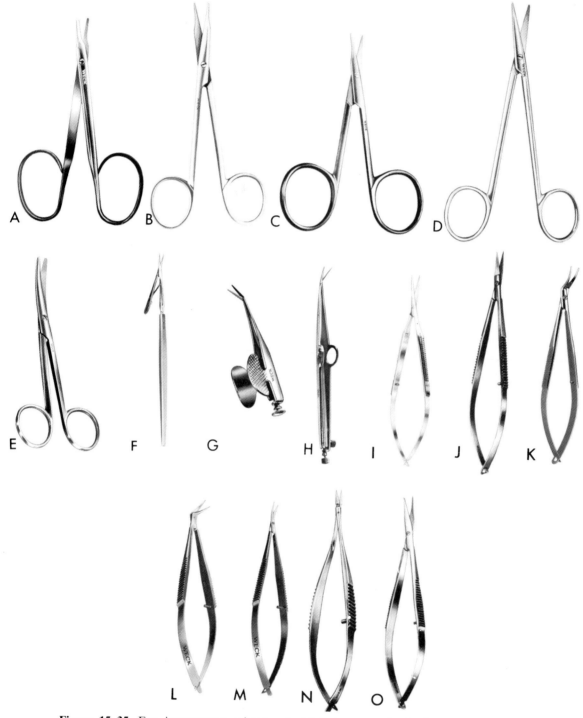

Figure 15–35. Eye instruments: scissors. *A.* McGuire corneal. *B.* Stevens tenotomy, standard size. *C.* Stevens tenotomy, short. *D.* Strabismus. *E.* Enucleation. *F.* Moyes iridectomy. *G.* Barraquer. *H.* DeWecker iridectomy. *I.* Iris. *J.* Fine stitch. *K.* Troutman conjunctiva and suture. *L.* Castroviejo corneal. *M.* Castroviejo corneal, miniature. *N.* Vannas capsulotomy. *O.* Westcott tenotomy. (Courtesy of Edward Weck and Company, Inc., Princeton, NJ.)

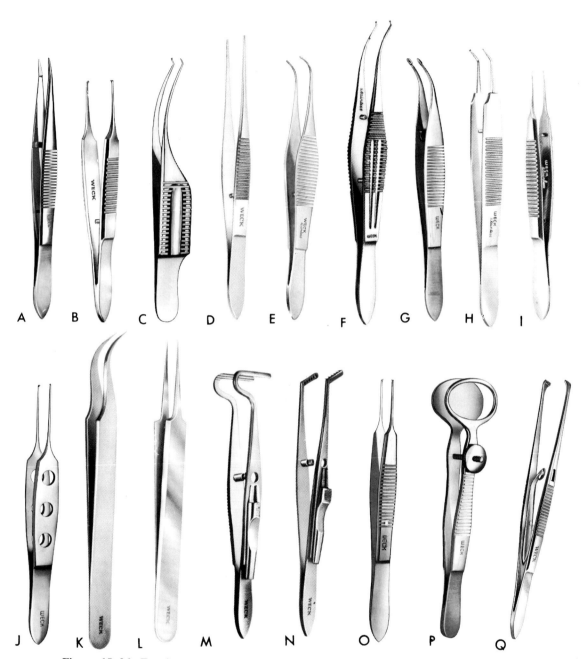

Figure 15–36. Eye instruments: forceps. *A.* Barraquer cilia. *B.* Graefe iris. *C.* Colibri corneal, utility. *D.* Dressing. *E.* Schweiger extracapsular. *F.* Hyde corneal. *G.* Arruga capsule. *H.* Castroviejo suturing. *I.* McPherson corneal. *J.* Bishop-Harman. *K.* Jeweler's No. 7. *L.* Jeweler's No. 5. *M.* Berke ptosis. *N.* Jameson muscle, right. *O.* Lester fixation. *P.* Desmarres chalazion. *Q.* Graefe fixation. (Courtesy of Edward Weck and Company, Inc., Princeton, NJ.)

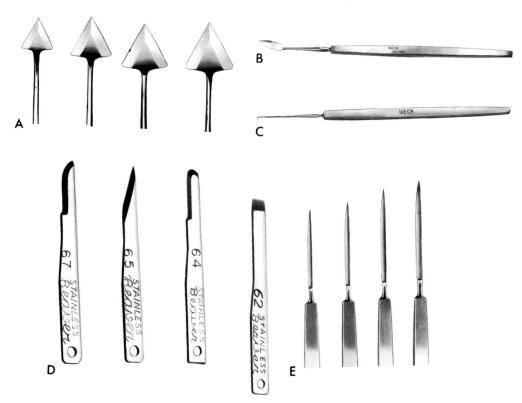

Figure 15–37. Eye instruments: knives, keratomes. *A.* Jaeger keratomes. *B.* Castroviejo keratome. *C.* Graefe cystotome. *D.* Beaver Mini-Blades. *E.* Graefe cataract knives. (Courtesy of Edward Weck and Company, Inc., Princeton, NJ.)

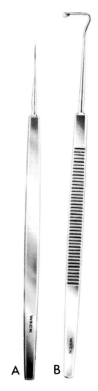

Figure 15–38. Eye instruments: hooks. *A.* Tyrrell iris hook. *B.* Jameson muscle hook. (Courtesy of Edward Weck and Company, Inc., Princeton, NJ.)

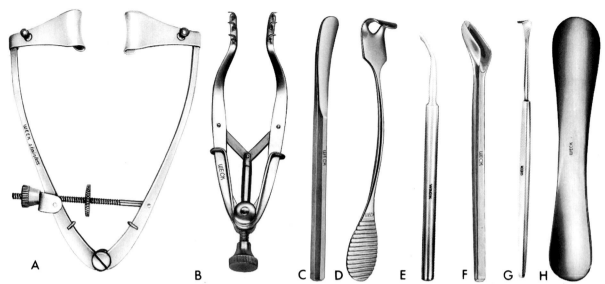

Figure 15–39. Eye instruments: retractors. *A.* McPherson speculum. *B.* Stevenson lacrimal sac retractor. *C.* Lid expressor. *D.* Berens lid elevator. *E.* Rosenbaum iris retractor. *F.* Arruga glove retractor. *G.* Conway lid retractor. *H.* Jaeger retractor. (Courtesy of Edward Weck and Company, Inc., Princeton, NJ.)

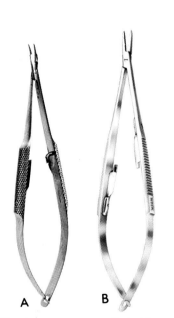

Figure 15–40. Eye instruments: needle holders. *A.* Barraquer. *B.* Castroviejo. (Courtesy of Edward Weck and Company, Inc., Princeton, NJ.)

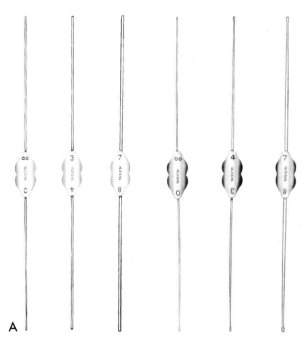

Figure 15–41. Eye instruments: miscellaneous. *A.* Bowman lacrimal probes.

Illustration continued on following page

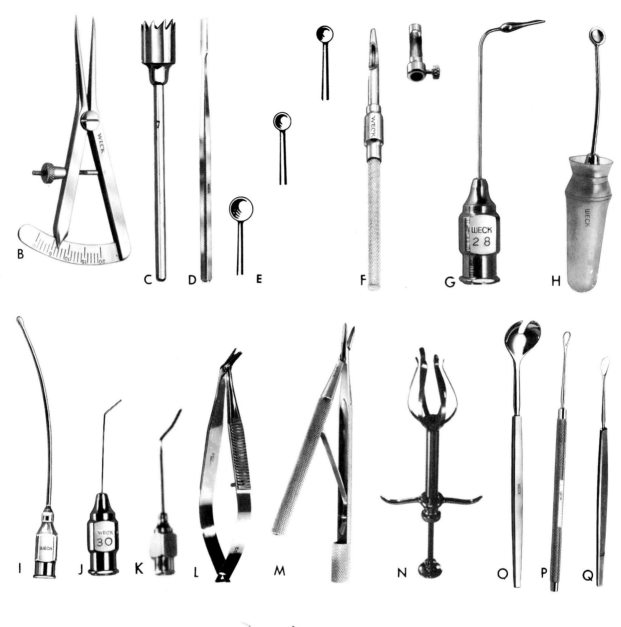

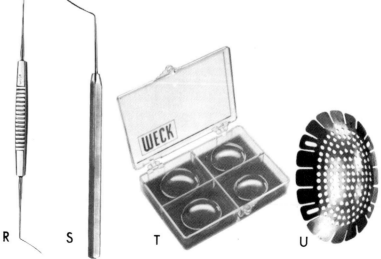

Figure 15–41 *Continued.* *B.* Castroviejo caliper. *C.* Arruga lacrimal trephine. *D.* West lacrimal chisel. *E.* Chalazion currettes. *F.* Grieshaber trephine. *G.* Tulevech lacrimal cannula. *H.* Bell erisophake. *I.* Troutman alpha-chymotrypsin cannula. *J.* Air injection cannula. *K.* Cyclodialysis cannula. *L.* Castroviejo corneoscleral punch. *M.* Castroviejo blade breaker. *N.* Sphere introducer. *O.* Wells enucleation spoon. *P.* Kirby lens loop. *Q.* New Orleans lens loop. *R.* Castroviejo cyclodialysis spatula. *S.* Troutman iris spatula. *T.* Universal conformers. *U.* Eye shield. (Courtesy of Edward Weck and Company, Inc., Princeton, NJ.)

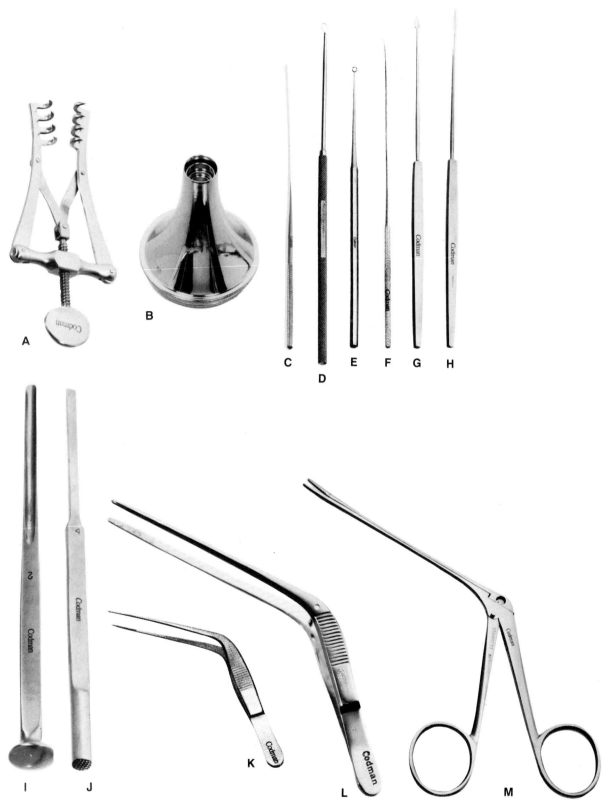

Figure 15–42. Ear instruments. *A.* Mastoid retractor. *B.* Ear specula. *C.* Farrell applicator. *D.* Ear loops. *E.* Ear curette. *F.* Day ear hook. *G.* Sexton ear knife. *H.* Politzer ear knife. *I.* Mastoid gouge. *J.* Mastoid chisel. *K.* Blake ear forceps. *L.* Wilde ear forceps. *M.* Hartmann ear forceps.

Illustration continued on following page

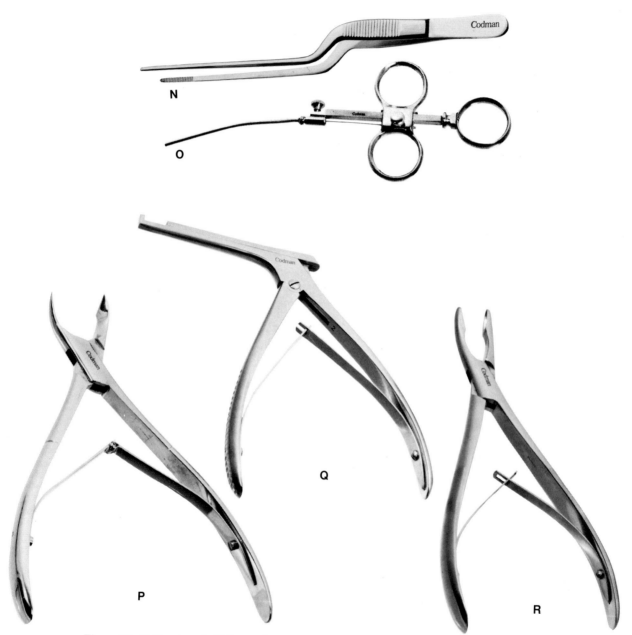

Figure 15–42 *Continued.* *N.* Lucae forceps. *O.* Krouse ear snare. *P.* Dean mastoid rongeur. *Q.* Kerrison mastoid rongeur. *R.* Bane mastoid rongeur. (Courtesy of Codman & Shurtleff, Inc., Randolph, MA.)

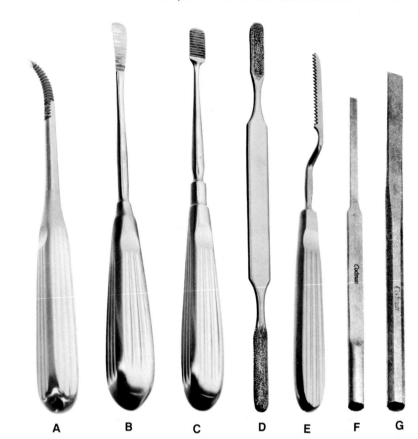

Figure 15-43. Nasal instruments: rasps, chisels, saws. *A.* Wiener antrum rasp. *B.* Aufricht rasp. *C.* Lewis rasp. *D.* Fomon rasp. *E.* Joseph saw, bayonet shank. *F.* Sheehan nasal chisel. *G.* Cottle chisel. (Courtesy of Codman & Shurtleff, Inc., Randolph, MA.)

A   B   C   D   E   F   G

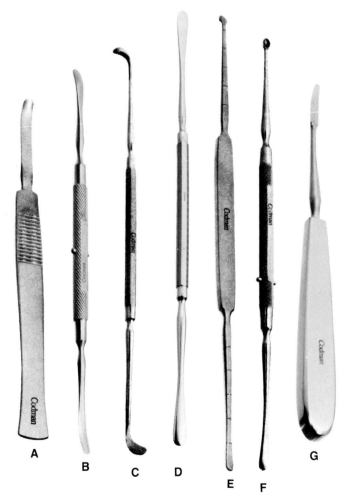

A   B   C   D   E   F   G

Figure 15-44. Nasal instruments: elevators. *A.* MacKenty septal elevator. *B.* Freer double-ended septal elevator. *C.* Pennington septum elevator. *D.* Ballenger septal elevator. *E.* Cottle graduated elevator. *F.* Carter elevator and curette. *G.* Joseph periosteal elevator. (Courtesy of Codman & Shurtleff, Inc., Randolph, MA.)

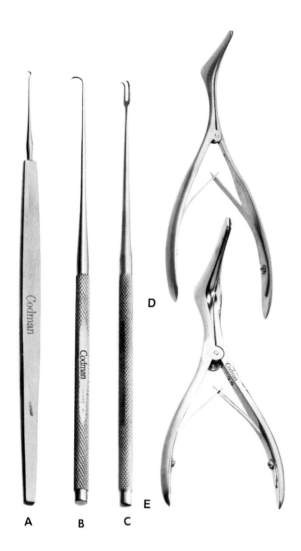

Figure 15–45. Nasal instruments. *A.* Gillies skin hook. *B.* Joseph single prong hook. *C.* Double prong hook. *D.* Vienna speculum. *E.* Killian speculum. (Courtesy of Codman & Shurtleff, Inc., Randolph, MA.)

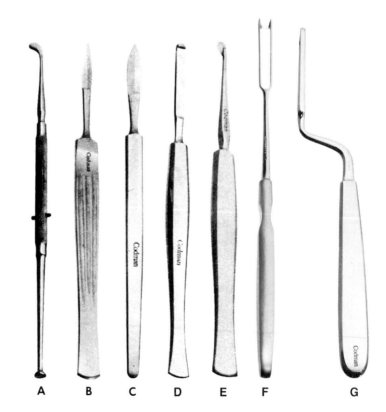

Figure 15–46. Nasal instruments. *A.* Freer septal knife. *B.* Joseph knife. *C.* Cottle knife. *D.* Joseph button knife. *E.* Freer mucosa knife. *F.* Ballenger swivel knife. *G.* Ballenger swivel knife, bayonet shaped. (Courtesy of Codman & Shurtleff, Inc., Randolph, MA.)

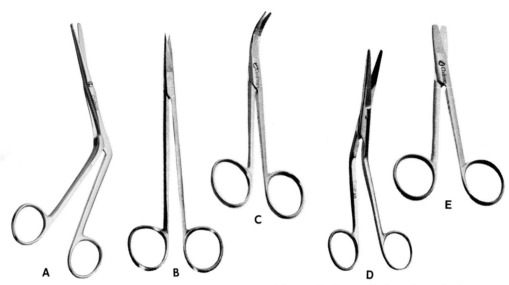

Figure 15–47. Nasal instruments: scissors. *A.* Knight nasal scissors. *B.* Joseph nasal scissors. *C.* Fomon upper lateral scissors. *D.* Cottle dorsal scissors. *E.* Cottle bulldog scissors. (Courtesy of Codman & Shurtleff, Inc., Randolph, MA.)

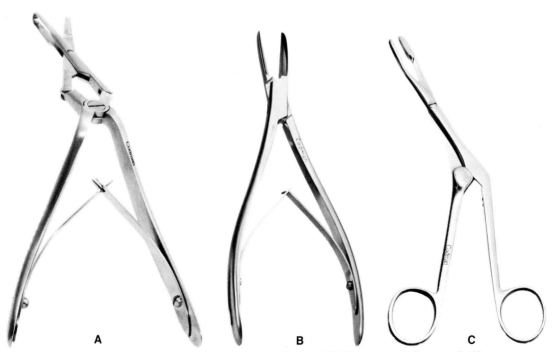

Figure 15–48. Nasal instruments: forceps. *A.* Jansen-Middleton septal forceps. *B.* Kazanjian nasal hump forceps. *C.* Knight septum-cutting forceps. (Courtesy of Codman & Shurtleff, Inc., Randolph, MA.)

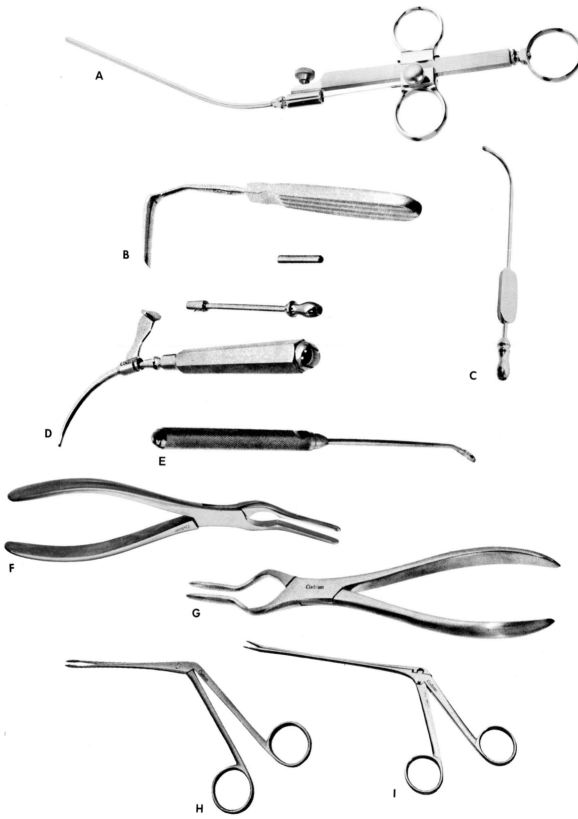

Figure 15–49. Nasal instruments: miscellaneous. *A.* Krause nasal snare. *B.* Aufricht retractor. *C.* Killian antrum cannula. *D.* Coakley antrum trocar. *E.* Nasal curettes. *F.* Asch nasal-straightening forceps. *G.* Walsham septum-straightening forceps. *H.* Hartmann nasal-dressing forceps. *I.* Noyes nasal-dressing forceps. (Courtesy of Codman & Shurtleff, Inc., Randolph, MA.)

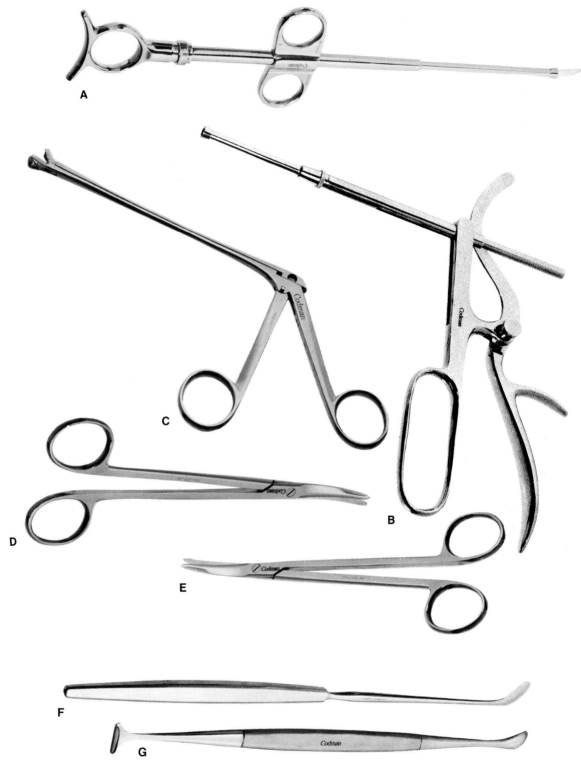

Figure 15–50. Tonsil and adenoid instruments. *A.* Eves tonsillar snare. *B.* Beck-Schenck tonsil snare. *C.* Schmeden tonsillar punch. *D.* Dean tonsillar scissors. *E.* Prince tonsillar scissors. *F.* Fisher tonsil knife (hockey stick). *G.* Hurd tonsil dissector and pillar retractor.

Illustration continued on following page

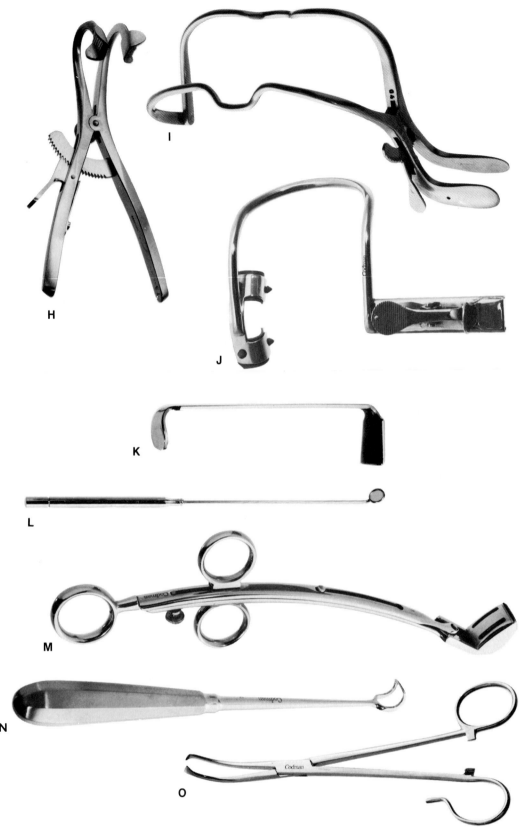

Figure 15–50 *Continued. H.* Denhardt mouth gag. *I.* Jennings mouth gag. *J.* Davis mouth gag. *K.* Davis tooth plate. *L.* Laryngeal mirror. *M.* LaForce adenotome. *N.* Barnhill adenoid curette. *O.* White tonsil-seizing forceps.

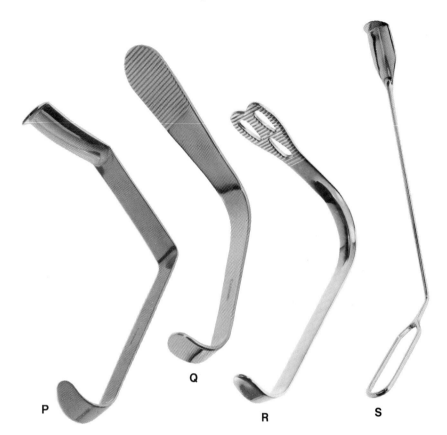

Figure 15–50 *Continued.* *P.* Love uvula retractor. *Q.* Andrews tongue depressor. *R.* Weder tongue depressor (cloverleaf retractor). *S.* Lothrop uvula retractor. (Courtesy of Codman & Shurtleff, Inc., Randolph, MA.)

During Surgery

1. Handle instruments gently.
2. Do not throw instruments into basins.
3. Keep the sharp surfaces of cutting instruments away from other metal surfaces that could dull them.
4. Do not soak or rinse instruments in saline solution. Saline causes corrosion.
5. When feasible, wipe blood from instruments. Avoid allowing blood to cake and dry on the instrument.
6. Use the correct instrument for the job at hand. Heavy needles mounted on delicate needle holders will damage the jaws and ratchets of the instrument. Hemostats are designed for use on delicate vessels and should never be used for prying or pulling at hard objects. Wire sutures must be cut with wire cutters, not suture scissors. Use towel clips and not hemostats for securing drapes.

After Surgery

1. Decontaminate instruments in the washer-sterilizer as soon as possible (see Chapter 6). Do not allow blood to dry and cake on the instruments.
2. Use accepted techniques when sterilizing instruments.
3. Separate sharp or delicate instruments from others when processing.
4. Process all instruments from a surgical case, whether or not they have been used.

HOW TO MEMORIZE INSTRUMENT NAMES

One of the greatest challenges to the student technologist or nurse is to memorize the names of surgical instruments. However, as in most disciplines, if a method is used, the task will be easier. The following are some helpful guidelines:

1. Do not try to memorize more than a *few* instrument names in one sitting. Develop a goal to memorize five to ten instruments a day and then follow through with this plan. It is better to memorize a few instruments well than many whose names you will be unsure of.
2. Review daily those instruments that you memorized in the previous session. Those whose names you are still unsure of must be added to the new list. Reduce the number of instruments in the new list to accommodate those that must be repeated.
3. Do not try to memorize instruments out of context. In other words, do not try to memorize the name of an orthopedic retractor along with that of a cardiovascular clamp. If the memorization groups are pictured together, such as in this chapter, it is easier to have a mental picture of the instruments and remember the names.
4. Try to remember the nicknames given to instruments used in your hospital. These help in memorization because they often describe the instrument in an anecdotal way.
5. If you find that you are unable to memorize a given number of instruments in one sitting, reduce the

number. Some persons are more adept at memorization than others. Do what you can do comfortably.

6. One of the quickest ways to memorize instruments is to assist in the assembly of instrument trays. Do not pass up an opportunity to take advantage of this valuable learning activity.

7. As a student, you will encounter many instruments with which you are unfamiliar. During surgery, do not become frustrated or upset that you do not know the names of each instrument. They will become familiar to you with time and exposure.

8. Memorization experts tell us that *association* is the surest method to memorize something. Try to associate the name of an instrument with an object, phrase, or acronym that is familiar. For example, you might remember the *B*eckman retractor because it is used in *B*ack surgery.

9. Many surgeons identify instruments by their type only. For example, few would ask for a "Lahey thyroid tenaculum," especially if it is the only tenaculum in the thyroid tray. In many cases, it is sufficient to know the generic name of instruments (in this case, the surgeon would probably request a "thyroid retractor"). Familiarity with your hospital's instrument trays and the surgeons' own particular methods of identification will make memorization easier.

Surgical Routines and Emergencies

Learning Objectives

After reading this chapter, you should be able to

♦ *Understand* the sequence of events in a surgical procedure.
♦ *Demonstrate* teamwork and courtesy in professional relationships.
♦ *Respond appropriately* to different types of surgical emergencies.
♦ *Understand* why a registered nurse must fulfill the role of circulator during all surgical procedures.

Key Terms

Bovie cleaner: Small, rough-surfaced pad used to clean the electrocautery tip during surgery.
case assignments: Written schedule of each team member's assigned surgical cases for the day.
code blue: Alert signal given during cardiopulmonary arrest anywhere in the hospital.
code red: Alert signal given when a fire occurs in thechospital.
endotracheal tube fire: A fire that occurs within the patient's endotracheal tube during laser surgery that causes immediate and severe trauma to the lungs.
lavage: Irrigation of body cavities. During malignant hyperthermia, cold saline is used to lower the patient's temperature.
malignant hyperthermia: Anesthetic-related phenomenon that causes the patient's temperature to rise suddenly and become critically high. Emergency procedures are initiated during this crisis.
specimen: Any tissue, foreign body, prosthesis, or fluid that is removed from the patient.
surgeon's preference card: File card that contains information pertaining to suture materials, equipment, or special instruments used by a particular surgeon.
teamwork: Cooperation in working toward a common goal by giving the goal the highest priority.

triage: Classification system used during major disasters such as earthquakes, air accidents, or industrial explosions. Victims are classified according to the severity of their condition and are treated in a corresponding order.

The clinical rotation that takes place in the student technologist's or nurse's teaching institution can, at first, be daunting. The purpose of this chapter is to combine the practical skills discussed in previous chapters and place them in a time-oriented sequence. The description of a routine surgical procedure, its flow and direction from start to finish, places events and the skills required by operating room personnel in their proper order. This will help to prioritize duties and thereby increase efficiency. Also included in this chapter are events that disrupt that flow—emergency situations. During any emergency in any workplace, the outcome of the emergency may depend largely on how persons react to the situation. By understanding the source or cause of the emergency, and by knowing what, if any, are the specific duties of each person involved, personnel are better able to help bring the situation under control safely and efficiently. In an operating room the behavior expected of personnel during both routine cases and emergencies may vary according to each institution's policies.

PREPARATION FOR THE DAY'S WORK

When surgical personnel enter the operating room they do so through the employee locker or changing rooms. After properly donning surgical attire, they may proceed to the restricted areas of the department and receive their case assignments for the day.

Case Assignments

Case assignments are made by the nurse manager. These decisions are based on the availability of staff,

each person's expertise, and the estimated duration of each procedure. The assignment of cases takes time and consideration and is not a topic of dispute or disagreement. All team members should accept their assignments willingly and proceed to work. The technologist and nurse receive their assignments from the *surgical schedule*. The schedule is first written in a scheduling book or entered in a computer when the surgeon or office nurse "books" the case. Each evening the schedule may then be transferred to a large board near the nurse manager's office. Posted on the board are the patient's name and age, the time the procedure will start, the procedure to be performed, and the suite in which the procedure will take place. Also included is the type of anesthesia to be administered. A typical schedule might look like the one presented in Table 16–1.

Gathering Supplies

Once the technologist or scrub nurse has noted his or her assignment, he or she locates the *surgeon's preference card* (Fig. 16–1). Preference cards are usually kept alphabetically in a file box in the workroom or in some other convenient location. These cards describe the surgeon's preference for suture material and special instruments, his or her glove size, and other information that the technologist or scrub nurse and circulator need to know. Preference cards must be updated whenever a surgeon changes his or her routine so that the next team to use the card is ready for the case. Cards must always be returned to the file as soon as possible because they contain valuable information that must be accessible to all personnel.

Next, the technologist or circulator (or both) gathers

Table 16–1. SURGERY SCHEDULE

Suite	Time	Patient	Age	Procedure	Surgeon(s)	Anesthetic	Anesthesiologist	Room Team
1	7:45	Brown, Sally	24	Repeat C-Section/BTL	Gabbs/Smith	Spinal	C	R/J
1	TF	Peters, John	57	Repair Ing. Hernia	Moser/Jones	Gen.	C	B/W
1	TF	Finch, Susan	42	Cholecystectomy	Gallo/Jones	Gen.	C	B/W
2	7:45	Morrel, Jack	31	Arthroscopy/Poss. Meniscectomy Rt. Knee	Rudkin/Welch	Gen.	B	D/M
2	9:00	Thomas, Bill	92	Open Reduction Rt. Hip	Rudkin/Welch	Spinal	B	D/M
2	1:00	Taylor, Mary	90	Débridement Decubitus Ulcer Lt. Foot	Wolf/Raney	Spinal	B	R/J
3	7:45	Martin, Toni	5	T & A	Marshall	Gen.	R	A/P
3	8:45	Wilson, Nina	78	Exc. Cataract Lt.	Wells/Briston	Local		A/P
3	TF	Olsen, Martha	56	Exc. Rt. Breast Mass, F.S., Poss. Rt. Radical Mastectomy	Jackson/Jones	Gen.	R	A/P

Abbreviations: BTL, bilateral tubal ligation; TF, to follow; Ing., inguinal; Poss., possible; Rt., right; Lt., left; Exc., excision; F.S., frozen section; T & A, tonsillectomy and adenoidectomy.

SURGEON: *Dr. Hawkins*	PROCEDURE: *Ventral Hernia*
GLOVE SIZE: *8*	POSITION OF PATIENT: *Supine*
SKIN PREP: *Betadine scrub and paint*	DRAPES: *Towels, lap sheet*

SUTURES AND NEEDLES	INSTRUMENTS AND EQUIPMENT
TIES: *3-0 Dexon* PERITONEUM: *0 Chromic atr. #924* FASCIA: *0 Dexon - lg. Mayo needles* SUB-CU: *3-0 Dexon lg. Ferg. needles* SKIN: *4-0 silk atr. Keith needle* RETENTION: *#2 Nylon uses rubber* OTHER: *bolsters* *0 Dexon atr. if mesh is inserted*	BASIC: *Major linen pack* *Major basin pack* *Lap instruments* SPECIAL: *Bovie, suction, plastic drape #1050* *Extra allis clamps!* *Irrigates sub-cu after closure.* *Stands on pt's. right*
DRESSINGS: *Telfa, 4x4's - Paper tape only (doesn't like silk tape)*	

Figure 16–1. Surgeon's preference card. (Reproduced by permission of Ethicon, Inc., Somerville, NJ.)

supplies needed for the case. In many hospitals the instruments and supplies for the first cases of the day are "picked" (or "pulled") the previous afternoon or evening by the previous shift's personnel. Because supplies are often located in different areas of the operating room, they are loaded onto a cart or table. Later, after the supplies are gathered, they are brought into the suite designated for the case. If a case cart system is in use (see Chapter 6), most of the supplies will arrive by way of the clean corridor or a dumbwaiter. The supplies should be checked off against the surgeon's preference card well in advance of the procedure so that if an item is missing it can be received from the central processing department in time.

"Opening" the Case

Supplies are opened after the operating suite has been damp dusted with a hospital-grade antiseptic (see Chapter 6). Linen packs are opened first onto the back table (instrument table) so that a large sterile field is available on which the other supplies can be opened. Individual supplies are opened randomly or according to operating room policy. Care should be taken that supplies are not placed so that they lie precariously on the edge of the table. Any wrapped supplies that are accidentally dropped onto the floor must not be opened onto the sterile field. If an item is dropped, regardless of whether it is still wrapped, it must be resterilized. Knife blades

that are dangerously sharp should be opened so that they are conspicuous; they must never lie hidden under other supplies where they might injure the scrub technologist or nurse as the supplies are arranged. The scrub technologist's or nurse's drying towel, gown, and gloves are placed in a conspicuous location on top of other supplies or on a separate table. Ideally, after the supplies are opened someone should stay in the room to protect them from accidental contamination. Once the supplies are set up, the scrub assistant proceeds to the scrub sink while the circulator reviews the patient's chart to verify identity, site and side of procedure, and completion of preoperative orders. The sequence of these events may vary from hospital to hospital. In some operating rooms, the nurse manager or supervisor checks in the patient while the supplies are being opened.

Table Set-up

One of the more difficult operating room skills is the ability to set up the back table quickly and neatly. The back table may be piled high with instruments, drapes, suction tubing, suture materials, electrocautery equipment, sponges, and many more items. The key to an orderly and efficient table and Mayo stand set-up is to *follow a routine.* Every scrub assistant can develop his or her own routine; and if this routine is followed faithfully, speed and efficiency will be increased. As the technologist performs the set-up, he or she should mentally rehearse the operative procedure by asking *what* is needed and *in what order* it is required. After gowning and gloving, the following tasks need to be done:

1. Arrange draping materials, gowns, and gloves in order of use.

2. Drape the Mayo stand (Fig. 16–2). Select and arrange instruments that are frequently used or those that will be needed at the beginning of the case on the Mayo stand.

3. Prepare suture materials.

4. Uncoil electrocautery pencils and suction tubing and place them with drapes. (These items are placed on the sterile field as soon as draping has been completed.)

5. Mount knife blades on handles.

6. Prepare any accessory supplies (e.g., bone wax, topical hemostatics).

7. Arrange basins and cups in an orderly fashion on the back table. Place them near the edge of the table so that the circulator has easy access to them.

8. Participate in the sponge, needle, and instrument counts. (The procedure for sponge, needle, and instrument counts is discussed in detail in Chapter 13.)

While the scrub assistant is arranging instruments and preparing supplies, the anesthesiologist has usually entered the room with the patient, and the circulator must be available to assist him or her. The circulator must stand by during induction of anesthesia and remain at the patient's side until the anesthesiologist no longer needs assistance.

Teamwork With Circulator

If the technologist is the scrub assistant in a surgical case, the circulator is his or her partner. The technologist is dependent on the circulator for all supplies needed after the case has started, and the circulator is the technologist's ally in case of emergency. As the technologist completes his or her work, he or she must be aware of the circulator's responsibilities. The technologist should not ask the circulator for items while the

circulator is assisting the anesthesiologist or occupied with setting up a complex piece of equipment. A sense of timing and courtesy is important. Before insisting that the circulator dash to the other end of the department for an instrument, the technologist should decide whether the item is really needed now or if the circulator can get it later when activities have subsided. Likewise, the circulator should recognize when the technologist is at a stopping point in the table set-up and when it is convenient to take the first sponge, needle, and instrument counts. Instead of making several requests at different times for equipment, the technologist should make a mental note of needed items so that the circulator can obtain all the items at one time. Remember that *teamwork is cooperation toward a common goal.* Additionally, courtesy is always appreciated.

Gowning and Gloving the Surgeons and Draping the Patient

When the surgeons enter the operating room suite, the technologist greets them and offers each a sterile towel. The scrub assistant then gowns and gloves each surgeon. The surgeon in first authority is gowned and gloved first and then his or her assistant is gowned and gloved. After gloving, the technologist offers the surgeon a moist towel so that glove powder can be wiped off. This towel must then be discarded away from the surgical field. Draping of the patient follows immediately. In most hospitals, the scrub technologist assists in draping by handing the drapes to the surgeons in order and assisting in their proper placement. Once the patient is draped, the electrocautery pencil and suction tubing are clamped to the procedure (top) drape, close to the surgical site. When placing these items, the technologist must make certain that there is enough slack to allow access to all points on the surgical site. For most procedures, the Mayo stand is then positioned below the surgical site, opposite the surgeon. The Mayo stand must not touch the patient at any point. The technologist should stand opposite the surgeon, at the Mayo stand, unless told otherwise. Two sponges are placed near the

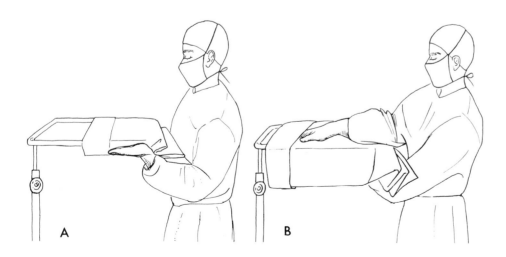

Figure 16–2. *A* and *B*. Technique for draping the Mayo stand. Note that the hand is cuffed to prevent its contamination. (From Ginsberg F, et al: A Manual of Operating Room Technology. Philadelphia, JB Lippincott, 1966.)

A

B

surgical site. The team is now ready to begin the procedure.

INTRAOPERATIVE ROUTINES

The technologist's primary functions during the procedure are to watch the field, listen to the surgeon's requests, and anticipate the need for specific instruments or other supplies. It is his or her duty to keep the field clear of instruments. Soiled sponges are dropped into the kick bucket, and fresh ones are supplied to the surgeons. The technologist guards the field from contamination and notifies the surgeons in case they contaminate their gown or gloves. The technologist handles the instruments as little as possible. Additional responsibilities are to keep the electrocautery pencil clean by scraping the debris *away* from the wound with the blunt side of a scalpel blade or other instrument or Bovie cleaner and to clear the suction of blood clots by occasionally running some saline solution or water through it.

INSTRUMENTATION

Anticipation of the need for instruments requires general knowledge of surgical technique and specific understanding of the procedure itself. Most instrumentation is quite logical. For example, when the surgeon requests a suture or free tie, he or she will need scissors to cut the suture or a clamp to tag the ends. When a bleeding vessel is encountered, the electrocautery pencil or a clamp is handed to the surgeon.

Hand Signals

Many surgeons use hand signals to indicate which instrument is needed. The signal for a hemostat (clamp) is shown in Figure 16–3. The technologist judges what size clamp to pass according to his or her knowledge of the depth and strength of the tissue to be clamped. *This knowledge comes with practice and experience.* The

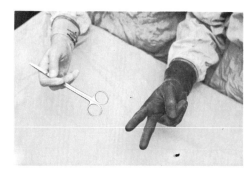

Figure 16–4. Hand signal for scissors. (From Nealon TF: Fundamental Skills in Surgery, 3rd ed. Philadelphia, WB Saunders, 1979.)

signal for scissors is illustrated in Figure 16–4. When requesting the scalpel (knife), the surgeon positions his or her hand as if holding the knife. The technologist passes it with the blade down and the handle pointed toward the surgeon's hand (Fig. 16–5). The surgeon will grasp it between the thumb and index finger. When passing the knife, the technologist must be certain that the surgeon has it firmly before releasing it; otherwise, the knife could fall onto the patient and cause injury. When passing thumb forceps, the technologist should grasp the end and place it between the surgeon's thumb and index finger, as shown in Figure 16–6. When a suture is needed, the surgeon may make a fist and turn it in a half-circle, simulating the motion required to suture (Fig. 16–7). The technologist then passes the needle holder with the suture and needle attached so that it is ready for immediate use, without having to be repositioned by the surgeon. When the surgeon needs a free tie, he or she simply holds his or her hand out, palm down, since this is the position of the hand while tying the blood vessel. The technologist grasps the tie by its ends and brings it in firm contact with the surgeon's palm, as shown in Figure 16–8.

The technologist should pass an instrument with a firm and definite motion. Thus, the surgeon knows that he or she has received the instrument and will not have to look up from the wound. Painfully hard slapping of instruments must be avoided. Efficient passing will produce a gentle, sharp snap as the instrument contacts the surgeon's palm. Heavy instruments such as retractors

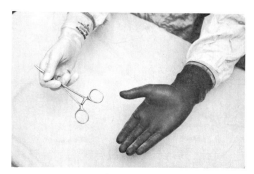

Figure 16–3. Hand signal for a hemostat. (From Nealon TF: Fundamental Skills in Surgery, 3rd ed. Philadelphia, WB Saunders, 1979.)

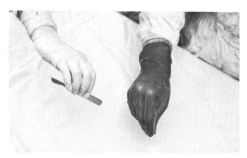

Figure 16–5. Hand signal for the scalpel. (From Nealon TF: Fundamental Skills in Surgery, 3rd ed. Philadelphia, WB Saunders, 1979.)

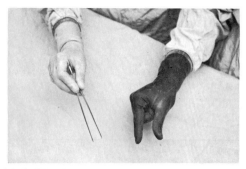

Figure 16–6. Hand signal for forceps. (From Nealon TF: Fundamental Skills in Surgery, 3rd ed. Philadelphia, WB Saunders, 1979.)

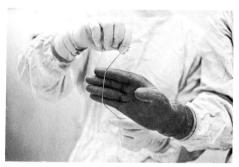

Figure 16–8. Hand signal for a free tie. (From Nealon TF: Fundamental Skills in Surgery, 3rd ed. Philadelphia, WB Saunders, 1979.)

and orthopedic instruments should be handed over gently.

Selection of Long or Short Instruments

It seems obvious that if the surgeon is working deep within the abdomen or chest, he or she will need instruments that are long enough to reach into the wound. However, the decision of when to use long instruments (general surgery instruments that are longer than usual) may not be straightforward. For example, many cholecystectomy procedures require long instruments because of the position of the gallbladder in the abdomen. If, however, the patient is very thin and small, long instruments will usually be unnecessary. It is wise to observe the patient when he or she is brought into the operating room in case the need arises for long instruments or extra-large retractors.

If the surgeon requests a clamp while working deep within the abdomen or chest, he or she probably wants a long hemostatic clamp, such as a Mixter or Péan clamp. However, a shorter clamp may be needed, such as a Kelly or Crile, to tag suture ends. By *watching* the wound site, the technologist can deduce the length of the clamp that is actually needed.

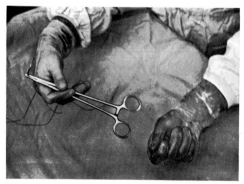

Figure 16–7. Hand signal for suture. (From Nealon TF: Fundamental Skills in Surgery, 3rd ed. Philadelphia, WB Saunders, 1979.)

SPECIMENS

As the procedure continues, the surgeon may announce "specimen." This means that a specimen, either tissue or fluid, is about to be delivered to the technologist. A sterile basin is made available and the specimen is placed on the back table. The specimen can be passed on to the circulator *only* after the surgeon has granted permission for its removal from the sterile field. (He or she may wish to examine it later during the case.) Specimens are always sent to the pathology department after the case. Some specimens for determination of suspected malignancy require immediate examination by the pathologist. In these cases the pathologist enters the surgical suite and performs a *frozen section*. To do this, the pathologist freezes a small amount of tissue and passes it through a slicing device called a *microtome*. The thin slices are placed on a glass slide, stained, and examined under the microscope. The surgeons are then informed whether the tissue is malignant. They may decide that additional surgery is needed. Because the pathologist is available to perform tissue examination during the procedure, the patient is spared a second procedure and anesthetic at a later date.

Routine handling of specimens requires some basic guidelines. All team members should study the following rules and adjust them to hospital policy, as needed.

1. Never hand the specimens over on a surgical sponge. The sponge might be taken out of the room, thus confusing the table count, or the specimen might be thrown away accidentally.

2. Specimens should be kept moistened (not soaking, unless specifically requested by the surgeon) in saline solution until ready for permanent preservation.

3. In some cases, multiple specimens are handed over to the technologist for frozen section. Each specimen must be carefully labeled and identified by both the technologist or scrub nurse and the circulator. Multiple specimens usually indicate the perimeter of a cancerous lesion. If a mistake is made in identification, the surgeon may dissect away tissue that is not diseased, causing unnecessary trauma or disfigurement to the patient.

4. A preservative such as formalin is often used to store permanent specimens. Tissue bound for frozen

section must *never* be placed in formalin since this substance reacts with the tissue, thus affecting the pathologist's diagnosis.

5. Kidney stones are never placed in formalin because their chemical composition (useful as a diagnostic tool) is changed by the preservative. Stones are sent to the pathology department in a dry container.

6. *All* tissue and foreign matter that come from the patient's body during surgery must be sent to pathology for examination. This includes items such as orthopedic implants (e.g., screws, plates, wires) and also foreign bodies (e.g., bullets).

7. If more than one specimen is obtained, each must be placed in a separate container and properly labeled as to type and location (left or right and exact region of the body).

8. *The technologist and nurse are both legally responsible for the proper handling of tissue specimens.*

9. The outside of the specimen containers, if touched by the surgical team, must be decontaminated before being sent to the pathology department.

COMMUNICATION

Because talking during surgery presents a threat of wound contamination and because excessive talking can distract and annoy team members, communication during surgery should be almost exclusively nonverbal. The technologist usually communicates with the circulator with his or her eyes and hands. Sometimes the surgeon communicates the possibility of an emergency situation. An alert technologist and nurse may note the surgeon's change in tone and manner. The surgeon may simply be having difficulty with the procedure, or there may be a dangerous situation arising.

It is important at all times that verbal communication be heard *the first time*. Voices muffled behind masks are drowned out by suction, electrocautery, respirator, and other equipment. Requests to the circulator should be made politely and audibly.

COMPLETION OF THE PROCEDURE—FINAL COUNT

When the procedure is completed (except for wound closure), the surgeon requests suture for the first tissue layer. As soon as the technologist has passed the suture to the surgeon and suture scissors to the assistant, a sponge and needle count must be taken. If a sponge or needle is missing, the technologist or nurse informs the surgeon immediately. The surgeon may choose to halt any further closure until the item is found. If the surgeon is quite certain that the missing object is not within the wound, he or she will continue to close. In many cases the item is found before closure has been completed. Sponges are often "lost" between the folds of the drapes or caught between the surgeon's waist and table. Needles are also often found stuck to the bottom of one

of the team member's shoes, on the floor, or beneath a basin on the back table. If the item is *not* found, a radiograph of the operative site is ordered. This may take place during wound closure or in the post-anesthesia care unit, according to the surgeon's request. The incident must be documented whether or not the item is found within the patient or even if it is never located. Lost items are a serious matter. Even if the item is found within the patient or in another location, the patient is charged for the radiograph, an expense possibly resulting from carelessness.

Following operating room policy, the third count is taken before skin closure. If all sponges and needles are accounted for, the circulator should announce to the surgeons that the final count is correct. At this time the circulator distributes the wound dressings to the technologist. After skin closure, the technologist assists in cleaning the wound site with wet and dry sponges. The dressings are placed over the incision and the drapes removed. The circulator or surgeon then applies nonsterile tape to the dressings. The technologist should not contaminate the Mayo stand until the patient has left the room.

At the completion of the case, it is the responsibility of the entire team to remain in the room until the patient is prepared for transfer to the post-anesthesia care unit. The patient is first transferred to a stretcher by the team; at least four persons are needed for the transfer. The patient may be raised by the draw sheet and lifted onto the stretcher, or a special (Davis) roller may be employed to complete the transfer. Refer to Chapter 10 for a complete discussion of patient transfer. The circulator then accompanies the anesthesiologist and patient to the post-anesthesia care unit.

The technologist stays in the room to disassemble all instruments and supplies. Sharp items such as needles and scalpel blades are separated from the other supplies and placed in a receptacle designated for such items. Specimens are logged into a specimen book and taken to an assigned area so that laboratory personnel can transfer them to the pathology department. Soiled instruments are taken to the workroom or transferred to a central processing area. Terminal decontamination is performed according to Universal Precautions. All disposable items are placed in the garbage, and linen is gathered and placed in the linen hamper where it will be removed by housekeeping personnel. The technologist should not remove his or her protective attire until there is no longer contact with soiled equipment and linen.

EMERGENCIES IN THE OPERATING ROOM

Emergencies, by their very nature, disrupt the usual flow of activities in the operating room. Hence, during any emergency the following guidelines are critical:

1. *Know ahead of time, as much as possible, what to do in an emergency.* For example, the scrub assistant

would not be expected to extinguish a fire occurring outside the department, However, it *is* his or her job to know where fire exits are and how to safely convey patients there. All hospitals publish emergency procedures that apply to every person working there. The technologist must read and memorize these procedures so that he or she is not caught off guard when one occurs.

2. *Follow directions.* During an emergency, usually one or more persons are responsible for directing personnel in either their activities or their movement. The technologist should follow these directions and not dispute or question those who are in charge.

3. *Remain alert.* The technologist must be thinking and aware of surroundings and the situation to be able to help.

4. *Unless in personal danger, do not leave the work area.* The technologist's assistance is needed in the emergency, and his or her absence could cause others to worry needlessly (such as during a fire).

5. *Do one's best.* Persons react in many different ways to an emergency. When under extreme stress a person can only be expected to do the best he or she can.

6. *The patient is the first priority.* In all situations the safety of the patient is given top priority. Whatever the technologist's specific role is in the situation, this priority must be kept foremost in mind.

Massive Hemorrhage

Serious traumatic hemorrhage is a risk whenever large blood vessels are close to or within the surgical wound. The cause of the hemorrhage is unimportant compared with the need for quick action on the part of *all* team members. During massive hemorrhage, three things must be done if the patient is to survive. The surgeon must *expose* the exact site of hemorrhage, *arrest* the bleeding, and *correct* the blood loss. Exposure is essential because the bleeding cannot be stopped until its origin is located. The bleeding may be severe enough to fill the wound completely. Therefore, the technologist must have additional retractors, sponges, and extra suction tubing available. The circulator, once alerted to the situation, will supply the needed equipment. Sponges may be brought to the field *uncounted* to save precious minutes because the patient can die quickly of severe hemorrhage.

Once the bleeding site is located, the surgeon will need clamps and suture material. The surgeon may use his or her hand to place pressure on the site until the clamps are available. Correction of blood loss is the anesthesiologist's responsibility. The circulator assists in starting additional intravenous sites and pumping blood or blood replacers forcibly through the intravenous tubing.

Malignant Hyperthermia

Malignant hyperthermia is a sudden and extreme increase in body temperature that certain patients ex-

perience during general anesthesia. It is associated with gas-vaporized anesthetics and requires immediate action, as it is life threatening. The patient's body temperature may rise to over 109°F. The cause of this condition is believed to be a heritable defect in the cell membrane that allows an abnormal rise of calcium within striated muscle cells. When this occurs, the anesthetic agent in use is immediately interrupted. During surgery, of course, this may mean interruption of the procedure. After the cessation of the gas anesthetic, the anesthesiologist may administer a conscious sedative to the patient to allow the surgeons to close the wound quickly. In all cases, however, all immediate attention is focused on lowering the patient's temperature. This is accomplished with massive amounts of iced saline used to irrigate body cavities (called *lavage*) or given intravenously. Surface cooling is accomplished with a cooling mattress. The only known therapeutic agent that counteracts the effects of malignant hyperthermia is sodium dantrolene (Dantrium), a drug that blocks calcium release by the skeletal muscle cell. Other emergency medical treatments include management of acidosis and kidney function, which are adversely affected during a malignant hyperthermia crisis.

The scrub technologist must first assist the surgeons in closing the operative wound, if applicable, or assist with the cold lavage. It is important to maintain a sterile environment as long as the surgical wound is open unless otherwise directed by the surgeons. Depending on the course of action taken by the surgeons, the scrub assistant's role will be to follow the surgeon's directions implicitly and without question.

Endotracheal Tube Fire

An endotracheal tube fire may occur any time lasers are in use during surgery when the patient is intubated and maintained on mechanical ventilation equipment. The fire, caused by the ignition of free oxygen within the airway, may be either small and "candle-like" or a shooting flame that emerges from the tube's opening. The result is that hot gases are forced into the patient's lungs, causing immediate and severe trauma. Special endotracheal tubes are available to help prevent endotracheal tube fire, but these are not completely effective. During endotracheal tube fire, the following steps are immediately initiated:

1. The breathing circuit is severed from the endotracheal tube. All ties or tapes that anchor the tube to the patient are cut.

2. The endotracheal tube is removed. It is then handed to team personnel to be extinguished.

3. The patient's airway is re-established and ventilated with air until it is determined that nothing is burning in the patient's throat. Oxygen is then administered through the airway.

4. The patient is treated medically according to his or her condition.

5. The endotracheal tube is saved for subsequent evaluation and documentation.

During endotracheal tube fire, the scrub assistant must stand by for instructions from the surgeons. Because surgery is interrupted, consequent actions will vary from case to case. The technologist should remain sterile unless directed otherwise or unless he or she is in personal danger from fire.

The registered nurse circulator will direct technical staff in their actions unless superseded by the anesthesiologist or surgeons. The staff should follow directions implicitly and without question.

Cardiopulmonary Arrest

If the patient suffers a cardiopulmonary arrest, the anesthesiologist and surgeon will administer cardiopulmonary resuscitation (CPR) immediately. If the heart is exposed, the surgeon may initiate open-heart massage while the anesthesiologist maintains a patent airway and administers oxygen. All hospital employees are required to know the techniques of CPR. If arrest occurs when the surgeon or anesthesiologist is not present, two persons must start CPR immediately. Most modern surgical suites are equipped with a special code switch or foot pedal that sets off an alarm indicating an arrest and the room in which it has occurred. Within seconds, additional personnel will be available to aid in resuscitation. It is imperative that all surgical personnel attend a current course in CPR and repeat the course every year. A thorough course and one that medical personnel should attend involves the use of an artificial dummy on which the student can practice.

In the event that the patient dies during surgery, the surgeon makes the decision whether to pronounce death in the operating room or maintain the patient on artificial devices and thus delay death. All hospitals have written policies concerning the handling of the deceased patient, including responsibility for handling the body and preparation of an incident report. All personnel should be familiar with their hospital's guidelines in the event of a patient's death.

Power Failure

When a power failure occurs in surgery, the lights and all other electrical equipment cease to operate. All hospitals are equipped with an alternative power source in case of power failure. However, there are usually a few moments or, in some circumstances, a few minutes of darkness before the alternate source is activated. All team members should know the location of high-intensity flashlights kept in the department for use during a power failure. The circulator is responsible for directing the flashlight beam into the surgical wound.

Fire

Whenever a fire occurs in the hospital, the switchboard operator will announce a fire alert code over the public address system that is familiar to all employees. The most common fire alert code is "Code Red, Code Red," and the location of the fire is given. If the fire is near the operating room, the surgeons are notified immediately. They may elect to stop the procedure, close the patient's wound quickly, and evacuate the area, or they may continue to operate. If the surgeon chooses to continue the procedure, he or she is alerted every few minutes as to the proximity of the fire. As in all hospital emergencies, the hospital has policies that govern the actions of personnel during the crisis. Duties must be carried out quickly and calmly. If the fire is in the operating room, patients are quickly evacuated from the department, the in-line gas valves are closed, and all doors are shut. The supervisor will then direct the nurses and technologists to assist in evacuation procedures outside the department, if necessary.

Major Disaster: Triage

Whenever there is a major disaster near a hospital, such as an aircraft accident, earthquake, or major explosion, victims are brought to the hospital and given a *triage* classification. This places victims into one of three categories so as to make the most efficient use of the medical personnel available to meet the crisis. The three classifications are (1) victims who would live without therapy, (2) those who would survive if given adequate care, and (3) those who would die regardless of what was done.

According to hospital policy, the fire department, and/or the police or sheriff's department, every hospital employee has a certain duty or station during triage. This may be ascertained by reading the hospital's disaster plan. In addition, designated areas of the hospital are assigned for specific purposes, such as a place in which to classify victims, a place for the deceased, and a place for spiritual comfort. Most cities have disaster plan drills at least once a year so that those involved can "practice" in case of a real emergency. During these practice sessions, "victims" (actually play-acting) are sometimes used to help make the practice more realistic. The practice sessions involve the entire personnel of the hospital, including surgery personnel, the fire department, and the police department. These can be successful only if taken seriously. All surgery personnel should study the hospital's disaster plan carefully so as to be prepared for a disaster *before* it occurs.

Questions for Study and Review

1. Where are case assignments posted in your hospital?

2. Who is responsible for damp dusting the operating room before a case set-up in your hospital?

3. How can you increase the efficiency and shorten the time needed to do a case set-up?

4. What area of the set-up takes you the most time? What have you done to increase efficiency?

5. Under what circumstances should a sponge, needle, and instrument count be omitted?

6. What are the characteristics of the person who gets along best with everyone in the operating room?

7. Under what circumstances does the relationship between the circulator and the scrub assistant become strained?

8. List four reasons why you believe that a registered nurse should be in the room to act as a circulator at all times?

9. What is malignant hypothermia?

10. What are the duties of the scrub assistant during massive hemorrhage?

11. What supplies or equipment do you think would be needed in the event of cardiac arrest during surgery?

12. Name four different types of specimens (i.e., gallstones, hernia sac) and describe how they should be handled before being sent to the pathologist.

13. Name the three triage classifications.

Bibliography

Association of Operating Room Nurses: Recommended Practices for Documentation of Perioperative Nursing Care, Denver, 1991.

Association of Operating Room Nurses: Recommended Practices for Sanitation in the Surgical Practice Setting, Denver, 1992.

Koener M, et al: Communicating in the operating room. AORN J 36(1), 1982.

Reducing the risk of endotracheal tube fires. Todays OR Nurse January 1991, p. 39.

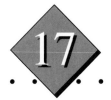

Communicating with the Surgical Patient

Learning Objectives

After reading this chapter you should be able to

♦ *Understand* what patient care plans are and why they are developed by the registered nurse.
♦ *Discuss* the common psychological concerns of the surgical patient.
♦ *Understand* the special needs of the pediatric patient.
♦ *Understand* the special needs of the elderly patient.
♦ *Become aware of* certain cultural and ethnic differences that affect the surgical patient.

Key Terms

alienation: The patient's emotional and physical separation from home, loved ones, work environment, and community.
compassion: Expression of care and support given by surgical team members.
patient care plan: Extensive written plan that outlines the patient's physical, social, psychological, and spiritual needs.
patient fears: Fears shared by many surgical patients, including fear of death or mutilation and fear of anesthesia, pain, and exposure.
perioperative nursing: Nursing care of the patient before, during, and after surgery.
physical restrictions: The patient's inability to move freely in his or her environment. The patient is required to stay within the limits of his or her unit, room, and bed. These restrictions can be very distressing.

THE ROLE OF THE NURSE AND TECHNOLOGIST IN PATIENT COMMUNICATION

The scope, depth, and quality of patient care have advanced tremendously in the past decade. These advances have followed the discovery of new diagnostic techniques, improvements in equipment, and developments in pharmacology. Along with these changes, the nursing profession has developed a new role associated with the care of the surgical patient—*perioperative nursing*. This discipline encompasses the total care of the surgical patient before, during, and after surgery. Included in the duties of the perioperative nurse is the development and implementation of a *preoperative patient care plan*. This plan is based on information collected from the patient's record, other health care workers, patient interviews and observations, and the patient's family.

The development of a patient care plan requires extensive training and practice in psychosocial behavior and in physical and physiologic assessment. The result of these heightened professional standards and skills is that the surgical patient is better equipped to understand, adjust to, and accept both the anticipated and the true outcome of his or her surgery. In addition, the psychological and physical assessment of the preoperative patient is now almost exclusively delegated to the registered nurse. The technologist must strive to preserve these standards of patient care by developing skills in patient interaction. The technologist's functions do not include the formulation of care plans. However, it is important that the technologist understand some common feelings that most surgical patients share.

PSYCHOLOGICAL CONCERNS OF THE SURGICAL PATIENT

Resentment

If the patient is ambulatory or even if he or she is restricted to bed rest through disease or injury, the hospital environment requires that he or she be assigned to a unit, a room, and a bed. These restrictions on their environment can be very disturbing to many patients. Loss of independence causes some patients to feel resentment and anger that may be directed toward those who care for them.

Anxiety

Almost all patients feel anxious about their physical condition and especially about pending surgery. Lack of understanding about the condition or about the surgery itself can contribute greatly to these feelings. The patient may not necessarily question certain procedures, but this is not an indication that he or she is at ease with the procedures. Questions concerning the procedure should be answered clearly and honestly. However, any questions concerning the *outcome of the procedure* or those that touch on the medical aspects of the patient's condition must be referred to the physician.

Fear

Fear of death, exposure, mutilation, and pain are some of the common threats felt by patients. These fears are especially strong in children, who may not have the intellectual capacity to understand the hospital environment. Trust in those caring for the patient and confidence in the level of care often helps to alleviate these fears. Every effort should be made to instill this trust in the patient. The technologist must answer questions that are within the scope of his or her knowledge. If the answer to a question is not known, or if it involves topics that are outside the person's scope of practice, then the nurse should tell the patient so.

Alienation

Many patients, especially children, feel extremely anxious over their separation from family and loved ones. The nurse, technologist, and other care givers in the hospital environment are temporary replacements for those persons who are emotionally prominent in each patient's life. It is very important, therefore, to offer comfort and security to help ease the feelings of abandonment that many patients experience.

SPECIAL NEEDS OF THE PEDIATRIC PATIENT

Interaction with the pediatric patient presents a particular challenge. Young children do not understand the surgical environment, and team members must approach children with an awareness of their fears to protect them from an experience that may be emotionally damaging.

Anxiety due to separation from the family is the child's most overwhelming feeling. He or she may feel abandoned permanently (Fig. 17–1). To combat these feelings, the technologist or nurse who greets and cares for the child during his or her stay in the operating room should reassure the child that he or she will be reunited with his or her parents and loved ones soon after surgery. Sometimes anxiety can be reduced if the child is allowed to bring a familiar object such as a stuffed toy into surgery. If a toy is brought into surgery, an identification tag should be attached to it so that it is not lost. Loss of the toy could be very distressing to the young patient. As soon as it can be removed from the patient, it should be taken to the post-anesthesia care unit or the patient's room. Extensive preoperative care plans include the nurse's visit to the child before surgery. During these visits the child is allowed to see the nurse in operating room attire (Fig. 17–2). This sometimes helps prevent fears.

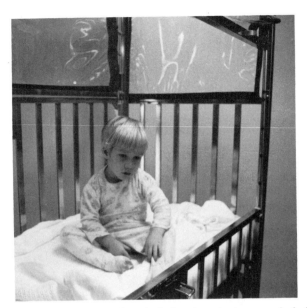

Figure 17–1. Many children feel abandoned, alone, and afraid while awaiting surgery.

Fear of anesthesia is very strong in children. They do not understand the state of unconsciousness and often equate it with death. Since the development of intravenous, intramuscular, and rectal anesthetic agents, children are now spared a long induction period, during which many children are prone to fight or resist the rubber anesthesia mask. Patients younger than the age of 2 years may be held and cradled during induction. All pediatric patients should be dealt with truthfully about injections and pain because many children recognize deception quickly and may lose trust in those who care for them. Most children respond positively when encouraged to be brave.

SPECIAL NEEDS OF THE ELDERLY PATIENT

Because of technologic advances in medicine, an increasing number of elderly patients are now safely admitted to the hospital for surgery. However, because of normal physical and psychological changes that accompany the aging process, many elderly patients require extra care and patience during the entire perioperative period. All patients, no matter what age, have the right to be treated with dignity and respect.

Although there is no proof that intelligence declines with increasing age, some elderly patients may become disoriented or confused when under stress. Compensation must be made under these circumstances, but no patient should be treated in a manner that is condescending or patronizing. Many elderly patients experience depression when taken away from their familiar surroundings and loved ones. Because of this, extra efforts should be made to comfort and orient the patient in the hospital environment. This is especially true in surgery, where the environment is extremely foreign.

Although some patients may have lost some sensory ability with age, not all experience difficulty in hearing or have lost the ability to see and feel. It is sometimes necessary to speak up slightly when addressing an elderly patient, but it is inappropriate and discourteous to shout at every patient who is older than age 60. For those whose hearing is impaired, it is more effective to speak slowly than loudly. The nurse should stay within the patient's sight when speaking to him or her. When caring for an elderly patient the nurse may need to leave his or her mask off when entering the operating room so that the patient can understand instructions and explanations.

Because of their frail tissue, many elderly patients require extra care during transportation and positioning. Because of decreased skeletal mobility, it is important to avoid sudden movements that may harm delicate bones and joints. When elderly patients are transferred to the stretcher or operating table, the transfer should be done slowly and if necessary, extra personnel should be present to complete the move. Particular attention must be given to the protection of prominent skeletal structures. Serious nerve and circulatory trauma can result from inadequate padding during surgery in the older patient whose circulatory system may already be compromised. Particular attention should be paid to evidence of pressure sores, which may be further aggravated by improper positioning or inadequate padding.

CULTURAL INFLUENCES

Differences in language and culture among patients can greatly influence their interactions with medical personnel. Language barriers require that health care personnel use alternative means of communication, such as hand signals. A comforting touch is universal. Cultural variations that occur in a number of ethnic groups are described in Table 17–1.

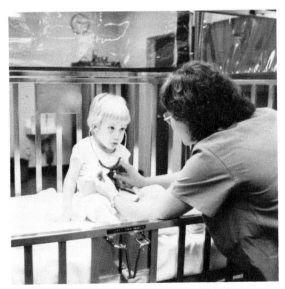

Figure 17–2. The nurse prepares the child for surgery by explaining each step to be taken. Here the nurse allows the patient to see and handle the stethoscope.

Table 17–1. CULTURAL VARIATIONS RELATED TO HEALTH CARE

Ethnic/Culture Group	Social Network	Nutritional Patterns	Health Beliefs and Practices	Folk Medicine and Healers	Unique Illnesses
African Americans	Strong kinship bonds; several generations may live in one household. Strong religious beliefs. This is an important source of psychological support in dealing with stresses associated with illness.	"Soul food" named from a feeling of kinship. Salt pork as a seasoning is key to vegetables, especially black-eyed peas, chicken, and pork. Food is usually boiled or fried.	Relates to African American belief about life and nature of being. Life is a process rather than a state. All things living or dead influence each other. Health is harmony with nature, whereas illness is a state of disharmony. Traditional African Americans view health, mind, body and spirit as one entity.	Roots, herbs, potions, oils, powders, tokens, and rituals are important. Predominately "self-treatment" is used under the direction of the "old lady" spiritualist, voodoo priest, and root doctors.	Sickle cell anemia Hypertension Dermatitides (keloids, vitiligo) Socioenvironmental diseases
Raza/Latina Americans	Close family ties. Courtesy and respect shown toward elderly and adults. Value modesty and privacy. Retain first language and take pride in speaking and reading Spanish.	Food is a form of socialization and consists of what they can afford: usually corn, beans, potatoes, rice, green bananas, and chilies.	Family planning is not discussed and birth control is not used. Diseases are related to spiritual punishment, hot/cold imbalances, witchcraft, dislocation of human organs, natural disease and mental/emotional origin. They use herbs and prayers.	Use herbs and potions as stimulants. Copper bracelets used to treat rheumatoid arthritis. Folk healers are (Curandero) spiritualists, folk chiropractors, midwives, and herbalists.	Anemia in females Parasites Lactose intolerance Lead poisoning Tuberculosis Diabetes Obesity High infant mortality related to malnutrition
Filipino Americans	Family has high value. Inter-dependency among family members stressed. Resources pooled with entire family. Children encouraged to develop modesty, industry, and respect toward elderly.	Hot and cold concepts influence diets. Mothers believe that what they eat affects their infant's health. Diet is influenced by religion. Rice, fish, and vegetables are staples.	Diseases attributed to natural and supernatural causes. Overwork, excessive exposure to cold, heat, and rain, anxiety, excessive eating, and poor living conditions contribute to illness. Curses come from spirits, the dead, witches, and evil persons.	Flushing, heating, and protection are important concepts. Flushing is to rid the body of debris. Heating means that hot and cold in the body must balance. Religious articles are worn to drive evil forces away.	Hyperuricemia Coccidioidomycosis Cardiovascular-renal disease Diabetes mellitus Tuberculosis Cancer of the liver

Table 17–1. CULTURAL VARIATIONS RELATED TO HEALTH CARE *Continued*

Ethnic/Culture Group	Social Network	Nutritional Patterns	Health Beliefs and Practices	Folk Medicine and Healers	Unique Illnesses
Native Americans	Extended family very important and has economic as well as a social function. Family plays a significant role during illness. Many tribes are matrilineal and this requires that decisions for surgery or treatment be discussed with the elder female family members.	Corn, squash, and beans. Corn is used in religious ceremonies. Navajo women drink blue cornmeal gruel after childbirth. They believe that it will increase the supply of milk. Food restrictions are frequently followed for 1 year after delivery of a child. Some persons do not eat certain foods for cultural and religious reasons.	Health is defined as a person's state of harmony with nature and the universe. If a person harms himself or herself, he or she also harms the earth. Forces that prevent persons from achieving harmony put them in a vulnerable and unhealthy state. All ailments have a supernatural aspect. Many persons carry objects to guard against witchcraft.	There are six types of medicine men: 1. Positive role: can transform self into another form 2. Good and evil: can perform negative acts against the enemy 3. Diviner and diagnostician: can diagnose, define cause, and indicate cure but cannot implement treatment 4. Specialist medicine person: can implement treatment 5. Care for the soul: takes care of the spiritual needs 6. Singers: cures by song and laying on of hands	High infant mortality Trachoma Tuberculosis Alcoholism Diabetes mellitus Liver disease Heart disease
Chinese Americans	Close family ties with extended family is very prevalent. Traditionalists have a tendency to cluster around Chinatown. Chinese heritage is preserved. Children are taught to respect elders and have filial piety toward parents.	Rice, tofu, soup, and Chinese vegetables. Food is usually stir-fried. Soy sauce and monosodium glutamate are used as condiments.	Chinese medicine is based on the theory of yin/yang and the five elements. Healing is aimed at re-establishing the balance. Health practices emphasize moderation to avoid excesses that bring on illness. The concept of disease is based on wind and poison. Wind enters the body and causes illness. Poison is used to describe disease conditions.	Herbalists, acupuncturists, and bone setters are all important. Herbs are used to balance the body and prevent illnesses. Soups and teas are used to increase energy, sedate the "hot" condition, and tone the "cold" condition.	Lactose intolerance Alcohol intolerance Tuberculosis Dermatitis

Table continued on following page

Table 17–1. CULTURAL VARIATIONS RELATED TO HEALTH CARE *Continued*

Ethnic/Culture Group	Social Network	Nutritional Patterns	Health Beliefs and Practices	Folk Medicine and Healers	Unique Illnesses
Japanese Americans	The person is seen in relation to the group. The extended family includes the work group, neighborhood and community. Behaviors and all aspects of life are interwoven within the group. Outsiders are not brought in to help solve problems since the group feels responsible for the members. Persons worship ancestors and think about the past.	Tea, fish, vegetables, beef, pork, and poultry. Soy sauce, monosodium glutamate, and miso sauce are used as condiments. Diet is low in total fat, cholesterol, animal protein, and sugar, high in carbohydrates and salt, and very rich in linoleic acid.	Disease is thought to be caused by person coming into contact with polluting agents such as blood, corpses, and skin diseases. Herbal purgatives are used to cleanse the body. Health is achieved through harmony and balance between self and society. Disharmony with society or not taking care of the body results in disease.	Acupuncture, acupressure, massage and moxibustion are used to restore the flow of energy by the use of needles, pressure, or heat at strategic locations along the affected meridians. Natural herbs are also used to help restore equilibrium to the body.	Alcohol intolerance Lactase deficiency Hypertension Cardiovascular accident Cancer of the esophagus, stomach, liver and biliary system Ulcers Colitis Psoriasis
Vietnamese Americans	Strong family-centered culture Emphasis on harmony in social relations. Family interests are first over persons. There is no word for "I" in their language. Kinship system is patrilineal, but females are not relegated to a low status; they share in major decisions.	Rice and fish are cooked in pungent sauce called nuoc-man. Vegetables, fruits, spices, noodle soups, sweets made from rice gluten and coconut. Drinking during meals is rare. Naps follow the noon meal.	Diseases are caused by natural and physical phenomena. Belief that life has been predisposed toward certain events by cosmic forces; therefore, they use astrology and fortune telling to determine these forces. They also believe that mental illnesses are caused by bad spirits that must be exorcised by a sorcerer. Concept of yin/yang is also important.	Health depends on maintaining a balance of bodily elements. Cure is dependent on restoring the balance. Foods and illness are believed to be related to hot and cold. Women avoid eating some hot and cold foods during pregnancy so the body's balance is not disturbed and they will not be susceptible to illness. They also avoid visiting shrines believed to be inhabited by bad spirits due to affects on the unborn child. Healers are generalists or specialists. Generalists have powers from supreme being. They use talismans, magic cloths, prayers and Sino-Vietnamese medical practices. Specialists treat certain ailments and particular patients.	Tuberculosis Intestinal parasites Anemia Malnutrition Skin diseases Malaria Hepatitis Dental problems

Table 17–1. CULTURAL VARIATIONS RELATED TO HEALTH CARE *Continued*

Ethnic/Culture Group	Social Network	Nutritional Patterns	Health Beliefs and Practices	Folk Medicine and Healers	Unique Illnesses
Gypsies	Romany language spoken. Close-knit family and ethnic unit. Extended families live together. Marriage between second cousins is ideal. After marriage couple lives with groom's parents. First-born grandson raised by paternal grandparents. Strong wanderlust contributes to lack of formal education. Maintain private society with an internal moral code and legal system. Home dominated by male. Woman's role to encounter outside world. Very distrustful of non-gypsies (Gaje).	Highly seasoned High in salt and sugar Meats high in fat (pork/beef) Tobacco use high	Hospitalization very turbulent—fear of being away from other gypsies. Therefore, members gather to support the sick. Hospitals are considered to be polluted. Seek "important" (well known) physicians. Distrust "free" clinics. Family elders may try to shield patient from facts of illness. When death occurs they freely scream, pull out clumps of hair, and hurl their bodies against the wall and floor. Refuse autopsy. Very wary of medical personnel, will change physicians frequently if experience is unfavorable. "Crises care": use emergency facilities freely. Poor preventive or follow-up care. Share medications with family. Few immunizations or prenatal care. Body below waist is considered "polluted," especially women. Menstruating women may not prepare food. Upper body is "pure". Measles called "God's rose".	Wise female is the elder administrator. Complex set of values containing evil spirits and demons. Special saints are for good luck. Traditional remedies are administered with a ceremony and include Mold/algae for hemorrhage or epilepsy Love potions of menstrual blood Alopecia ointment of hog lard and chrysarobin Garlic compresses Tea with crushed strawberries	Hypertension Diabetes Occlusive coronary or peripheral vascular diseases Elevated triglycerides or cholesterol levels Obesity

Adapted from Groah L: Operating Room Nursing: Perioperative Practice, 2nd ed. Norwalk, CT, Appleton & Lange, 1991.

Questions for Study and Review

1. What are some common fears that surgical patients have?

2. What is the main fear of the pediatric patient?

3. How can you alleviate the fears of a child in surgery?

4. How is the preoperative visit important?

5. What are some of the communication difficulties in the elderly patient?

6. How should you best communicate with the surgical patient who has difficulty hearing?

7. What are some of the health beliefs of cultural or ethnic groups in your community?

Bibliography

Dellasega C, et al: Perioperative nursing care for the elderly surgical patient. Todays OR Nurse 13(6), 1991.

Groah L: Operating Room Nursing: Perioperative Practice, 2nd ed. Norwalk, CT, Appleton & Lange, 1991.

Koener M, et al: Communicating in the operating room. AORN J 36(1), 1982.

Saylor E: Understanding presurgical anxiety. AORN J 22:624, 1975.

Laser Technology and Use

Learning Objectives

After reading this chapter, you should be able to

- *Describe* the three types of lasers.
- *Understand* how the laser works in simple terms.
- *Describe* all safety precautions taken with laser use.
- *Define* the role of the scrub assistant when the laser is used.
- *Define* the role of the circulator when the laser is used.

Key Terms

ablation: Removal by erosion or vaporization, usually due to intense heat.

anodized: Metal coated with a very thin layer of another metal, usually applied by electrolysis, used to give a colored or nonglare finish.

coagulation: Clotting of blood.

gas: Matter in its least dense state; air at room temperature is a gas.

infrared: That portion of the electromagnetic spectrum just below visible light. All warm objects give off infrared radiation.

laser: *L*ight *a*mplification by *s*timulated *e*mission of *r*adiation; a device that generates a beam of extremely bright light of a single color.

nanosecond: One billionth (10^{-9}) of 1 second.

photodynamic: Caused by the motion or influence of photons (light).

photon: The smallest particle of light. A photon is massless and travels at the speed of light.

semiconductor: A material, such as silicon, that is neither a conductor of electricity nor an insulator. Its electrical properties can be changed by adding minute amounts of other elements. Semiconductors are the basis of transistors and computer chips.

solid: Matter in a rigid state, not liquid or gaseous.

solid-state: Using the electrical properties of solid components (such as transistors) instead of vacuum tubes.

HISTORY OF THE LASER

The laser is found in many phases of our lives. We find the laser's application in national defense (missile guidance), printing (newspapers), and entertainment (holograms). Lasers are also used in astronomy to measure the distances between the Earth and other planets and in physics to simulate the interior of stars. Applied laser technology has created abundant energy resources.

Laser is an acronym for the description of how a laser works—*l*ight *a*mplification by *s*timulated *e*mission of *r*adiation. *Stimulated* is the key word to understanding lasers. Light waves stimulate molecules to generate additional light waves, which, if allowed to continue, generate millions of similar waves until an intense beam of light is created.

Albert Einstein theorized the process of stimulated light. His theory stated that photons stimulating photons could make light act as if it were matter. This theory became fact with the invention of the ruby laser (maser).

In 1950, Charles Townes, Nikolai Bason, and Alexander Prokhorov amplified microwaves through their work in quantum electronics. Theodore Maiman built the first ruby laser in 1960. Others quickly followed with argon, dye, carbon dioxide, helium-neon, and metal-vapor lasers:

1960	Ruby laser	Maiman
1961	Helium-neon (HeNe) laser	Javan
1961	Neodymium: yttrium-aluminum-garnet (Nd:YAG) laser	Johnson
1962	Argon (Ar) laser	Bennett
1964	Carbon dioxide (CO_2) laser	Patel

The first application of lasers to medicine and surgery was in the treatment of eye disease. L'Esperance researched the ruby laser beam's application to retinopathy and demonstrated to the health care community the potential lasers would have in retinal therapy. While several different types of lasers were being developed, new medical research centers were established across the country, each determined to discover the applications to photocoagulation and photoradiation therapy.

Although the laser was invented in the United States, Israel and Japan quickly turned the invention into mass production. Israel recognized the military value and developed multiple military applications. Japan, known for its ability to copy technology and produce mechanically superior products, immediately developed devices capable of delivering this light beam in a multitude of ways.

Leaders in medicine and surgery continued to research projects that ultimately gave us thermal vaporization and coagulation at a microscopic level. Isaac Kaplan, Leon Goldman, Leonard Cerullo, Joseph Bellina, Daniele Aron-Rosa, John Dixon, and many others are the pioneers of laser medicine and surgery. These visionaries took the basic concepts and rudimentary machinery and applied it to some of the most precious and delicate targets of the human body: the eye, brain, spinal cord, fallopian tubes, and digestive tract. These pioneers are highly respected for their contributions to medicine because they took risks during a time when risk-taking and experimentation in health care were not readily approved.

TYPES OF LASERS

Lasers are distinguished by the *medium*—the element or compound—used to create photons. The medium can be liquid, solid, gas, or a semiconductor. The types of laser may be summarized as follows: gas, solid, semiconductor, excimer, solid-state, and dye. Lasers are further distinguished by the functional or biophysical reaction created in the target tissue. The two types of reactions are thermal dissolution and photodynamic destruction. Those lasers found in hospitals, ambulatory care centers, clinics, and physicians' offices are the thermal reactive types and include the carbon dioxide, argon, krypton, and neodymium:yttrium-aluminum-garnet lasers. Table 18–1 is a list of the types of lasers and their uses. Essentially, all the lasers described in Table 18–1 are similar in construction. They all have (1) an optical resonator or optical cavity, usually a glass tube; (2) the lasing medium; (3) reflective mirrors, located at each end of the optical cavity; and (4) a pumping source, which stimulates the photons to create more photons (electricity, heat, or light). The main components of a laser are shown in Figure 18–1.

The Carbon Dioxide Laser

The CO_2, laser medium is actually a combination of helium, nitrogen, and carbon dioxide, and the beam is invisible to the human eye. A helium-neon (HeNe) laser beam (visible, red) is used in conjunction with the CO_2 beam so that surgeons can see where the CO_2 beam contacts the tissue. The HeNe beam is frequently referred to as the "pilot light" because of its guiding function.

The CO_2 laser beam is absorbed by water; thus it reacts with all animal tissue. The density of water in tissue determines how rapidly the beam is absorbed. For example, fat tissue will absorb the beam quickly, whereas bone takes a long time to absorb the beam. Because of this characteristic, the CO_2 laser has broad application to soft tissue lesions but little to bone resection. Its ready absorption by water makes the CO_2 laser a poor tool for use in the bladder, and it is therefore not generally used in urology.

Biophysical functions of the CO_2 laser include vaporization, coagulation, sealing, ablation, cutting, and drilling.

Table 18–1. TYPES OF LASERS

Laser Medium	Wavelength (Microns)	Significant Properties and Action	Medical Use	Delivery System
Argon	0.48	Absorbed by pigmented tissue (red-brown) Coagulation, sealing	Ophthalmology Dermatology Gastroenterology Otology	Hollow tube with mirrors or fiberoptic cable
Ruby	0.69	Pigment specific Coagulation, sealing		
Nd:YAG	1.06	Nonspecific absorption Deep coagulation	Gastroenterology Pulmonology Ophthalmology Urology Gynecology	Fiberoptic cable
CO_2	10.6	Highly absorbed by water Vaporization, coagulation, sealing, drilling	Gynecology Rhinolaryngology Neurosurgery Dermatology	Hollow tube with mirrors Fiberoptic cable

The Argon Laser

The gas medium of argon produces a visible blue-green beam that is absorbed by red-brown pigmented tissue (hemoglobin). It is absorbed readily by blood, red-brown tissue, and melanin. The argon beam is not absorbed by clear or translucent tissue; thus it can pass through the cornea, vitreous, and lens of the eye without creating a thermal effect.

Biophysical functions of the argon laser include coagulation and sealing.

The Neodymium:Yttrium-Aluminum-Garnet Laser

This solid medium has crystals that are similar to artificial diamonds. The beam is infrared and thus invisible to the human eye. As with the CO_2 laser, a HeNe beam is used to allow the surgeon to see the location of the Nd-YAG beam.

The thermal energy of the Nd:YAG laser beam is absorbed by pigmented and nonpigmented tissue. It is less absorbed by blood than the argon but is more absorbed by water than is the argon. The Nd:YAG laser is best known for its deep penetration into tissue.

Biophysical functions of the Nd:YAG laser include vaporization, deep coagulation, and ablation.

HOW THE LASER WORKS

When photons (light beams) exit the optical cavity, an intense stream of light is emitted. This light has three basic characteristics that make it different from any other type of light. These characteristics are illustrated in Figure 18–2.

The reaction of this light to biologic tissue varies according to absorption propensities, power settings, time of exposure, and size of the target tissue. The sum total of these factors is called the *radiant exposure* and is measured by the depth the laser beam will travel into the target tissue. When the laser beam touches the tissue, the cells heat to incredible temperatures, explode, and change into steam and carbon (Fig. 18–3). This vaporization and coagulation process allows the

MONOCHROMATIC:
All waves have exactly the same wavelength (one color)

PARALLEL:
All waves move in columns

Ordinary light

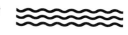

Laser light

COHERENT:
All waves are exactly in step with each other (space and time)

Laser beam

Figure 18–2. Basic characteristics of a laser.

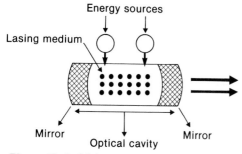

Figure 18–1. Main components of a laser.

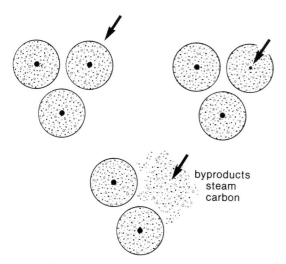

Figure 18–3. Tissue reaction to a laser.

surgeon to treat tumors, abnormal cells, strictures, burns, and decubitus and gastrointestinal ulcers.

MEDICAL AND SURGICAL APPLICATIONS OF LASERS

Gynecology

The CO_2 and Nd:YAG lasers are the most common types used by the gynecologist. Conditions treated with the CO_2 laser include condylomata acuminata, cervical intraepithelial neoplasia, cervical stenosis, endocervical polyps, herpes lesions, vaginal intraepithelial neoplasia, Bartholin's duct abscess, and endometriosis.

Laryngology

The Ar, CO_2, and Nd:YAG lasers have all been used to treat problems of the head, neck, oral cavity, and throat. These conditions include benign tumors of the tongue, leukoplakia, hemangiomas, nasopharyngeal stenosis, nasopharyngeal carcinoma, vocal cord nodules, laryngeal papillomas, laryngeal polyps, anterior commissure lesions and webs, subglottic and tracheal stenosis, and cavernous hemangiomas.

Neurosurgery

The ability of the CO_2 laser to vaporize abnormal central nervous tissue growths has been invaluable to corrective neurosurgery. Some neurologic conditions that are treated with the laser include tumors of the brain (acoustic neuromas), tumors of the spinal cord, arterial venous malformations, aneurysms, angiomatous lesions, and peripheral nerve lesions (neuroma amputations).

Cardiovascular Surgery

The application of Nd:YAG, argon, and CO_2 laser beams to atherosclerotic vessels is under great scrutiny at this time. Many research projects are examining the reaction of all three beams to plaque and vessel walls. *Excimer lasers,* which produce short, intense bursts of cool ultraviolet light, are now in use. Current laser energy can perforate the artery too easily and produce heat, which damages surrounding tissue, and plaque tends to reaccumulate on the remaining rough surface on the artery wall.

With the aid of a new technology of glass magnetic switches, the excimer laser produces a uniform beam of energy that can be controlled and pulsed from 10 to 200 nanoseconds in an extremely short period of time. One pulse cuts away microns of tissue with great precision. In experiments, blocked coronary arteries have been cleared in 2 minutes. In addition, the excimer laser does not damage surrounding tissue.

The fiberoptic delivery system used in conjunction with the excimer laser is a 1.5-mm catheter that not only carries the energy to the site but also produces a video image of the blockage that the physician can look at as he works. One group of fibers carries the laser beam while another shines a light on the tip of the catheter. A third group of fibers has a lens on the tip that provides video pictures of the field. A clear liquid is flushed through the catheter to push back blood and allow a clear view. The fibers are thin enough to be threaded through smaller arteries where plaque accumulates.

Gastrointestinal Surgery

The Nd:YAG laser is proving to be an invaluable tool for vaporizing obstructive lesions of the digestive tract. This laser's ability to control gastric, peptic, and esophageal bleeding is also being carefully studied. Endoscopic delivery of the Nd:YAG fiberoptic cable allows the physician to treat lesions along the entire intestinal tract.

Ophthalmology

The ruby laser was first used to treat retinopathy (bleeding vessels behind the retina); however, the argon laser is the instrument of choice today. Other uses of the argon laser include treatment of glaucoma, ocular histoplasmosis, and senile macular degeneration.

The Nd:YAG laser has been found valuable for posterior capsulotomies, preoperative anterior capsulotomy, anterior adhesions, and vitreous bands.

SAFETY PRECAUTIONS

The laser is a powerful and potentially dangerous tool. The following safety precautions for laser use should be studied and reviewed often.

1. *Protect the eyes.* When the CO_2 laser is used, clear safety glasses *with side wings* must be worn. The patient under local anesthesia must also wear protective glasses. If a general anesthetic is to be administered, the patient's eyes are protected with wet eye pads and tape and the face is covered with a wet absorbent towel.

The Nd:YAG laser requires the use of blue-green safety goggles and the argon laser, orange-colored eyewear.

2. *Do not use alcohol-based prepping solutions.* The laser beam is analogous to a flame. All flammable liquids such as alcohol must be kept away from the field.

3. *Keep sterile saline and an irrigating syringe on the field.* Although a rare occurrence, dry drapes, 4 × 4–inch sponges, and towels have been inadvertently ignited by the CO_2 laser beam or a "hot" fiberoptic cable. Sterile saline may be used to fill cavities such as the abdomen or cranium to absorb the energy of the CO_2 beam in areas not intended for laser application.

4. *Have extra lap tapes available.* These may be used as backdrops behind tissue to be lased.

5. *Use a smoke evacuating suction device.* The evacuating device should have appropriate connectors and correctly fitting tubes. Instruments that help to evacuate smoke, such as speculums with a second portal for suctioning or endoscopes with additional evacuation portals, should be used.

6. *Post warning signs on entry doors.* Whenever the laser is in use, appropriate signs should be placed on entry doors. A pair of protective glasses may be hung next to the sign so that anyone entering the laser area can put them on before opening the door.

7. *Use the "standby" or "stop" mode whenever the laser beam is not needed.* This is the duty of the registered nurse circulator.

8. *Wear masks whenever the laser is in use.* Personnel should always wear masks when the CO_2 or Nd:YAG laser is in use. This prevents inhalation of steam or carbon produced when tissue is lased.

9. *Only the physician should have control of the foot pedal, and he or she should have only one pedal.* Assistants should activate all other pedals such as the bipolar or electrosurgery unit. If the physician must use other foot pedals, such as that controlling the microscope, that pedal should be placed behind him or her.

10. *If the gloved hand is inadvertently burned with the laser beam, remove the glove immediately.* The latex melting into the skin may retard healing.

11. *Personnel operating the laser must keep in mind the electrical hazards related to high-wattage equipment.* Routine safety precautions must always be followed when high-wattage equipment, including the laser, is in use.

Safety is the most critical factor related to the use of any type of laser. Because the *laser beam destroys tissue,* it can injure patients and personnel if precautions are not taken. A laser safety program should be comprehensive and include the establishment of a laser safety committee. The committee should establish policies related to its composition, purpose, and scope of responsibility.

THE ROLE OF THE SCRUB ASSISTANT IN LASER SURGERY

Planning is a critical feature of any surgery and is even more important when high technology tools such as the laser will be used during the surgical procedure. The scrub assistant should have specific information regarding the type of laser to be used, accessory equipment for operating the laser, and safety supplies that will be needed on the field. If, for example, the CO_2 laser is to be used for lysis of the adhesions surrounding the fallopian tubes, the scrub assistant should ask the following questions:

1. How is the laser to be used?
2. What delivery system is needed?
3. If the CO_2 is used free-hand with the articulating arm (hollow tube with mirrors), the handpiece must be sterile. How, then, will the draping proceed to cover the remaining portion of the arm?
4. If the microscope is to be attached, has the adaptor been cleaned, and what lenses are necessary on both the laser and the microscope? What draping technique will prevent contamination of the field and wound site during the procedure?
5. As the safety guidelines have indicated, the surgeon will have only the laser foot pedal. What foot pedal will the scrub assistant control, and where is it best located for easy access without inadvertent activation?

Instrument planning is also very important. Are there new instruments to be used? What sizes are needed, and do they have special safety surfaces? Quartz and titanium rods are added to the Mayo stand for gynecology laser surgery. Wet tongue blades, anodized instruments, laser smoke suctioning devices, and specialized laser beam–resistant instruments should be available. As in all procedures, the surgeon's preference card (discussed in Chapter 16) should be consulted to conclude instrument planning.

The CO_2 laser beam will reflect off any shiny instrument surface. Protective supplies, such as wet laparotomy sponges, should be available. An additional suction should be used to eliminate smoke and debris that accumulate from the lasing process.

During the procedure, the primary function of the scrub assistant is to observe the field (through safety goggles). In addition to guarding the field against contamination, the scrub assistant must keep sponges wet and in position, remove ignitable items out of the CO_2 beam's path, and assist with the suctioning of smoke so as to provide a clear visual field for the surgeon. A basin of sterile saline with an irrigating syringe ready and full should always be available. Saline may be needed to cool thermally involved tissue or to extinguish any inadvertent heating of supplies. The scrub assistant must stay vigilant, watch each application of the beam, and anticipate any need for protective supplies or special equipment or instruments.

Regardless of the patient position, if field drapes are applied they need to be protected with wet towels or lap sponges. All drapes will adversely alter the impact of the laser beam or heat of the delivery system. The scrub assistant must be sure that the addition of wet towels does not cause strikethrough contamination.

THE ROLE OF THE CIRCULATOR DURING LASER USE

It is the job of the circulator to help prepare all laser equipment to be used during surgery and to plan for and provide emotional support to the patient.

Before surgery, the laser coordinator or circulator should test the laser *before the patient arrives in the surgery suite.* A wet tongue blade is used as the target. The CO_2 or Nd:YAG laser is placed at 10 watts of power, and the foot pedal is activated. The tip of the handpiece or fiber should be within focal distance of the tongue blade. Alignment is measured. Is the red (HeNe) beam illuminating at the same point as the burn on the tongue blade? If not, the beam is out of alignment. The laser will need maintenance before it can be used.

The circulator should double check all special supplies. Is the smoke evacuator functional? Are there enough protective goggles for everyone involved in the procedure? Are the electrical connections safe (no loose wires), and have all maintenance policies been enforced? Is there a fire extinguisher available in the room? A backup supply of operational gases (for CO_2) should be readily available. The circulator should always exercise caution when handling the cylinder. He or she should make sure that it is securely mounted and be careful not to drop the cylinder and not to use it if it does not connect easily to the gauge. The cylinder head should never be struck with a blunt instrument to disengage coupling devices.

It is the circulator's duty to always prepare and protect patients who are undergoing laser surgery. Patients under local anesthesia need instructions and reassurance periodically during the procedure. The circulator can calm them and stay with them mentally. Movement of the patient who is undergoing a gynecologic procedure under local anesthesia should be prevented. This can be done by placing a draw sheet over the hips and abdomen and tucking it under the operating table mattress. The patient should be reminded during the procedure that she should remain as still as possible.

In addition to the scrub and circulating personnel, a third person should be assigned to any procedure when the laser is in use. The roles of the scrub assistant and circulator are full-time jobs. The laser is new enough to everyone to justify a third person to monitor its function.

At the close of the procedure, the circulator or laser coordinator, in addition to his or her routine functions, should return the laser lock key to the supervisor's office or other secure location.

OPERATING ROOM POLICY REGARDING LASER USE

All operating rooms should have written policies regarding the use of lasers. These policies ensure that the laser is used within the safe and efficient bounds for which it is intended. See the sample policy in the box. *All operating room personnel should read and frequently review this type of written policy so that the safety of the patient and personnel is protected at all times.*

Sample Policy

Title: Laparoscopy With Carbon Dioxide Laser

Scope: Nursing Service OR Personnel, OB-Gyn Staff, Anesthesia Chief, Surgery Chief—Ambulatory Surgery

Purpose: To protect patients and personnel from laser hazards

Policy Statements:
1. The carbon dioxide laser will be used by gynecologists who have approved laser credentials.
2. Personnel assigned to operate the laser will have been trained:
   a. Inservice program on operations of laser by manufacturers
   b. Attended a CO_2 laser safety course Documentation of training will be in each staff member's personnel file.
3. All persons present during CO_2 laser applications will wear clear protective eyewear.
4. Signs shall be posted on doors leading into CO_2 laser treatment areas. The sign will warn of danger, display the radiation symbol, state that protective eyewear is needed, and display the type of laser being used.
5. The (brand name) smoke evacuator will be used on all CO_2 laser procedures.
6. The key to the laser shall be locked in the narcotic cabinet when the laser is not being used.
7. The operational checklist is attached to the CO_2 laser cabinet and is followed when the laser is operationalized.
8. Applications of the CO_2 laser will be documented on the Intraoperative Patient Record and will include the following:
   Type laser used
   Operator's name
   Tissue type applied to
   Power settings
   Time durations
   All safety measures used for the patient

Equipment Needed:
CO_2 laser
Laparoscope
Laparoscope coupling lens
Smoke evacuator
Sterile suction tubing
Drape for laser arm
Insufflator and high-pressure valve
Scope light source and cable
Instrumentation for laparoscopy
Laparoscopy drape pack
Basin for saline with Asepto syringe
Wet absorbent towels
4×4-inch radiopaque sponges

Questions for Study and Review

1. What color eye protection should be used for each of the common types of laser: CO_2, argon, and Nd:YAG?

2. Why should alcohol-based prepping solutions *not* be used before laser surgery.

3. How should a CO_2 or Nd:YAG laser be tested before surgery?

4. Why should the surgeon have access to only the laser foot pedal and not pedals for other equipment?

5. What is the purpose of safety surfaces on instruments used during laser surgery?

6. For what purpose is the argon laser used?

7. Can you see a CO_2 laser beam when it is in use?

8. What warnings and safety equipment should be placed *outside* the door of a room where laser surgery is taking place?

Bibliography

Bellina J: Lasers in gynecology. World J Surg 7:692, 1983.

Carruth JA: The role of lasers in otolaryngology. World J Surg 7:719, 1983.

Dixon J: Surgical Application of Lasers. Chicago, Year Book Medical Publishers, 1983.

Kirschner R, Unger M: Symposium on Laser Surgery. Surg Clin North Am 16:839–1024, 1984.

Pfister J, Kneedler J: A Guide to Lasers in the OR. Denver, Education Design/Editorial Consultants, 1983.

Polanyui TG: Laser Physics. Otolaryngol Clin North Am 16:753–774, 1983.

SECTION II
PRACTICE: SURGICAL PROCEDURES

◆ The following chapters on surgical procedures (Chapters 19 through 29)

• emphasize the role of the scrub technologist or nurse. One of the major

• difficulties in teaching and learning operative procedures is the wide variation in

• the approach, choice of instrumentation, sutures, and specific techniques.

• Variations occur according to (1) where and how the surgeon was taught, (2)

• available instrumentation, (3) the patient's specific disease problem, and (4) the

• surgeon's expertise. Each procedure, however, does have a purpose, direction,

• and final goal, and these principles are the basis for the procedures presented.

• The specific choice of procedures is meant to teach the scrub assistant

• techniques that can be applied to additional procedures of that specialty.

• Surgical techniques are inseparable from the regional anatomy. Therefore,

• each chapter begins with a basic anatomic review of that system. Although not

• intended to provide the student's entire education in anatomy, the reviews serve

• as quick reference, should questions arise during study.

SURGICAL SUFFIXES AND PREFIXES

The following list of suffixes and prefixes includes those used to describe surgical processes or conditions. These suffixes and prefixes are encountered as part of the description of a surgical procedure. It is extremely important for the technologist or nurse to learn to recognize and use these suffixes and prefixes.

-ectomy: To remove surgically. For example, *appendectomy* means the appendix (append-) is removed.

Colectomy means that a portion of the colon (col-) is removed.

-otomy: To surgically open or make an incision into. For example, *thoracotomy* means the chest cavity (thora-) will be opened. *Pyloromyotomy* means that the pylorus (pylor-) muscle (myo-) is cut into or opened.

-ostomy: To create an opening or passageway. When this suffix is preceded by the name of one structure, such as in *colostomy*, it means that an opening is created in that structure that leads to the outside of the body. In this example, a new passage is made to the outside of the abdomen. When the suffix is preceded by two structures, such as in *dacryocysto-rhinostomy*, it means that a new passageway is created between the two structures. If the components of this example are separated, its exact meaning can be extracted easily. *Dacryocysto* means "tear sac" and refers to the tear sac or duct of the eye. *-rhin* refers to the nose. Thus, *dacryocystorhinostomy* means the surgical creation of a new passageway between the tear sac and the nose. *Jejunojejunostomy* means that two separate sections of the jejunum are joined together to form a new passageway.

-scopy: When preceded by the name of an anatomic structure, this suffix refers to the examination of that structure through a *lensed* instrument. The instrument could be a fiberoptic instrument or simply an instrument lighted by a conventional light source. For example, *pelviscopy* is the examination of the pelvic contents through a fiberoptic laparoscope. *Sigmoidoscopy* means the examination of the sigmoid colon (terminal section of the colon) through the lighted sigmoidoscope.

auto-: "Self." When this prefix is followed by a procedure or other root word, it refers to the source itself. For example, an *autologous* tissue graft is one that is both taken from and implanted into the patient's own body. *Autotransfusion* means transfusion of the patient's own blood.

Key Terms

anastomosis: The surgical formation of a passageway between two spaces, hollow organs, or lumens. *End-to-end anastomosis of the small bowel* means that two sections of bowel are joined together to form a continuous passageway. The suture line that forms the union is also referred to as the anastomosis. To anastomose means to create the union or passageway.

appose: To bring two structures together. *The surgeon apposes the tissue edges* means that he or she draws them together so that their edges or sides are touching.

approximate: To bring body parts or tissues together by sutures or other means. In surgery, this commonly refers to two tissue edges that are sutured. *The surgeon approximates the wound edges* means that he or she sutures the wound edges together.

blunt dissection: The separation of tissues or tissue planes with an instrument that has no cutting ability. For example, during hernia repair, the surgeon often uses his or her fingers or a rough sponge to separate the tissue planes of the inguinal area. The tissues are gently peeled away from each other.

communicate: When two structures or organs connect. *The surgeon makes an incision around the fistula where it communicates with the skin* refers to the area where the fistula passes through or connects with the skin.

deflect: To peel or retract back and away but not detach. *The surgeon deflects the septum.* The *deflection* is the process of peeling back tissue.

divide: To cut or sever. *The surgeon divides the tissues* means that he or she separates the tissues by cutting them.

excise: To remove by cutting out. *The tumor is excised* means that the tumor has been cut away from its location in the body. *Excision* is the surgical process of cutting away a structure or diseased area.

exposure: The anatomic area that the surgeon can see and thus operate on. *The subcostal incision allows the surgeon adequate exposure of the gallbladder* means that the incision is large enough to bring the gallbladder into view. To *expose* means to create this anatomic area. *The surgeon then incises the peritoneum to expose the abdominal contents.*

incise: To cut or sever with a cutting instrument. *The surgeon incises the skin* means the surgeon cuts the skin making an *incision*.

resect: To cut out and remove a section of tissue. This term usually refers to the removal of a major portion of tissue. *The surgeon resects the large intestine* means that he or she removes a linear portion of the intestine. *Resection* refers to the partial removal of tissue. *Resection of the stomach* means the surgical removal of a portion of the stomach.

retract: To pull tissues back or away to expose a structure or other tissue. *The assistant retracts the wound edges to expose the abdominal contents.* Retraction is the performance of this action. *Retraction is needed at the wound edges.*

transect: To cut *across* an organ or section of tissue. *The surgeon transects the vessel* means that he or she cuts across the vessel perpendicular to its length. *Transection* refers to the result of this action. *The bowel transection is performed with fine scissors* means that cross-cutting of the bowel is performed with scissors.

General Surgery

General surgery encompasses operations of the gastrointestinal tract, biliary system, spleen, pancreas, liver, hernias of the abdominal wall, and procedures of the rectum and breast. Also included are surgery of the thyroid gland and associated structures. A specialist is not needed in these areas of surgery, although the general surgeon may specialize in one of these areas.

Most of the procedures require similar instrumentation, as well as special items in rectal, breast, and thyroid procedures. The gastrointestinal instruments are used interchangeably for various procedures of the stomach and intestine.

SURGICAL ANATOMY

Abdominal Incisions

The most common incisions encountered in general surgery of the abdomen (Fig. 19–1A) are the midline, upper paramedian, subcostal, McBurney (appendix), and oblique inguinal (hernia). The Pfannenstiel incision is used almost exclusively for gynecologic surgery and is discussed in Chapter 21.

Midline

The midline incision is the simplest and most common abdominal incision used by the general surgeon. It offers a nearly bloodless field and adequate exposure of nearly all structures of the abdominal cavity. The layers of the midline incision from ventral to dorsal sides of the body are as follows:

1. Skin
2. Subcutaneous fat
3. Fascia
4. Abdominal peritoneum

Refer to Figure 19–1. In this illustration, note that the midline incision lies directly over the *linea alba* ("white line") of the abdominal wall. There are no muscle fibers in the path of this incision, hence the nearly bloodless field. However, if the surgeon makes the incision slightly left or right of this line, the rectus abdominus muscles are encountered.

Upper Paramedian

This incision is used primarily to expose the stomach, duodenum, and pancreas. It allows the surgeon to enter the abdominal cavity with a minimum of bleeding and the incision can be extended in a superior or inferior direction to meet the needs of the procedure. The tissue layers include the following:

1. Skin
2. Subcutaneous fat
3. Anterior rectus muscles (retracted laterally, not severed)
4. Rectus fascia
5. Abdominal peritoneum

Subcostal

The right subcostal incision is used to expose the gallbladder and its associated structures. It is occasionally used for operations of the pancreas. The left subcostal incision may be used to expose the spleen, although its limited exposure precludes its use in splenic trauma cases in which a midline incision would allow the surgeon to do a more complete exploration of the abdominal cavity.

This incision follows the lower costal (rib) margin in a semi-curved shape. Because the rectus muscles are severed, this incision is more painful postoperatively than the midline incision. The tissues encountered are as follows:

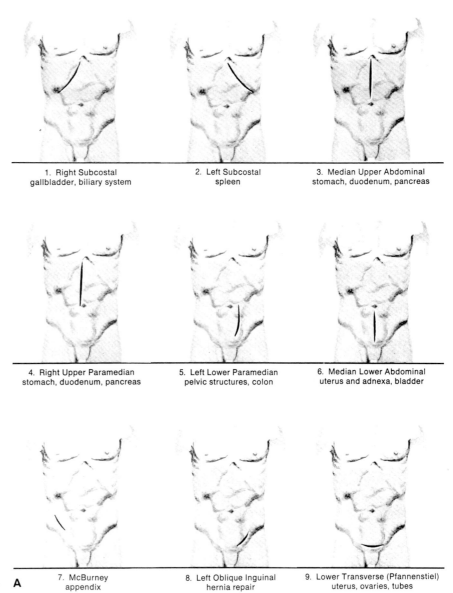

1. Right Subcostal
gallbladder, biliary system

2. Left Subcostal
spleen

3. Median Upper Abdominal
stomach, duodenum, pancreas

4. Right Upper Paramedian
stomach, duodenum, pancreas

5. Left Lower Paramedian
pelvic structures, colon

6. Median Lower Abdominal
uterus and adnexa, bladder

7. McBurney
appendix

8. Left Oblique Inguinal
hernia repair

9. Lower Transverse (Pfannenstiel)
uterus, ovaries, tubes

Figure 19–1. *A.* Common abdominal incisions. (From Ethicon, Inc.: Nursing Care of the Patient in the O.R. Somerville, NJ, Ethicon, Inc.)

Illustration continued on following page

A

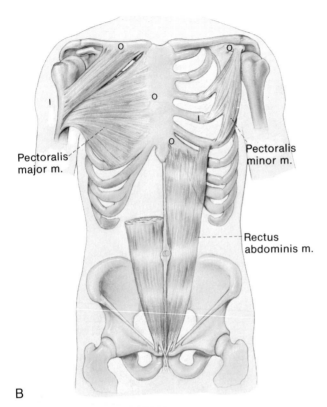

B

Figure 19–1 *Continued. B.* Anterior abdomen showing rectus abdominis muscles. The midline incision is made between the two muscles. (From Jacob S, Francone C, Lossow WJ: Structure and Function in Man, 5th ed. Philadelphia, WB Saunders, 1982.)

1. Skin
2. Subcutaneous fat
3. Rectus muscles
4. Fascia
5. Abdominal peritoneum

McBurney (Appendix)

The McBurney incision is used for exploration and removal of the appendix. It is made on the right side, at an oblique angle below the umbilicus, across the flank. This incision is called a *muscle-splitting incision*, because the muscle fibers are split manually, not severed. The exposure offered is very limited, and the incision cannot be lengthened easily. The tissue layers of this incision include the following:

1. Skin
2. Subcutaneous fat
3. Fascia
4. Oblique and transversalis muscle
5. Abdominal peritoneum

Oblique (Inguinal)

The right and left oblique inguinal incision is used for inguinal hernia repair. This incision gives excellent exposure to the two common types of inguinal hernias: the direct hernia and the indirect hernia. The muscle

layers of this incision converge at the hernia site and are illustrated in Figure 19–2.

Structures of the Abdominal Cavity

The structures of the abdominal cavity include those of the gastrointestinal tract, the liver, gallbladder, pancreas, and spleen. Each of the structures is interrelated, and it is important to visualize them as *integral parts* of a whole system rather than as isolated organs. Each structure is related to other structures and connected by vessels, ducts, enveloping tissues, and protective coverings.

Esophagus

The esophagus is a tubular structure that extends from the pharynx to the stomach. It conveys food throughout its length by a combination of voluntary and involuntary muscle fibers. The esophagus enters the abdominal cavity at the level of the diaphragm. In the adult, it measures approximately 10 inches.

Stomach

The stomach (Fig. 19–3) lies just under the diaphragm in the upper abdomen. This organ serves to mix and liquefy food material so that it can be broken down into usable nutrients by the intestines. The stomach is composed of three major sections; these are the *fundus* (upper portion), *body* (central area), and *antrum* (lower portion, closest to the duodenum). These portions are

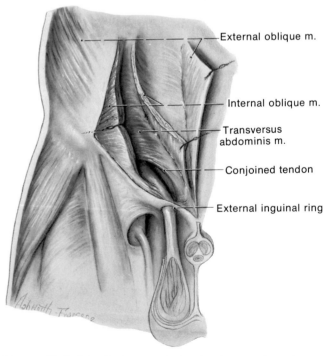

Figure 19–2. Muscle layers of the inguinal region. (From Jacob S, Francone C, Lossow WJ: Structure and Function in Man, 5th ed. Philadelphia, WB Saunders, 1982.)

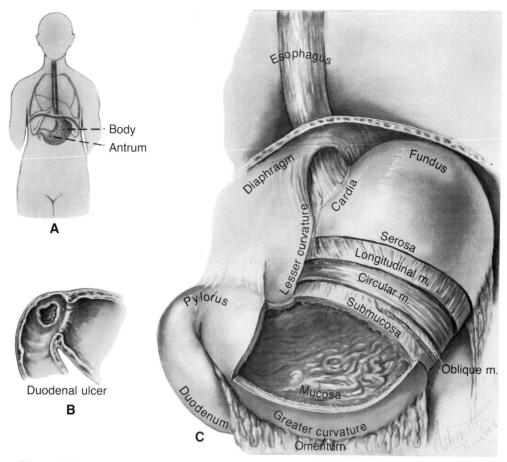

Figure 19–3. *A.* Location of the stomach. *B.* Site of duodenal ulcer. *C.* Layers and sections of the stomach. Note the location of the diaphragm. (From Jacob S, Francone C, Lossow WJ: Structure and Function in Man, 5th ed. Philadelphia, WB Saunders, 1982.)

continuous with one another and are spoken of only as landmarks, not as distinct anatomic sections.

The wall of the stomach contains an outer layer of delicate tissue called the *serosa,* two inner layers of smooth (involuntary) muscles, and an inner layer called the *submucosa.* The two orifices of the stomach, located at each end, are the *cardia* (superior or upper end) and the *pylorus* (inferior or lower end). The cardia is located between the esophagus and the stomach, and the pylorus is located between the stomach and the duodenum, the first section of small intestine.

The *omentum,* an extension of the abdominal peritoneum, is a sheet of tissue that extends from the greater and lesser curvature of the stomach (Fig. 19–4).

Small Intestine

The small intestine is the first or proximal portion of the entire intestine. It extends from the pylorus of the stomach to the cecum or proximal end of the large intestine.

The *duodenum,* the first section of small intestine, is an important anatomic structure because the pancreatic duct (duct of Wirsung) and the common bile duct from the liver drain their contents into this section of intestine.

The *jejunum* and *ileum* are the second and third sections of the small intestine. These sections are suspended from the abdominal wall by a sheet of vascular tissue called the *mesentery,* which supplies blood and lymph to the lower sections of the small intestine. It is this sheet of tissue that must be resected, and each vessel must be clamped and ligated any time portions of the jejunum or ileum are removed.

The tissue layers (Fig. 19–5) of the small intestine are similar to those of the stomach and the large intestine. The inner surface of the small intestine contains small fingerlike projections called *villi.* These increase the surface area of the lumen and contain blood and lymphatic vessels.

The small intestine terminates at the *cecum,* the first portion of the large intestine.

Large Intestine

The large intestine (Fig. 19–6) extends from the distal end of the small intestine, the ileum, to the rectum and is divided into five distinct sections. These sections are the *ascending colon, transverse colon, descending colon, sigmoid colon,* and *rectum.* The entire large intestine measures about 1.5 meters in the adult.

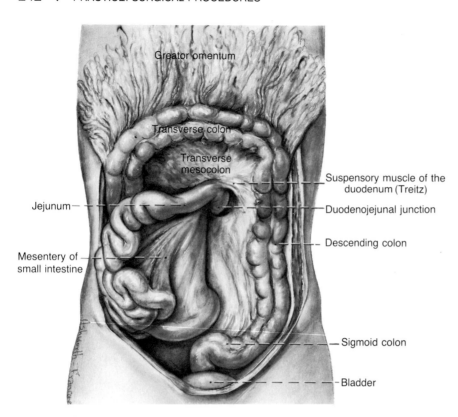

Figure 19–4. Anterior view of the intestine with the greater omentum raised. (From Jacob S, Francone C, Lossow WJ: Structure and Function in Man, 5th ed. Philadelphia, WB Saunders, 1982.)

The first portion of the large intestine, called the *cecum,* is actually a long pouch where a small thin hollow tube called the *appendix* lies. The appendix occasionally becomes infectious because its blind end becomes the site of obstruction. The ascending colon extends upward toward the liver and lies just behind the right lobe of this organ. The transverse colon then crosses the abdomen to the left, below the stomach. The descending colon extends downward on the left side of the abdomen and terminates at the sigmoid colon, which lies in the pelvic cavity. The sigmoid colon ends at the rectum (Fig. 19–7), which rests near the sacrum and coccyx. The anal canal extends from the rectum to the outside of the body. Near the outside orifice, the muscular fibers form both *internal* and *external sphincters.* These sphincters contain large veins that may become engorged, enlarge, and are then called *hemorrhoids.*

Liver

The liver (Fig. 19–8) is a large, vascular organ that aids in digestion and filtration of toxic substances from the body. It is located in the upper abdomen just under the diaphragm. The liver is divided into four distinct lobes. The right and left lobes are separated by a ligament called the *falciform ligament.* The right lobe is then divided into subsections called the *right lobe proper, quadrate lobe,* and *caudate lobe.* The liver contains a complicated network of blood vessels and blood sinusoids (small cavities). The vessels communicate with the large hepatic artery and portal vein, which lie near the center of the organ. Small *bile canaliculi* (channels that convey bile) are interspersed among the liver cells. These canaliculi communicate with larger ducts that convey bile (fluid that aids in the digestion of fat) into the *hepatic duct.* From this duct, the bile leaves the organ through the *cystic duct* and on to the *common bile duct,* where it is deposited into the duodenum. The exact location of this exit into the duodenum is called *ampulla of Vater.* The pancreatic duct shares this location, where it also deposits digestive fluid.

Gallbladder

The gallbladder is a pouch located at the inferior surface of the liver where it attaches (see Fig. 19–8). This structure is a reservoir for bile, which is conveyed to the duodenum through the cystic and common bile ducts. These two ducts converge below the gallbladder (Fig. 19–9). The gallbladder is subject to infection and may contain stones, which sometimes must be surgically removed.

Pancreas

The pancreas is a lobulated gland that is elongated and lies inferior to the liver, behind the stomach. This organ has two landmarks: the head and the tail. The head, which is the broader portion of the gland, lies in the curve of the duodenum and is connected to that portion of the small intestine. The pancreatic duct, or *duct of Wirsung,* the central duct of the pancreas, communicates with the duodenum at the *ampulla of*

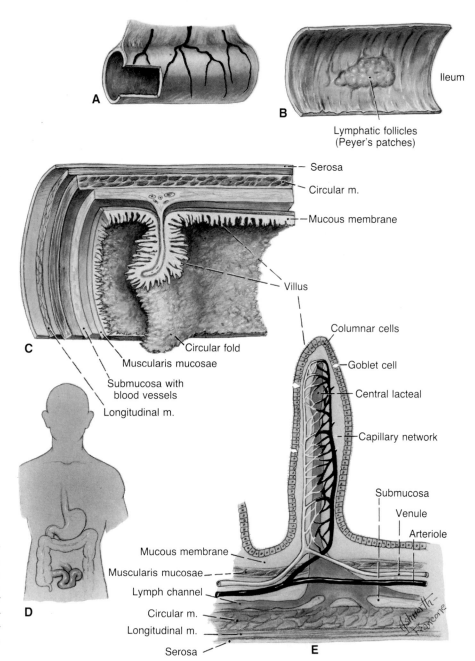

Figure 19–5. *A.* Segment of small intestine. *B.* Interior of intestine. *C.* Layers composing intestinal wall. *D.* Anatomic position of small intestine. *E.* Single villus showing blood supply and intestinal tissue layers. (From Jacob S, Francone C, Lossow WJ: Structure and Function in Man, 5th ed. Philadelphia, WB Saunders, 1982.)

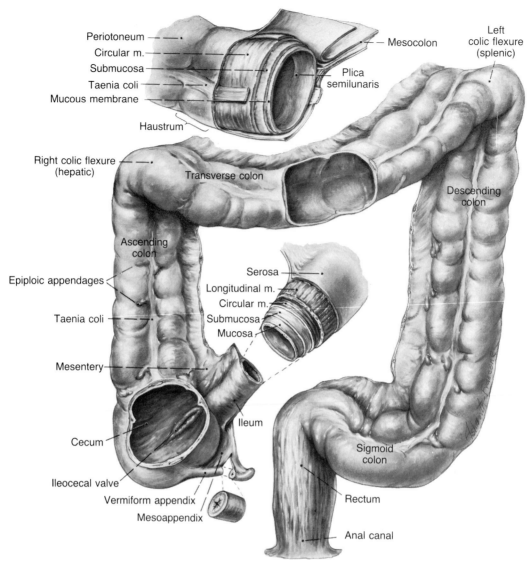

Figure 19–6. Structure and segments of the large intestine. The walls have been cut away to show the tissue layers. (From Jacob S, Francone C, Lossow WJ: Structure and Function in Man, 5th ed. Philadelphia, WB Saunders, 1982.)

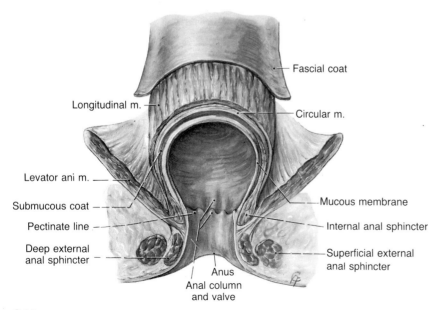

Figure 19–7. Anal canal and layers of the rectum. (From Jacob S, Francone C, Lossow WJ: Structure and Function in Man, 5th ed. Philadelphia, WB Saunders, 1982.)

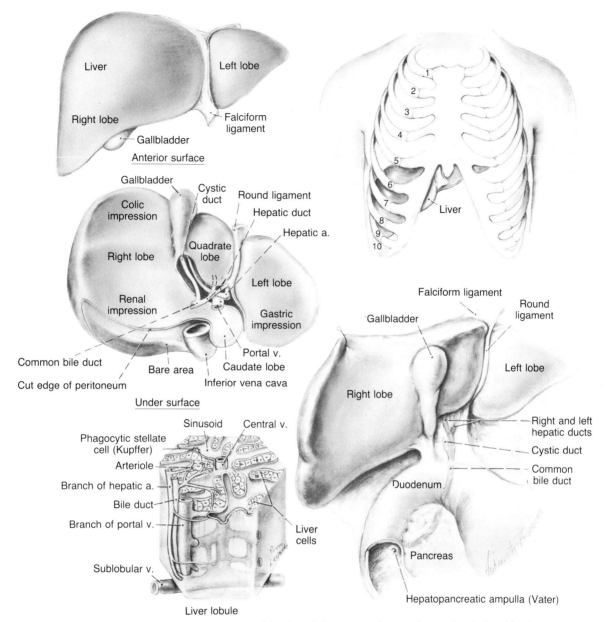

Anterior surface

Under surface

Liver lobule

Figure 19–8. The liver, its position in the abdomen, various units, and relationship to other organs. (From Jacob S, Francone C, Lossow WJ: Structure and Function in Man, 5th ed. Philadelphia, WB Saunders, 1982.) (Liver lobule courtesy of Lederle Laboratories.)

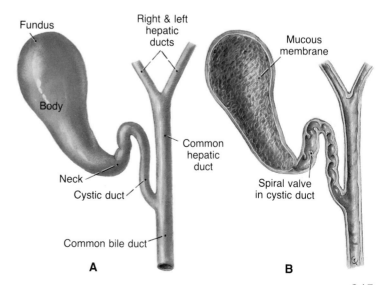

Figure 19–9. *A.* Gallbladder showing right and left hepatic ducts coming from the liver, common hepatic duct, cystic duct, and common bile duct. *B.* Internal structure. (From Jacob S, Francone C, Lossow WJ: Structure and Function in Man, 5th ed. Philadelphia, WB Saunders, 1982.)

Vater, a location shared with the common bile duct. The tail of the pancreas lies near the hilus of the spleen. The pancreas produces *insulin* and *glucagon,* which aid in the digestion of carbohydrates. The relationship of the pancreas to other organs is shown in Figure 19–10.

Spleen

The spleen (Fig. 19–11) is a kidney-shaped organ that is extremely vascular and relatively soft. It lies under the diaphragm in the left upper abdomen. This organ functions to destroy aged red blood cells, store blood, and filter microorganisms from the blood and plays a major role in the immune system of the body. The spleen is supplied by two major blood vessels: the splenic vein and artery. Because of its vascularity and location, the spleen is subject to trauma by direct blow during vehicular and other accidents. The spleen can be safely removed without harm to body function; this procedure is indicated whenever splenic hemorrhage becomes life threatening.

GASTROINTESTINAL AND ABDOMINAL SURGERY

Laparotomy

Definition

Laparotomy is the term used to describe an incision made through the abdominal wall to perform an operation on the abdominal contents. If the surgeon performs a laparotomy as a diagnostic procedure, without knowing the exact nature of the patient's condition or disease, it is called an *exploratory* laparotomy. Once the abdomen is opened, a particular procedure can be initiated depending on the specific conditions that are discovered. An exploratory laparotomy may be performed following trauma to the abdomen or when the patient has abdominal pain and the cause cannot be determined by diagnostic studies.

Routines that are followed during every abdominal procedure are discussed here only to avoid repetition for each separate procedure.

Highlights

1. An incision is made through the abdominal tissues.
2. The wound is explored.
3. The wound is closed.

Description

The patient is placed in supine position, prepped, and draped for a specific abdominal incision. Once draping is completed, the technologist moves the Mayo stand up to the field below the wound site. The cautery and suction tubing are clamped to the top drape by the technologist or surgeon. The technologist places two dry lap sponges on the field and passes a No. 10 or No. 20 knife blade to the surgeon. This knife will hereafter be referred to as the *skin knife* and is designated for use *only on the skin.* Most surgeons believe that the skin knife carries bacteria from the skin into deeper layers, although some surgeons dispute this.

The skin incision (Fig. 19–12) exposes the subcutaneous or fatty layer that lies just under the skin. This layer is usually incised with the cautery pencil or knife (Fig. 19–13). The surgeon clamps large bleeding vessels in this layer with Kelly or Crile hemostats and ligates them with absorbable suture, size 3-0 (Fig. 19–14), or he or she may simply cauterize them.

The incision is carried through to the next layer, the fascia. At this level, the technologist should have small Richardson or U.S. retractors available for the assistant. The surgeon incises the layer with a No. 10 or No. 20 knife blade. This knife is then referred to as the *deep knife.* As lap sponges become soiled, the technologist must replace them with clean ones. The exchange of clean lap sponges continues throughout the entire procedure.

The surgeon may lengthen the fascial incision with the cautery pencil or may use curved Mayo scissors. If the incision is on the midline, no muscle tissue is encountered. If, however, the incision lies off the midline, there will be a layer of muscle tissue that the surgeon will separate manually or with the scalpel. In preparation for entrance into the abdomen, the technologist should have available several lap sponges and a self-retaining retractor such as a Balfour retractor. The lap sponges are dipped in *warm* (not hot) saline solution and wrung as dry as possible. If small 4 × 4-inch sponges have been used before the opening of the peritoneum, the technologist must remove them from the field immediately. They may not be used again (unless mounted on a sponge forcep) until the subcutaneous layer has been closed. The surgeon and assistant each pick up the peritoneum with hemostats and elevate it. The surgeon then nicks the peritoneum with the deep knife and extends the incision with Metzenbaum scissors (Fig. 19–15).

The abdominal contents are now exposed. From this point on, to protect the abdominal contents from injury, *only saline-moistened sponges are allowed on the field.* The technologist passes the moistened sponges to the surgeon, who covers the tissue edges to protect them from the self-retaining retractor. The Balfour retractor is now placed in position by the surgeon and assistant. At this time the surgeon explores the wound for evidence of disease. When the area of disease has been located, the surgeon packs the abdominal contents away from the diseased area with several lap sponges. A specific surgical procedure can then be initiated.

During the procedure, the technologist's duties are to

1. Keep the field clear of instruments not in use.
2. Keep the cautery pencil free of tissue debris.
3. Exchange soiled sponges for clean ones.
4. Keep loose items such as needles, small dissecting sponges, and suture wrappers off the Mayo stand. Needles and sponges go on the field or Mayo tray *only* when mounted on the appropriate clamp.
5. Protect the field from contamination.

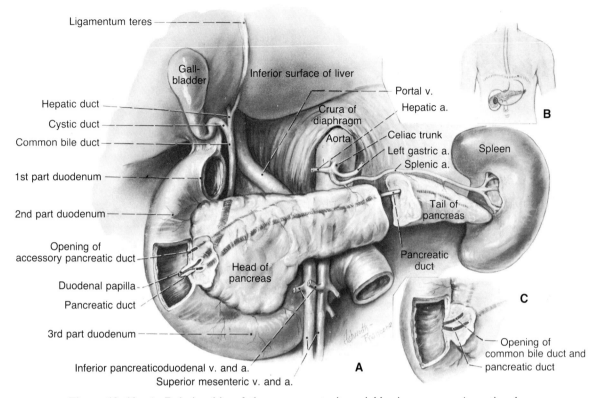

Figure 19–10. *A.* Relationship of the pancreas to its neighboring organs. A section has been cut away from the pancreatic head to show the pancreatic duct where it joins the duodenum. *B.* Anatomic position of the pancreas. *C.* A common variation of the ducts. (From Jacob S, Francone C, Lossow WJ: Structure and Function in Man, 5th ed. Philadelphia, WB Saunders, 1982.)

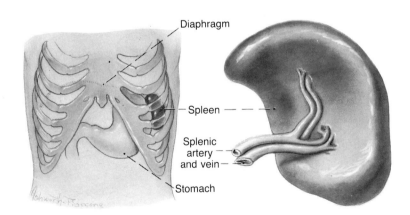

Figure 19–11. The spleen and its anatomic position. (From Jacob S, Francone C, Lossow WJ: Structure and Function in Man, 5th ed. Philadelphia, WB Saunders, 1982.)

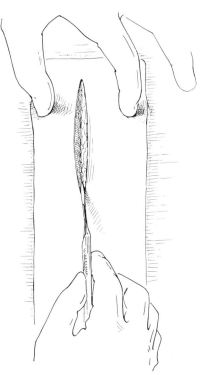

Figure 19–12. Laparotomy. Skin incision. (From Parsons L, Ulfelder H: Atlas of Pelvic Operations, 2nd ed. Philadelphia, WB Saunders, 1968.)

6. Anticipate the needs of the surgeon.

7. Notify the surgeons of a break in aseptic technique, if one should occur.

8. Notify the circulator when the surgeon needs his or her brow wiped.

9. Participate in sponge counts at the appropriate time.

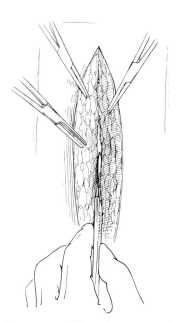

Figure 19–13. Laparotomy. The subcutaneous layer is incised with the deep knife. (From Parsons L, Ulfelder H: Atlas of Pelvic Operations, 2nd ed. Philadelphia, WB Saunders, 1968.)

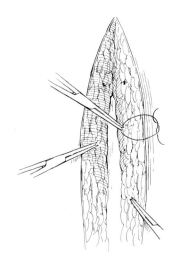

Figure 19–14. Laparotomy. Small bleeders in the subcutaneous layer are ligated with fine absorbable sutures. (From Parsons L, Ulfelder H: Atlas of Pelvic Operations, 2nd ed. Philadelphia, WB Saunders, 1968.)

During the procedure, the surgeon may request that the patient be tipped into the Trendelenburg position. As soon as this request is made, the technologist should immediately raise the Mayo stand to prevent injury to the patient's legs and feet. The Mayo stand must never be allowed to rest on the patient.

Many surgeons irrigate the wound with warm saline solution just before the abdomen is closed. The technologist must check the saline to be sure that it is not too hot; it should feel comfortable to the touch.

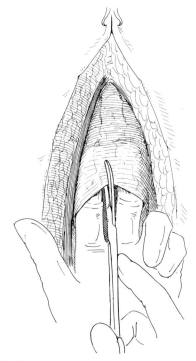

Figure 19–15. Laparotomy. The incision in the peritoneum is lengthened with Metzenbaum scissors. (From Parsons L, Ulfelder H: Atlas of Pelvic Operations, 2nd ed. Philadelphia, WB Saunders, 1968.)

Following irrigation, the wound is closed. The surgeon and assistant remove all sponges and instruments from the abdomen and grasp the edges of the peritoneum with several Mayo clamps. The peritoneum is usually closed with absorbable suture swaged to a taper needle, size 0 or 2-0. Next, the fascia is closed with any of a variety of materials—silk, Dacron, and Dexon are commonly used. Because the fascia is the strongest layer of the abdominal wall and the integrity of the closure depends on its strength, interrupted sutures are most often used to close it. Size 2-0 suture is most commonly used, although size 0 may be used if the patient is very large or obese. The suture may be mounted on a taper or cutting needle, according to the surgeon's preference. During fascia closure, the assistant retracts the skin and subcutaneous layer with U.S. or Richardson retractors. The subcutaneous layer is closed next with interrupted sutures of 3-0 Dexon, chromic catgut, or plain catgut. Fine tapered needles are used. After the subcutaneous layer is closed, the assistant may choose to leave. If this occurs, the technologist must step up to take his or her place and assist in skin closure by cutting the suture ends once the surgeon has tied them in place.

At the completion of skin closure, the technologist or surgeon places the dressings over the wound. The drapes are then removed, and tape is applied to the dressings by the circulator or surgeon.

Partial Gastrectomy With Gastroduodenostomy

Definition

This procedure involves removal of part of the stomach and creation of a new opening between the stomach and duodenum. Partial gastrectomy is performed for chronic gastric ulcer, perforating ulcer, or tumor.

Highlights

1. The abdomen is entered.
2. The stomach is mobilized.
3. The duodenum is mobilized.
4. The duodenum is divided and closed.
5. The stomach is anastomosed to the duodenum.
6. The wound is closed.

Description

The surgeon enters the abdomen through an upper midline incision and examines the abdominal contents to determine the extent of disease and to choose a site for anastomosis. After the exact line of anastomosis is determined, the surgeon mobilizes the stomach from the ligaments, vessels, and omentum that attach to the greater and lesser curvature of the stomach. The technologist must be ready with numerous Mayo clamps, Metzenbaum scissors, and silk ties, sizes 2-0 and 3-0. Additional ties of absorbable suture such as 2-0 and 3-0 Dexon and one or two suture ligatures of silk mounted

on fine tapered needles should also be available. The suture ligatures will be used to ligate the large vessels of the stomach.

The surgeon begins mobilization by grasping the surface of the stomach with Allis or Babcock clamps. The assistant offers traction on these instruments. Dissection is begun on the attachments to the greater curvature. The surgeon places two Mayo clamps for each small segment of tissue to be divided. After double-clamping the segments, he or she divides the tissue between the clamps with Metzenbaum scissors or the cautery pencil. Each section is then tied with silk or Dexon. The lesser curvature of the stomach is divided from its attachments in a similar fashion.

Once the stomach is mobilized, the duodenum is resected from the stomach. The surgeon places two intestinal clamps such as Kocher or Allen-Kocher clamps across the duodenum. The duodenum is divided from the stomach by cutting between the two clamps with knife or cautery pencil.

The duodenal stump is now closed. A running suture of silk, chromic catgut, or Dexon on a fine tapered needle is used to close the stump.

To begin the gastroduodenal anastomosis, the surgeon aligns the stomach and duodenum at the proposed junction site. Silk traction sutures are placed at each end of the site to hold the stomach and duodenum in alignment. The surgeon uses a continuous or interrupted suture swaged on a fine tapered needle, size 3-0 or 4-0, to form the first row of sutures. At the completion of this row, the surgeon makes two incisions, one on each side of the suture line. This exposes the inner surfaces of the stomach and duodenum; they are then joined with fine interrupted sutures (Fig. 19–16). The wound is then irrigated and closed in routine fashion.

Related Procedures

Gastrojejunostomy
Esophagogastrostomy (Fig. 19–17)

Gastrostomy

Definition

This is an incision made into the stomach to allow the insertion of a synthetic feeding tube. One end of the tube is brought out through the skin. This procedure is performed when the patient is unable to ingest food normally because of stricture or lesion of the esophagus.

Highlights

1. The abdomen is entered.
2. The stomach is incised.
3. The feeding tube is placed inside the stomach and secured.
4. The wound is closed.

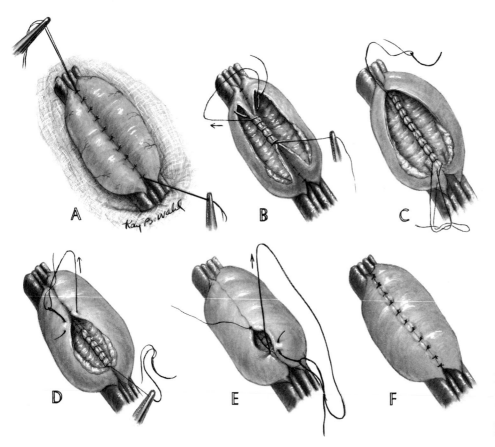

Figure 19–16. Gastrointestinal anastomosis. (From Higgins GA: Orr's Operations of General Surgery, 4th ed. Philadelphia, WB Saunders, 1968.)

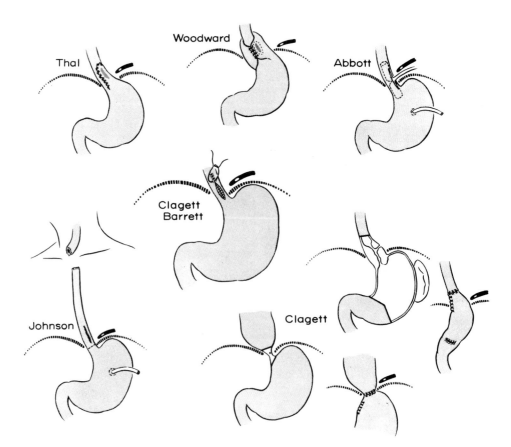

Figure 19–17. Techniques of esophagogastrostomy. (From Schwartz SI, et al: Principles of Surgery, 2nd ed. New York, McGraw-Hill, 1974. Used with the permission of McGraw-Hill Book Company.)

Description

The surgeon enters the abdomen through a short left upper paramedian incision (Fig. 19–18). The surgeon identifies and grasps the stomach with Babcock or Allis clamps and delivers it into the wound site. The assistant retracts the abdominal wall edges with medium Richardson retractors. The surgeon then places a pursestring suture in the stomach where the feeding tube is to be inserted. A small incision in the center of the pursestring suture is then made with the knife or cautery pencil. The technologist should be ready to suction the contents of the stomach as soon as the incision is made.

The feeding tube is now placed inside the stomach through the incision, and the pursestring suture is tied tightly around it (Fig. 19–19). Before closing the abdomen, the surgeon may suture the tube to the peritoneum to secure it in place (Fig. 19–20). The wound is then closed in routine fashion.

Pyloromyotomy

Definition

This is an incision made into the pylorus to release a stenosis. Pyloric stenosis is a congenital defect in which the muscle fibers of the structure are hypertrophied (enlarged) and form fibrous bands, causing the stricture (stenosis) within the pylorus. Pyloromyotomy is performed to allow ingested food to pass easily into the duodenum.

Highlights

1. The abdomen is entered.
2. The pylorus is identified.

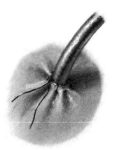

Figure 19–19. Gastrostomy. Pursestring suture is placed around feeding tube. (From Higgins GA: Orr's Operations of General Surgery, 4th ed. Philadelphia, WB Saunders, 1968.)

3. Longitudinal incisions are made into the pylorus.
4. The wound is closed.

Description

The abdomen is entered through a right upper paramedian incision. The surgeon may insert a baby Balfour retractor or may have the assistant retract the abdominal walls with small hand-held retractors. The pylorus is identified. The surgeon then makes an incision into the pylorus, over the defect, with a No. 10 or No. 15 knife blade (Fig. 19–21). Hemostasis is maintained with the electrocautery pencil on a very low setting. The incision is deepened with a fine Kelly clamp. Using Metzenbaum scissors, the surgeon incises the circular muscle fibers to the depth of the inner mucosa, thus releasing the stricture (Fig. 19–22). The incisions are not sutured but are left to heal in their newly released position.

The wound is closed in routine fashion with fine sutures.

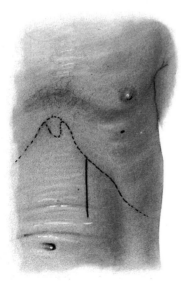

Figure 19–18. Gastrostomy. Line of incision. (From Higgins GA: Orr's Operations of General Surgery, 4th ed. Philadelphia, WB Saunders, 1968.)

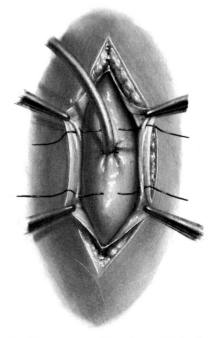

Figure 19–20. Gastrostomy. The stomach tube is secured to the peritoneum. (From Higgins GA: Orr's Operations of General Surgery, 4th ed. Philadelphia, WB Saunders, 1968.)

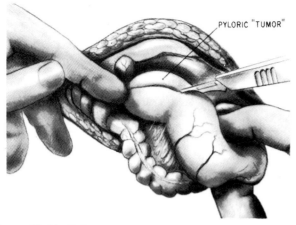

Figure 19–21. Pyloromyotomy. Incision in pylorus. (From Schwartz SI, et al.: Principles of Surgery, 2nd ed. New York, McGraw-Hill, 1974. Used with the permission of McGraw-Hill Book Company.)

Vagotomy

Definition

This is resection of portions of the vagus nerve near the stomach at the level of the esophagus. This procedure is performed in conjunction with gastric resection. The goal of the surgery is to decrease the amount of gastric juices by severing the nerves that control their release.

Highlights

1. The abdomen is entered.
2. The esophagus is mobilized.
3. The left (posterior) and right (anterior) vagus nerves are resected.
4. The wound is closed.

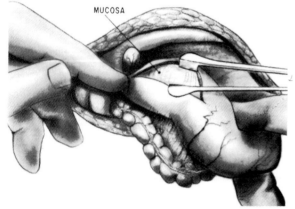

Figure 19–22. Pyloromyotomy. Herniation of the mucosa after the stricture is released. (From Schwartz SI, et al.: Principles of Surgery, 2nd ed. New York, McGraw-Hill, 1974. Used with the permission of McGraw-Hill Book Company.)

Description

The abdomen has already been entered for gastric resection. The esophagus is exposed by the assistant as he or she retracts the liver upward using a Weinberg ("Joe's hoe") retractor. The operating lights are aimed upward into the wound. Using long Metzenbaum scissors and long fine tissue forceps, the surgeon divides the esophagus from the attached peritoneal membrane. Once it has been exposed completely, the esophagus is retracted to the side with a long Penrose drain that has been dipped in saline solution by the technologist.

The surgeon then catches a portion of the vagus nerve with a long nerve hook. Two long right-angled clamps are placed over the nerve. The surgeon cuts the section of nerve lying between the clamps and passes it to the technologist. The surgeon announces "right" or "left" because the technologist must keep each side separate. This can be done by simply placing the specimens on the right and left side of a small basin. The sections of nerve will be sent to the pathologist to confirm that the specimen is nerve tissue. The severed edges of the nerve are then clamped with ligation clips or ligatures. The procedure is repeated on the other side of the esophagus.

The wound is closed in routine fashion.

Anastomosis of the Small Intestine: End-to-End and Side-to-Side Techniques

Definition

Following resection of the small intestine for conditions such as cancer, torsion, diverticulosis, ulcer, or obstruction, the continuity of the intestine is restored. Two techniques, end-to-end and side-to-side, are commonly employed. A third technique that closely resembles these is the end-to-side.

Highlights

1. The abdomen is entered.
2. The lesion is located and the intestine is isolated.
3. The diseased intestine is removed.
4. The healthy intestine is anastomosed.
5. The wound is closed.

Description

Following prepping and draping, the surgeon enters the abdominal cavity through an upper midline incision. To identify diseased portions of the intestine, the surgeon passes the loops of intestine through his or her fingers, examining each segment. Once the surgeon is satisfied that the diseased area has been located, the area between the proposed site of anastomosis must be isolated from the attached mesentery. In preparation for isolation, the technologist must have available many Mayo clamps and silk and Dexon sutures, in both sizes

2-0 and 3-0. The surgeon will use these sutures to tie off the mesenteric tissue and vessels. Using Metzenbaum scissors, the surgeon makes a small incision in an avascular area of the mesentery (Fig. 19–23).

Resection of the diseased segment is begun. The surgeon places Mayo clamps over a section of mesentery, divides it with the knife or cautery pencil between the two clamps, and ligates the segments. Whenever large mesenteric arteries are encountered, the surgeon uses suture ligatures to occlude the vessels. The surgeon continues to dissect the mesentery from the intestine until the diseased portion and anastomosis site are completely isolated.

Two intestinal clamps are placed at each end of the isolated segment, and the tissue is divided with the cautery pencil or knife (Fig. 19–24). The specimen is then passed to the technologist.

End-to-End Technique

The assistant aligns the two cut ends of the bowel in close approximation, turning the clamps slightly outward (Fig. 19–25). In preparation for the anastomosis, the technologist must have an ample supply of fine gastrointestinal sutures available. Most commonly used are 3-0 or 4-0 silk swaged to suture-release needles. The surgeon places the first row of interrupted sutures, leaving the two end sutures long for traction. The clamps are then removed and the next layer of sutures placed. As shown in Figure 19–26, this layer joins the two intestinal lumens. Chromic catgut is often used for this. The layer is continued around the two segments until they are joined. A final layer of interrupted silk sutures is placed through the outside layer of the intestine (Fig. 19–27). The final step in the procedure is to approximate the edges of the mesentery (Fig. 19–28). The surgeon uses fine silk to suture the edges.

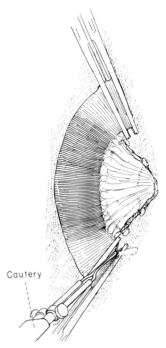

Figure 19–24. Anastomosis of the small intestine: end-to-end technique. To divide the intestine, the surgeon places two intestinal clamps at each end of the area to be resected. The intestine is divided between the clamps with the cautery pencil. (From Parsons L, Ulfelder H: Atlas of Pelvic Operations, 2nd ed. Philadelphia, WB Saunders, 1968.)

Side-to-Side Technique

To begin the side-to-side anastomosis, the surgeon first closes the two intestinal stumps with a continuous suture of 3-0 or 4-0 silk or chromic catgut (Fig. 19–29). The suture line may be reinforced with interrupted 3-0 silk sutures. The assistant then aligns the two segments side to side (Fig. 19–30), and the first layer of interrupted fine silk sutures is placed, with the first and last suture left long for traction. The surgeon makes double incisions into the bowel, one on each side of the suture line (Fig. 19–31). A running suture is placed around the edges of the two bowel limbs to join them (Fig. 19–32). A final layer of interrupted silk sutures is placed over the previous suture line. Using 3-0 silk on fine needles,

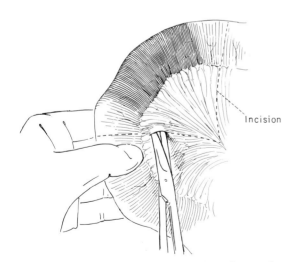

Figure 19–23. Anastomosis of the small intestine: end-to-end technique. To begin the procedure the surgeon makes a small incision in the mesentery. Dotted lines indicate the area of resection. (From Parsons L, Ulfelder H: Atlas of Pelvic Operations, 2nd ed. Philadelphia, WB Saunders, 1968.)

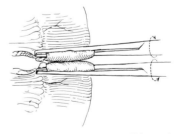

Figure 19–25. Anastomosis of the small intestine: end-to-end technique. The two ends of the severed bowel are brought in close approximation and rotated slightly outward. (From Parsons L, Ulfelder H: Atlas of Pelvic Operations, 2nd ed. Philadelphia, WB Saunders, 1968.)

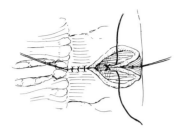

Figure 19–26. Anastomosis of the small intestine: end-to-end technique. The bowel is anastomosed. (From Parsons L, Ulfelder H: Atlas of Pelvic Operations, 2nd ed. Philadelphia, WB Saunders, 1968.)

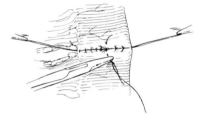

Figure 19–27. Anastomosis of the small intestine: end-to-end technique. Final running suture in the anastomosis. (From Parsons L, Ulfelder H: Atlas of Pelvic Operations, 2nd ed. Philadelphia, WB Saunders, 1968.)

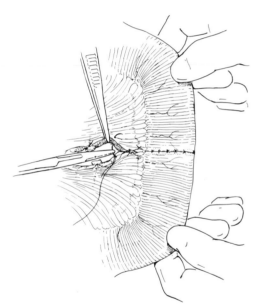

Figure 19–28. Anastomosis of the small intestine: end-to-end technique. The mesentery is approximated. (From Parsons L, Ulfelder H: Atlas of Pelvic Operations, 2nd ed. Philadelphia, WB Saunders, 1968.)

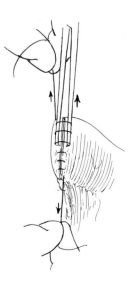

Figure 19–29. Anastomosis of the small intestine: side-to-side technique. The two intestinal stumps are closed. (From Parsons L, Ulfelder H: Atlas of Pelvic Operations, 2nd ed. Philadelphia, WB Saunders, 1968.)

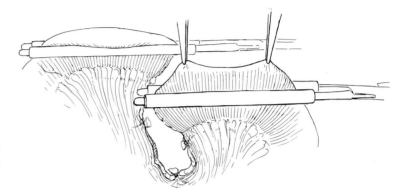

Figure 19–30. Anastomosis of the small intestine: side-to-side technique. The assistant aligns the two bowel segments side to side. (From Parsons L, Ulfelder H: Atlas of Pelvic Operations, 2nd ed. Philadelphia, WB Saunders, 1968.)

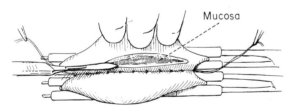

Figure 19–31. Anastomosis of the small intestine: side-to-side technique. After placing an initial layer of interrupted sutures, the surgeon makes two incisions, one on each side of the suture line. This exposes the intestinal mucosa, which is then approximated. (From Parsons L, Ulfelder H: Atlas of Pelvic Operations, 2nd ed. Philadelphia, WB Saunders, 1968.)

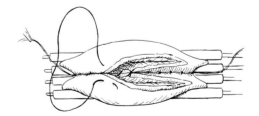

Figure 19–32. Anastomosis of the small intestine: side-to-side technique. A final layer of sutures joins the two intestinal limbs. (From Parsons L, Ulfelder H: Atlas of Pelvic Operations, 2nd ed. Philadelphia, WB Saunders, 1968.)

the surgeon closes the mesentery (Fig. 19–33). The wound is then irrigated and closed in routine fashion.

Related Procedures

Ileostomy
Resection of duodenal ulcer

Colon Resection and Anastomosis

Definition

In this procedure a section of the large intestine is removed and its continuity is restored. It is performed to remove cancerous lesions or to correct other conditions, such as ulcerative colitis or diverticula of the colon. In all procedures involving the large intestine, special precautions are taken to prevent contamination of the field by the bowel contents. Once the bowel has been opened, all contaminated instruments, sponges, and other equipment are kept separate from equipment that is used for closure. Many technicians set up a separate closure stand with the needed suture materials and instruments. This equipment is not touched until the bowel has been closed and the team has been regloved and regowned according to the operating room policy manual.

Highlights

1. The abdomen is entered.
2. The diseased portion of the bowel is identified and isolated.
3. The bowel is cross-clamped and divided.
4. An end-to-end anastomosis is performed.
5. The wound is closed.

Description

According to the location of the lesion, the surgeon enters the abdomen through an appropriate incision. However, a midline incision is usually chosen to give the best exposure to all segments of the bowel. Once the abdomen is entered, the surgeon explores loops of

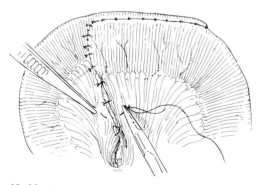

Figure 19–33. Anastomosis of the small intestine: side-to-side technique. The surgeon completes the procedure by approximating the mesentery. (From Parsons L, Ulfelder H: Atlas of Pelvic Operations, 2nd ed. Philadelphia, WB Saunders, 1968.)

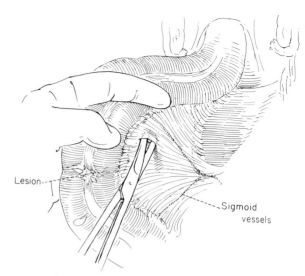

Figure 19–34. Colon resection and anastomosis. Immobilization of the bowel by sharp dissection. (From Parsons L, Ulfelder H: Atlas of Pelvic Operations, 2nd ed. Philadelphia, WB Saunders, 1968.)

intestine to identify the portion to be removed. A wide margin of intestine on either side of the lesion is also removed if the lesion is cancerous.

To free the bowel from its peritoneal and mesenteric attachments, the surgeon dissects them with Metzenbaum scissors (Fig. 19–34). The technologist should have available an ample supply of Mayo clamps and ties of the surgeon's choice. Sizes 2-0 and 3-0 silk are usually used. Portions of mesentery are double-clamped, divided, and ligated. Large vessels are controlled with suture ligatures. The surgeon completes the mobilization procedure along the full length of bowel to be resected. Many surgeons sling a soft rubber Penrose drain around the loop of bowel for retraction.

Once the bowel is isolated, the segment is double-clamped at each end with intestinal clamps. Using the cautery pencil, the surgeon divides the bowel between each set of clamps and passes the specimen to the technologist. At this point the bowel is open and the potential for fecal contamination is present. To help prevent this, the surgeon may place two lap sponges around the base of the intestinal stumps or use rubber bands to seal off the openings of the stumps.

The anastomosis begins as the assistant places the two bowel ends in close approximation (Fig. 19–35). The first layer of interrupted sutures is placed. Fine silk suture-release needles are commonly used. The technologist should take care to place *returned* needles on a magnetic needle board or other such device *as soon as* the surgeon discards the needle. These needles are very small and may be easily lost in the rapid exchange between the surgeon and the technologist. The first and last sutures of the initial suture layer are left long to be used in traction.

After making double incisions in the bowel, the surgeon places a second layer of interrupted chromic catgut sutures, size 3-0, swaged to a fine gastrointestinal needle (Fig. 19–36). The surgeon continues the interrupted

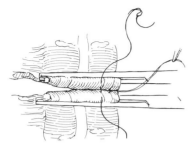

Figure 19–35. Colon resection and anastomosis. To begin the anastomosis, the assistant holds the two ends of the severed bowel in close approximation while the surgeon places the first layer of interrupted sutures. (From Parsons L, Ulfelder H: Atlas of Pelvic Operations, 2nd ed. Philadelphia, WB Saunders, 1968.)

sutures until the two intestinal lumens are joined (Fig. 19–37). The intestinal clamps are then removed and a final reinforcing suture layer of interrupted silk is placed (Fig. 19–38).

The final step in the procedure is closure of the mesentery. Interrupted sutures of silk or chromic catgut, size 3-0, are used (Fig. 19–39).

Following accepted bowel technique, the technologist is now responsible for directing the changeover from a possibly contaminated field to a sterile one. He or she should remove all lap sponges from the wound, remove the suction and cautery pencil from the field, and pull the "dirty" Mayo stand away from the field. The circulator removes each team member's gloves and gown and distributes clean gowns and gloves to the technologist. The technologist dons the new sterile gown and gloves and proceeds to gown and glove the surgeons. A sterile procedure (laparotomy) drape is placed directly over the contaminated one on the patient, and a new suction tubing and electrocautery pencil are clamped to it. Usually, to save time, the surgeon will assist the technologist in this. It is important to note that some hospitals and surgeons are stricter than others in the extent to which they perform the changeover. Some surgeons simply change gloves, while others order a complete changeover. Occasionally the decision is left to the technologist. Since the relative cost of a complete changeover is minimal and certainly will not *harm* the patient, it is recommended.

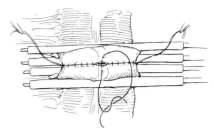

Figure 19–37. Colon resection and anastomosis. Continuation of second suture row. (From Parsons L, Ulfelder H: Atlas of Pelvic Operations, 2nd ed. Philadelphia, WB Saunders, 1968.)

The technologist distributes fresh lap sponges on the field, and the wound is irrigated (in some operating rooms this is done *before* the changeover) and closed in routine fashion.

Related Procedure

Total colectomy

Ileotransverse Colostomy

Definition

This is the surgical removal of a portion of the ileum and transverse colon and a side-to-side anastomosis between the ileum and colon. This procedure is performed for lesions such as those caused by cancer, diverticulosis, or obstruction of the large intestine in an area close to the cecum.

Highlights

1. The abdomen is entered.
2. The lesion is identified.
3. The portion of bowel to be resected is mobilized.
4. The bowel is cross-clamped and divided.
5. The blind stump of the ileum is closed.
6. The ileum is anastomosed to the transverse colon.
7. The wound is closed.

Description

Following routine prepping and draping, the surgeon enters the abdomen through a right paramedian or

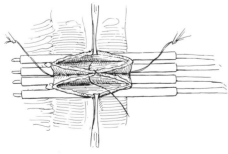

Figure 19–36. Colon resection and anastomosis. Second row of interrupted sutures that approximate the inner surfaces of the bowel. (From Parsons L, Ulfelder H: Atlas of Pelvic Operations, 2nd ed. Philadelphia, WB Saunders, 1968.)

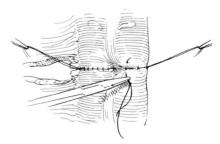

Figure 19–38. Colon resection and anastomosis. Final outside row of interrupted sutures. (From Parsons L, Ulfelder H: Atlas of Pelvic Operations, 2nd ed. Philadelphia, WB Saunders, 1968.)

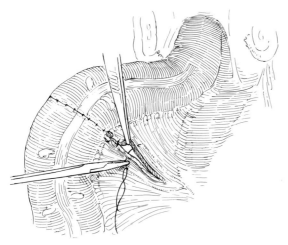

Figure 19–39. Colon resection and anastomosis. The surgeon completes the procedure by approximating the mesentery with interrupted sutures. (From Parsons L, Ulfelder H: Atlas of Pelvic Operations, 2nd ed. Philadelphia, WB Saunders, 1968.)

median incision. Once the wound is open, the surgeon examines loops of intestine to locate the exact position of the bowel lesion. The surgeon begins the procedure by isolating the bowel segment from the mesentery. Using Metzenbaum scissors, the surgeon locates an avascular area in the mesentery and incises a small portion (Fig. 19–40). As in most intestinal procedures, Mayo clamps are used to double-clamp sections of mesentery. The surgeon divides the tissue between the two clamps with the knife, scissors, or cautery pencil. The tissue sections are then ligated with silk or Dexon ties. Large mesenteric vessels are ligated with suture ligatures as described for previous intestinal procedures.

Once the bowel is completely free of its mesenteric attachments, the surgeon cross-clamps the ileum at the

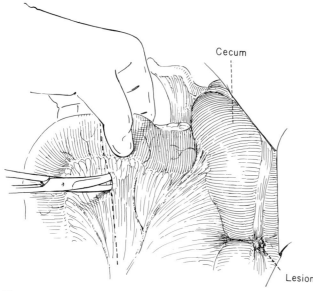

Figure 19–40. Ileotransverse colostomy. Mobilization of the bowel with Metzenbaum scissors. Dotted lines indicate area of resection. (From Parsons L, Ulfelder H: Atlas of Pelvic Operations, 2nd ed. Philadelphia, WB Saunders, 1968.)

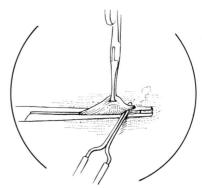

Figure 19–41. Ileotransverse colostomy. Using the cautery pencil, the surgeon removes a small section of tissue from the colon. (From Parsons L, Ulfelder H: Atlas of Pelvic Operations, 2nd ed. Philadelphia, WB Saunders, 1968.)

proposed site of anastomosis with two intestinal clamps. The ileum is then divided between the two clamps with the knife or cautery pencil. The surgeon closes the blind (distal) stump of the ileum in two layers. The first layer is a running catgut suture, size 3-0, swaged to a fine gastrointestinal needle. The second layer is composed of interrupted silk sutures of the same size or smaller. Suture-release needles may be used for this layer.

The surgeon prepares the colon for anastomosis by grasping the area of proposed anastomosis with one or two Allis clamps. A Kocher, Allen, or similar intestinal clamp is placed in a longitudinal plane beside the Allis clamp. The colon is then incised with the cautery pencil (Fig. 19–41). The incised portion of colon is passed to the technologist, who isolates it from sterile instruments or equipment. (It must be remembered that accepted bowel technique must be observed, since the large intestine is now open and the field may be contaminated.)

The surgeon begins the anastomosis by placing interrupted sutures of 3-0 or 4-0 silk to join the two bowel segments. The assistant holds the two Kocher clamps close together as the surgeon places the sutures (Fig. 19–42). As soon as the first layer is completed, the surgeon places the second layer using interrupted sutures

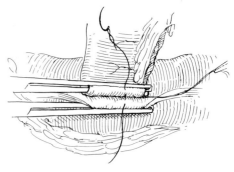

Figure 19–42. Ileotransverse colostomy. While the assistant holds the severed ileum and colon in close approximation, the surgeon begins the anastomosis. (From Parsons L, Ulfelder H: Atlas of Pelvic Operations, 2nd ed. Philadelphia, WB Saunders, 1968.)

of chromic catgut on a fine needle. The layer is continued around the two structures until they are joined (Fig. 19–43). A final layer of interrupted silk is placed through the outer tissue layers, completing the anastomosis (Fig. 19–44). The mesentery is sutured to the posterior peritoneum using 3-0 interrupted silk sutures. The wound is irrigated and closed in routine fashion.

Loop Colostomy

Definition

A loop of large intestine is brought out through a small abdominal incision, sutured to the skin, and opened. The resulting *colostomy* serves as a temporary channel for the evacuation of fecal material. A colostomy is performed to give the bowel a rest following colon resection. The procedure may also be performed in the presence of inflammatory disease or obstruction of the colon. The loop colostomy is closed when fecal diversion is no longer needed.

Highlights

Opening

1. The abdomen is entered.
2. A small portion of transverse colon is mobilized.
3. The mobilized bowel is brought out through the incision.
4. A colostomy rod is inserted under the loop.
5. The wound is closed.
6. The loop is incised 24 to 48 hours after the procedure.

Closure

1. The skin edges around the colostomy are incised.
2. Dissection is carried to the peritoneum.
3. The colostomy edges are trimmed and sutured together.
4. The loop is allowed to retract into the abdomen.
5. The wound is closed.

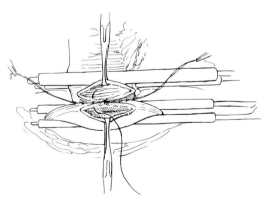

Figure 19–43. Ileotransverse colostomy. The second row of sutures joins the inner lumens. (From Parsons L, Ulfelder H: Atlas of Pelvic Operations, 2nd ed. Philadelphia, WB Saunders, 1968.)

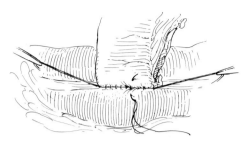

Figure 19–44. Ileotransverse colostomy. Final row of sutures in the anastomosis. (From Parsons L, Ulfelder H: Atlas of Pelvic Operations, 2nd ed. Philadelphia, WB Saunders, 1968.)

Description

Opening

The abdomen is entered through a short transverse upper paramedian incision. The assistant retracts the abdominal wall with a medium Richardson retractor. Using one or more Babcock clamps, the surgeon grasps a loop of transverse colon and brings it forward into the wound.

The surgeon begins to mobilize the bowel from its attachments to the omentum with Metzenbaum scissors (Fig. 19–45). An avascular area of the omentum is chosen for the mobilization. However, if blood vessels are encountered, the surgeon grasps the tissue with Mayo clamps, divides the tissue between the clamps, and ligates it with 3-0 silk or Dexon ties.

When mobilization is complete, the loop of intestine is brought out of the abdomen and a glass or plastic colostomy rod is placed under the loop to prevent it from retracting back into the abdomen (Fig. 19–46). The wound is then closed in standard fashion around the loop (Fig. 19–47).

Closure

After prepping and draping of the patient, the surgeon initiates the procedure by placing a gauze sponge at the opening of the colostomy. This prevents gross contamination of the wound by fecal material. The surgeon then incises the skin around the edges of the colostomy (Fig. 19–48). The incision is carried through the subcutaneous and fascial layer (Figs. 19–49 and 19–50). The peritoneum is dissected free of the colostomy with Metzenbaum scissors (Fig. 19–51). To prevent contamination of the peritoneal cavity, the colostomy is surrounded with one or two lap sponges. The surgeon then trims the skin from the edges of the colostomy (Fig. 19–52).

The surgeon closes the colostomy by inserting two layers of suture through the colostomy edges. The first layer is closed with running or interrupted chromic catgut, size 3-0, swaged to a fine needle (Fig. 19–53). A second layer of interrupted silk, size 3-0 or 4-0, is placed over the chromic suture line.

The bowel is then allowed to slide back into position in the peritoneal cavity, and the wound is closed in routine fashion.

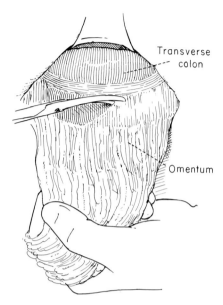

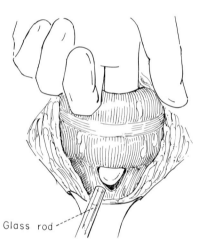

Figure 19–45. Loop colostomy. Mobilization of the colon from the omentum. (From Parsons L, Ulfelder H: Atlas of Pelvic Operations, 2nd ed. Philadelphia, WB Saunders, 1968.)

Figure 19–46. Loop colostomy. Insertion of colostomy rod under mobilized colon loop. This prevents the loop from retracting back into the abdomen. (From Parsons L, Ulfelder H: Atlas of Pelvic Operations, 2nd ed. Philadelphia, WB Saunders, 1968.)

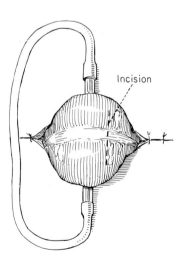

Figure 19–47. Loop colostomy. The line of incision in the colostomy. The colostomy is usually opened 24 to 48 hours after it has been brought out of the wound. (From Parsons L, Ulfelder H: Atlas of Pelvic Operations, 2nd ed. Philadelphia, WB Saunders, 1968.)

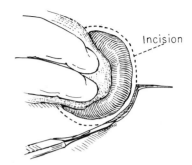

Figure 19–48. Loop colostomy. Closure of colostomy. The surgeon makes an incision around the colostomy. (From Parsons L, Ulfelder H: Atlas of Pelvic Operations, 2nd ed. Philadelphia, WB Saunders, 1968.)

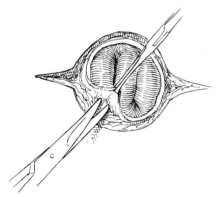

Figure 19–49. Loop colostomy. The incision is carried to the subcutaneous layer. (From Parsons L, Ulfelder H: Atlas of Pelvic Operations, 2nd ed. Philadelphia, WB Saunders, 1968.)

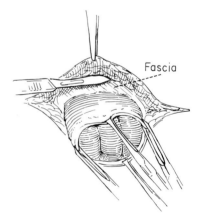

Figure 19–50. Loop colostomy. Allis clamps are placed on the edge of the colostomy for retraction. (From Parsons L, Ulfelder H: Atlas of Pelvic Operations, 2nd ed. Philadelphia, WB Saunders, 1968.)

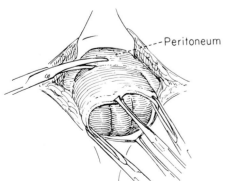

Figure 19–51. Loop colostomy. The peritoneum is incised with Metzenbaum scissors. (From Parsons L, Ulfelder H: Atlas of Pelvic Operations, 2nd ed. Philadelphia, WB Saunders, 1968.)

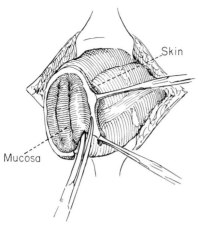

Figure 19–52. Loop colostomy. The surgeon excises the skin from the edges of the colostomy. (From Parsons L, Ulfelder H: Atlas of Pelvic Operations, 2nd ed. Philadelphia, WB Saunders, 1968.)

Abdominoperineal Resection of the Rectum

Definition

Through combined abdominal and perineal incisions, the anus, rectum, and sigmoid colon are removed en bloc. This procedure is performed to treat cancer of the rectum. The obliteration of the rectum necessitates the formation of a permanent colostomy in the abdominal wall for drainage of bowel contents.

Highlights

1. The abdomen is entered.
2. The lesion is located and the bowel is mobilized.
3. The colon is divided in an area proximal to the lesion.

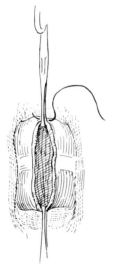

Figure 19–53. Loop colostomy. The colostomy is closed with two layers of sutures. (From Parsons L, Ulfelder H: Atlas of Pelvic Operations, 2nd ed. Philadelphia, WB Saunders, 1968.)

4. A colostomy is performed and the abdomen is closed.
5. Through a perineal incision, the lower sigmoid colon, rectum, and anus are mobilized and removed.
6. The perineal incision is closed.

Description

Abdominoperineal resection is often performed as two simultaneous procedures, with one team operating on the abdominal region and a second on the perineal portion. When the operation is performed in this manner, the patient is placed in the lithotomy position. Because the abdominal team has restricted space in which to work, the technologist on the team must stand slightly behind the assistant rather than next to him or her, as is the usual practice during abdominal procedures. The technologist must take special care to avoid contamination while standing in this awkward position. During simultaneous procedures, the technologist on the lower team stands next to the surgeon, as for vaginal procedures. The surgeon usually performs the procedure while sitting. Both technologists must keep in mind that there is usually only one circulator to assist both teams. Much confusion and aggravation can be avoided if the technologists anticipate the need for equipment before the procedure so that the circulator is not unduly stressed in performing his or her duties.

To avoid confusion, the procedure is discussed here as if performed by one team. The surgeon enters the abdomen through a long midline incision. The intestine is examined and the line of resection is determined.

Mobilization of the colon involves isolation of the mesenteric tissue and omentum that contain diseased lymph nodes. The surgeon frees the colon from its attachments by double-clamping the tissue with Mayo clamps. The tissue between the clamps is then divided with Metzenbaum scissors or a cautery pencil, and the sections are ligated with silk or Dexon ties. As mobilization continues, longer instruments will be needed. The technologist must have an ample supply of Péan clamps, long right-angled clamps, and small sponge dissectors. Both smooth and toothed long tissue forceps are also required. Large blood vessels are clamped with right-angled or Péan clamps and ligated with suture ligatures. The technologist should have one or two suture ligatures ready at all times during the dissection.

Dissection and mobilization are continued through the pelvic floor to the level of the levator muscles. At this point the abdominal dissection is halted, because the depth of the incision is too great for the surgeon to work on comfortably. The surgeon places two intestinal clamps across the bowel at the proximal end of the mobilized area. The bowel between the clamps is divided, and the distal end is placed in the pelvis. The proximal end of the divided bowel may be temporarily ligated with heavy silk. To reconstruct the pelvic floor, a portion of the omentum may be sutured to it.

To prepare a site for the colostomy, the surgeon incises a small circle in the abdomen using the skin knife. The incision is deepened to the inner abdomen with cautery. The small disk of tissue is then passed to the technologist as a specimen. The proximal end of the bowel is brought through the circular incision and temporarily clamped in place while the abdominal incision is closed in routine fashion.

To create the colostomy, the surgeon everts the edges of the bowel stoma and sutures the edges of the skin using interrupted sutures of 3-0 chromic catgut on a fine cutting needle.

Surgery from the perineal end begins as the surgeon places a heavy silk pursestring suture through the anus to occlude it (Fig. 19–54) and the perineum is incised (Fig. 19–55). The incision is deepened with the cautery pencil. Large bleeding vessels are double-clamped and ligated with silk or Dexon. As the incision becomes deeper, Péan clamps are used to grasp the bowel attachments, as described in the abdominal portion of the procedure. Stick sponges and suction should be available at all times during the mobilization and dissection.

Dissection is continued until the surgeon reaches the previously mobilized area of the bowel. The entire specimen is delivered through the perineal incision (Fig. 19–56). The surgeon then irrigates the wound, using an Asepto syringe.

In the past, surgeons packed the wound with a large sheet of rubber (rubber dam) rather than closing it with sutures. The present trend, however, is to obliterate the "dead space" with many interrupted sutures. One or two Penrose drains are placed in the wound, which is then closed with size 0 chromic catgut or Dexon. The skin is approximated with the surgeon's choice of nonabsorbable material and dressed with a bulky abdominal pad and gauze sponges.

Appendectomy

Definition

This is removal of the appendix, a blind, narrow, elongated pouch attached to the cecum. It is removed when acutely infected to prevent peritonitis, which will occur if it should rupture. Many surgeons perform an appendectomy as a prophylactic (preventive) procedure when operating in the abdomen for other reasons. The procedure is then called an *incidental appendectomy*.

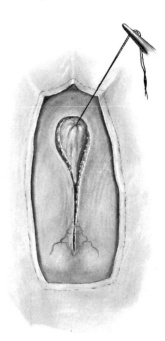

Figure 19–55. Abdominoperineal resection. Area of incision around the rectum. (From Higgins GA: Orr's Operations of General Surgery, 4th ed. Philadelphia, WB Saunders, 1968.)

Highlights

1. The abdomen is entered.
2. The appendix is isolated from the mesoappendix.
3. The appendix is ligated and removed.
4. A pursestring suture is placed around the stump of the appendix.
5. The wound is closed.

Description

The abdomen is entered through a McBurney's incision. The surgeon's assistant retracts the wound edges

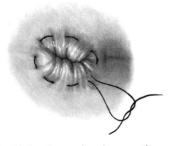

Figure 19–54. Abdominoperineal resection. The surgeon places a heavy pursestring suture around the anus to occlude it. (From Higgins GA: Orr's Operations of General Surgery, 4th ed. Philadelphia, WB Saunders, 1968.)

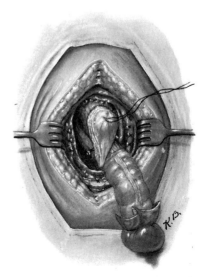

Figure 19–56. Abdominoperineal resection. The colon and rectum are delivered through the perineal incision. (From Higgins GA: Orr's Operations of General Surgery, 4th ed. Philadelphia, WB Saunders, 1968.)

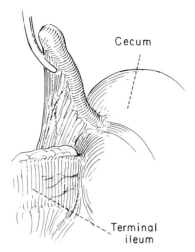

Figure 19–57. Appendectomy. The surgeon grasps the tip of the appendix with a hemostat. (From Parsons L, Ulfelder H: Atlas of Pelvic Operations, 2nd ed. Philadelphia, WB Saunders, 1968.)

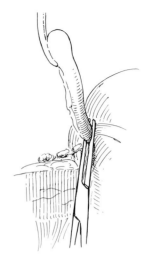

Figure 19–59. Appendectomy. The base of the appendix is clamped with a small straight hemostat. (From Parsons L, Ulfelder H: Atlas of Pelvic Operations, 2nd ed. Philadelphia, WB Saunders, 1968.)

with a Richardson or similar retractor. The surgeon grasps the appendix with Babcock clamps and delivers it into the wound site. The tip of the appendix may then be grasped with a Mayo or Kelly clamp to hold it up (Fig. 19–57). A moist lap sponge is placed around the base of the appendix to prevent contamination of the wound with bowel contents, in case any spill out during the procedure. During an appendectomy or other bowel procedure, all instruments that come into contact with the inner surface of the bowel must be isolated from other clean instruments, drapes, and equipment. The technologist must have a square pan or kidney basin designated as "dirty" to receive the contaminated instruments and specimen. This pan can be kept on the back table and brought up to the Mayo stand when needed.

The surgeon isolates the appendix from its attachments to the bowel (mesoappendix). Using Metzenbaum scissors, the surgeon makes a small hole in an avascular area of the mesoappendix near its base. By taking small

bits of tissue along the appendix, the surgeon double-clamps the mesoappendix and ligates it with free ties of 3-0 silk or absorbable suture until the appendix is completely mobilized (Fig. 19–58).

The base of the appendix is grasped with a straight Kelly clamp (Fig. 19–59). The technologist should have a free tie for the base and a pursestring suture available. The base tie is usually size 0 and can be any of a variety of materials, depending on the surgeon's preference. The pursestring suture should be silk or cotton, size 3-0 or 4-0, on a fine needle such as a French-eye. The surgeon ligates the base of the appendix. The assistant then places a straight Kelly clamp close to the knot and the surgeon cuts the suture ends directly above the clamp. The appendix is now ready for amputation, and the technologist should bring up the "dirty" pan. Using the knife, the surgeon amputates the appendix (Fig. 19–60) and delivers it into the "dirty" pan. The pursestring suture is placed around the appendix stump (Fig. 19–

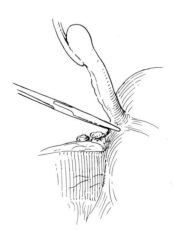

Figure 19–58. Appendectomy. The appendix is freed from its attachments. (From Parsons L, Ulfelder H: Atlas of Pelvic Operations, 2nd ed. Philadelphia, WB Saunders, 1968.)

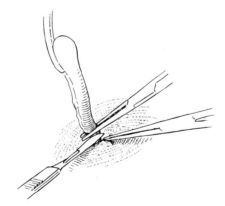

Figure 19–60. Appendectomy. The surgeon amputates the appendix with the knife. This should be discarded in a "dirty" pan, along with the appendix and all other instruments that come in contact with the inside of the appendix. (From Parsons L, Ulfelder H: Atlas of Pelvic Operations, 2nd ed. Philadelphia, WB Saunders, 1968.)

61). The assistant then pushes the appendix stump against the cecum while the surgeon ties the pursestring suture. The stump is thus buried (Fig. 19–62). The straight clamp is withdrawn and discarded in the dirty pan. The wound is irrigated with warm saline solution and the abdomen is closed in routine fashion.

Cholecystectomy

Definition

This is surgical removal of a diseased gallbladder. In acute cholecystitis, the normally bluish green gallbladder becomes distended and inflamed due to obstruction by one or more gallstones. In removing the gallbladder, the common bile duct is left unimpaired so that it becomes a functional passageway through which bile can enter the duodenum.

Highlights

1. The abdomen is entered.
2. The bile ducts are identified and isolated.
3. The cystic artery is identified and ligated.
4. The cystic duct is ligated.
5. The gallbladder is dissected from the liver bed.
6. The wound is closed.

Description

The patient is placed in the supine position with a small pad or gallbladder lift placed under the right upper quadrant. This facilitates exposure of the gallbladder and associated structures. The abdomen is entered through a right subcostal or right paramedian incision. If the patient is very obese, an upper midline incision may be used. Once the abdomen is entered, the liver is covered with moist lap sponges and retracted gently upward by the assistant. A Deaver or Harrington retractor is used.

If the gallbladder is greatly distended, the surgeon may drain it of bile. The technologist passes a gallbladder trocar to the surgeon. The trocar is fitted to the

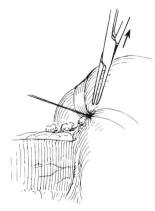

Figure 19–62. Appendectomy. The assistant pushes the appendix stump into the cecum while the surgeon ties the pursestring suture. The clamp is then withdrawn and discarded into the "dirty" pan. (From Parsons L, Ulfelder H: Atlas of Pelvic Operations, 2nd ed. Philadelphia, WB Saunders, 1968.)

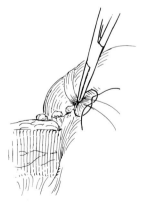

Figure 19–61. Appendectomy. A pursestring suture is placed around the appendix stump. (From Parsons L, Ulfelder H: Atlas of Pelvic Operations, 2nd ed. Philadelphia, WB Saunders, 1968.)

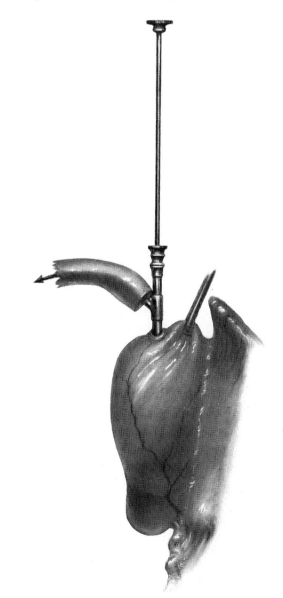

Figure 19–63. Cholecystectomy. The surgeon drains the gallbladder with a trocar. (From Higgins GA: Orr's Operations of General Surgery, 4th ed. Philadelphia, WB Saunders, 1968.)

suction and thrust into the gallbladder, allowing it to drain (Fig. 19–63). A Mayo clamp is then placed over the hole made by the trocar. The trocar should be handed off the field to the circulator.

To identify the cystic duct, cystic artery, and common bile duct, the surgeon removes a thin peritoneal layer from these structures. This is done with both blunt and sharp dissection. Metzenbaum scissors, long fine-toothed forceps, and small sponge dissectors are used. The surgeon then identifies the vessels. Using right-angled clamps, the surgeon double-clamps the cystic duct, which is then divided and ligated with a long 2-0 silk tie on a passer (Fig. 19–64). The cystic artery is clamped and ligated similarly (Fig. 19–65).

The dissection of the gallbladder from the undersurface of the liver is carried out with Metzenbaum scissors and right-angled clamps. The surgeon continues the dissection until the gallbladder is completely mobilized. The specimen is then passed to the technologist. The removal of the gallbladder leaves a raw surface on the liver. This surface may be sewn over with 3-0 or 4-0 chromic catgut swaged to a fine needle, but many surgeons believe that the surface heals just as well without sutures.

The wound is irrigated with warm saline solution, and the operative site is examined for small bleeders. The surgeon lays one or two Penrose drains into the wound and brings them to the outside of the abdomen through a stab incision near the original abdominal incision. The wound is then closed in routine fashion.

Operative Cholangiography: Exploration of the Common Bile Duct

Definition

The biliary vessels are injected with dye and radiographs are taken to determine the presence of stones or stricture. Once a stone or group of stones is located on the radiograph, the stones are removed and the ducts are dilated. These procedures are generally performed in conjunction with a cholecystectomy. Many surgeons perform cholangiography routinely with a cholecystectomy.

Highlights

1. The abdomen is entered.
2. The gallbladder is drained of bile.

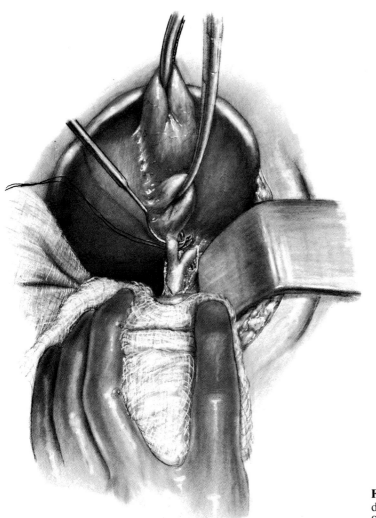

Figure 19–64. Cholecystectomy. Ligation of the cystic duct. (From Higgins GA: Orr's Operations of General Surgery, 4th ed. Philadelphia, WB Saunders, 1968.)

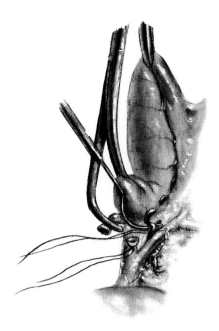

Figure 19–65. Cholecystectomy. The cystic artery is ligated and divided. (From Higgins GA: Orr's Operations of General Surgery, 4th ed. Philadelphia, WB Saunders, 1968.)

3. An incision is made in the common bile duct and a biliary catheter is introduced.
4. Radiographs are taken.
5. The ducts are explored.
6. A T-tube is inserted.
7. The wound is closed.

Description

The patient is prepped, draped, and positioned as for a cholecystectomy. The abdomen is entered through a right subcostal or upper midline incision. The assistant retracts the liver upward with a Deaver or Harrington retractor. In many cases the gallbladder is distended and must be drained; this is performed as previously described for a cholecystectomy. Once the gallbladder is drained, the trocar is passed back to the technologist, who places it in a basin. During the case, this basin will receive all instruments contaminated with bile.

The base of the gallbladder is explored using Metzenbaum scissors, right-angled clamps, and small sponge dissectors. The surgeon separates the common bile duct from nearby structures. If there is doubt as to whether the common duct has been identified correctly, the surgeon may wish to aspirate the vessel with a needle. A 30-mL syringe and 18-gauge needle are suitable for this. Once the surgeon has identified the common duct, two traction sutures of 3-0 silk are placed through the wall of the duct. An incision is then made between the sutures with a No. 15 or No. 11 knife blade or Potts scissors (Fig. 19–66).

The technologist should have a catheter for insertion into the duct, radiopaque dye, and a 30- or 50-mL syringe available. The dye should be prepared by the technologist *before* the surgeon actually needs it to avoid delay. The dye is prepared using the following guidelines:

1. According to the surgeon's preference card or verbal orders, the circulator distributes dye in the surgeon's desired strength to the technologist. Many surgeons prefer the dye to be diluted with saline solution. If so, the technologist receives injectable saline from the circulator and mixes it with the proper amount of dye. At least 30 mL of solution should be prepared, which is then aspirated into the syringe, which is then attached to the biliary catheter.

2. *All air bubbles must be removed* from both the syringe and catheter. To do this, the technologist holds the syringe upright and injects a tiny amount of dye solution through the catheter. Tapping the syringe gently should cause the bubbles to rise to the top of the syringe, where they can be ejected out of the catheter.

3. The technologist places a Kelly clamp across the catheter, near its tip, to prevent air from backing up into the syringe. If any air bubbles remain, they will appear as stones on the radiograph. The syringe, catheter, and its attaching clamp are then passed to the surgeon.

The surgeon threads the tip of the catheter through the incision in the common duct. He or she may wish to tie it in place with a strand of 0 or 2-0 silk. Before radiographs are taken, the wound should be protected with a towel from contamination by the overhead x-ray machine. All team members except the surgeon leave the field to stand behind a lead x-ray shield brought into the room by the circulator. (The surgeon remains behind to inject the dye.)

Once the radiographs have been taken and returned and the stones are identified on the films, the common duct exploration may proceed. During exploration, the exact instruments and the order in which they are used will vary according to the size and location of the stones. Randall stone forceps, toothed forceps, and gallbladder scoops are used to remove the stones (Fig. 19–67). The surgeon may also elect to use a special biliary irrigation

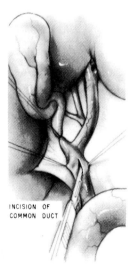

INCISION OF COMMON DUCT

Figure 19–66. Cholangiography. The surgeon incises the common bile duct. (From Schwartz SI, et al: Principles of Surgery, 2nd ed. New York, McGraw-Hill, 1974. Used with the permission of McGraw-Hill Book Company.)

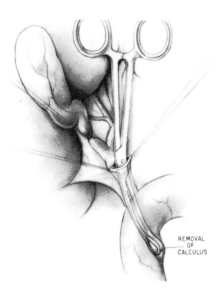

REMOVAL
OF
CALCULUS

Figure 19–67. Cholangiography. The biliary stones are removed with Randall stone forceps. (From Schwartz SI, et al: Principles of Surgery, 2nd ed. New York, McGraw-Hill, 1974. Used with permission of McGraw-Hill, 1974. Used with the permission of McGraw-Hill Book Company.)

catheter (Fig. 19–68). Special biliary probes (Fig. 19–69) are also available for stone removal. The catheter probe is advanced beyond the level of the stone, the balloon is inflated, and the catheter is withdrawn, bringing the stone with it. As the stones are removed, the technologist should retrieve them as specimens. Additional films may be taken to ensure that the bile ducts are patent (open). If a cholecystectomy is to be performed, it is done at this time.

After exploration, the surgeon may wish to dilate the biliary ducts using Bakes dilators. The scrub assistant should hand the dilators to the surgeon one at a time, starting with a small one and progressing to larger ones.

At the close of the procedure, a T-tube is inserted into the common duct (Fig. 19–70). The surgeon will state which size tube is preferred. The tube is inserted using fine tissue forceps such as Cushing forceps. The ductal incision is then closed with size 3-0 or 4-0 silk on a fine tapered needle (Fig. 19–71). The long end of the T-tube is brought out from the wound and later attached to a special "bile bag," which collects bile while the wound heals. The wound is irrigated with warm saline solution and is closed in standard fashion.

Choledochoduodenostomy

Definition

This is establishment of a new connection between the common bile duct and duodenum. It is performed in conjunction with a cholecystectomy when the normal opening into the duodenum is obstructed by a cancerous lesion or stricture. The duodenum can be completely bypassed when the common bile duct is anastomosed to the jejunum (choledochojejunostomy).

Highlights

1. The abdomen is entered.
2. The common bile duct and duodenum are identified and exposed.
3. The duodenum is mobilized.
4. The common bile duct and duodenum are anastomosed.
5. The wound is closed.

Description

The patient is prepped and draped as for a cholecystectomy. The surgeon enters the abdomen through a right subcostal or upper right paramedian incision. The surgeon then examines the biliary structures and determines the area of anastomosis on the duodenum (Fig. 19–72). The assistant retracts the liver upward with a

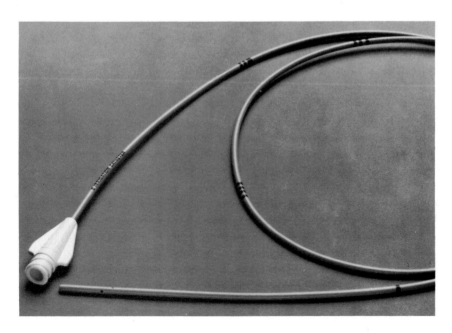

Figure 19–68. Fogarty irrigation catheter. (Courtesy of Edwards Laboratories.)

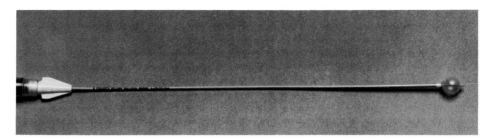

Figure 19–69. Fogarty biliary probe. The catheter is threaded past the stone, the balloon is inflated, and the catheter is withdrawn. (Courtesy of Edwards Laboratories.)

large Deaver or Harrington retractor. The surgeon dissects the common duct free from surrounding structures using Metzenbaum scissors and long fine tissue forceps. There may be bands of scar tissue over the duct, which are removed with sharp and blunt dissection.

A small area of duodenum is mobilized. The surgeon places one row of fine sutures to connect the duodenum and common duct. Two small incisions are then made, one on each side of the suture line (Fig. 19–73). The anastomosis is completed with an additional layer of fine silk sutures (Fig. 19–74). The abdomen is irrigated and closed as for a cholecystectomy.

Related Procedure

Choledochojejunostomy

Splenectomy

Definition

This is surgical removal of the spleen. Indications for splenectomy are serious traumatic injury to the organ and certain blood disorders. The procedure is often performed in an emergency, and the technologist must remain alert and attentive. If splenectomy is performed for a blood disorder, accessory spleens are also sought and removed.

Highlights

1. The abdomen is entered.
2. The spleen is mobilized.
3. The splenic artery and vein are clamped and ligated.
4. The spleen is removed.
5. The wound is closed.

Description

The surgeon enters the abdomen through an upper midline or left subcostal incision. In cases in which the spleen is greatly enlarged, a combined thoracoabdominal incision may be used. The technologist must have suction available as soon as the procedure begins, since during traumatic injury the abdomen is often filled with blood. As soon as the abdomen is entered and retractors are inserted, the surgeon explores the abdomen for the site of injury. The technologist should place a large basin on the field to receive blood clots. The surgeon and assistant manually remove large clots from the abdomen. Suction is used continuously during the exploration and removal of clots.

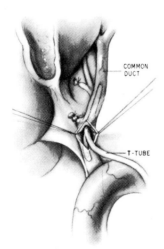

Figure 19–70. Cholangiography. A T-tube is inserted into the common duct following the procedure. (From Schwartz SI, et al: Principles of Surgery, 2nd ed. New York, McGraw-Hill, 1974. Used with the permission of McGraw-Hill Book Company.)

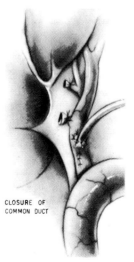

Figure 19–71. Cholangiography. The surgeon closes the ductal incision with fine interrupted sutures. (From Schwartz SI, et al: Principles of Surgery, 2nd ed. New York, McGraw-Hill, 1974. Used with the permission of McGraw-Hill Book Company.)

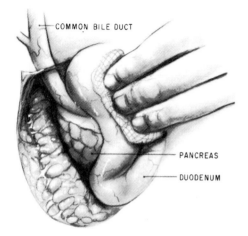

COMMON BILE DUCT

PANCREAS

DUODENUM

Figure 19–72. Choledochoduodenostomy. The surgeon examines the biliary structures to determine the area of anastomosis. (From Schwartz SI, et al: Principles of Surgery, 2nd ed. New York, McGraw-Hill, 1974. Used with the permission of McGraw-Hill Book Company.)

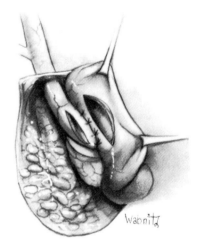

Figure 19–73. Choledochoduodenostomy. After placing a single row of sutures between the common bile duct and the duodenum, the surgeon makes one incision on each side of the suture line. (From Schwartz SI, et al: Principles of Surgery, 2nd ed. New York, McGraw-Hill, 1974. Used with the permission of McGraw-Hill Book Company.)

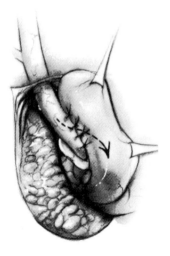

Figure 19–74. Completed anastomosis. Dotted line indicates flow of bile. (From Schwartz SI, et al: Principles of Surgery, 2nd ed. New York, McGraw-Hill, 1974. Used with the permission of McGraw-Hill Book Company.)

To begin the procedure, the surgeon must free the spleen from its attachments to the abdominal viscera. The attachments are composed of ligaments and blood vessels. Using sharp dissection with Metzenbaum scissors, the surgeon begins to free the spleen. When blood vessels are encountered, the technologist passes right-angled (Mixter) clamps to the surgeon and his or her assistant. The vessels are double-clamped, divided, and ligated with 2-0 or 3-0 silk mounted on passers. During mobilization, the assistant retracts the stomach with a Deaver retractor.

Once the spleen is mobilized, the splenic artery and vein are identified. The surgeon places two or three Mayo clamps, large right-angled pedicle clamps, or a vascular clamp across the two structures. The vessels may also be clamped individually. The surgeon applies a heavy silk tie to the clamped vessels and ligates them (Fig. 19–75). The vessels are then severed, thus freeing the spleen. The surgeon delivers the spleen to the technologist, who receives it in a basin.

The wound is then irrigated with warm saline solution and further explored for bleeding vessels. After complete hemostasis is maintained, the wound is closed in routine fashion.

Pancreaticojejunostomy (Whipple's Procedure)

Definition

The stomach, duodenum, head of the pancreas, and common bile duct are resected. Gastrointestinal continuity is then restored. This radical procedure is performed for the treatment of early cancers of the pancreas.

Highlights

1. The abdomen is entered.
2. A portion of the stomach, all of the duodenum, a portion of distal common bile duct, and all or part of the pancreas are removed.
3. A choledochojejunostomy is performed.
4. A gastrojejunostomy is performed.
5. A pancreaticojejunostomy is performed.
6. The wound is closed.

Description

The procedure is initiated through a midline incision. Techniques for the choledochojejunostomy (anastomosis of the common bile duct and jejunum) are nearly identical to those discussed for a choledochoduodenostomy. The gastrojejunostomy (anastomosis of the stomach and jejunum) has also been previously described. The pancreaticojejunostomy (anastomosis of the pancreas and jejunum) is a simple end-to-end anastomosis, as for anastomosis of the small intestine. Often the pancreaticojejunostomy procedure is omitted and the remaining end of the pancreas is oversewn. The main

pancreatic duct is ligated in this case. The completed anastomoses and variations of the procedure are shown in Figure 19–76.

Related Procedure

Excision of pancreatic cyst

Wedge Resection of the Liver

Definition

This entails removal of a small wedge of liver tissue for biopsy. The procedure is often performed to determine the presence of metastatic carcinoma. It may be performed in conjunction with other abdominal procedures.

Highlights

1. The abdomen is entered.
2. A wedge is cut from the edge of the liver.
3. The incised edges are closed.
4. The wound is closed.

Description

The surgeon enters the abdomen through an upper midline incision. A wedge is then incised from the liver edge using the deep knife or cautery pencil. The specimen is passed to the technologist.

The edges of the liver may be approximated with chromic catgut, size 2-0 or 3-0, swaged to a blunt needle. To control bleeding on the surface of the liver, a small strip of Surgicel gauze or a small amount of Avitene may be placed over the suture line. Some surgeons avoid suturing the liver and, by using the coagulating current of the cautery pencil, control bleeding from the raw liver edges. When oozing has stopped, the wound is closed in routine fashion.

Liver Transplantation

Liver transplantation represents one of the successful transplant procedures under current investigation. Potential recipients in end-stage liver disease are screened for the following criteria:

1. Whether the disease is life threatening or reversible
2. Whether the disease is correctable by transplant
3. Age
4. Previous abdominal surgery (kind and type)
5. Psychological and psychosocial considerations
6. Physical status

Organ procurement is through the United Network for Organ Sharing (Richmond, VA), which matches recipient and donors when an organ becomes available. Liver transplants are very tedious owing to the complexity of the anatomy, the friable nature, and the

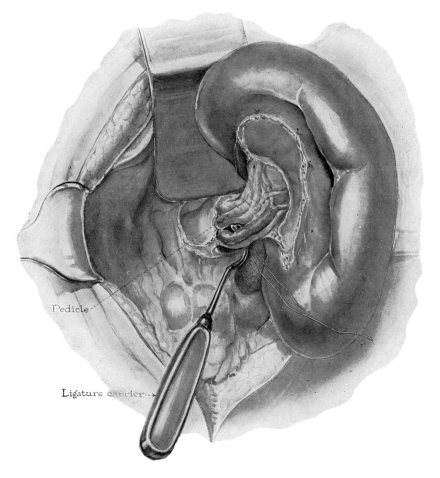

Pedicle

Ligature carrier

Figure 19–75. Splenectomy. Ligation of the splenic vessels. (From Hanrahan, Vincent: Lewis WF Practice of Surgery, Vol VI. Prior Co.)

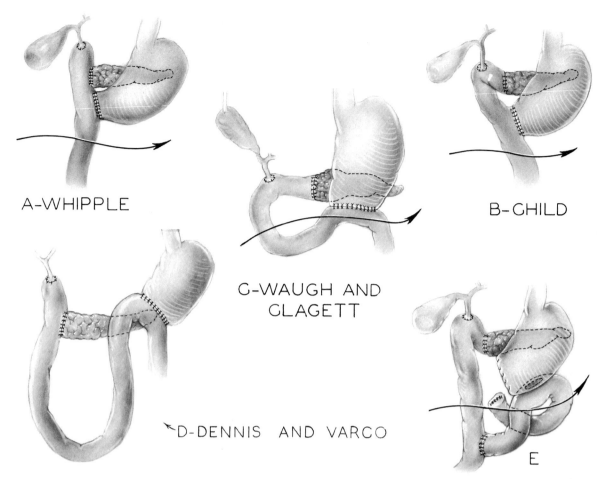

A-WHIPPLE

C-WAUGH AND CLAGETT

B-CHILD

D-DENNIS AND VARCO

E

Figure 19–76. Methods of pancreaticoduodenostomy. (From Higgins GA: Orr's Operations of General Surgery, 4th ed. Philadelphia, WB Saunders, 1968.)

vascularity of the liver. Extensive dissection is required as well as ligation of vessels to avoid postoperative hemorrhage. Implanting a donor liver requires reanastomosis of the suprahepatic vena cava, infrahepatic vena cava, portal vein, hepatic artery, and biliary reconstruction with end-to-end anastomosis of donor and recipient common bile ducts.

Transabdominal Repair of Hiatal Hernia

Definition

This is repair of a defect that occurs in the phrenoesophageal membrane attached to the esophagus at the level of the diaphragm. The defect causes the esophagus and upper stomach to slide upward into the thoracic cavity. The goal of surgical repair is to reduce the herniated stomach and its fatty tissue and to repair the defect. The hiatal hernia may be approached from the thoracic cavity as well as abdominally.

Highlights

1. The abdomen is entered.
2. The esophagus is mobilized.
3. The hernia is reduced.
4. The hernia defect is sutured.
5. The wound is closed.

Description

The surgeon enters the abdomen through an upper midline or left subcostal incision, with the patient in the supine position. Before beginning the hernia repair, the surgeon examines the abdominal contents for disease or conditions other than a hernia. Sometimes the patient's complaints are due not only to the hernia but also may arise from another condition, such as cancer. When the surgeon is satisfied that the hernia is the only cause of the patient's discomfort, the procedure is begun.

The assistant retracts the liver upward using a Weinberg retractor, while the surgeon carefully dissects the esophagus free from its attachments to the liver. The technologist must have long right-angled clamps and small sponge dissectors available. The dissection is carried out very cautiously, since the large vessels nearby could be damaged, which would cause severe bleeding that is difficult to control. Exposure of the hernia is a major technical difficulty in this procedure. As the dissection is continued, the patient may be tipped into the Trendelenburg position so that the overhead operating lights can be directed up into the wound.

Once the esophagus is mobilized, the technologist passes a long Penrose drain mounted on a right-angled clamp to the surgeon. The technologist should dip the drain in saline solution before passing it to the surgeon. The surgeon slings the drain around the esophagus and clamps the ends with a Mayo clamp. The assistant can then use the drain to retract the esophagus. The surgeon pulls the herniated stomach and adherent fatty tissue downward, thus reducing the hernia. Once it is reduced, the surgeon repairs the hernia defect using nonabsorbable sutures of size 2-0 on a small taper needle (Fig. 19–77). Interrupted sutures are used to close the defect around the esophagus and diaphragm (Fig. 19–78). The wound may be irrigated with saline and is then closed in routine fashion.

SURGICAL STAPLING PROCEDURES OF THE GASTROINTESTINAL SYSTEM

Because of recent technologic advances in the field of surgical stapling, the surgeon can now perform anastomoses, resections, and bypass operations in a fraction of the usual time. The instruments discussed in this chapter contain cartridges containing a prescribed number of noncrushing stainless steel or titanium staples. The staples are fired in single, double, triple, or quadruple lines and replace the traditional fine suture lines used in procedures of the gastrointestinal systems. Depending on the type of instrument used, a precision-made knife may simultaneously divide the tissue between staple lines. When the surgeon chooses surgical stapling instruments over traditional suture techniques, it is the duty of the scrub technologist or nurse to properly load and unload the staple cartridges at the surgical field. Complete instructions for these techniques and further information on the instruments are provided in Chapter 12.

The instruments described in this chapter are manufactured by the United States Surgical Corporation (Norwalk, CT). These particular instruments were chosen for discussion because of their *widespread use and* reliability. Surgical stapling instruments are available from a number of other manufacturers, and the choice of instruments presented here in no way implies the inferiority of any other manufacturer's products.

Esophagogastrectomy

Definition

This is the resection of the lower esophagus and upper stomach (fundus).

Highlights

1. The abdomen is entered.
2. The distal esophagus is mobilized.
3. The fundus is stapled.
4. A gastrotomy is performed.
5. The distal esophagus and stomach are anastomosed.
6. The wound is closed.

Stapling Instrumentation

The surgical stapling instruments used in this procedure are shown in Figure 19–79.

Description

The patient is prepped and draped for an abdominal incision. After incising the abdomen, the surgeon mobilizes the distal esophagus and proximal stomach using the LDS instrument to ligate and divide the omental vessels. The gastric fundus is stapled with two applications of the TA 90. The stomach is then divided between the two double staple lines with the knife (Fig. 19–80).

The GIA is used to incise the stomach and provide hemostasis of the cut edges (Fig. 19–81). To do this, the surgeon makes a stab wound in the gastric wall at the level of the gastrotomy. He or she inserts the anvil fork of the GIA instrument into the lumen of the stomach and places the cartridge fork on the serosal

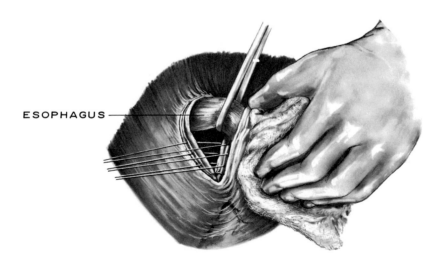

ESOPHAGUS

Figure 19–77. Transabdominal repair of hiatal hernia with interrupted sutures. The surgeon uses his or her hand to retract the stomach downward. Note Penrose drain used for traction on the esophagus. (From Higgins GA: Orr's Operations of General Surgery, 4th ed. Philadelphia, WB Saunders, 1968.)

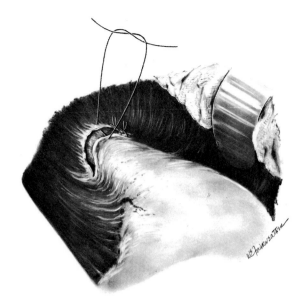

Figure 19–78. Transabdominal repair of hiatal hernia. The defect in the esophagus and diaphragm is repaired with interrupted sutures. (From Higgins GA: Orr's Operations of General Surgery, 4th ed. Philadelphia, WB Saunders, 1968.)

surface. The instrument is then closed, and the staples are fired.

To begin the anastomosis between the stomach and esophagus, the surgeon grasps the proximal stomach with Allis clamps. He or she then applies a pursestring suture to this area, using the pursestring instrument shown in Figure 19–82A. The EEA instrument is used to create the anastomosis. This is introduced, without the anvil, into the gastric incision. The pursestring instrument is removed, and the center rod is passed through the gastric wall (Fig. 19–82B). The surgeon then ties the pursestring suture and places the anvil on the center rod.

The pursestring instrument is placed around the esophagus just above the area of transection. A pursestring suture is placed here and the esophagus incised (Fig. 19–83A). The pursestring instrument is removed, and the anvil is introduced into the esophagus (Fig. 19–83B). The surgeon then ties the pursestring suture and divides the esophagus, which releases the specimen (Fig. 19–83C).

To complete the anastomosis, the surgeon closes the EEA instrument and fires the staples. The gastrotomy incision may then be closed with the TA 90 (Fig. 19–84A). The completed anastomosis is shown in Figure 19–84B. The wound is irrigated and closed in routine fashion.

Gastroduodenostomy (Billroth II Operation)

Definition

In this procedure, a portion of the stomach is removed and a new opening between the stomach and jejunum

is created. The name "Billroth II" refers to the anastomosis sites.

Highlights

1. The abdomen is entered.
2. The stomach is mobilized.
3. The duodenum is closed and divided.
4. The stomach is divided.
5. The gastrojejunostomy is created.
6. The wound is closed.

Stapling Instrumentation

The stapling instruments used in this procedure are illustrated in Figure 19–85.

Description

The patient is positioned, prepped, and draped for an abdominal incision. After the abdomen is entered, the surgeon mobilizes the stomach using the LDS instrument. Two staples automatically ligate the tissue, and the instrument's knife blade divides the tissue between the staples (Fig. 19–86).

The duodenum is closed with the TA 55 instrument. Before removing the instrument, the surgeon places a bowel clamp across the specimen side of the duodenum. The duodenum is then divided with the knife (Fig. 19–87). The gastric pouch (the portion of the stomach that will remain functional following the surgery) is closed with the TA 90. The surgeon places a clamp across the stomach on the specimen side. He or she then divides the stomach between the TA 90 and the clamp (Fig. 19–88).

In preparation for the gastrojejunostomy, the surgeon makes two stab wounds—one in the stomach and one in the jejunum. These wounds will be the sites of entry for the GIA instrument forks (Fig. 19–89A). The GIA is inserted into the stab wounds, and the staples are fired (Fig. 19–89B). Two double-staggered rows of staples join the two organs simultaneously, and the knife blade in the instrument cuts between the two double staple lines. This creates the new opening between the two organs. To close the two stab wounds, the surgeon places several traction sutures at their edges and trims away excess tissue (Fig. 19–90). The stab wounds are then closed with the TA 55 instrument. The completed anastomosis is shown in Figure 19–91.

Gastric Bypass

Definition

In this procedure, a large portion of the stomach is bypassed and a new gastric pouch is created. The anastomosis between the pouch and the jejunum substantially decreases the amount of food absorbed by the patient's gastrointestinal system. This surgery is performed to treat patients who suffer from morbid (life-threatening) obesity.

Text continued on page 289

INSTRUMENT	CLINICAL APPLICATION
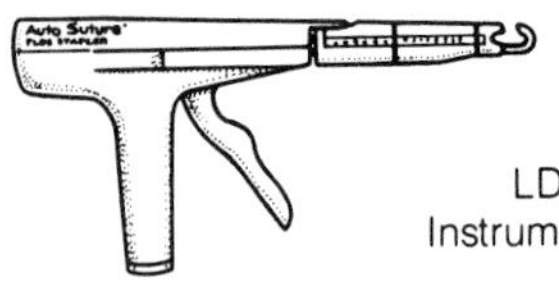 LDS™ Instrument	Ligation and division of the omental vessels and vagus nerves.
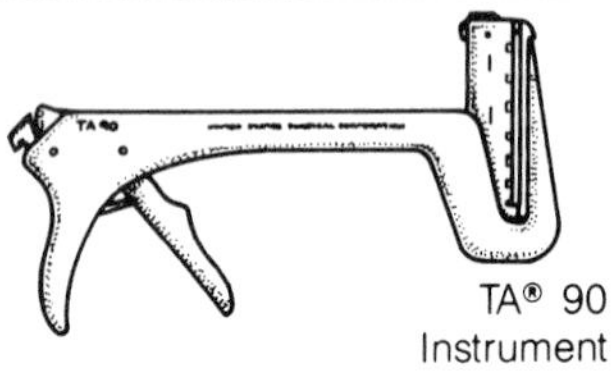 TA® 90 Instrument	Closure of the gastric fundus.
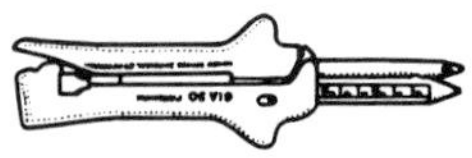 GIA™ Instrument	Creation of the gastrotomy. Alternate technique: Anastomosis of the esophagus to the stomach.
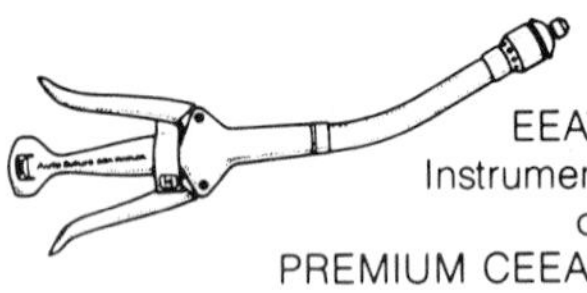 EEA™ Instrument or PREMIUM CEEA™ Instrument	Anastomosis of the esophagus to the stomach.
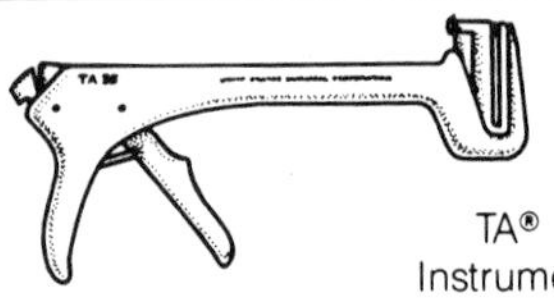 TA® 55 Instrument	Closure of the gastrotomy. Closure of the pyloroplasty incision.
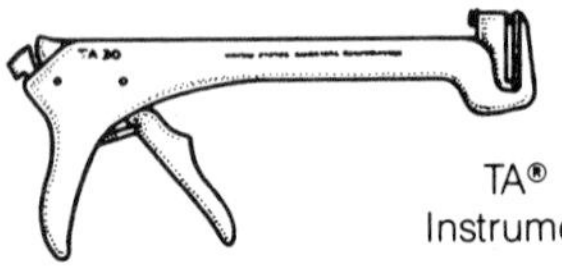 TA® 30 Instrument	Alternate technique: Closure of the esophagus and the gastric stab wound.
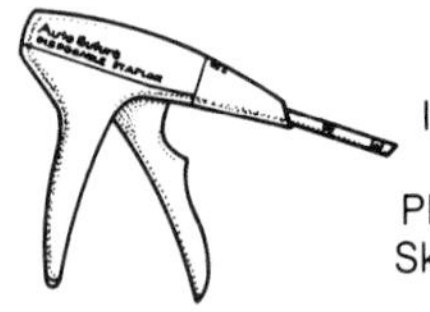 DFS™ Instrument and PREMIUM® Skin Stapler	Closure of fascia and skin.

Figure 19–79. Surgical stapling instruments used during esophagogastrectomy. (Copyright © 1974, 1980, 1988 United States Surgical Corporation. All rights reserved. Reprinted with the Permission of United States Surgical Corporation, Norwalk, CT.)

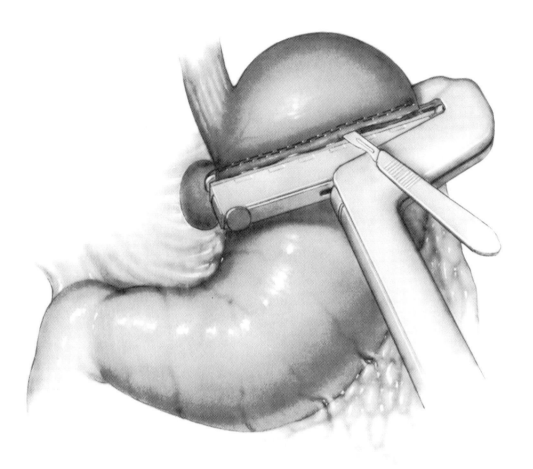

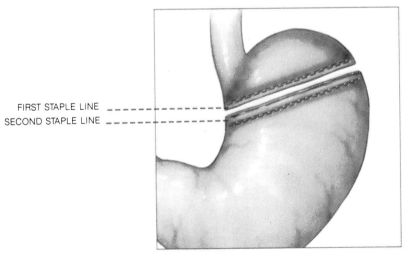

FIRST STAPLE LINE
SECOND STAPLE LINE

Figure 19–80. Esophagogastrectomy. The gastric fundus is stapled with two applications of the TA 90. The stomach is divided between the two staple lines. (Copyright © 1974, 1980, 1988 United States Surgical Corporation. All rights reserved. Reprinted with the Permission of United States Surgical Corporation, Norwalk, CT.)

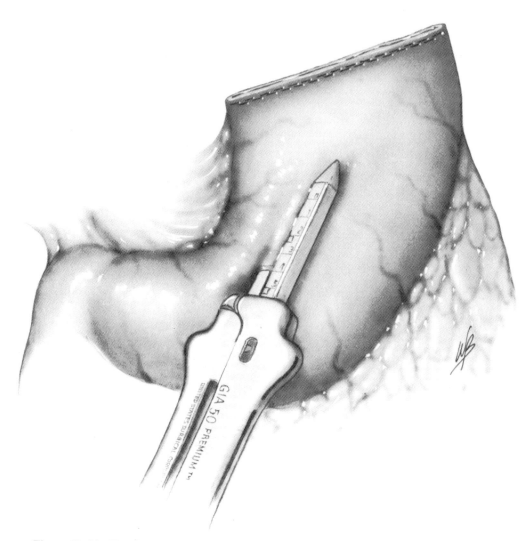

Figure 19–81. Esophagogastrectomy. The GIA is used to incise the stomach and provide hemostasis of the cut edges. (Copyright © 1974, 1980, 1988 United States Surgical Corporation. All rights reserved. Reprinted with the Permission of United States Surgical Corporation, Norwalk, CT.)

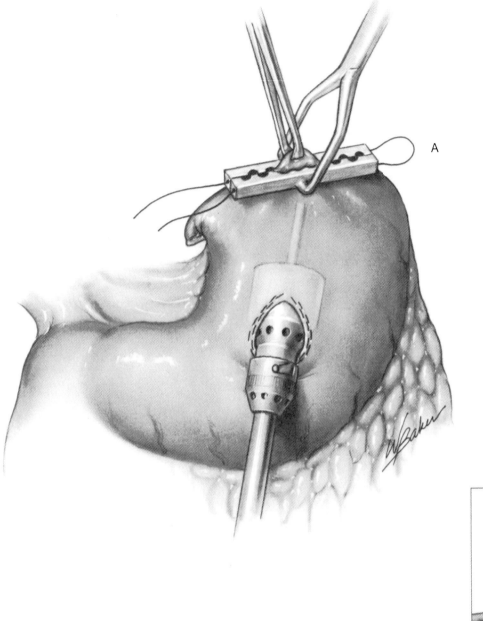

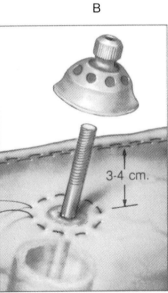

Figure 19–82. Esophagogastrectomy. *A.* A pursestring instrument is placed over the anastomosis area. The EEA instrument is introduced into the gastric incision. *B.* The pursestring instrument is removed, and the center rod is passed through the gastric wall. (Copyright © 1974, 1980, 1988 United States Surgical Corporation. All rights reserved. Reprinted with the Permission of United States Surgical Corporation, Norwalk, CT.)

A

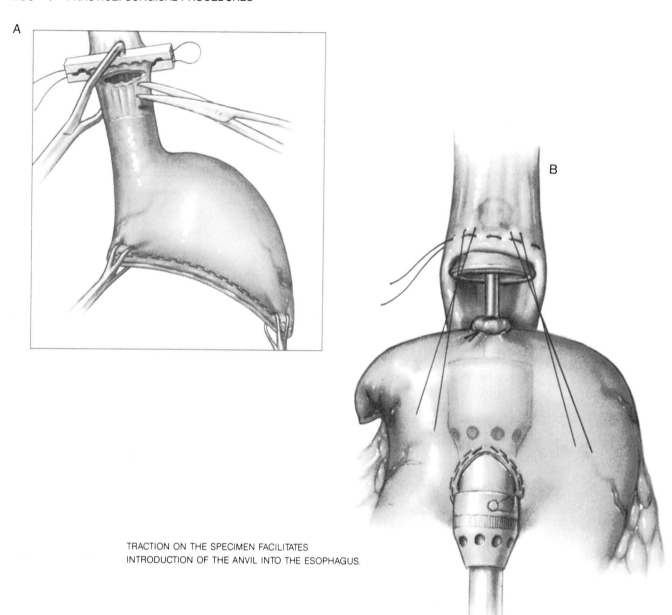

TRACTION ON THE SPECIMEN FACILITATES
INTRODUCTION OF THE ANVIL INTO THE ESOPHAGUS.

C

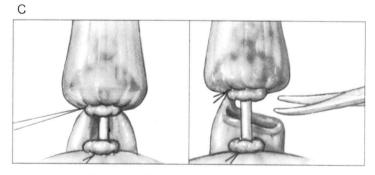

Figure 19–83. Esophagogastrectomy. *A.* A pursestring suture is placed around the esophagus just above the area of transection. The esophagus is incised. *B.* The pursestring instrument is removed, and the anvil is introduced into the esophagus. *C.* The surgeon ties the pursestring and divides the esophagus. (Copyright © 1974, 1980, 1988 United States Surgical Corporation. All rights reserved. Reprinted with the Permission of United States Surgical Corporation, Norwalk, CT.)

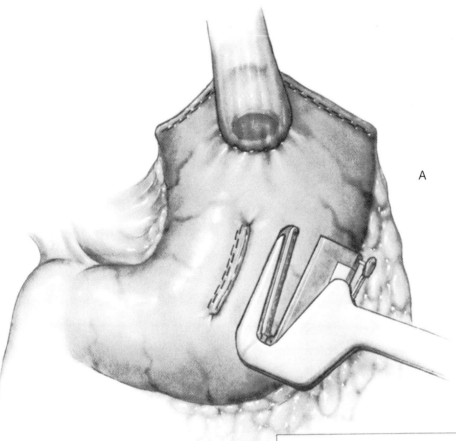

A

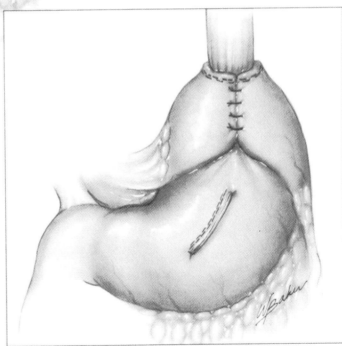

B

Figure 19–84. Esophagogastrectomy. *A.* The gastrotomy incision is closed with the TA 55. *B.* The completed anastomosis. (Copyright © 1974, 1980, 1988 United States Surgical Corporation. All rights reserved. Reprinted with the Permission of United States Surgical Corporation, Norwalk, CT.)

INSTRUMENT	CLINICAL APPLICATION
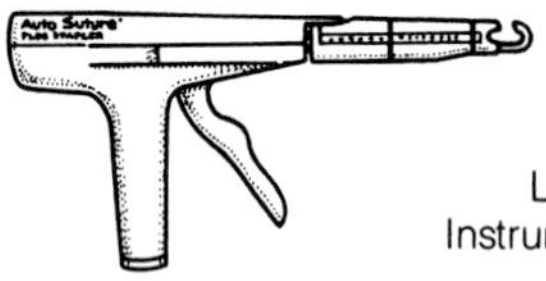 LDS™ Instrument	Ligation and division of the omental vessels.
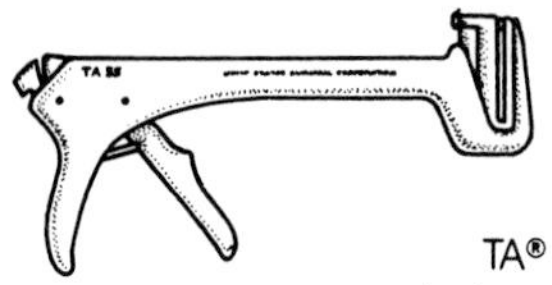 TA® 55 Instrument	Closure of the duodenum. Closure of the gastrojejunal stab wound. Closure of the jejunojejunal stab wound for the Roux-en-Y. Alternate technique: Closure of the gastrotomy.
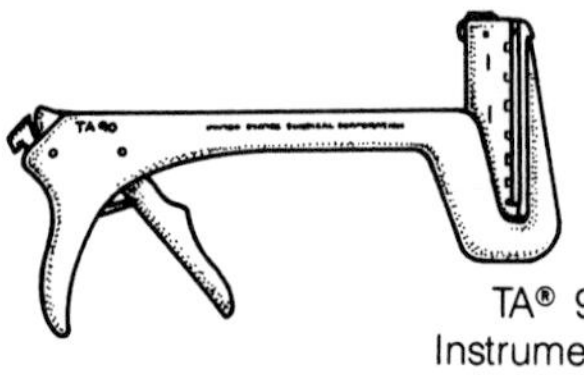 TA® 90 Instrument	Closure of the gastric pouch.
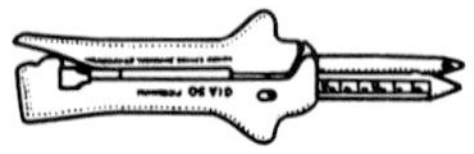 GIA™ Instrument	Anastomosis of the jejunum to the gastric pouch. Closure and transection of the jejunum and anastomosis of the proximal and distal jejunum for the Roux-en-Y. Alternate technique: Creation of the gastrotomy.
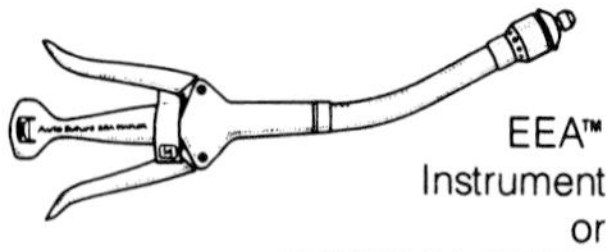 EEA™ Instrument or PREMIUM CEEA™ Instrument	Alternate technique: Anastomosis of the jejunum to the gastric pouch.
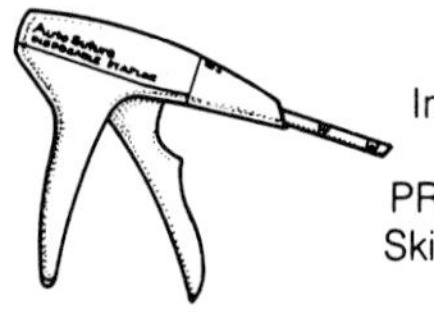 DFS™ Instrument and PREMIUM® Skin Stapler	Closure of fascia and skin.

Figure 19–85. Gastroduodenostomy. Surgical stapling instruments used during gastroduodenostomy. (Copyright © 1974, 1980, 1988 United States Surgical Corporation. All rights reserved. Reprinted with the Permission of United States Surgical Corporation, Norwalk, CT.)

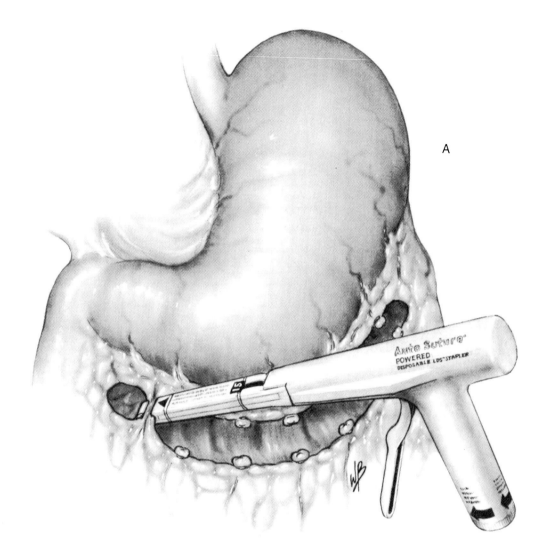

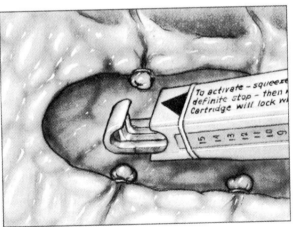

Figure 19–86. Gastroduodenostomy. *A.* Mobilization of the stomach using the LDS instrument. *B.* Two staples automatically ligate the tissue, and the instrument's knife blade divides the tissue between the staples. (Copyright © 1974, 1980, 1988 United States Surgical Corporation. All rights reserved. Reprinted with the Permission of United States Surgical Corporation, Norwalk, CT.)

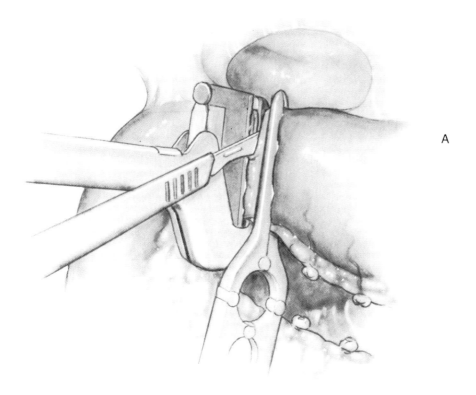

A

B

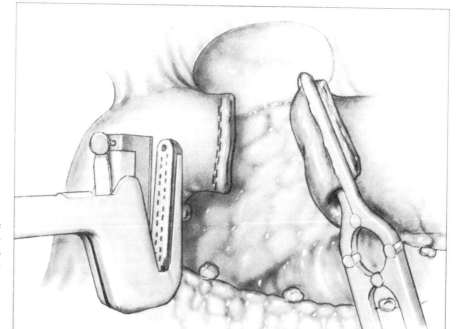

Figure 19–87. Gastroduodenostomy. The duodenum is closed. *A.* Before the instrument is removed, a bowel clamp is placed across the specimen side of the duodenum. *B.* The duodenum is then divided with the knife. (Copyright © 1974, 1980, 1988 United States Surgical Corporation. All rights reserved. Reprinted with the Permission of United States Surgical Corporation, Norwalk, CT.)

A

B

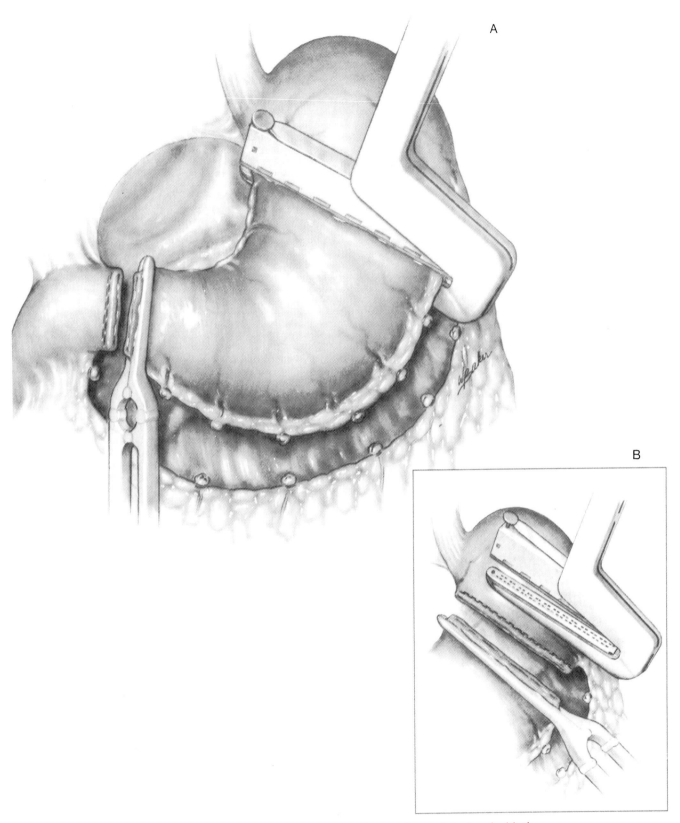

Figure 19–88. Gastroduodenostomy. *A.* The gastric pouch is closed with the TA 90. A clamp is placed across the stomach on the specimen side. *B.* The stomach is divided between the TA 90 and the clamp. (Copyright © 1974, 1980, 1988 United States Surgical Corporation. All rights reserved. Reprinted with the Permission of United States Surgical Corporation, Norwalk, CT.)

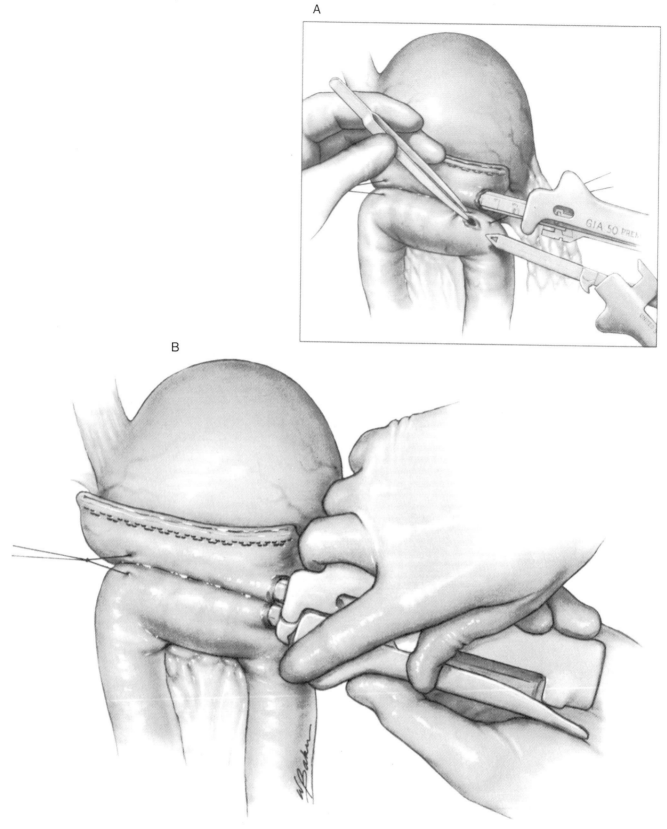

Figure 19–89. Gastroduodenostomy. *A.* Entry sites for the GIA are created in the stomach. *B.* The GIA is inserted in the stab wounds, and the staples are fired. (Copyright © 1974, 1980, 1988 United States Surgical Corporation. All rights reserved. Reprinted with the Permission of United States Surgical Corporation, Norwalk, CT.)

A

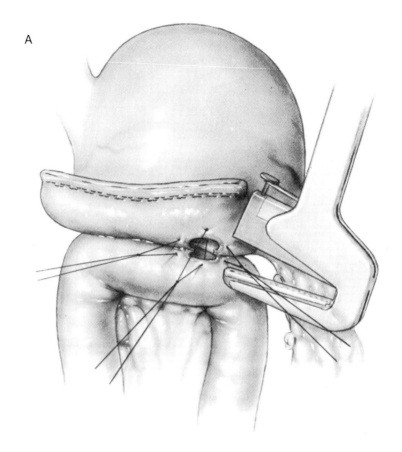

B

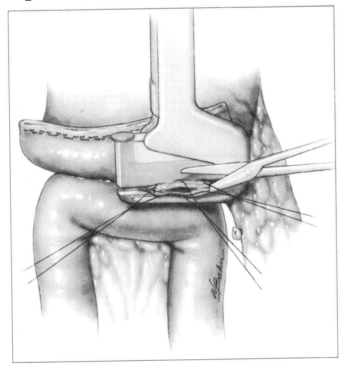

Figure 19–90. Gastroduodenostomy. *A*. Two double-staggered rows of staples join the two organs simultaneously, and the knife blade in the instrument cuts between the two double staple lines. Traction sutures are placed at the tissue edges. The stab wounds are closed with the TA 55. *B*. Excess tissue is trimmed away. (Copyright © 1974, 1980, 1988 United States Surgical Corporation. All rights reserved. Reprinted with the Permission of United States Surgical Corporation, Norwalk, CT.)

A

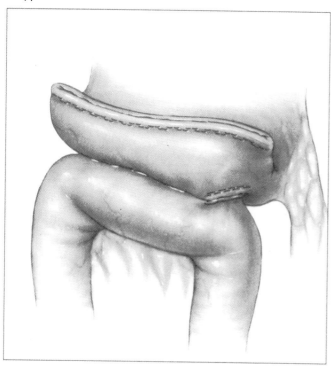

B

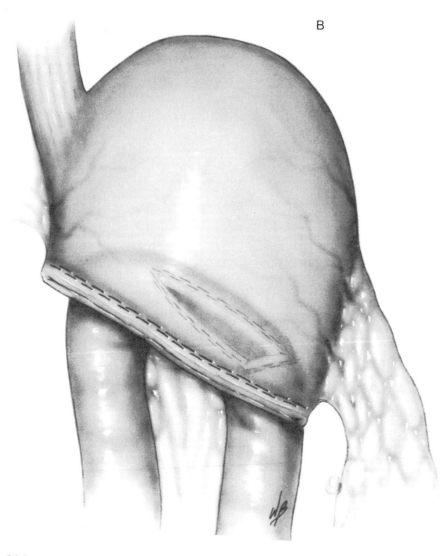

Figure 19–91. Gastroduodenostomy. *A.* Completed anastomosis. *B.* Cutaway view of anastomosis. (Copyright © 1974, 1980, 1988 United States Surgical Corporation. All rights reserved. Reprinted with the Permission of United States Surgical Corporation, Norwalk, CT.)

Highlights

1. The abdomen is entered.
2. The gastric pouch is created.
3. The jejunum is transected.
4. A gastrojejunostomy is created.
5. A jejunojejunostomy (Roux-en-Y anastomosis) is performed.
6. The wound is closed.

Stapling Instrumentation

The surgical stapling instruments used in this procedure are illustrated in Figure 19–92.

Description

The patient is positioned, prepped, and draped for an abdominal incision.

After the abdomen is entered, the surgeon makes a small hole in the lesser omentum at the level of the proposed partition. The TA 90 instrument is placed across the stomach at the partition site, and the staples are fired (Fig. 19–93). The GIA is used to close and transect the jejunum (Fig. 19–94).

To provide a new opening between the jejunum and the stomach, the surgeon makes two stab wounds to accommodate the forks of the GIA. The GIA is inserted into the stab wounds, and the staples are fired (Fig. 19–95A). Silk sutures may be used to close the stab wounds (Fig. 19–95B). The Roux-en-Y (jejunojejunostomy) anastomosis is performed with the GIA instrument (Fig. 19–96A). The common opening between the two portions of jejunum is then closed with the TA 55 (Fig. 19–96B). The wound is irrigated and closed in routine fashion.

End-to-End Bowel Anastomosis

Definition

This is the re-establishment of continuity in the large intestine following resection.

Highlights

1. The abdomen is entered.
2. The large intestine is mobilized.
3. The anastomosis is created.
4. The wound is closed.

Stapling Instrumentation

Surgical stapling instruments used in this procedure are illustrated in Figure 19–97.

Description

The patient is positioned, prepped, and draped for an abdominal incision. After the abdomen is entered, the diseased bowel is located and the area of resection is determined. The LDS instrument is used to mobilize the bowel along the area of resection (Fig. 19–98A). The bowel is then resected in the usual fashion as described for Colon Resection and Anastomosis in this chapter. The surgeon then positions the serosal layers of the severed bowel ends face to face with traction sutures (Fig. 19–98B). The Roticulator 55 instrument is used to join one side of the anastomosis (Fig. 19–98C). The margin of tissue remaining outside the instrument is then removed with the knife (Fig. 19–99). A second set of staples is fired over the anastomosis, and excess tissue is removed to complete it (Fig. 19–100A). Note the location of the traction sutures, which are used to elevate the tissue margins during the anastomosis. The completed anastomosis is shown in Figure 19–100B.

The wound is irrigated and closed in routine fashion.

Right Hemicolectomy

Definition

This is the removal of a diseased portion of the right colon. Bowel continuity is re-established by an anastomosis between the colon and the ileum.

Highlights

1. The abdomen is entered.
2. The right colon is mobilized.
3. An ileocolostomy is performed.
4. The wound is closed.

Surgical Stapling Instrumentation

The surgical stapling instruments used in this procedure are illustrated in Figure 19–101.

Description

The patient is positioned, prepped, and draped for an abdominal incision. After the abdomen is entered, the right colon is mobilized in the area of disease and is transected in the usual manner (see Colon Resection and Anastomosis). The EEA instrument is used to perform the ileocolostomy. The terminal ileum is first prepared with a pursestring suture, and the diameter of the lumen is determined. The instrument is introduced into the severed end of the colon, without the anvil. The center rod is advanced through the colon through a stab wound, around which a pursestring suture has been placed (Fig. 19–102A). The surgeon then ties the rod suture, places the anvil on the center rod, and introduces the anvil into the ileum (Fig. 19–102B). The pursestring suture is closed, and the EEA staples are fired (Fig. 19–103A). The stump of the colon is then closed with the TA 55 (Fig. 19–103B). The completed anastomosis is shown in Figure 19–103C.

The wound is closed in routine fashion.

Text continued on page 301

INSTRUMENT	CLINICAL APPLICATION
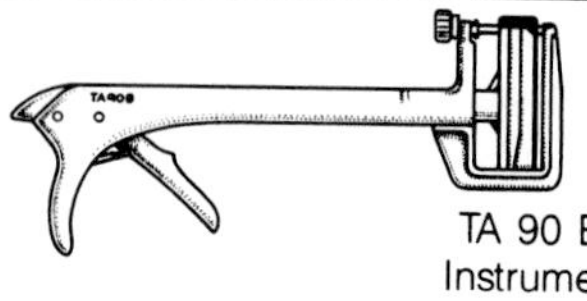 TA 90 B™ Instrument	Closure of the gastric pouch.
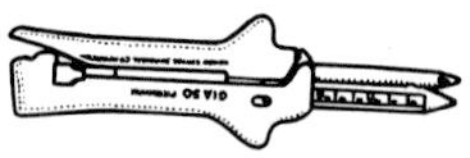 GIA™ Instrument	Closure and transection of the jejunum. Anastomosis of the distal jejunum to the gastric fundus. Anastomosis of the proximal and distal jejunum.
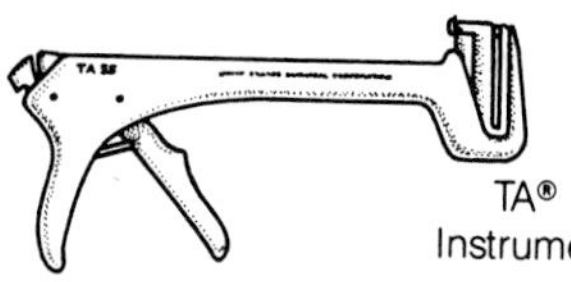 TA® 55 Instrument	Closure of the jejunal stab wounds.
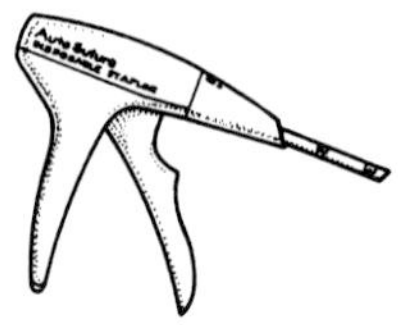 DFS™ Instrument and PREMIUM® Skin Stapler	Closure of fascia and skin.

Figure 19–92. Gastric bypass. Surgical stapling instruments used during the procedure. (Copyright © 1974, 1980, 1988 United States Surgical Corporation. All rights reserved. Reprinted with the Permission of United States Surgical Corporation, Norwalk, CT.)

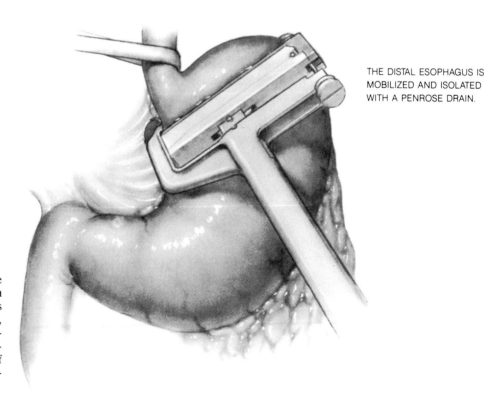

THE DISTAL ESOPHAGUS IS MOBILIZED AND ISOLATED WITH A PENROSE DRAIN.

Figure 19–93. Gastric bypass. The TA 90 is placed across the stomach at the partition site, and the staples are fired. (Copyright © 1974, 1980, 1988 United States Surgical Corporation. All rights reserved. Reprinted with the Permission of United States Surgical Corporation, Norwalk, CT.)

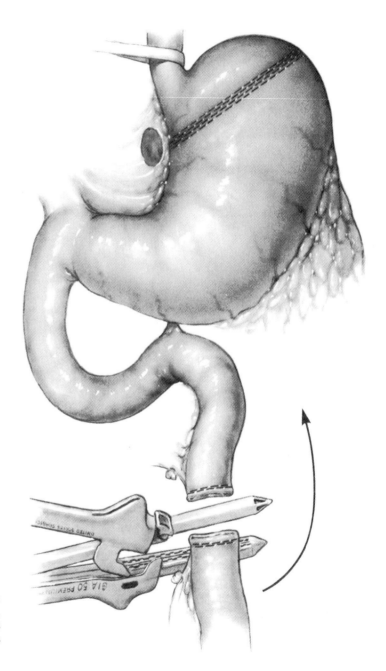

Figure 19–94. Gastric bypass. The GIA is used to close and transect the jejunum. (Copyright © 1974, 1980, 1988 United States Surgical Corporation. All rights reserved. Reprinted with the Permission of United States Surgical Corporation, Norwalk, CT.)

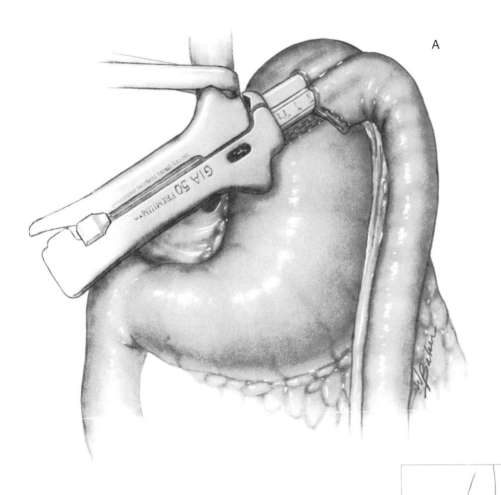

A

B

Figure 19–95. Gastric bypass. *A.* The GIA is inserted into stab wounds in both organs. The instrument is inserted, and the staples are fired. *B.* Silk sutures are used to close the stab wounds. (Copyright © 1974, 1980, 1988 United States Surgical Corporation. All rights reserved. Reprinted with the Permission of United States Surgical Corporation, Norwalk, CT.)

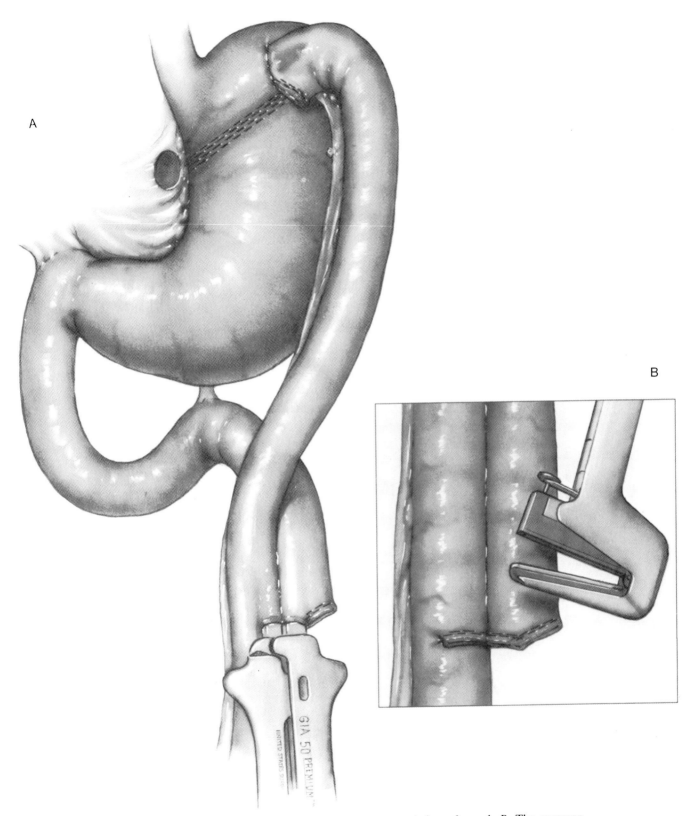

Figure 19–96. Gastric bypass. *A*. Roux-en-Y anastomosis is performed. *B*. The common opening between the two portions of jejunum are closed with the TA 55. (Copyright © 1974, 1980, 1988 United States Surgical Corporation. All rights reserved. Reprinted with the Permission of United States Surgical Corporation, Norwalk, CT.)

INSTRUMENT	CLINICAL APPLICATION
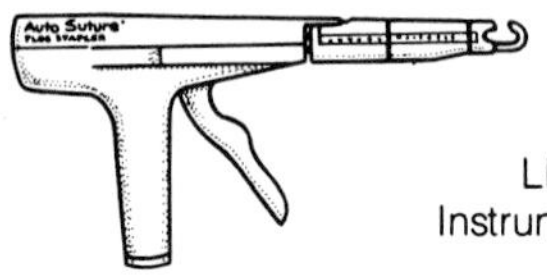 LDS™ Instrument	Ligation and division of the mesenteric vessels.
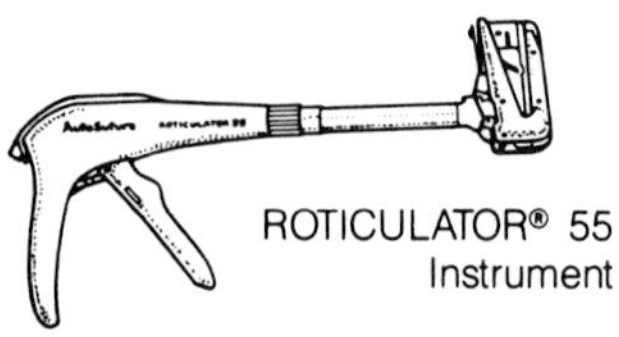 ROTICULATOR® 55 Instrument	Anastomosis of the proximal and distal large bowel.
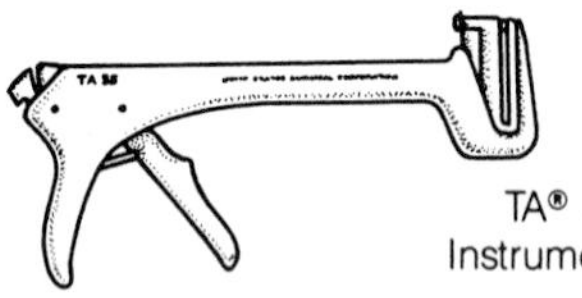 TA® 55 Instrument	Anastomosis of the proximal and distal large bowel.
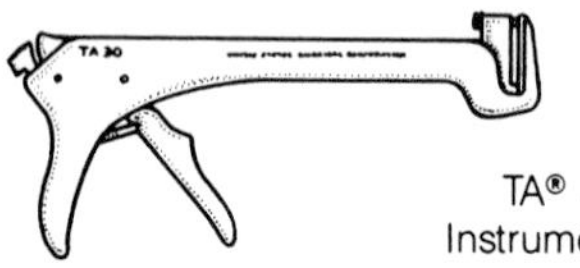 TA® 30 Instrument	Anastomosis of the proximal and distal small bowel.
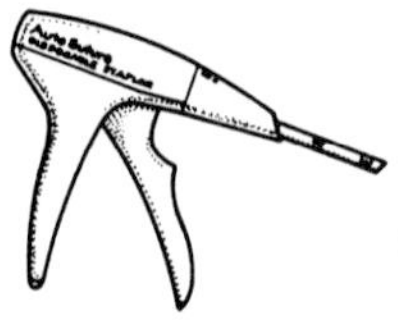 DFS™ Instrument and PREMIUM® Skin Stapler	Closure of fascia and skin.

Figure 19–97. End-to-end bowel anastomosis. Surgical stapling instruments used in this procedure. (Copyright © 1974, 1980, 1988 United States Surgical Corporation. All rights reserved. Reprinted with the Permission of United States Surgical Corporation, Norwalk, CT.)

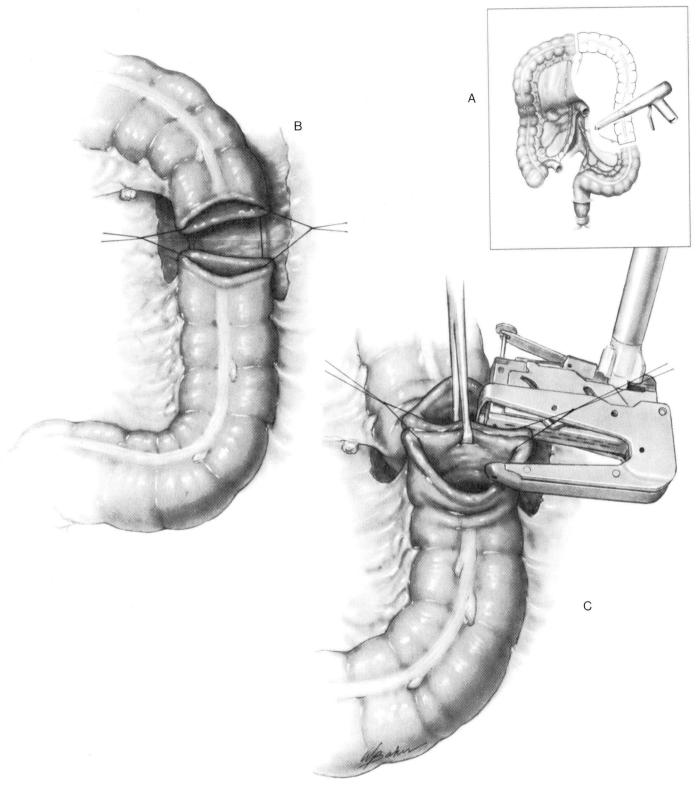

Figure 19–98. End-to-end bowel anastomosis. *A.* The area of resection is mobilized using the LDS instrument. *B.* After resection, the serosal layers are positioned face to face with traction sutures. *C.* The Roticulator 55 instrument is used to join one side of the anastomosis. (Copyright © 1974, 1980, 1988 United States Surgical Corporation. All rights reserved. Reprinted with the Permission of United States Surgical Corporation, Norwalk, CT.)

A

B

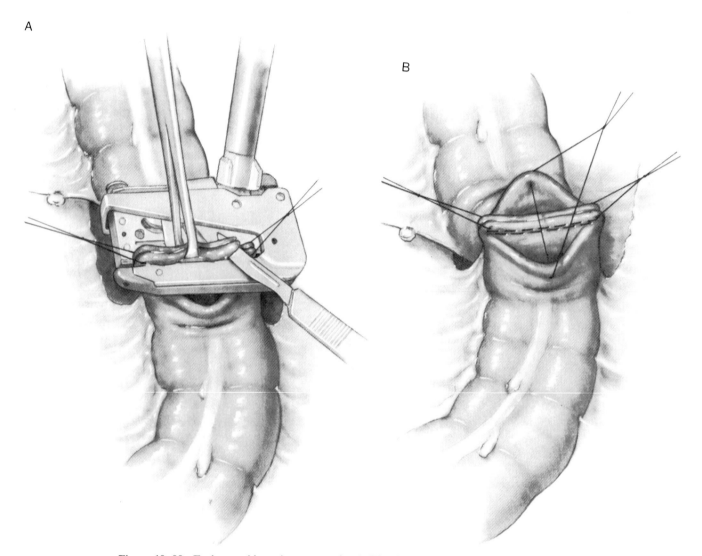

Figure 19–99. End-to-end bowel anastomosis. *A.* The tissue margin is incised. *B.* Resulting double triangles. (Copyright © 1974, 1980, 1988 United States Surgical Corporation. All rights reserved. Reprinted with the Permission of United States Surgical Corporation, Norwalk, CT.)

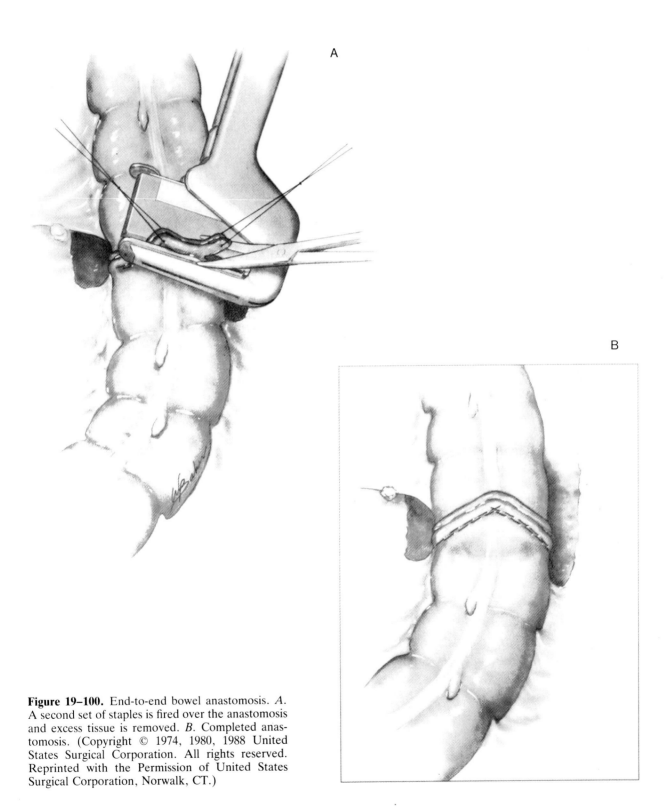

Figure 19–100. End-to-end bowel anastomosis. *A.* A second set of staples is fired over the anastomosis and excess tissue is removed. *B.* Completed anastomosis. (Copyright © 1974, 1980, 1988 United States Surgical Corporation. All rights reserved. Reprinted with the Permission of United States Surgical Corporation, Norwalk, CT.)

INSTRUMENT	CLINICAL APPLICATION
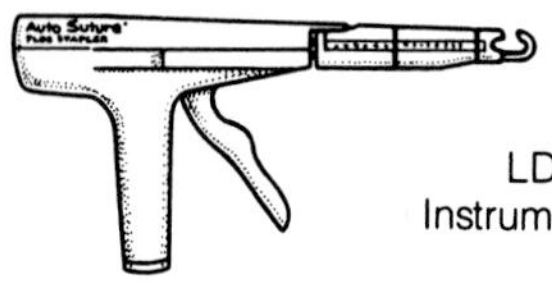 LDS™ Instrument	Ligation and division of the mesenteric vessels.
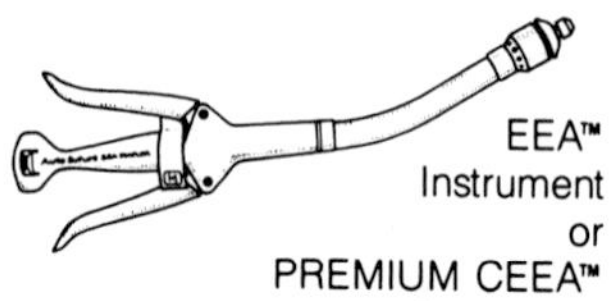 EEA™ Instrument or PREMIUM CEEA™ Instrument	Anastomosis of the ileum to the colon.
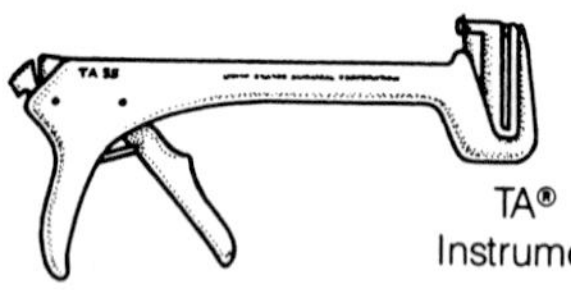 TA® 55 Instrument	Closure of the colon. Alternate technique: Closure of the common opening.
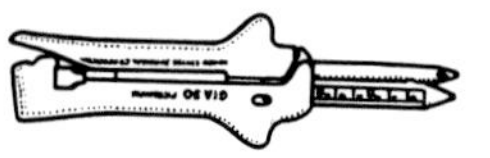 GIA™ Instrument	Alternate technique: Closure and transection of the ileum and transverse colon. Anastomosis of the ileum to the colon.
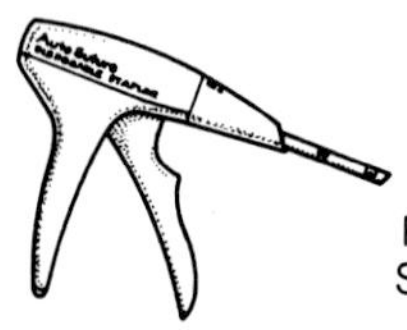 DFS™ Instrument and PREMIUM® Skin Stapler	Closure of fascia and skin.

Figure 19–101. Right hemicolectomy. Surgical stapling instruments used in this procedure. (Copyright © 1974, 1980, 1988 United States Surgical Corporation. All rights reserved. Reprinted with the Permission of United States Surgical Corporation, Norwalk, CT.)

A

B

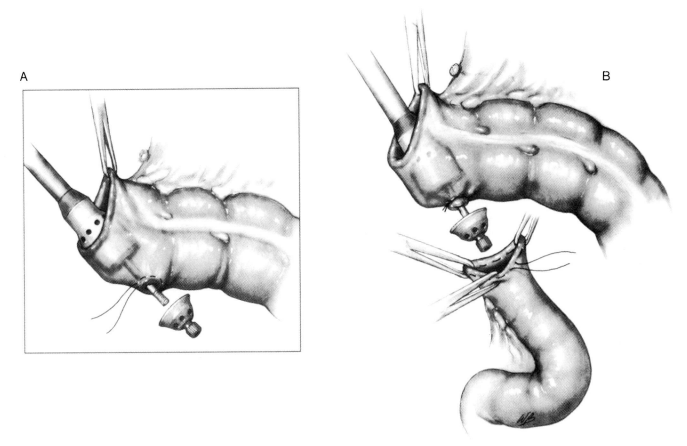

Figure 19–102. Right hemicolectomy. *A.* Following transection of the colon, the EEA instrument is used to perform the anastomosis. The center rod is advanced through the colon through a stab wound. *B.* The anvil is placed around the center rod. The center rod is introduced into the ileum. (Copyright © 1974, 1980, 1988 United States Surgical Corporation. All rights reserved. Reprinted with the Permission of United States Surgical Corporation, Norwalk, CT.)

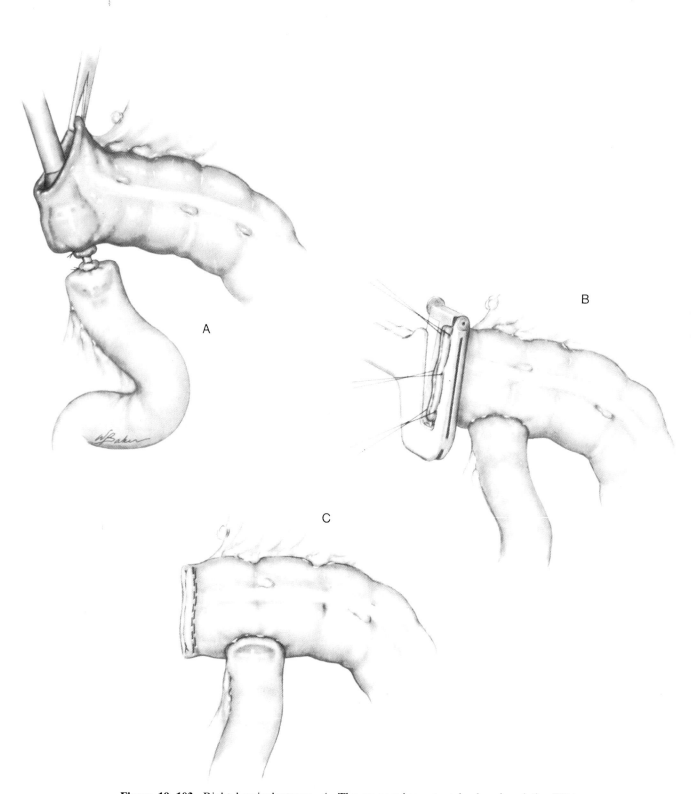

Figure 19–103. Right hemicolectomy. *A.* The pursestring suture is closed and the EEA staples are fired. *B.* The stump of the colon is closed with the TA 55. *C.* Completed anastomosis. (Copyright © 1974, 1980, 1988 United States Surgical Corporation. All rights reserved. Reprinted with the Permission of United States Surgical Corporation, Norwalk, CT.)

Low Anterior Resection (End-to-End Anastomosis)

Definition

This procedure is the removal of a portion of the distal large intestine. Continuity of the bowel is re-established through an anastomosis of the rectum and healthy colon tissue.

Highlights

1. The abdomen is entered.
2. The area of resection is mobilized.
3. The proximal colon is resected and closed.
4. The proximal rectum is resected.
5. An anastomosis is created between the proximal rectum and the distal colon.
6. The wounds are closed.

Surgical Stapling Instrumentation

The surgical stapling instruments used during this procedure are shown in Figure 19–104.

Description

In this procedure, the colon is mobilized through an abdominal incision. Once this is accomplished, the patient is repositioned into the lithotomy position and the procedure is completed transanally (through the anus). When only one team is available for the surgery, a complete change of instruments, drapes, gowns, and gloves is necessary between the two phases. When two teams are used, two separate operative set-ups must be used, and each team's equipment must be kept separated from the other's. A complete discussion of a double set-up is presented in the section on Abdominoperineal Resection of the Rectum. The procedure described here is performed by one team.

The patient is positioned, prepped, and draped for an abdominal procedure. After the abdomen is entered, the area of resection is determined and the colon is mobilized with the LDS instrument. The GIA is then used to close and transect the proximal colon (Fig. 19–105A). A pursestring instrument is applied around the proximal rectum, and the specimen is resected (Fig. 19–105B). Pursestring sutures are then placed around the proximal rectum (Fig. 19–105C). The operating team now changes its entire set-up to operate transanally. The patient is placed in lithotomy position, prepped, and draped. The Premium CEEA instrument is used to perform the anastomosis. The instrument is introduced transanally and advanced to the level of the pursestring instrument. The pursestring instrument is removed, and the CEEA is allowed to protrude from the proximal rectum (Fig. 19–106A). The pursestring suture is tied, and the pursestring instrument is placed around the previously stapled closure line in the colon (Fig. 19–106B). Excess tissue protruding from the pursestring suture is excised with a knife.

The pursestring instrument is removed, and the tissue edges are grasped with Allis clamps (Fig. 19–107). The anvil of the CEEA is introduced into the proximal colon, and the pursestring suture is tied (Fig. 19–108A). The stapling instrument is then closed, and the staples are fired, creating a new stoma (Fig. 19–108B). The CEEA is gently withdrawn (Fig. 19–109A). The completed anastomosis is shown in Figure 19–109B.

Kock Ileal Reservoir

Definition

The Kock ileal reservoir provides a pouch for the collection of urine following surgery to remove the bladder. The ileum is used to create the pouch, which the patient empties by self-catheterization through one of two nipples created at the abdominal skin edges. The ureters are anastomosed near the inflow valve, which prevents reflux of urine back into the kidneys. The outflow valve provides urinary continence. This procedure describes only the creation of the ileal pouch, using surgical stapling instruments. The section on creating an ileal conduit (see Chapter 22) includes a discussion of ureteral implantation.

Surgical Stapling Instrumentation

The surgical stapling instruments used in this procedure are illustrated in Figure 19–110.

Description

The terminal ileum is closed and transected using the GIA instrument. The proposed segment of ileum to be used for nipple valve construction is determined, and an opening is made in the mesentery. A portion of the mesentery is removed to reduce the bulk it would create during nipple construction (Fig. 19–111A).

To construct the ileal reservoir, the surgeon folds a bowel segment of about 30 cm in a U-shape, leaving a short segment for the nipple and stoma. Parallel stab wounds are made in the apposed bowel segments, as shown in Figure 19–111B. The GIA instrument is used with the SGIA loading unit, which contains no knife in the assembly (Fig. 19–112A). Four parallel rows of staples are fired. Before removal of the GIA, the forks are used as a cutting guide to incise the bowel walls for the length of the staple line (Fig. 19–112B).

With the use of a Babcock clamp, a short portion of bowel is intussuscepted (telescoped in on itself) at a distal segment (Fig. 19–113). The intussusception will be constructed into a nipple. Its shape is maintained with the GIA instrument with the SGIA loading unit (Fig. 19–114).

To separate the two nipple loops, the surgeon incises the afferent loop. The flat bowel segment is folded upon itself so that the serosal layers are face to face (Fig. 19–115). Both walls of the pouch are closed in an inverted fashion with the TA 90 (Fig. 19–116). The pouch is then

Text continued on page 308

INSTRUMENT	CLINICAL APPLICATION
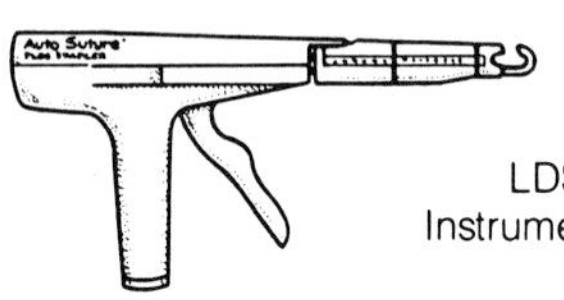 LDS™ Instrument	Ligation and division of the mesenteric vessels.
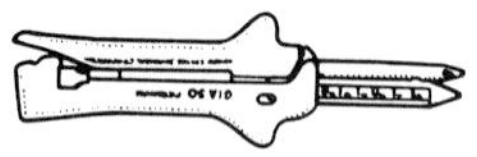 GIA™ Instrument	Closure and transection of the proximal colon.
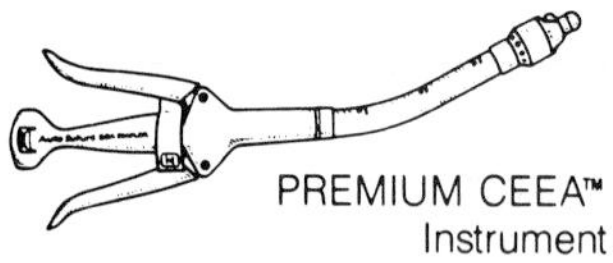 PREMIUM CEEA™ Instrument or EEA™ Instrument	Anastomosis of the proximal colon to the rectum.
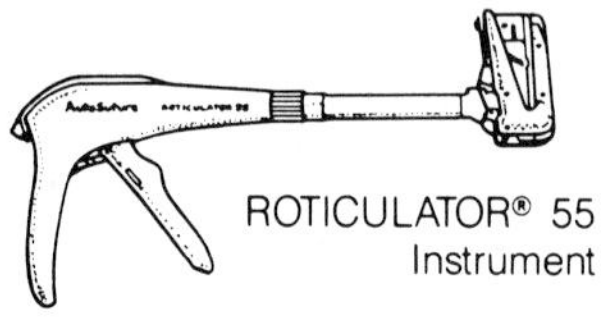 ROTICULATOR® 55 Instrument	Alternate technique: Closure of the rectum.
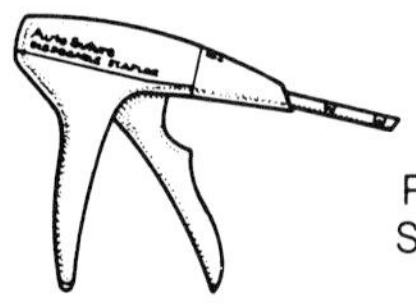 DFS™ Instrument and PREMIUM® Skin Stapler	Closure of fascia and skin.

Figure 19–104. Low anterior resection. Surgical stapling instruments used during the procedure. (Copyright © 1974, 1980, 1988 United States Surgical Corporation. All rights reserved. Reprinted with the Permission of United States Surgical Corporation, Norwalk, CT.)

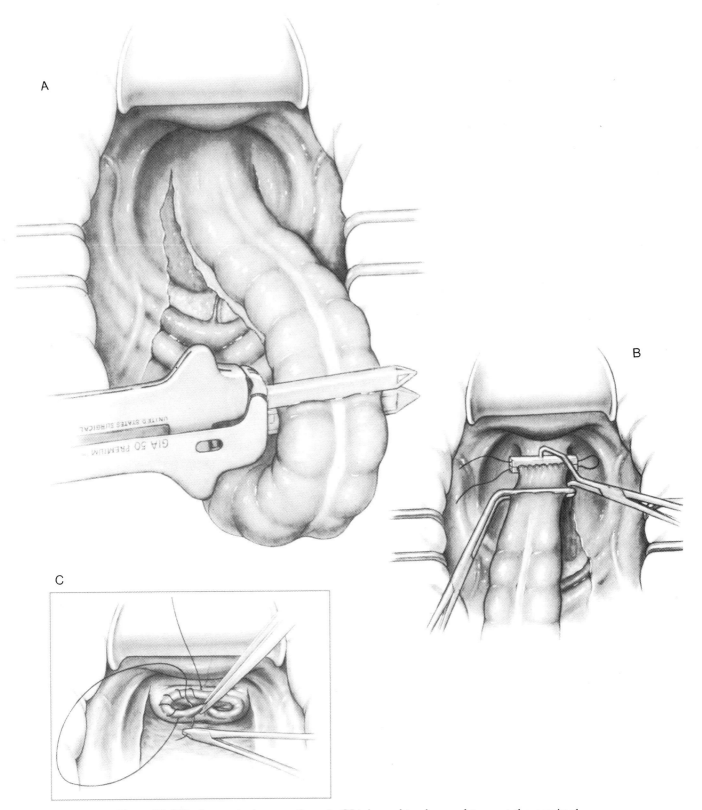

Figure 19–105. Low anterior resection. *A.* GIA is used to close and transect the proximal colon. *B.* A pursestring instrument is applied around the proximal rectum, and the specimen is resected. *C.* Pursestring sutures are placed around the proximal rectum. (Copyright © 1974, 1980, 1988 United States Surgical Corporation. All rights reserved. Reprinted with the Permission of United States Surgical Corporation, Norwalk, CT.)

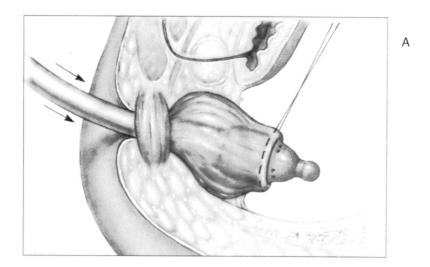

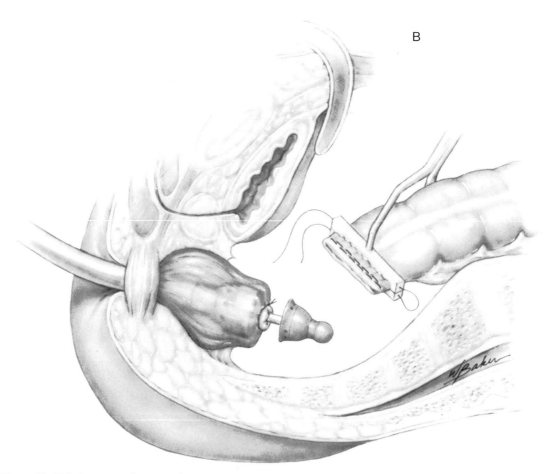

Figure 19–106. Low anterior resection. *A.* The patient is now in lithotomy position (note the position of the sacrum). The CEEA is introduced transanally to the level of the pursestring. *B.* The pursestring is tied, and the pursestring instrument is placed around the previously stapled closure line. (Copyright © 1974, 1980, 1988 United States Surgical Corporation. All rights reserved. Reprinted with the Permission of United States Surgical Corporation, Norwalk, CT.)

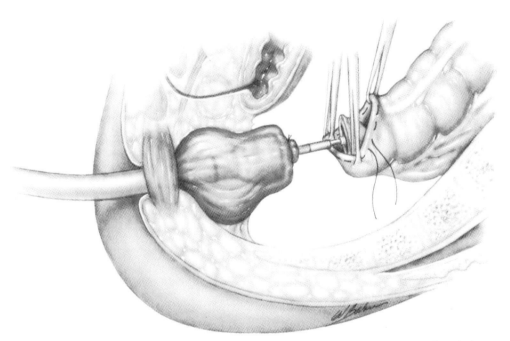

Figure 19–107. Low anterior resection. The pursestring instrument is removed and the tissue edges are grasped with Allis clamps. (Copyright © 1974, 1980, 1988 United States Surgical Corporation. All rights reserved. Reprinted with the Permission of United States Surgical Corporation, Norwalk, CT.)

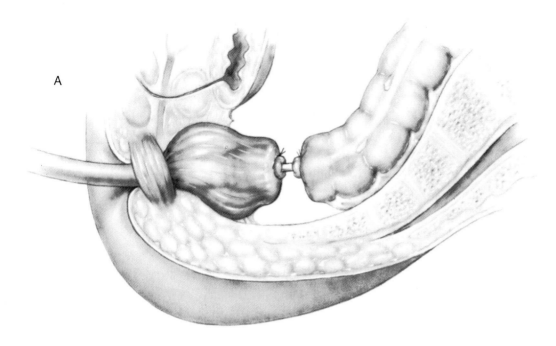

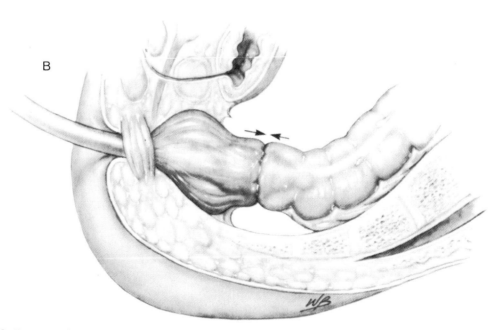

Figure 19–108. Low anterior resection. *A.* The anvil of the CEEA is introduced into the proximal colon, and the pursestring suture is tied. *B.* The stapling instrument is closed and the staples are fired, creating continuity. (Copyright © 1974, 1980, 1988 United States Surgical Corporation. All rights reserved. Reprinted with the Permission of United States Surgical Corporation, Norwalk, CT.)

A

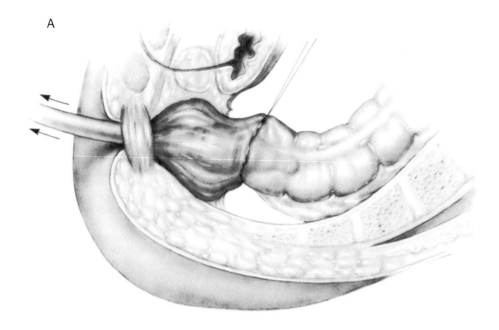

B

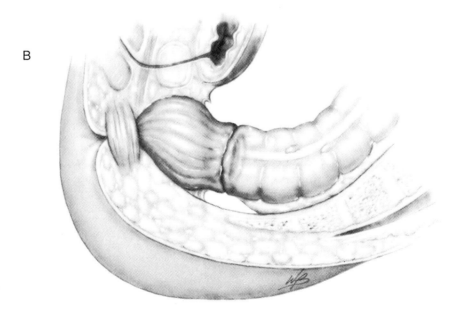

Figure 19–109. Low anterior resection. *A.* The CEEA is withdrawn. *B.* Completed anastomosis. (Copyright © 1974, 1980, 1988 United States Surgical Corporation. All rights reserved. Reprinted with the Permission of United States Surgical Corporation, Norwalk, CT.)

INSTRUMENT	CLINICAL APPLICATION
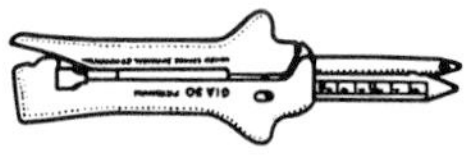 GIA™ Instrument	Closure and transection of the terminal ileum. Creation of the posterior wall of the pouch. Secure shape of the nipple.
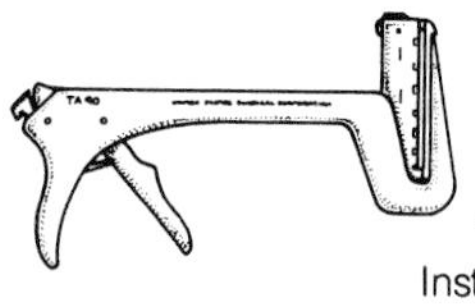 TA® 90 Instrument	Closure of the lateral walls of the pouch.
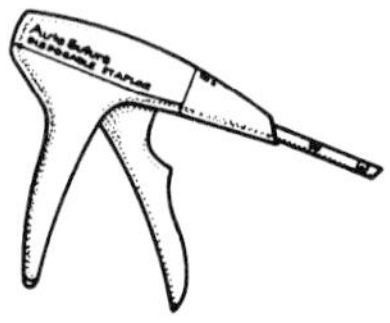 DFS™ Instrument and PREMIUM® Skin Stapler	Closure of fascia and skin.

Figure 19–110. Kock ileal reservoir. Surgical stapling instruments used in this procedure. (Copyright © 1974, 1980, 1988 United States Surgical Corporation. All rights reserved. Reprinted with the Permission of United States Surgical Corporation, Norwalk, CT.)

turned right-side out to assume its final shape (Fig. 19–117).

The anterior bowel edges extending between the nipple and afferent bowel are closed with a running absorbable suture reinforced with interrupted silk sutures (Fig. 19–118A). The nipple is anchored externally with interrupted silk sutures (19–118B). The pouch is positioned and secured, and the stoma is created.

The wound is irrigated with warm saline and closed in routine fashion.

HERNIA REPAIR

Repair of Inguinal Hernia

Definition

This is repair of a herniation (protrusion) of abdominal contents caused by a defect in the abdominal wall in the groin area of the male. Two types of inguinal hernias are encountered. A *direct* hernia is the result of stress on the abdominal wall, which causes the peritoneum to bulge through the fascia in the groin area. The peritoneal bulge (sac) may contain abdominal viscera. An *indirect* hernia is caused by a congenital defect in the internal abdominal ring, which causes the peritoneum to bulge along the spermatic cord. This sac may also contain abdominal viscera. The goal of surgery is to strengthen the abdominal layers in the groin and close the defect.

Highlights

1. Layers of the abdominal wall are incised.
2. The spermatic cord is identified and dissected free.
3. The hernia sac is identified.
4. The sac is ligated and removed.
5. Layers of the wound are closed individually.

Description

The patient is placed in the supine position and prepped and draped as for an abdominal procedure, with the groin area on the affected side exposed. The surgeon begins the procedure by incising the groin. The area of the incision is shown in Figure 19–119. The incision is deepened using Metzenbaum scissors and the cautery pencil. Small bleeders are controlled with the cautery pencil. Both blunt and sharp dissection are used to gain access to the hernia. After incising the fascia that lies over the spermatic cord (Fig. 19–120), the surgeon places several hemostats on the edge of the incised fascia. These can then be used to retract the fascial layer.

When the spermatic cord has been identified, the surgeon separates it from the surrounding tissue. The technologist must have a moistened Penrose drain available at this time. The drain is mounted on a Mayo clamp and passed to the surgeon, who slings it around the cord for retraction (Fig. 19–121). Dissection is continued until the hernia is located. If the hernia is direct, the surgeon will begin to suture the defect using interrupted sutures, size 2-0. Various types of suture material can be used.

If the hernia is indirect, the surgeon dissects the sac away from the cord using Metzenbaum scissors. The sac is opened and the edges are grasped with many hemostats. The surgeon then pushes the contents of the sac back toward the abdomen with a finger or a small sponge. If it is small, the sac may simply be ligated (Fig. 19–122). For large sacs, a pursestring suture is used to close the sac. The sac is closed near the abdominal wall

Text continued on page 317

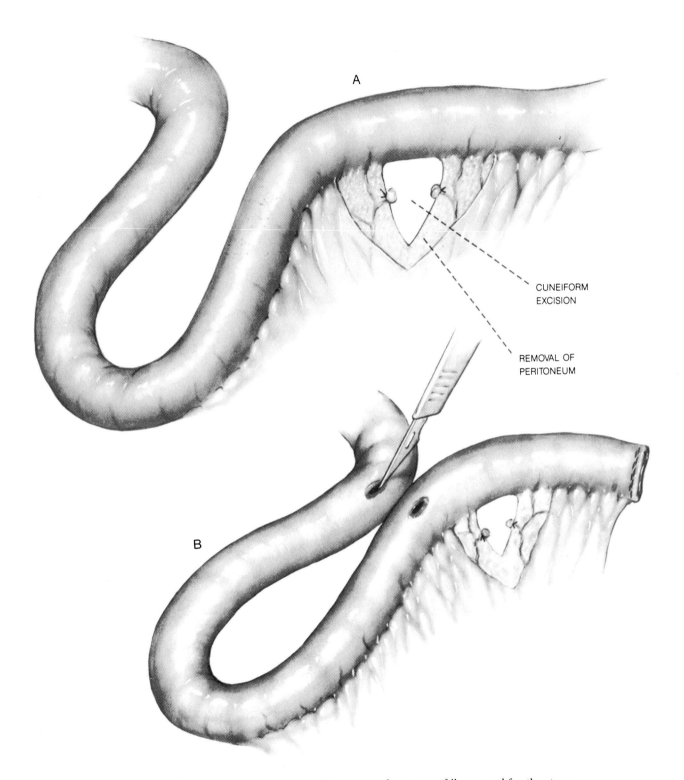

A

CUNEIFORM
EXCISION

REMOVAL OF
PERITONEUM

B

Figure 19–111. Kock ileal reservoir. *A.* The proposed segment of ileum used for the stoma is determined and an opening is made in the mesentery. A small portion of the mesentery is removed to reduce the bulk at the site. *B.* The segment of bowel is folded and parallel stab wounds are made in the segments. (Copyright © 1974, 1980, 1988 United States Surgical Corporation. All rights reserved. Reprinted with the Permission of United States Surgical Corporation, Norwalk, CT.)

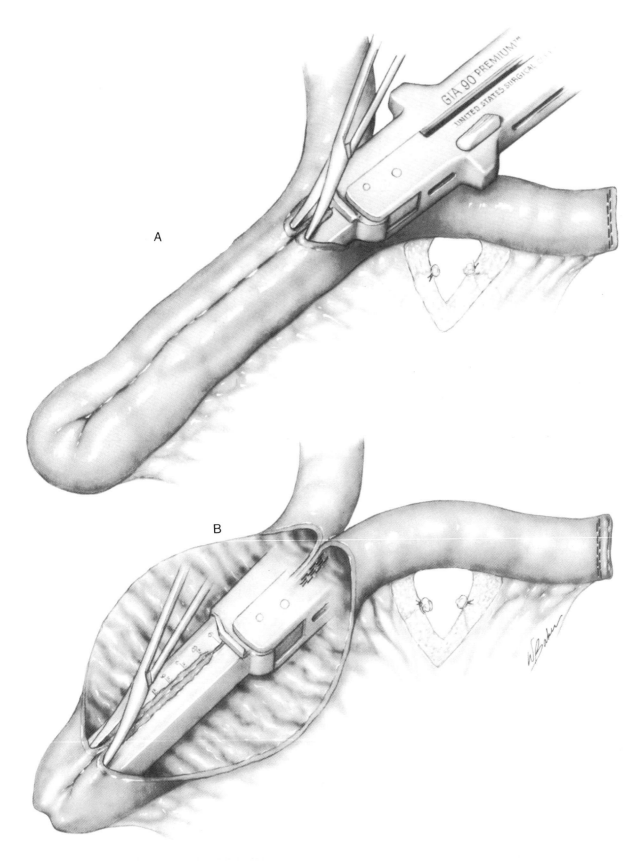

Figure 19–112. Kock ileal reservoir. *A.* The GIA is used with the SGIA loading unit. *B.* Four parallel rows of staples are fired and the bowel walls are incised. (Copyright © 1974, 1980, 1988 United States Surgical Corporation. All rights reserved. Reprinted with the Permission of United States Surgical Corporation, Norwalk, CT.)

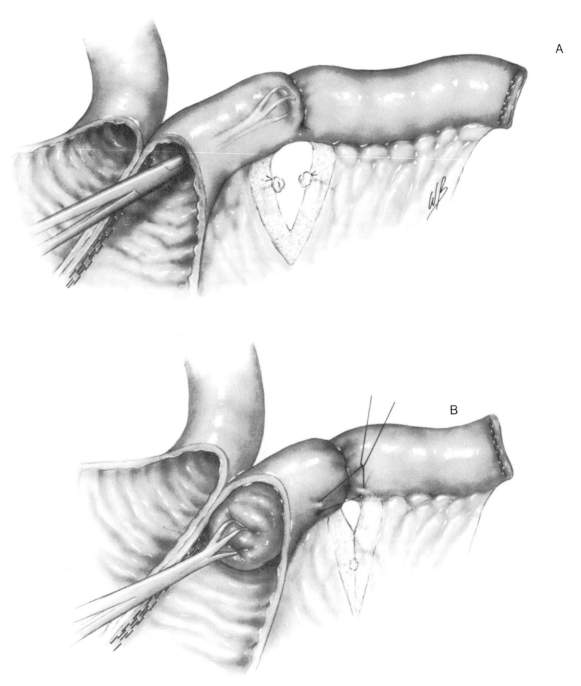

Figure 19–113. Kock ileal reservoir. *A.* A Babcock clamp is used to grasp the distal segment of bowel. *B.* The end is intussuscepted. (Copyright © 1974, 1980, 1988 United States Surgical Corporation. All rights reserved. Reprinted with the Permission of United States Surgical Corporation, Norwalk, CT.)

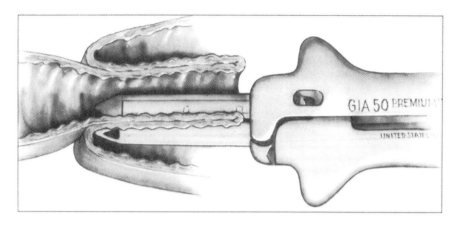

Figure 19–114. Kock ileal reservoir. The shape of the stoma is maintained with the GIA and SGIA loading unit. (Copyright © 1974, 1980, 1988 United States Surgical Corporation. All rights reserved. Reprinted with the Permission of United States Surgical Corporation, Norwalk, CT.)

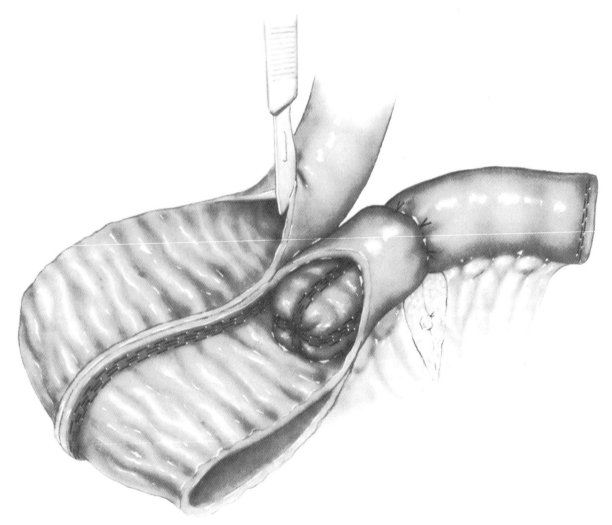

Figure 19–115. Kock ileal reservoir. The flat bowel segment is folded upon itself so that the serosal layers are face to face. (Copyright © 1974, 1980, 1988 United States Surgical Corporation. All rights reserved. Reprinted with the Permission of United States Surgical Corporation, Norwalk, CT.)

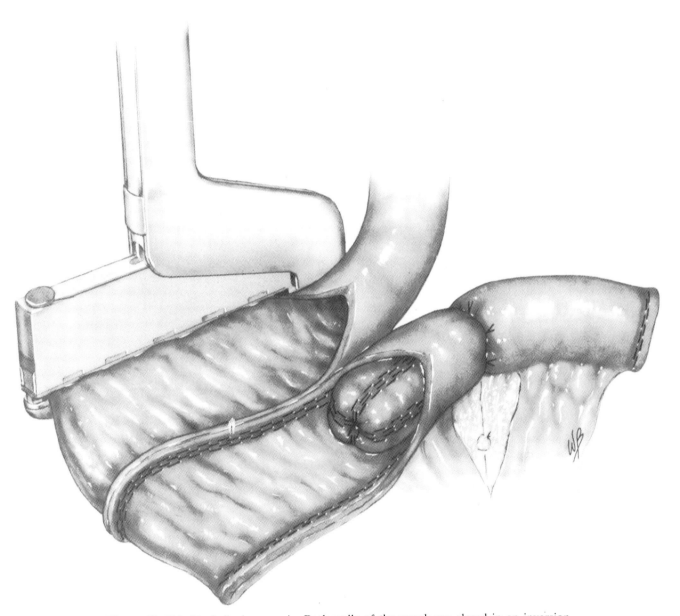

Figure 19–116. Kock ileal reservoir. Both walls of the pouch are closed in an inversion with the TA 90. (Copyright © 1974, 1980, 1988 United States Surgical Corporation. All rights reserved. Reprinted with the Permission of United States Surgical Corporation, Norwalk, CT.)

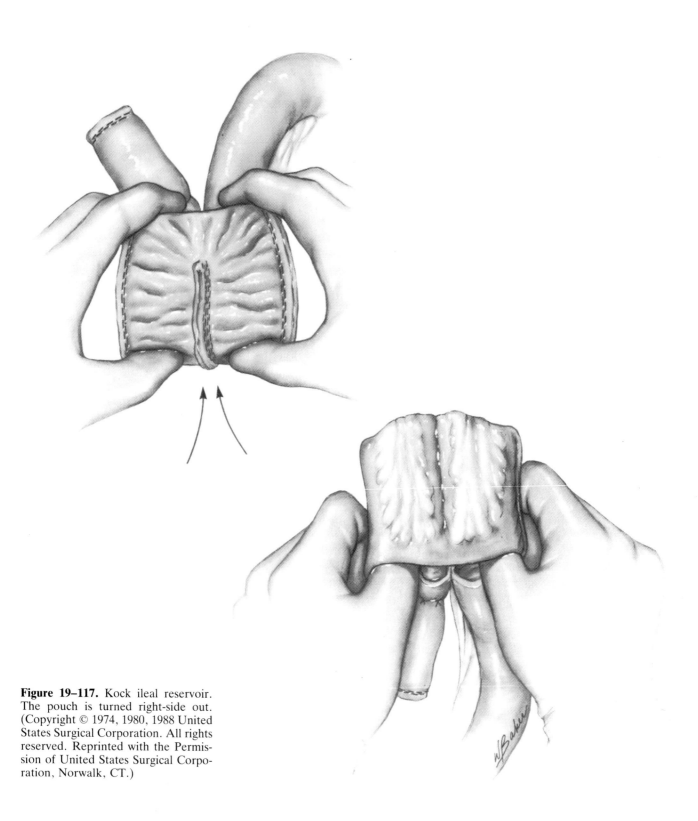

Figure 19–117. Kock ileal reservoir. The pouch is turned right-side out. (Copyright © 1974, 1980, 1988 United States Surgical Corporation. All rights reserved. Reprinted with the Permission of United States Surgical Corporation, Norwalk, CT.)

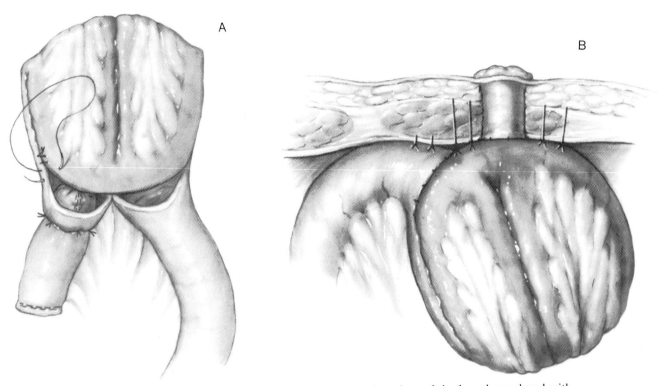

Figure 19–118. Kock ileal reservoir. *A.* The anterior edges of the bowel are closed with sutures. *B.* The completed stoma is anchored externally with interrupted silk sutures. (Copyright © 1974, 1980, 1988 United States Surgical Corporation. All rights reserved. Reprinted with the Permission of United States Surgical Corporation, Norwalk, CT.)

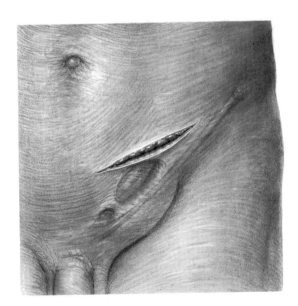

Figure 19–119. Repair of inguinal hernia. Incision for inguinal hernia. (From Higgins GA: Orr's Operations of General Surgery, 4th ed. Philadelphia, WB Saunders, 1968.)

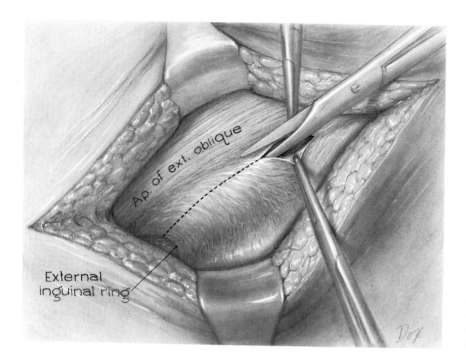

Figure 19–120. Repair of inguinal hernia. The surgeon divides the fascia over the spermatic cord. (From Higgins GA: Orr's Operations of General Surgery, 4th ed. Philadelphia, WB Saunders, 1968.)

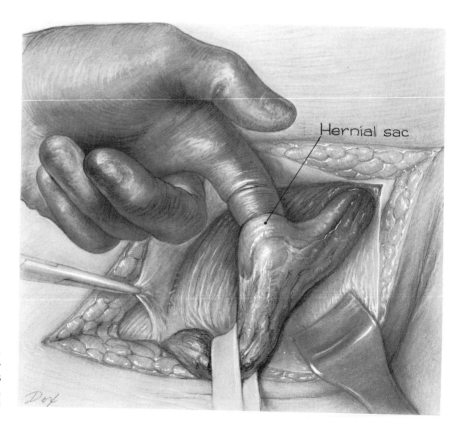

Figure 19–121. Repair of inguinal hernia. A Penrose drain is passed under the spermatic cord for traction. (From Higgins GA: Orr's Operations of General Surgery, 4th ed. Philadelphia, WB Saunders, 1968.)

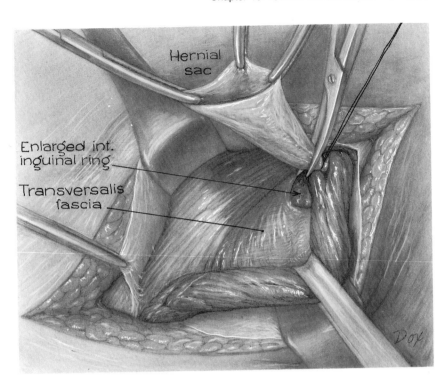

Figure 19–122. Repair of inguinal hernia. Ligation of the hernia sac. (From Higgins GA: Orr's Operations of General Surgery, 4th ed. Philadelphia, WB Saunders, 1968.)

and its edges removed; it is then passed to the technologist as a specimen.

The wound is closed in individual layers. Fascial layers are approximated with size 2-0 nonabsorbable suture (Fig. 19–123). If the fascia is very weak, the surgeon may reinforce it with a strip of synthetic mesh, such as Marlex, which is sewn directly to the fascia edges (Fig. 19–124). Subcutaneous and skin layers are closed in routine fashion.

Repair of Incisional Hernia

Definition

This is repair of an incisional hernia caused by a weakening in the abdominal wall due to previous abdominal surgery. The hernia may involve one or more of the abdominal layers. In some instances there is a peritoneal sac that is dissected free; if the hernia is severe, there may be a loop of intestine contained within the sac.

Highlights

1. A previous abdominal scar is removed.
2. The abdomen is entered to the level of the defect.
3. The wound is closed.

Description

The patient is placed in the supine position, prepped, and draped as for an abdominal procedure. The surgeon's assistant grasps the edges of the abdominal scar with Allis clamps while the surgeon incises the edges of the scar using the skin knife and fine tissue forceps. The

scar is then removed and passed to the technologist. If nonabsorbable sutures have been placed during the previous surgery, the surgeon removes the knots using a straight hemostat. The technologist should place a folded towel on the field on which the surgeon may place the knots. Since the knots constitute a foreign body, they must not be allowed to fall back into the wound.

Once the incision has been deepened to the herniation (usually at the fascia), the surgeon grasps the edges of the tissue with Allis clamps. Using the deep knife, the surgeon incises the weakened edges. Synthetic mesh is often used as a bridge over a large defect; the mesh is sewn directly to the edges of the fascia. The wound is then closed in routine fashion.

Related Procedure

Repair of umbilical hernia

Repair of Femoral Hernia

Definition

This is correction of a hernia in the groin area, which presents through the femoral canal inferior to (below) the inguinal ligament. The hernia sac is ligated and removed.

Highlights

1. The groin area is incised on the affected side.
2. The sac is identified and opened.
3. The sac is ligated and removed.
4. The wound is closed.

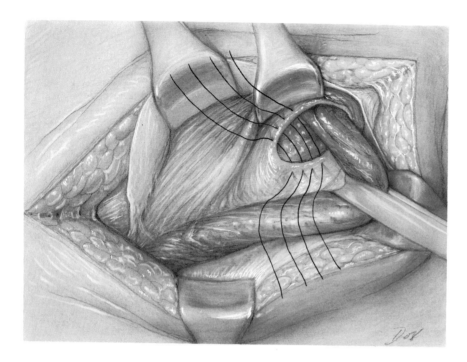

Figure 19–123. Repair of inguinal hernia. The surgeon closes the fascia with interrupted sutures. (From Higgins GA: Orr's Operations of General Surgery, 4th ed. Philadelphia, WB Saunders, 1968.)

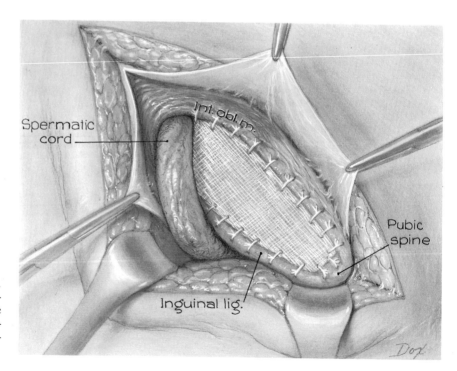

Figure 19–124. Repair of inguinal hernia. If the fascia is particularly weak, the surgeon may use synthetic mesh to close the tissue. (From Higgins GA: Orr's Operations of General Surgery, 4th ed. Philadelphia, WB Saunders, 1968.)

Description

The patient is placed in the supine position, prepped, and draped as for an abdominal procedure with the groin exposed. Using the skin knife, the surgeon incises the groin area (Fig. 19–125). The incision is deepened using the cautery pencil or deep knife. Sharp dissection is continued. Once the fascial layers have been incised, the hernia sac becomes visible (Fig. 19–126). The assistant elevates the sac using hemostats. The sac is then nicked with the knife and opened fully with Metzenbaum scissors. Because the sac may contain a portion of intestine, the surgeon carefully explores it with a finger (Fig. 19–127). The surgeon places additional Kelly or Crile clamps on the edges of the sac. A pursestring suture of synthetic material, size 2-0 or 3-0, is then placed around the neck of the sac close to the abdominal wall (Fig. 19–128). The surgeon now amputates the sac and passes it to the technologist as a specimen. The layers of the groin are closed individually in routine fashion.

RECTAL SURGERY

Hemorrhoidectomy

Definition

This is removal of painful dilated veins of the anus and rectum. Hemorrhoids are classified as *internal* (inside the rectum) or *external* (outside the rectum). Hemorrhoids are generally acquired by those whose occupations require sitting most of the day, or they may accompany pregnancy.

Highlights

1. The rectum is dilated.
2. The hemorrhoid is clamped and excised.
3. The base of the vein is ligated.

Description

The patient is placed in the Kraske or lithotomy position. Before beginning the scrub prep of the patient,

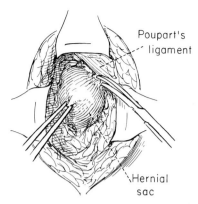

Figure 19–126. Repair of femoral hernia. Small hernia sac. (From Parsons L, Ulfelder H: Atlas of Pelvic Operations, 2nd ed. Philadelphia, WB Saunders, 1968.)

the circulator tapes the patient's buttocks apart by placing 4-inch adhesive tape on each side of the anus and attaching the ends to the operating table frame. Only a minimal scrub prep is performed.

Before beginning the operative procedure, many surgeons perform a sigmoidoscopy. Following the internal examination, the surgeon dilates the rectum with a rectal dilator (Fig. 19–129). This is done slowly since the musculature can be severely damaged if the dilation is hurried. Following satisfactory dilation, the surgeon inserts a rectal speculum. The technologist may be required to hold the speculum in place. The hemorrhoid is then grasped with a Pennington, Allis, or Kocher clamp, according to the surgeon's preference. Using the knife or cautery pencil, the surgeon amputates the vessel, excising a small amount of rectal mucosa at the same time (Fig. 19–130). To ligate the vein, a suture ligature of 2-0 or 3-0 chromic suture on a fine needle is used. The mucosa may be loosely approximated or left open. It is not sutured tightly because this would cause an abscess to form. Each hemorrhoid is removed in a similar manner.

At the close of the procedure, the surgeon may examine the rectum digitally to be sure that the sutures have not constricted the rectal lumen. The anus is then

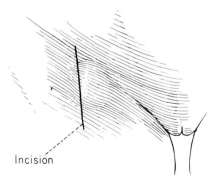

Figure 19–125. Repair of femoral hernia. Incision for femoral hernia. (From Parsons L, Ulfelder H: Atlas of Pelvic Operations, 2nd ed. Philadelphia, WB Saunders, 1968.)

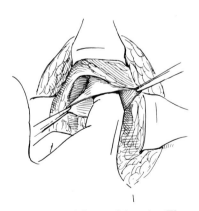

Figure 19–127. Repair of femoral hernia. The surgeon uses his or her finger to reduce the contents of the hernia sac. (From Parsons L, Ulfelder H: Atlas of Pelvic Operations, 2nd ed. Philadelphia, WB Saunders, 1968.)

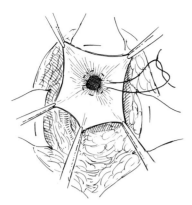

Figure 19–128. Repair of femoral hernia. The sac is closed with a pursestring suture. (From Parsons L, Ulfelder H: Atlas of Pelvic Operations, 2nd ed. Philadelphia, WB Saunders, 1968.)

dressed with packing impregnated with an antibiotic or antiseptic, such as Adaptic packing.

Related Procedures

Excision of venereal warts
Rectal polypectomy

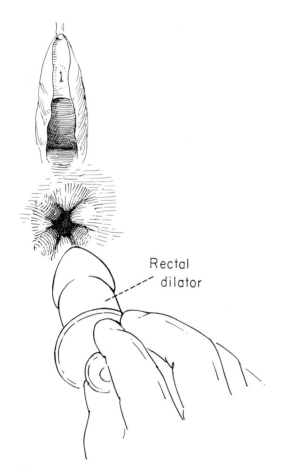

Figure 19–129. Hemorrhoidectomy. Before beginning the procedure, the surgeon dilates the rectum. (From Parsons L, Ulfelder H: Atlas of Pelvic Operations, 2nd ed. Philadelphia, WB Saunders, 1968.)

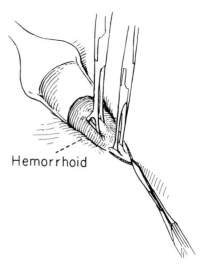

Figure 19–130. Hemorrhoidectomy. The surgeon excises the hemorrhoid with the knife. (From Parsons L, Ulfelder H: Atlas of Pelvic Operations, 2nd ed. Philadelphia, WB Saunders, 1968.)

Excision of Pilonidal Cyst

Definition

This is removal of a pilonidal cyst, which is caused by a congenital defect that allows epithelial tissue to be trapped below the surface of the skin in the area of the sacrum and coccyx. The cyst is removed when it causes recurrent infection of the area. A sinus tract (channel leading to an abscess) is often present.

Highlights

1. The skin is incised in a circle around the sinus.
2. The incision is carried to the sacrum and the tissue is removed en bloc.
3. The wound is closed.

Description

The patient is placed in the Kraske position and the buttocks are taped apart as for a hemorrhoidectomy.

The surgeon begins the procedure by placing a probe into the sinus tract, if one exists. The probe identifies the exact location of the sinus and the cyst itself. The surgeon may wish to inject dye into the sinus tract. If so, the technologist should have a blunt needle, syringe, and methylene blue dye available.

The area around the sinus is then incised with the skin knife. The technologist will be required to retract the skin with rake retractors as the surgeon deepens the incision. Using the cautery pencil or deep knife, the surgeon incises the subcutaneous layer. The incised tissue mass is then grasped with a Kocher or Allis clamp for traction. The dissection continues until the sacrum is exposed and the mass is removed. Bleeding vessels are controlled with cautery or ties of 3-0 Dexon or catgut.

The wound is then closed. Some surgeons prefer to place a very loose closure, while others close in routine fashion. The subcutaneous tissue is closed with absorbable suture, size 3-0. The skin is closed according to the surgeon's preference. When active infection is present, the wound is not sutured but is left open. If the wound is not sutured, it may be packed with iodophor-impregnated packing. Otherwise it is dressed with gauze and tape.

Excision of Anal Fistula

Definition

This is excision of tissue surrounding a draining sinus tract in the area of the anus. The fistula is continuous from the anus to the skin. The goal of surgery is to expose healthy tissue around the fistula so that the tract can heal.

Highlights

1. The extent of the fistula is determined.
2. The tract is incised around its circumference.

Description

The patient is placed in the Kraske position and prepared as for a hemorrhoidectomy. The surgeon dilates the rectum and inserts a rectal retractor. A malleable probe is then inserted into the fistula to determine its exact location and depth. Since the fistula may have more than one passageway, the surgeon identifies these also.

Once the extent of the fistula has been determined, the surgeon makes a circular incision around the fistula where it communicates with the skin. The incision is deepened with the cautery pencil and carried along the full length of the fistula. The incised tissue is removed as a specimen.

The wound is not sutured but is dressed with Adaptic packing or a similar material.

BREAST SURGERY

Excision of Breast Mass

Definition

This is removal of a suspicious breast mass for biopsy and confirmation of a diagnosis. When the surgeon is relatively certain that a breast mass is benign, the procedure is scheduled *without* a frozen section. If there is significant doubt that the mass is benign, the procedure is scheduled as a "breast biopsy with possible mastectomy." A simple breast biopsy without frozen section may be performed under local anesthesia.

Highlights

1. The breast is incised over the mass.
2. The mass is grasped and dissected free.
3. The wound is closed.

Description

The patient is placed in the supine position, prepped, and draped with the affected breast exposed. The surgeon makes a small incision over the area of the mass with the skin knife. As soon as the skin is incised, the breast tissue, which consists of fatty and connective tissue, is exposed. The surgeon deepens the incision using the cautery pencil or dissecting scissors (Metzenbaum or Mayo). On a simple breast biopsy, the technologist acts as first assistant by retracting the tissue with small rake retractors. With the mass partially mobilized, the surgeon can grasp it with Allis or Kocher clamps. The clamps are then used to elevate the mass as dissection continues. Bleeders are cauterized or clamped and ligated with chromic catgut or Dexon, size 3-0.

The surgeon completes the dissection and passes the specimen to the technologist. Since the tissue may determine the need for mastectomy, the technologist must take particular care in handling it. Its loss or alteration might have disastrous effects for the patient.

The breast tissue is approximated with interrupted 3-0 chromic catgut or Dexon sutures. The skin suture is usually size 4-0 or 5-0 material of the surgeon's choice.

Simple Mastectomy

Definition

This is removal of a breast to halt the spread of cancer. In recent years there has been a trend away from radical treatment of breast cancer. The radical mastectomy, which in the past involved the removal of breast tissue, skin, muscle, fascia, and axillary lymph nodes, has been replaced by the simple mastectomy and the modified radical mastectomy.

Highlights

1. The breast is incised elliptically.
2. The incision is deepened to encompass the entire breast.
3. The breast is removed en bloc.
4. The wound is closed.

Description

The patient is placed in the supine position with a small sandbag or folded bath towel under the shoulder on the affected side. The arm on the affected side may be placed on an armboard and included in the scrub prep.

Because the electrocautery pencil is used frequently during this procedure, the surgeon may request that two cautery pencils be available on the field (while the surgeon uses one pencil, the technologist can be cleaning the other). *Caution must be observed when both pencils are attached to one power unit.* If the pencil not in use comes in contact with the patient's skin while the surgeon activates the power unit, the patient will be burned. When not in use, a pencil must be placed in a specially designed holder, or two separate power units may be used to prevent accidental injury.

If a breast biopsy has just been performed during the same procedure, all instruments used on the biopsy are removed, the patient is redraped, and the team changes gloves. This is done to prevent contamination of the wound by cancer cells released from the biopsy tissue.

The surgeon begins the procedure by incising the skin around the breast elliptically. The incision is deepened with the cautery pencil. The skin flaps are then elevated. Kocher or Allis clamps are placed along the skin edges and retracted up by the surgeon and assistant. The surgeon then dissects the skin from the underlying tissue with the cautery pencil.

Once the skin flaps have been raised, the breast is freed from the chest wall at the level of the fascia to which it adheres. Many surgeons perform the entire dissection with the cautery pencil. Large bleeding vessels are clamped and ligated with silk or Dexon suture. If the incision extends into the axilla, sharp dissection with Metzenbaum scissors is used to isolate large vessels from the breast tissue. Frequently a lymph node biopsy is performed in the axillary region to determine whether metastasis has occurred. The node is grasped with an Allis clamp and dissected free with the scissors or cautery pencil.

Once the breast is completely mobilized, it is removed en bloc and passed to the technologist. The wound is then irrigated with warm saline solution. Before closing the wound, the surgeon places a rubber drain or Hemovac tube in the wound. The drainage tubes are brought out of the skin flap through two stab wounds made with the Hemovac trocar. The skin is then closed and the drains anchored with the surgeon's choice of suture.

Modified Radical Mastectomy

Definition

This is removal of a breast and axillary lymph nodes to halt the spread of cancer. This is a slightly more radical procedure than the simple mastectomy.

Highlights

1. A mastectomy is performed.
2. Axillary lymph nodes are removed.
3. The wound is closed.

Description

A mastectomy is performed, as previously described. The surgeon extends the incision well into the axilla (Fig. 19–131). The assistant retracts the tissue layers with small or medium Richardson retractors. Using sharp dissection, the surgeon removes the axillary lymph nodes.

The wound is closed as previously described for a simple mastectomy.

THYROID SURGERY

Thyroidectomy

Definition

This is surgical removal of one or more lobes of the thyroid gland. This procedure is performed to treat various diseases of the thyroid, such as hyperthyroidism or cancer that cannot be treated by chemotherapy.

Highlights

1. The neck is incised.
2. The thyroid is mobilized and removed.
3. The wound is closed.

Description

The patient is placed in the supine position with the neck hyperextended. To achieve this, a rolled bath blanket is placed under the patient's neck and shoulders.

Before beginning the procedure, the surgeon marks the proposed incision line by grasping a length of suture and pressing it against the patient's neck. The resulting indentation will serve as a guideline for an incision that produces a nearly unnoticeable scar.

The surgeon incises the neck with a No. 10 blade. The subcutaneous tissue is incised with the cautery pencil, exposing the platysma muscle (Fig. 19–132). The assistant retracts the tissue layers with rake retractors. The surgeon then divides the muscle layer with the deep knife. Using both sharp and blunt dissection, the flaps of the incision are deepened above and below. The cautery pencil is used frequently to coagulate bleeders in the vascular tissue.

As the dissection continues, deeper retractors are used. A special thyroid (Green) retractor may be used, or, if the wound is very deep, U.S. retractors should be available.

When the thyroid gland is finally exposed, two Lahey spring (self-retaining) retractors are placed in the wound. The surgeon then grasps the gland with one or two Lahey tenaculi that are designed for thyroid procedures.

The thyroid gland is an extremely vascular structure and its attachments to the trachea consist of a bed of tissue that is rich with blood vessels. Therefore, to mobilize the gland, the surgeon successively double-

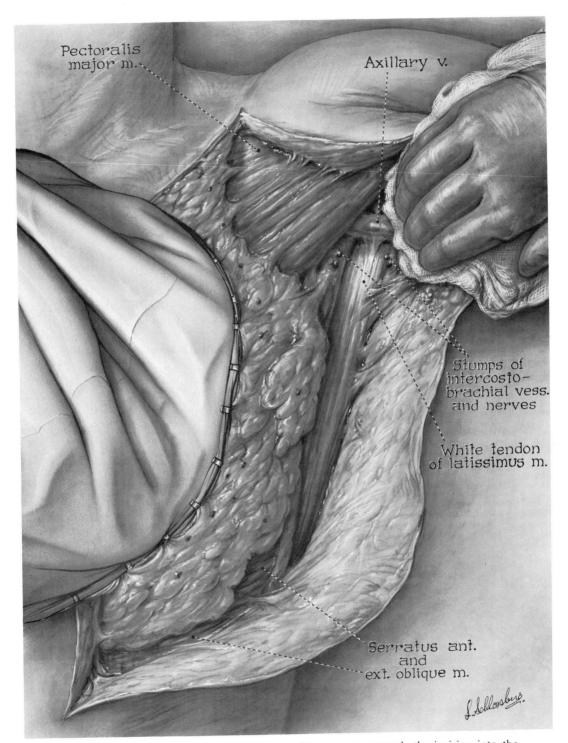

Figure 19–131. Modified radical mastectomy. The surgeon extends the incision into the axilla and removes the lymph nodes that drain the breast tissue. (From Haagensen CD: Diseases of the Breast, 3rd ed. Philadelphia, WB Saunders, 1986.)

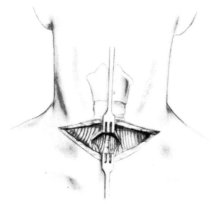

Figure 19–132. Thyroidectomy. Incision exposes the platysma muscle. Rake retractors are used to retract the wound edges. (From Schwartz SI, et al: Principles of Surgery, 2nd ed. New York, McGraw-Hill, 1974. Used with the permission of McGraw-Hill Book Company.)

clamps small sections of tissue, divides between the clamps, and ligates the stumps. Most surgeons prefer to use *straight* Kelly clamps or mosquito clamps for mobilization. The technologist should have at least 12 clamps available and may need as many as two dozen if the surgeon prefers to clamp and divide many sections before ligating the stumps and returning the clamps to the technologist. Mobilization is performed as described above. A No. 15 knife blade is used to divide the tissue sections, and sizes 3-0 and 4-0 silk sutures are used for ligation. Because the knife is used so frequently during mobilization, the surgeon may request that it be left on the field where he or she can pick it up rather than having the technologist hand it to him or her repeatedly. If left on the field, the knife should be placed on a folded towel to prevent accidental injury to the patient.

Large arteries of the thyroid are occluded with suture ligatures of 2-0 or 3-0 silk mounted on a fine (Ferguson or French-eye) needle (Fig. 19–133). When mobilization is complete, the gland is passed to the technologist. If

the tissue looks suspicious, the surgeon may order a frozen section to determine what type of disease is present.

The wound is irrigated, a small Penrose drain is inserted, and the layers of the neck tissue are closed individually. The surgeon uses interrupted silk sutures on a fine needle on muscle and fascial layers. Subcutaneous tissue is closed with fine interrupted absorbable sutures. The skin is closed with the surgeon's preferred material, or wound clips may be used.

The incision is dressed and the dressings are secured by passing a gauze strip around the patient's neck. Because of the danger of tracheal swelling and consequent obstructed airway, a tracheostomy tray is sent to the recovery room with the patient.

Related Procedure

Parotidectomy

FIBEROPTIC PROCEDURES

These procedures involve direct visualization of the inner surfaces of the gastrointestinal tract through a lighted scope. They are performed for diagnosis or biopsy. Many hospitals employ a special endoscopic team to assist the physician during the procedure, while others may request the assistance of surgery personnel. The techniques for all fiberoptic procedures of the gastrointestinal tract are similar. Patients are usually given a light sedative before the procedure, and most procedures are done on an outpatient basis.

Esophagogastroduodenoscopy

This procedure is performed to examine the esophagus, stomach, and duodenum. The scope (Fig. 19–134) is inserted with the patient in the lateral position. When

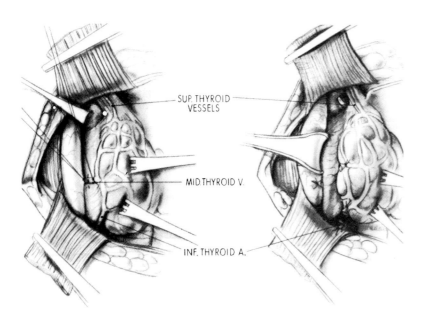

SUP. THYROID VESSELS

MID. THYROID V.

INF. THYROID A.

Figure 19–133. Thyroidectomy. Large arteries of the thyroid gland are ligated with suture ligatures. Note the divided strap muscles. (From Schwartz SI, et al: Principles of Surgery, 2nd ed. New York, McGraw-Hill, 1974. Used with the permission of McGraw-Hill Book Company.)

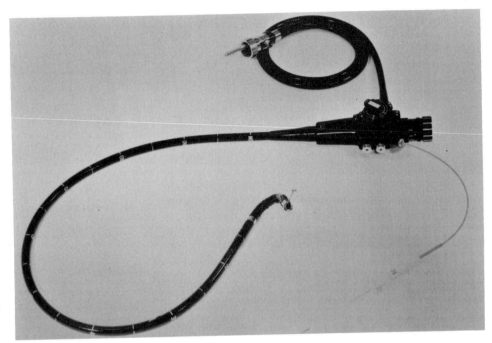

Figure 19–134. Fiberoptic gastroscope. (Courtesy of the Olympus Corporation, Lake Success, NY.)

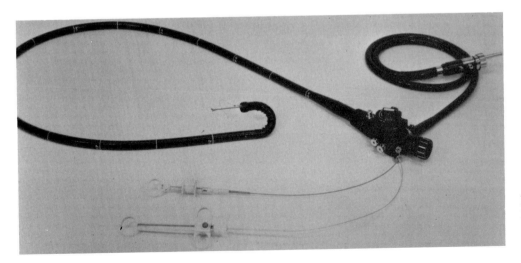

Figure 19–135. Fiberoptic colonoscope. (Courtesy of the Olympus Corporation, Lake Success, NY.)

cancer, ulceration, or other disease is suspected, the surgeon inserts the scope through the patient's mouth and systematically examines the tissue for a lesion. If one is found, a small biopsy specimen is obtained. The technologist hands the operator the biopsy forceps. As the operator threads the forceps through the biopsy channel of the scope, the technologist may be required to hold the scope in place to prevent it from sliding away from the area of the lesion. Once the forceps is withdrawn, tissue can be removed from the forceps with a hypodermic needle. The technologist scrapes the tissue into a small specimen cup or basin. The scope is withdrawn slowly to prevent damage to the tissues.

Sigmoidoscopy

This procedure is performed to examine tissue and/or obtain a biopsy specimen of the sigmoid colon and rectum. The patient is placed in the jackknife position, and the scope is introduced into the patient's rectum. Biopsy tissue can be obtained or rectal polyps removed with the aid of a rectal snare. Because this procedure is embarrassing and uncomfortable for the patient, the technologist should offer constant emotional support during the procedure. Unlike the gastroscope, the sigmoidoscope does not have a built-in suction and irrigation system; the technologist will therefore be required to hold the suction tip for the operator. When suction is required, the technologist threads the suction tip into the scope. Other accessory instruments, such as the electrocautery tip, are passed in the same way.

Colonoscopy

This procedure is performed to examine the lumen of the colon. The patient is placed in the jackknife or supine position with the knees slightly bent. The scope (Fig. 19–135) is introduced into the rectum and slowly advanced. This scope has a built-in suction and irrigation system. The technologist assists the operator by holding the scope in place during the biopsy and by passing needed accessory equipment such as the cautery pencil, forceps, or snare. Biopsy tissue is obtained in the same way as in an esophagogastroduodenoscopy.

Bibliography

Artz CP, Cohn I Jr, Davis JH Jr: A Brief Textbook of Surgery. Philadelphia, WB Saunders, 1976.

Berci G, et al: Laparoscopy Guideline for Nurses. Los Angeles, Cedars-Sinai Medical Center.

Gardner E, Gray D, O'Rahilly R: Anatomy: A Regional Study of Human Structure, 5th ed. Philadelphia, WB Saunders, 1986.

Haagensen CD: Diseases of the Breast, 3rd ed. Philadelphia, WB Saunders, 1985.

Jacob S, Francone C, Lossow WJ: Structure and Function in Man, 5th ed. Philadelphia, WB Saunders, 1982.

McVay C: Surgical Anatomy, 6th ed. Philadelphia, WB Saunders, 1984.

Sabiston DC Jr (ed): Davis-Christopher Textbook of Surgery, 14th ed. Philadelphia, WB Saunders, 1991

Schwartz SI, et al: Principles of Surgery, 2nd ed. New York, McGraw-Hill, 1974.

Taber's Cyclopedic Medical Dictionary. Philadelphia, FA Davis, 1973.

Zuidema GD: Shackelford's Surgery of the Alimentary Tract, 3rd ed (5 volumes). Philadelphia, WB Saunders, 1991.

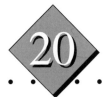

Minimal Access Surgery

Minimal access surgery—that is, surgery performed or assisted through a *laparoscope*—is one of the most dramatic surgical developments of the past few decades. The laparoscope is a lighted telescopic instrument that is inserted through a small abdominal incision. Surgery is performed with special instruments through one or more tubular sleeves that are passed through the abdominal wall at strategic locations within the viewing range of the laparoscope. The major advantages of minimal access surgery are those associated with minimal trauma:

- Shorter hospital stay
- Decreased postoperative pain
- Shorter recovery time

At the present time, a number of laparoscopic procedures are under investigation. These include intestinal resection, nephrectomy, tumor resection, and lymph node dissection. The risks associated with all laparoscopic procedures are compounded during complex operations. Many surgeons believe that some complex procedures are feasible, but their purpose as laparoscopic procedures may be questionable or they may result in complications. However, the success of a number of laparoscopic procedures has been established and well documented. These procedures are presented in this chapter.

All laparoscopic procedures require three distinct categories of equipment:

1. Equipment for visualization of the involved anatomy (laparoscope and video camera system)
2. Instruments for exposure of the anatomy
3. Instruments for hemostasis, dissection, and removal of tissue

VISUALIZATION

Laparoscope

The laparoscope (Fig. 20–1) is a delicate, lensed instrument that is inserted into the abdomen to enable the surgeon to view internal anatomy. This is one of many types of fiberoptic instruments used in surgery. The laparoscope lens is subject to scratching, chipping, or breaking. Thus, this instrument must be handled gently and carefully. The laparoscope is always handled by the eyepiece, and it or any one of its components is never placed near a table edge where it might fall to the floor and break. A discussion on the proper cleaning and sterilization of endoscopic equipment is presented in Chapter 7.

Fiberoptic Cable and Light Source

Fiberoptic refers to the cable that connects the laparoscope to its light source. A fiberoptic cable is composed of hundreds of very small, optical-quality glass tubes called *fibers*. Each glass fiber is coated on its surface with a special material that reflects light. This material causes the light to travel along the length of the fiber and emerge at its end. The combination of hundreds of these fibers results in an extremely intense light that is capable of rounding corners. The cable is connected to a fiberoptic light source, which is specially designed to transmit light to the cable.

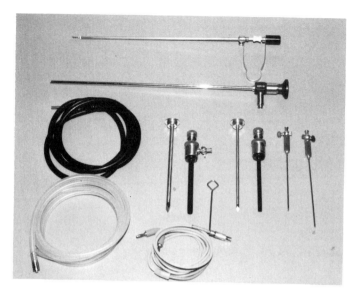

Figure 20–1. Laparoscope and accessories.

Care of the Fiberoptic Cable and Light Source

Because it is made of glass, the fiberoptic cable must be handled very gently. It should never be bent, pulled, or stretched because this could damage the fibers. Any sharp instrument that could puncture the cable, such as a towel clip, should never be used to secure the cable during surgery. In addition, the manufacturer's specifications for sterilization should always be followed.

The *fiberoptic light source* (Fig. 20–2) is operated by the circulating nurse. The light source regulates the intensity of the light by a rheostat. Before the light source is activated, the rheostat must be turned to "0". Failure to do this may result in a blown bulb. Following use, the light source fan should be allowed to run for a few minutes to cool the unit. When the light source is on, care must be taken that the light cable is not left in a position where it could cause injury or damage. The light cable produces an extremely intense source of light, which can heat up over time and may burn the patient or ignite drapes. When the cable is being removed from the light source, it should always be grasped by its fitting, because handling the cable can cause the fibers to break.

Video Camera System

The images projected by the laparoscope's effective viewing area are quite small. Thus, for surgery to be performed safely and efficiently, these images must be projected and enlarged. This is accomplished with a

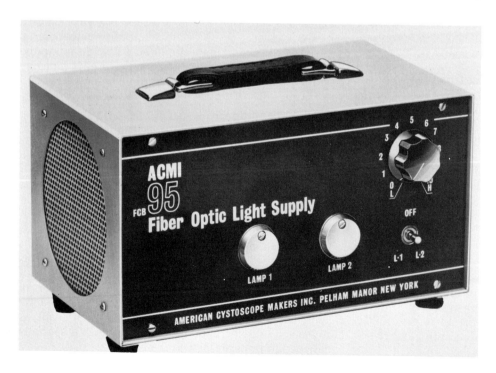

Figure 20–2. Fiberoptic light source.

video camera system (VCS). The VCS transmits the images that are viewed through the laparoscope to a video screen. The surgeon then operates by viewing the screen. The surgical assistant can anticipate the surgeon's need for instruments by watching the image.

The components of the VCS are somewhat complex, but the basic use, care, and handling of the components can be mastered by anyone who has the patience to learn. There are three components of the system: the camera, the control unit, and the monitor. Each of the components has individual parts that are important to learn. The following describes the fundamental parts of each component and how they work.

Camera

The camera is very small, about 3 inches long and 1 to 2 inches wide. There are two parts to the camera: the head and the cable. The camera head attaches to the endoscope with a small fitting called an endocoupler. The camera head cable is fitted between the camera head and the control unit. All camera heads have some type of marker on them that allows the operator to keep the camera oriented properly on the video screen. The zoom feature on some cameras enables the operator to enlarge the screen image without actually moving the endoscope. However, the zoom feature may create some loss of light in the projected image.

Camera Operation

Many operating rooms designate and train one or two persons as camera operators. The camera operator may be a technologist or nurse who shows interest and skill in this specialty. The operator must have a steady hand, good spatial orientation, and the ability to concentrate for long periods of time. The job is of utmost importance because it allows the surgeon to perform the tasks both quickly and efficiently. The functions of the camera operator are to move *with the surgeon* during the procedure. He or she must serve as the surgeon's eyes by adjusting the camera to keep both the instruments and the anatomic structures in clear view. He or she must also be completely familiar with the mechanics of the camera in the event a part must be replaced during surgery or adjustments must be made. The camera head cable is the most sensitive component of the entire system, and its failure rate is the highest. Thus, the camera operator must be familiar with both the tools and the procedure for replacing this part. In addition, the operator must know how to assemble all parts of the camera system and must know techniques used to maintain clarity of the image produced on the screen. Trouble-shooting suggestions for solving camera malfunctions are given in Table 20–1.

Camera Control Unit

The camera control unit enables the operator to adjust the image for color and light intensity. It also connects the camera to the video recorder monitor (screen).

One of the most important features of the control unit is the white balance. To understand white balance, it is necessary to know a little about light.

White Balance

Different sources of light, such as incandescent or fluorescent light or sunlight, produce wavelengths that vary in intensity and length. Each different wavelength produces a different color of light. Some of these colors (wavelengths) are more intense than others. When we perceive white light, we are actually seeing a composite of all the wavelengths. However, incandescent light, which is used in homes, makes objects look pinkish, and fluorescent light, which is used in office buildings, tends to make objects look greenish. This is because the wavelengths responsible for those color hues are more intense. Our eyes and minds have adjusted for these color intensities, but some still remain in our viewing perception. The white balance on the video camera has the same ability to adjust for these color or wavelength intensities. When we set the white balance, by focusing the camera on a white object, we are allowing the camera to store information about the wavelengths so that it can correct for the intensities—it "balances" the color. The most common cause of color distortion on the screen is caused by failure to set the white balance. Another cause is the use of an "off white" object for setting the white balance.

Because color intensity and wavelength are associated with the temperature of the source ("color temperature"), some control units automatically measure the light in degrees Kelvin and adjust it accordingly. However, if the lens is dirty or the fiberoptic light cable is cracked, this decreases the temperature rating, and the procedure for white balancing may be necessary.

The gain switch on the control monitor adjusts the intensity of the light. The light boost, used when sufficient light is unavailable, increases the quality of the screen image.

Monitor

The monitor is the screen component of the VCS (Fig. 20–3). It should have a higher resolution than the camera to ensure clarity. A 20-inch screen is used in most operating rooms.

Care of the Video Camera System Components

The VCS represents a substantial investment, and all components must be handled with extreme care. The camera may cost between $6,000 and $16,000 and is the most costly component of the system. Because it is used on the sterile field, it must be sterilized with a method that has been proven to be both effective and safe for the instrument. The Steris System, discussed in Chapter 7, is one method that is used to sterilize the camera head and cable. The camera manufacturer's specifications must be consulted before the camera is subjected

Table 20–1. TROUBLE-SHOOTING PROBLEMS OF VIDEO CAMERA SYSTEM

Problem	Possible Causes	Solutions
No power	1. Power switch off 2. Power cord not plugged in 3. Circuit breaker tripped	1. Turn power on. 2. Plug cord in. 3. Check circuit box.
No picture	1. No power 2. Equipment sequence incomplete 3. Camera placed on dark surface	1. See above. 2. System will not work unless all components have power. Check all components. 3. Turn face of camera up.
No sound	1. Microphone battery dead 2. Microphone switch off 3. Audio cables incorrectly connected	1. Replace battery. 2. Turn switch on. 3. Connect VCR audio "out" to monitor "in."
Poor light	1. Light bulb blown 2. Fiberoptic light cable damaged 3. Camera light sensor picking up glare from instruments	1. Replace light bulb. 2. Replace cable. 3. Reposition instruments.
Foggy picture	1. Tissue or condensation on lens 2. Smoke	1. Place tips of scope in warm water. 2. Use suction.
Picture will not focus	1. Cracked scope or camera lens 2. Coupling between eyepiece of scope and camera endocoupler loose	1. Send scope out for repair. 2. Tighten.
Picture grainy	1. Loose cable connections 2. Cable not grounded	1. Tighten all cables. 2. Remove any cables not in use.
Colors unnatural	1. Camera not white balanced 2. Camera white balanced with filter on 3. "Off white" object used to white balance camera 4. Monitor unbalanced	1. Follow procedure for white balancing. 2. Remove filter. 3. Use white object to white balance. 4. Use color bar switch on control unit or set to "reset."
Record button will not engage	1. No tape in VCR	1. Put tape in. Depress "record" and "play" simultaneously.
Insufflator alarm sounds	1. CO_2 tubing blocked	1. Check tubing. Crimped? Stopcock turned off?
CO_2 leakage	1. CO_2 tubing blocked 2. Stopcock partially closed 3. Incorrect size or faulty seals 4. Sleeve incorrectly reduced	1. Check tubing. 2. Open fully. 3. Check sizes and seals. 4. Check reducer.

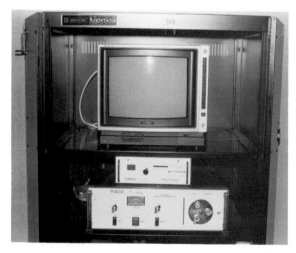

Figure 20–3. *Top.* Video monitor. *Middle.* Camera control unit. *Bottom.* Fiberoptic light source. (Courtesy of Raymond Lemaster, Alameda Hospital, Alameda, CA.)

to any sterilization system. The camera should never be pointed toward any high-intensity light source, such as the operating room lights, as this may permanently damage its light-sensing element.

The control unit and monitor should be kept clean and dust free. Solutions should never be placed near the control unit where they might accidentally spill or be splashed onto the unit. The monitor screen should be kept clean according to the manufacturer's specifications. All cables, connections, and cords should be routinely inspected for their integrity and stored in a manner that prevents them from kinking or bending.

EXPOSURE DURING THE SURGICAL PROCEDURE

To prevent injury to abdominal structures during surgery, the surgeon inflates the peritoneal cavity with carbon dioxide gas. This process is called a *pneumoperitoneum*. Certain instruments and equipment are necessary to establish pneumoperitoneum. Many of the instruments used in endoscopic procedures, including the establishment of pneumoperitoneum, are disposable and intended for single use only.

A long needle called an insufflation needle (Fig. 20–4) is inserted directly through the abdominal wall. Flexible tubing is attached to this needle, which is then connected to a carbon dioxide insufflator. The flow rate and pressure exerted in the abdominal wall are manually regulated by adjusting the insufflator controls. This is the responsibility of the registered nurse circulator. The normal flow rate is 6 L/min, and the intra-abdominal pressure is usually set at 14 mm Hg. The pressure must never exceed 20 mm Hg. A minimum of 8 mm Hg is needed for most procedures.

To further facilitate exposure, surgeons performing some gynecologic operations require the use of a uterine manipulator. This instrument is placed through the

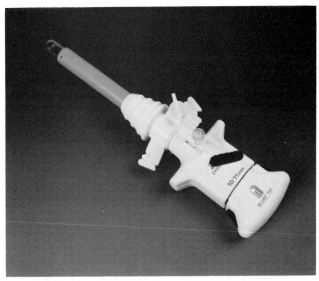

Figure 20–5. Trocar and sleeve. (Courtesy of Ethicon ENDO-Surgery, Inc., Somerville, NJ.)

cervix before the laparoscopic procedure and is used to rotate or flex the uterus and thereby bring nearby anatomic structures into view.

To introduce cutting, dissection, suction, and hemostasis instruments into the abdomen, the surgeon passes one or more *trocars and sleeves* (Fig. 20–5) through the abdominal wall during the operative procedure. Following the establishment of pneumoperitoneum, the trocar and sleeve are inserted as one unit. The trocar is then withdrawn, leaving the sleeve, through which the laparoscope or other instruments can be passed. Trocars are available in a variety of sizes and may be reusable or disposable. The disposable trocars are generally sharper than reusable ones, and their valves are more efficient in preventing the escape of gas. The choice of size depends on the diameter of the laparoscope and instruments to be used. Five- or 10-mm trocars are commonly used in general laparoscopic surgery. *Reducers* (Fig. 20–6) allow passage of a small instrument through a large opening without the loss of gas. For example, a 5-to-3 reducer allows passage of a 3-mm instrument through a 5-mm sleeve. Two types of trocars and sleeves are used.

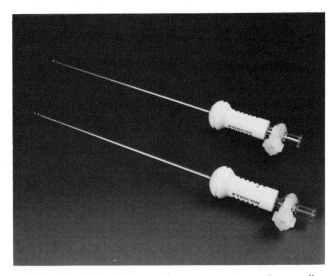

Figure 20–4. Insufflation (pneumoperitoneum) needles. (Courtesy of Ethicon ENDO-Surgery, Inc., Somerville, NJ.)

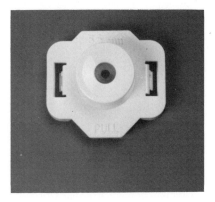

Figure 20–6. Trocar reducer. (Courtesy of Ethicon ENDO-Surgery, Inc., Somerville, NJ.)

For *open technique* a blunt trocar is introduced through a small incision. Some types of trocars may be sutured in place to prevent gas leakage. For *closed technique* a sharp, triangular, conical, or pyramidal tipped trocar is used. The closed technique trocar is self-piercing and requires no previous incision. Unless the procedure requires *only visualization* of the abdominal anatomy, more than one trocar and sleeve must be inserted. One sleeve accepts the laparoscope, and the others accept various instruments needed during the procedure. Some procedures require three or four separate sleeves. When two or more trocars and sleeves are used, the procedure is said to be two handed. After the initial trocar and sleeve are introduced and the laparoscope and camera are attached, the internal abdominal structures can be easily visualized on the television screen, and the other trocars can be safely introduced.

HEMOSTASIS, DISSECTION, AND TISSUE REMOVAL

Hemostasis can be achieved during laparoscopic surgery by one of several methods. Electrocautery is routinely used by many surgeons. Some laparoscopic instruments are coated with nonconductive material along their length so that inadvertent destruction of tissue is prevented. A complete discussion of electrocautery is found in Chapter 13. Some surgeons advocate the use of bipolar cautery as it prevents the arcing of current and accidental burning of nearby structures that are out of the visual field. A combination electrosurgery, suction/irrigation instrument is shown in Figure 20–7. The tip may be spatula shaped, hook shaped, or right angled.

The laser is frequently used during laparoscopic surgery, and many surgeons prefer its use over electrocautery. The laser allows a more precise area of treatment and may prevent inadvertent tissue destruction. A laser fiber may be passed through an irrigator-aspirator. Whenever the laser is used during laparoscopic surgery, all safety precautions must be strictly observed. A complete discussion of these safety standards is presented in Chapter 18.

Another type of hemostatic tool is the heater probe. This instrument generates heat at its tip to cauterize small vessels and is excellent for cauterizing capillary beds such as the surface of the liver. It does not use electric current as the source of heat; thus, there is no danger of arcing.

Ligatures used during laparoscopy are inserted through a snare-type instrument. An alternative to ligature is the use of absorbable, titanium, or stainless steel clips, which are placed over a vessel or duct before its division. Sutures are placed with an endoscopic needle holder. Alternatively, endoscopic staplers may be used. These instruments resemble the surgical stapling instruments discussed in Chapter 12.

Dissection, clamping, and cutting instruments are available in a variety of types and sizes. These instruments are extremely delicate and must be handled carefully. Disposable instruments are popular because they retain their cutting edge.

Two types of scissors (Fig. 20–8) are commonly used: hook-tipped scissors, which are strong enough for sutures and fibrous tissue, and microscissors, which are used on more delicate tissue.

Graspers (see Fig. 20–8) are used in the same way as forceps would be in open surgery. These are available in varying sizes and strengths.

Dissectors (see Fig. 20–8) are used to separate tissue planes. The tips may be straight, right angled, or curved.

The extractor (see Fig. 20–8) is used to grasp and hold structures.

Bowel instruments (Fig. 20–9) whose tips are the same as those used in open surgery are also used. These include bowel, right-angled, Babcock, and Allis clamps.

Thoracic instruments (Fig. 20–10) include lung forceps and Glassman clamps.

OPERATIVE PROCEDURES

Laparoscopy

Definition

This is direct visualization of the abdominal contents using the fiberoptic laparoscope. As a gynecologic procedure, laparoscopy may be performed for elective tubal ligation or to remove small ovarian cysts or adhesions. The description of this procedure (except for those sections of the text that discuss the uterine manipulator and patient position) applies to all laparoscopic procedures. These basic steps in laparoscopy are omitted from the discussions of laparoscopic appendectomy, laparoscopic cholecystectomy with operative cholangiography, and laparoscopic hernia repair.

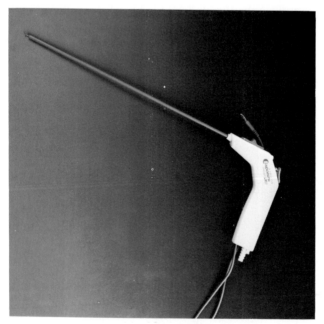

Figure 20–7. Combination electrosurgery probe, suction, and irrigation tip. (Courtesy of Ethicon ENDO-Surgery, Inc., Somerville, NJ.)

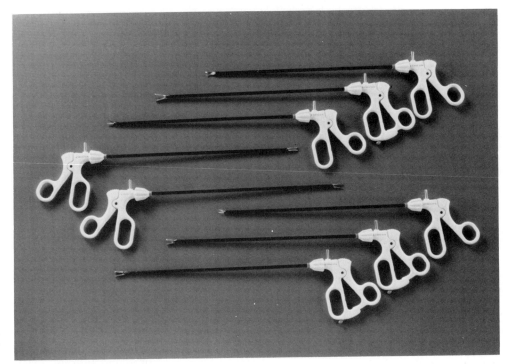

Figure 20–8. *Top to bottom*: Straight grasper, straight dissector, hook scissors, straight forceps, curved forceps, micro scissors, extractor, curved dissector. (Courtesy of Ethicon ENDO-Surgery, Inc., Somerville, NJ.)

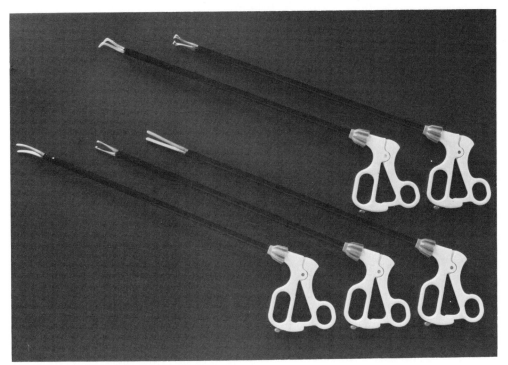

Figure 20–9. Bowel instruments. *Top to bottom*: Babcock clamp, right-angled clamp, bowel clamp, Allis clamp, Kelly clamp. (Courtesy of Ethicon ENDO-Surgery, Inc., Somerville, NJ.)

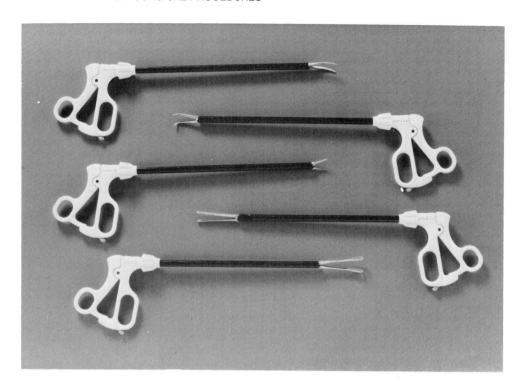

Figure 20–10. Thoracic clamps. *Top to bottom:* Kelly clamp, right-angled clamp, forceps, Glassman clamp, lung grasping clamp. (Courtesy of Ethicon ENDO-Surgery, Inc., Somerville, NJ.)

Highlights

1. The uterine manipulator is placed at the cervix.
2. Pneumoperitoneum is established.
3. A trocar and sleeve are introduced through the abdominal wall.
4. The laparoscope is inserted.
5. A specific procedure such as tubal ligation, ovarian cystectomy, or lysis of adhesions is performed.
6. The laparoscope is withdrawn, and the wound is closed.

Description

The patient is placed in the lithotomy position with the stirrups lowered for better access to the abdomen. The abdomen and entire perineal area, including the vaginal vault, are prepped. At the completion of the prep, the scrub assistant gloves the surgeon, who then inserts a uterine manipulator into the cervix. Two types of manipulators are available. One requires suction tubing that is attached to the manipulator (Fig. 20–11). Continuous suction on the cervix prevents the manipulator from dislodging during the procedure. A second type of manipulator is attached to a uterine tenaculum. Once the surgeon has inserted the manipulator, he or she removes the contaminated gloves and is gowned and gloved in routine fashion.

To begin the procedure, the surgeon makes a small nick in the abdominal wall, close to the umbilicus, with a No. 11 or No. 15 knife blade. To prevent the bowel or other abdominal structures from being injured by the scalpel, two towel clips may be used to grasp the abdominal wall and elevate it above the viscera. The scrub technologist may be required to elevate the towel clips once the surgeon has inserted them.

A pneumoperitoneum needle is inserted through the incision (Fig. 20–12). A 10-mL syringe filled with sterile saline solution is attached to the needle so that the surgeon can aspirate and verify that no blood vessels have been punctured. The insufflator tubing is attached to the needle. The other end of the tubing is then passed to the circulator, who connects it to the insufflator. The circulator switches the insufflator to the correct rate and pressure, and pneumoperitoneum is thus initiated. When the pressure has reached the desired operative level, the surgeon withdraws the needle and lengthens the abdominal incision slightly with the scalpel.

A large trocar and sleeve are then inserted through the incision (Fig. 20–13). The trocar is removed, leaving the sleeve to receive the fiberoptic laparoscope. The insufflator tubing is attached to the sleeve to maintain operative abdominal pressure. The laparoscope is then threaded into the sleeve, and a fiberoptic light cable is attached to it. The abdominal contents are examined for disease or injury.

If tubal ligation or excision of an ovarian cyst is to be performed, a second trocar and sleeve are inserted. The second incision is made directly below the umbilical incision at the symphysis. The surgeon will request

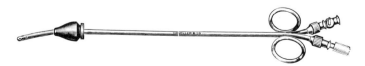

Figure 20–11. Uterine manipulator. (Courtesy of V. Mueller Co.)

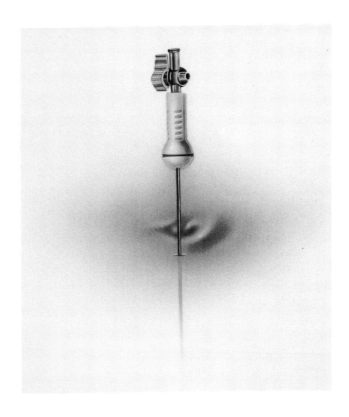

Figure 20–12. Laparoscopy. Insertion of pneumoperitoneal needle. (Reprinted from Techniques in Endosurgery: Appendectomy. Courtesy of Ethicon, Inc., Somerville, NJ.)

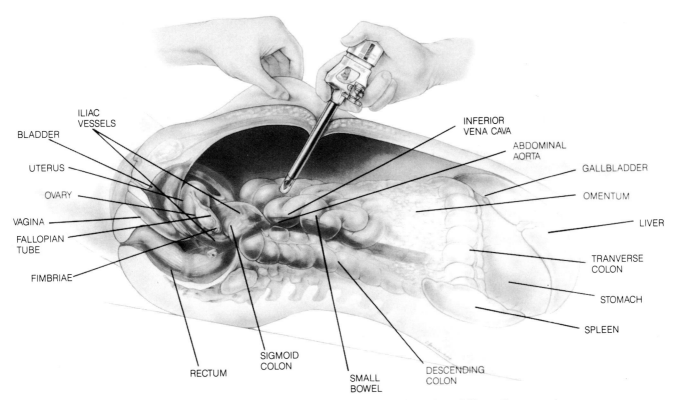

Figure 20–13. Laparoscopy. Placement of single trocar through umbilicus. Cutaway view of regional anatomy. (Courtesy of Ethicon ENDO-Surgery, Inc., Somerville, NJ.)

specific accessories, as needed. The scrub assistant may be asked to manipulate the uterus by gently retracting the manipulator to one side or the other while the surgeon continues the procedure.

At the completion of the procedure, the gas is allowed to escape through the sleeve, which is then withdrawn. The surgeon closes the incisions with subcuticular sutures of Dexon or chromic catgut, size 3-0 on a fine cutting needle, sterile strips, or skin staples. The wounds are then dressed with Band-Aids or adhesive strips.

Laparoscopic Appendectomy

Definition

Laparoscopic appendectomy is the removal of a diseased appendix with the aid of the fiberoptic laparoscope. The appendix is a blind, narrow, elongated pouch attached to the cecum (Fig. 20–14). The appendix is often inflamed and infected and must be removed to prevent its rupture and subsequent peritonitis.

Highlights

1. Pneumoperitoneum is established.
2. Accessory trocars are placed.
3. The appendix is divided from the mesoappendix.
4. A ligature is placed at the base of the appendix.
5. The appendix is divided and delivered from the wound.
6. The appendiceal stump is cauterized.

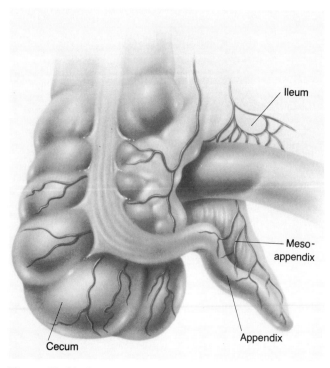

Figure 20–14. Laparoscopic appendectomy. Anatomic location of appendix—a blind, narrow, elongated pouch attached to the cecum. (Reprinted from Techniques in Endosurgery: Appendectomy. Courtesy of Ethicon, Inc., Somerville, NJ.)

Description

The patient is prepped and draped for an abdominal incision. Because there remains the possibility of an open procedure, the entire abdomen should be prepped. In this procedure, after the establishment of pneumoperitoneum, four trocars are placed (Fig. 20–15): a 10/11-mm umbilical trocar, two 5-mm accessory trocars, and a second 10/11-mm trocar, which is used for extraction of the appendix.

After placement of the trocars, a straight grasper is used to hold the cecum and pull it upward. This exposes the appendix. A second grasper is used to provide tension on the appendix so that it can be divided from the mesoappendix. The electrosurgery probe with a hook dissector is used to simultaneously cauterize and divide the appendix from the mesoappendix (Fig. 20–16). Dissection continues to the base of the appendix (Fig. 20–17). At this stage, the surgeon may ligate the tip of the appendix and use the ends of the ligature for more manageable traction.

As the assistant pulls upward on the tip of the appendix, the surgeon applies a suture to its base (Fig. 20–18). Two more ligatures are then applied (Fig. 20–19). The appendix is now ready to be severed from its base and delivered from the wound. This is accomplished with hook scissors (Fig. 20–20).

The appendix can be delivered directly through the 10/11-mm lateral trocar port (Fig. 20–21*A*), or a special specimen pouch can be used (Fig. 20–21*B*). The specimen and the trocar are removed simultaneously. The appendiceal stump is cauterized with the electrosurgery probe with hook dissector (Fig. 20–22). Ligating clips may be applied to any persistent bleeding vessels. At this time, the wound may be irrigated with warm normal saline. The pneumoperitoneum is released, and all trocars are removed. The trocar wounds are closed with sterile skin strips, skin staples, or individual skin sutures.

Laparoscopic Cholecystectomy With Operative Cholangiography

Definition

Laparoscopic cholecystectomy is the removal of a diseased gallbladder with the aid of the fiberoptic laparoscope. Operative cholangiography refers to the injection of radiopaque dye into the cystic duct, performed as part of the operative procedure, to determine the presence of gallstones.

Highlights

1. Pneumoperitoneum is established.
2. Trocars are placed.
3. The gallbladder is retracted upward.
4. The gallbladder is dissected free.
5. The cystic artery and duct are ligated.
6. The cystic duct is incised.
7. A cholangiogram catheter is threaded into the cystic duct and dye is injected. Radiographs are taken.

Text continued on page 341

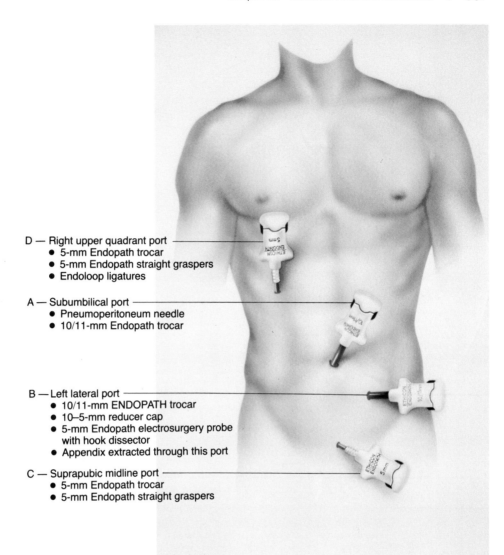

D — Right upper quadrant port
  ● 5-mm Endopath trocar
  ● 5-mm Endopath straight graspers
  ● Endoloop ligatures

A — Subumbilical port
  ● Pneumoperitoneum needle
  ● 10/11-mm Endopath trocar

B — Left lateral port
  ● 10/11-mm ENDOPATH trocar
  ● 10–5-mm reducer cap
  ● 5-mm Endopath electrosurgery probe
    with hook dissector
  ● Appendix extracted through this port

C — Suprapubic midline port
  ● 5-mm Endopath trocar
  ● 5-mm Endopath straight graspers

Figure 20–15. Laparoscopic appendectomy. Four trocars are inserted into the abdominal cavity. *A.* A 10/11-mm umbilical trocar. *B* and *C.* Two 5-mm accessory trocars. *D.* A second 10/11-mm trocar, used to extract the appendix. (Reprinted from Techniques in Endosurgery: Appendectomy. Courtesy of Ethicon, Inc., Somerville, NJ.)

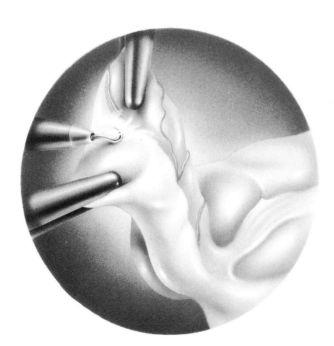

Figure 20–16. Laparoscopic appendectomy. The electrosurgical probe with hook dissector is used to simultaneously cauterize and divide the appendix from the mesoappendix. (Reprinted from Techniques in Endosurgery: Appendectomy. Courtesy of Ethicon, Inc., Somerville, NJ.)

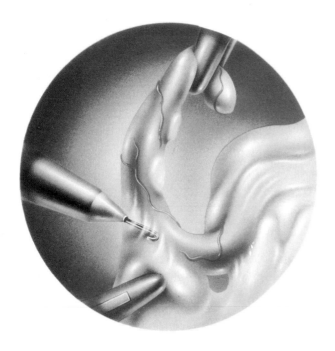

Figure 20–17. Laparoscopic appendectomy. Dissection of the mesoappendix continues to the base of the appendix. (Reprinted from Techniques in Endosurgery: Appendectomy. Courtesy of Ethicon, Inc., Somerville, NJ.)

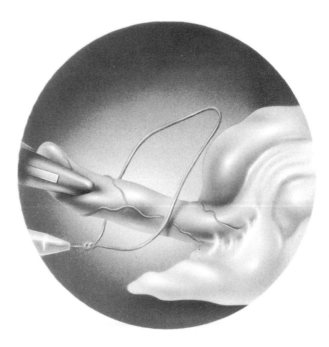

Figure 20–18. Laparoscopic appendectomy. A ligature is placed at the base of the appendix. (Reprinted from Techniques in Endosurgery: Appendectomy. Courtesy of Ethicon, Inc., Somerville, NJ.)

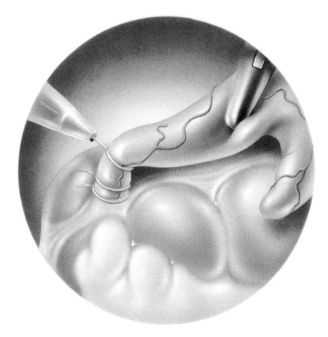

Figure 20–19. Laparoscopic appendectomy. Two additional sutures are used to ligate the base of the appendix. (Reprinted from Techniques in Endosurgery: Appendectomy. Courtesy of Ethicon, Inc., Somerville, NJ.)

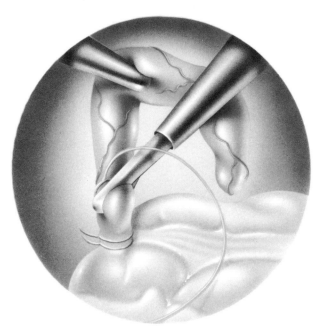

Figure 20–20. Laparoscopic appendectomy. Following placement of the ligatures, the surgeon dissects the appendix free with the hook scissors. (Reprinted from Techniques in Endosurgery: Appendectomy. Courtesy of Ethicon, Inc., Somerville, NJ.)

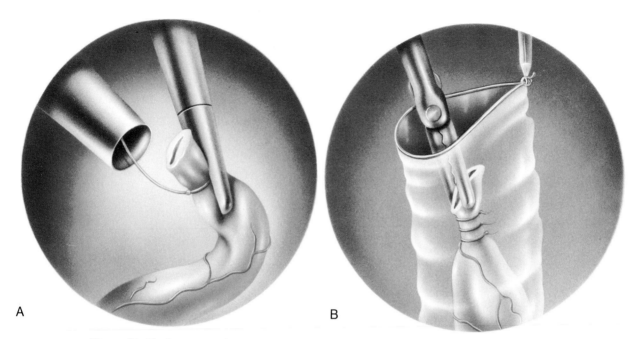

A

B

Figure 20–21. Laparoscopic appendectomy. *A.* The appendix is delivered through the 10/11 port. *B.* A special specimen pouch can be used to bring the appendix out of the wound. (Reprinted from Techniques in Endosurgery: Appendectomy. Courtesy of Ethicon, Inc., Somerville, NJ.)

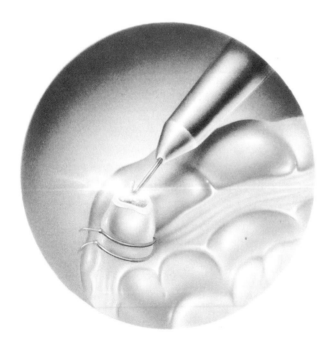

Figure 20–22. Laparoscopic appendectomy. The appendiceal stump is cauterized with electrosurgical probe with hook dissector. (Reprinted from Techniques in Endosurgery: Appendectomy. Courtesy of Ethicon, Inc., Somerville, NJ.)

8. Gallstones are removed.
9. The gallbladder is removed.

Description

The patient is placed in the supine position, and the entire abdomen is prepped and draped. In this procedure, four trocars are placed (Fig. 20–23): an umbilical 10/11-mm trocar, an additional 10/11-mm trocar at the midline, and two 5-mm trocars at the axillary line. This procedure may require the use of a 30-degree angled laparoscope to view the gallbladder, which lies high in the abdominal cavity. The laparoscope is inserted through the trocar. A straight locking grasper is inserted through one axillary trocar and used to apply upward traction on the gallbladder (Fig. 20–24). Some surgeons clip this grasper to the surgical drapes or patient's skin to free one of the assistant's hands.

The gallbladder, still retracted by the first grasper, is dissected from its surrounding tissue with an additional grasper (Fig. 20–25). When the cystic duct and artery have been identified, the surgeon may use the electrocautery hook to separate the tissues. The cystic artery is then ligated with a titanium clamp. An additional clip is placed over the cystic duct at the base of the gallbladder (Fig. 20–26).

In preparation for cholangiography, the surgeon makes a small incision in the cystic duct (Fig. 20–27). A cholangiogram or ureteral catheter is threaded into the duct through the incision (Fig. 20–28). The catheter may be held in place with a titanium clip or special cholangiography clamp. A 25% solution of radiopaque contrast medium is injected into the catheter, and radiographs are taken. If stones are located, the surgeon may extend the exploration by dilating the cystic duct with a balloon catheter. This is done by threading a guide wire through the cystic duct and into the common duct. The balloon catheter is then inserted over the guide wire and slowly inflated with saline solution. Once the cystic duct is dilated, a choledochoscope (fiberoptic telescope used to examine the common bile duct) is inserted over the guide wire and the duct is explored for additional gallstones. Stones can be removed through the scope's stone basket (Fig. 20–29A). The addition of the choledochoscope to the fiberoptic set requires that a second monitor be used to receive its images.

Stones can be collected in a retrieval bag (Fig. 20–29B) or removed with a grasper. A second cholangiogram may be taken at this time. If it is negative, the catheter is removed and the cystic duct occluded and divided. This may be done with titanium clips or with a suture ligature. The cystic artery is occluded and divided

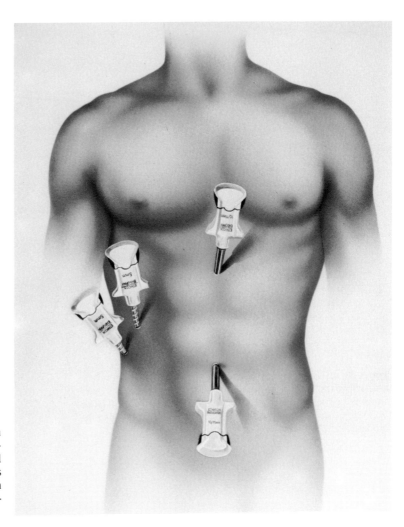

Figure 20–23. Laparoscopic cholecystectomy with operative cholangiography. Placement of four trocars. *A.* Umbilical 10/11-mm trocar. *B.* Additional 10/11-mm trocar at midline. *C.* Two 5-mm trocars at the axillary line. (Reprinted from Techniques in Endosurgery: Cholecystectomy. Courtesy of Ethicon, Inc., Somerville, NJ.)

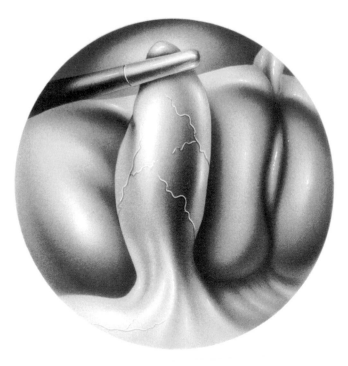

Figure 20–24. Laparoscopic cholecystectomy with operative cholangiography. A straight locking grasper is inserted through one axillary trocar and used to apply upward traction on the gallbladder. (Reprinted from Techniques in Endosurgery: Cholecystectomy. Courtesy of Ethicon, Inc., Somerville, NJ.)

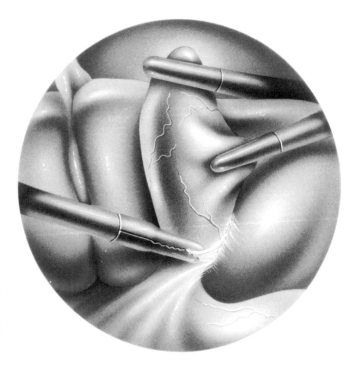

Figure 20–25. Laparoscopic cholecystectomy with operative cholangiography. The gallbladder is dissected from its surrounding tissue with an additional grasper. (Reprinted from Techniques in Endosurgery: Cholecystectomy. Courtesy of Ethicon, Inc., Somerville, NJ.)

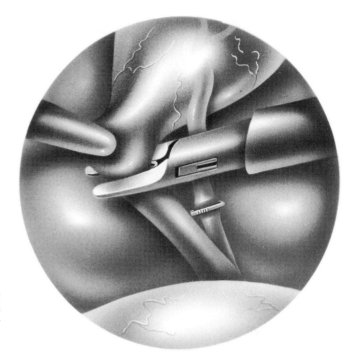

Figure 20–26. Laparoscopic cholecystectomy with operative cholangiography. The cystic artery is ligated with a titanium clip. An additional clip is placed over the cystic duct. (Reprinted from Techniques in Endosurgery: Cholecystectomy. Courtesy of Ethicon, Inc., Somerville, NJ.)

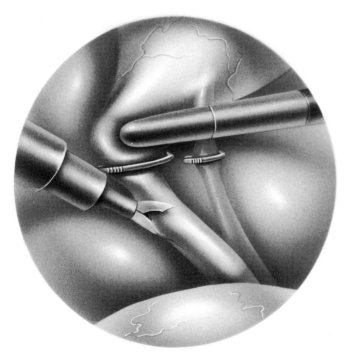

Figure 20–27. Laparoscopic cholecystectomy with operative cholangiography. In preparation for cholangiography, the surgeon makes a small incision in the cystic duct. (Reprinted from Techniques in Endosurgery: Cholecystectomy. Courtesy of Ethicon, Inc., Somerville, NJ.)

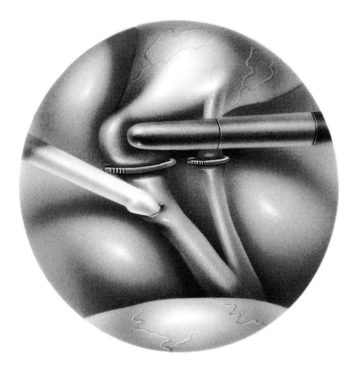

Figure 20–28. Laparoscopic cholecystectomy with operative cholangiography. A cholangiogram catheter is threaded into the cystic duct. If the duct is very small a ureteral catheter may be used instead. (Reprinted from Techniques in Endosurgery: Cholecystectomy. Courtesy of Ethicon, Inc., Somerville, NJ.)

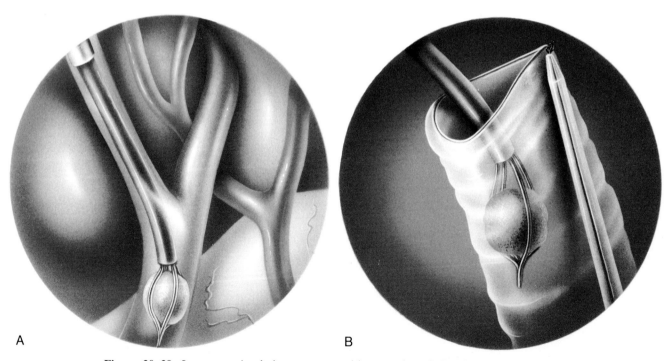

A   B

Figure 20–29. Laparoscopic cholecystectomy with operative cholangiography. *A.* After performing the cholangiography, small stones can be retrieved with a wire stone basket. *B.* Stone delivered through retrieval pouch. (Reprinted from Techniques in Endosurgery: Cholecystectomy. Courtesy of Ethicon, Inc., Somerville, NJ.)

with microscissors in the same manner. The gallbladder is then removed from the liver bed with the electrocautery hook (Fig. 20–30) and delivered from the wound in a retrieval bag, as shown in Figure 20–31.

Laparoscopic Hernia Repair

Definition

This is laparoscopic repair of a herniation (protrusion) of abdominal contents caused by a defect in the abdominal wall in the groin area of the male. A direct hernia results in a peritoneal bulge through the fascia layer. An indirect hernia is a genetic defect in the internal abdominal ring that causes the peritoneum to bulge along the spermatic cord. The regional anatomy is illustrated in Figure 20–32. In Figure 20–33 the exposed anatomy is shown as it is seen through the laparoscope. The procedure described here is an indirect hernia repair with polypropylene mesh.

Highlights

1. Pneumoperitoneum is established.
2. The trocars are placed.
3. The peritoneum is incised to expose the involved anatomy.
4. The hernia sac is removed from the cord structures.
5. Two layers of synthetic mesh are placed over the canal and secured.
6. The peritoneum is closed.

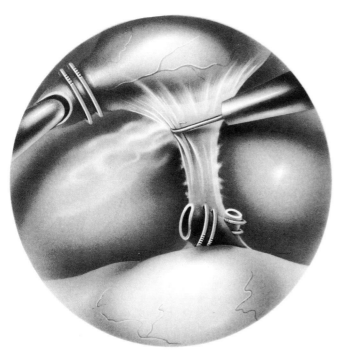

Figure 20–30. Laparoscopic cholecystectomy with operative cholangiography. The gallbladder is freed from the liver bed with the electrocautery probe with hook dissector. (Reprinted from Techniques in Endosurgery: Cholecystectomy. Courtesy of Ethicon, Inc., Somerville, NJ.)

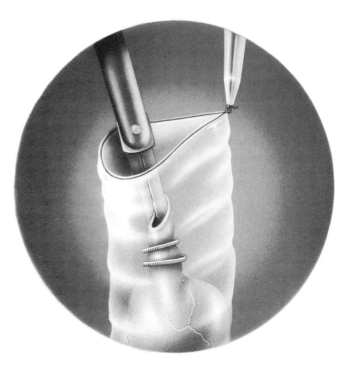

Figure 20–31. Laparoscopic cholecystectomy with operative cholangiography. The gallbladder is removed through a specimen retrieval bag. (Reprinted from Techniques in Endosurgery: Cholecystectomy. Courtesy of Ethicon, Inc., Somerville, NJ.)

Description

The patient is prepped and draped for a lower abdominal incision. This procedure requires three trocars, as shown in Figure 20–34. The size of these trocars depends on the surgeon's choice. Once the trocars are in place, the patient is tipped into Trendelenburg position to shift the abdominal viscera. This allows the surgeon to identify important anatomic landmarks—the vas deferens, external artery and vein, spermatic vessel, inferior epigastric artery and vein, and lateral umbilical ligament. The peritoneum is dissected using the laser, as shown in Figure 20–35. Once the peritoneum and fat have been pulled away from the muscle wall, the hernia sac is dissected from the spermatic cord structures (Fig. 20–36). A patch graft of polypropylene mesh is then placed into the canal (Fig. 20–37A). A second sheet of mesh is placed over the inguinal area and secured with surgical staples (Fig. 20–37B). The peritoneal closure using the Endopath EAS Endoscopic Articulating Stapler (Ethicon, Inc., Somerville, NJ) is shown in Figure 20–38. This instrument is also used to secure the mesh graft. The trocars are withdrawn, the pneumoperitoneum is released, and the wounds are closed in routine fashion.

Single-Puncture Pelviscopy

Single-puncture pelviscopy is laparoscopy performed for procedures of the female pelvic cavity. This approach

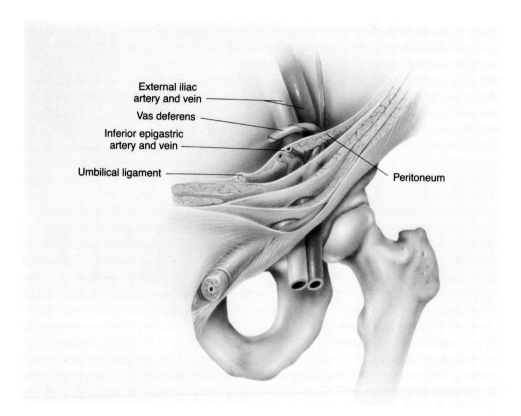

External iliac artery and vein

Vas deferens

Inferior epigastric artery and vein

Umbilical ligament

Peritoneum

Figure 20–32. Laparoscopic inguinal hernia repair. Regional anatomy of the groin area in the male. Note close proximity of the vas deferens to the inferior epigastric artery and vein. (Reprinted from Techniques in Endosurgery: Hernia Repair. Courtesy of Ethicon, Inc., Somerville, NJ.)

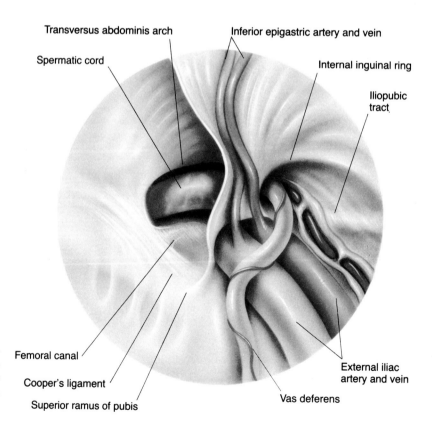

Transversus abdominis arch

Spermatic cord

Inferior epigastric artery and vein

Internal inguinal ring

Iliopubic tract

Femoral canal

Cooper's ligament

Superior ramus of pubis

Vas deferens

External iliac artery and vein

Figure 20–33. Laparoscopic inguinal hernia repair. Anatomy as viewed through the laparoscope. (Reprinted from Techniques in Endosurgery: Hernia Repair. Courtesy of Ethicon, Inc., Somerville, NJ.)

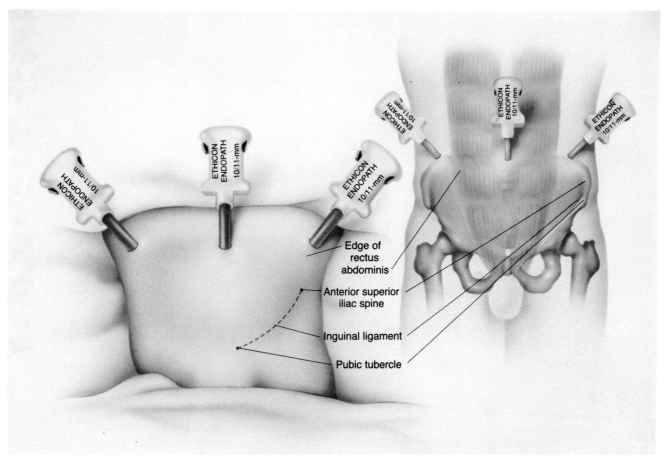

Figure 20–34. Laparoscopic inguinal hernia repair. Placement of trocars. (Reprinted from Techniques in Endosurgery: Hernia Repair. Courtesy of Ethicon, Inc., Somerville, NJ.)

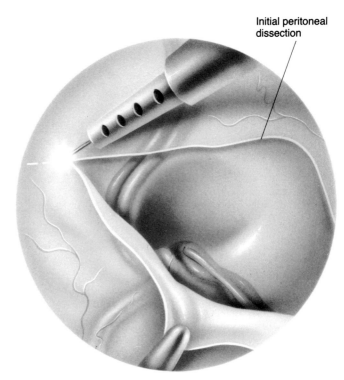

Figure 20–35. Laparoscopic inguinal hernia repair. Using the laser, the surgeon incises the peritoneum. (Reprinted from Techniques in Endosurgery: Hernia Repair. Courtesy of Ethicon, Inc., Somerville, NJ.)

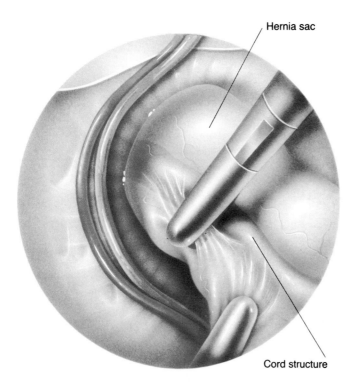

Hernia sac

Cord structure

Figure 20–36. Laparoscopic inguinal hernia repair. Once the peritoneum and fat have been pulled away from the muscle wall, the hernia sac is dissected from the spermatic cord structures. (Reprinted from Techniques in Endosurgery: Hernia Repair. Courtesy of Ethicon, Inc., Somerville, NJ.)

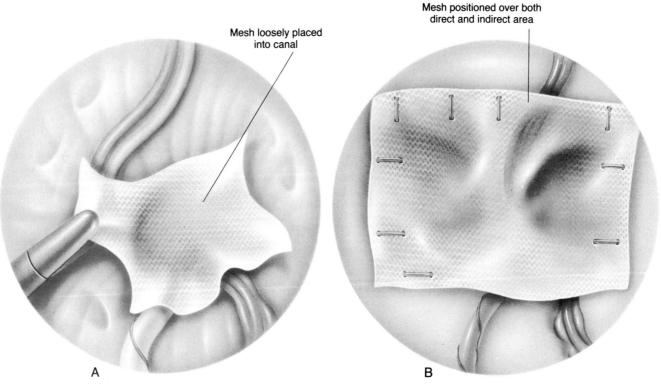

Mesh loosely placed into canal

Mesh positioned over both direct and indirect area

A

B

Figure 20–37. Laparoscopic inguinal hernia repair. *A.* A patch graft of polypropylene mesh is gently pushed into the inguinal canal. *B.* A second patch graft is placed over the first and secured with surgical staples. (Reprinted from Techniques in Endosurgery: Hernia Repair. Courtesy of Ethicon, Inc., Somerville, NJ.)

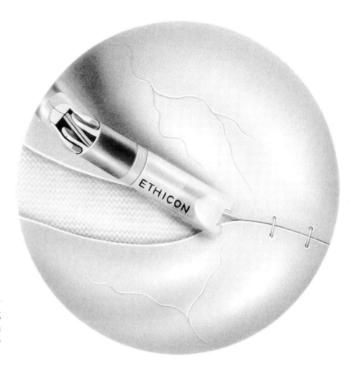

Figure 20–38. Laparoscopic inguinal hernia repair. The peritoneum is closed with surgical staples, and the remaining layers are closed individually. (Reprinted from Techniques in Endosurgery: Hernia Repair. Courtesy of Ethicon, Inc., Somerville, NJ.)

is almost identical to two-handed procedures, except that only one puncture site is made. The special laparoscope used for this procedure allows passage of both the fiberoptic telescope and the instruments used during the procedure. The single puncture is made transumbilically and has several advantages over multiple puncture procedures. These advantages include the following:

1. Complications associated with multiple puncture procedures such as hemorrhage, puncture of pelvic structures, wound infection, and hernia are avoided.

2. Recuperation is faster than with multiple puncture procedures.

3. The procedure can be performed with the use of local anesthesia.

Bibliography

Cooperman AM, Katz V, Zimmon D, Botero G: Laparoscopic colon resection: A case report. J Laparoendoscop Surg 1(4):221–224, 1991.

Fowler DL, White SA: Laparoscopy-assisted sigmoid resection. Surg Laparosc Endosc 1(3):183–188, 1991.

Jacobs M, Merdeja JC, Goldstein HS: Minimally invasive colon resection (laparoscopic colectomy). Surg Laparosc Endosc 1(3):144–150, 1991.

Lange V, Meyer G, Schardey MH, Schildberg FW: Laparascopic creation of a loop colostomy. J Laparoendoscop Surg 1(5):307–312, 1991.

Sackier JM: Future horizons of minimal access surgery. Probl Gen Surg 8(3):507–512, 1991.

Welenski M et al: The single puncture approach for advanced pelviscopy surgery. Todays OR Nurse 13:1, 1991.

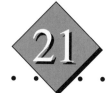

Obstetric and Gynecologic Surgery

Obstetric and gynecologic surgery involves the female reproductive structures, including the uterus, ovaries, fallopian tubes, vagina, and vulva. The procedures are categorized as abdominal or vaginal, with the position of the operating team members differing for the two types. Instrumentation is the same as that used in general surgery, with the addition of some specialized instruments.

SURGICAL ANATOMY

Internal Organs of Reproduction

Uterus

The uterus (Fig. 21–1) is a pear-shaped organ that lies in the anterior portion of the female pelvic cavity. This organ is approximately 3 inches long and 2 inches deep. It is composed of thick muscular tissue and is suspended in the pelvic cavity by a series of ligaments that form an envelope around it. On both sides of the uterus lie the fallopian tubes, which communicate directly with the interior of the uterus. The body or *corpus* of the uterus is the central landmark of the organ, and the upper portion is called the *fundus*. The *cervix* is the lowest portion and communicates directly with the vagina, which is the external passageway of the organ. The uterine body in normal position tilts forward, toward the front of the pelvis, although this position varies in some women. The various positions of the uterine body are illustrated in Figure 21–2.

Uterine Ligaments

The ligaments that surround the uterus (Fig. 21–3) are suspended from the pelvic cavity. These ligaments are called the *broad ligaments*. Above the broad ligaments, near the fallopian tubes, lie the *round ligaments*; these help suspend the uterus anteriorly. The *cardinal ligaments* lie below the broad ligaments and are the main supports for the uterus. The *uterosacral ligaments* curve along the bottom of the uterus to suspend the cervix and uterine body to the sacrum.

All the uterine ligaments appear as almost continuous sheets of strong elastic tissue and must be clamped and severed whenever the uterus is surgically removed. Within these sheets lie the blood vessels that supply the uterus.

Ovaries

Two ovaries, the organs of female reproduction and those responsible for the production of female hormones, lie on each side of the uterus in the upper portion of the pelvic cavity. The ovaries are suspended by the *mesovarium*—peritoneal tissue attached to the uterus by ovarian ligaments. Each ovary is approximately 1½ inches long and is oval. The ovary contains many follicles in which lie ova of various stages of development.

Fallopian Tubes

Two fallopian tubes, one for each ovary, extend from the body of the uterus toward the ovary and convey the

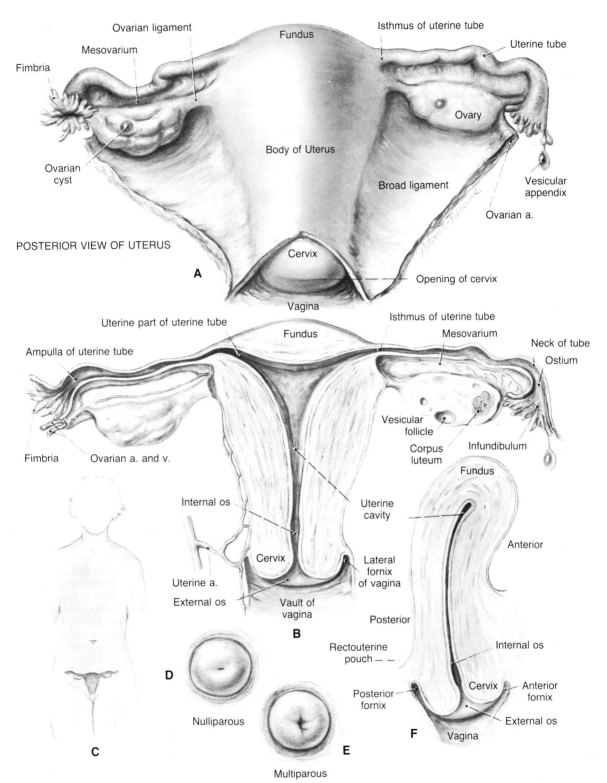

Figure 21–1. Female reproductive organs. *A.* Posterior view of uterus. *B.* Uterus cut away to show internal structure. *C.* Anatomic position. *D* and *E.* Cervix before and after childbirth. *F.* Side view cut away. (From Jacob S, Francone C, Lossow WJ: Structure and Function in Man, 5th ed. Philadelphia, WB Saunders, 1982.)

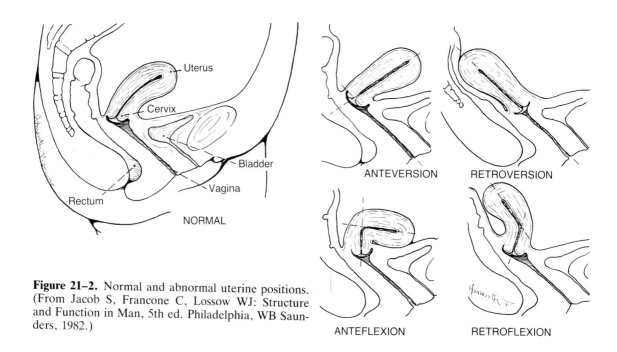

Figure 21–2. Normal and abnormal uterine positions. (From Jacob S, Francone C, Lossow WJ: Structure and Function in Man, 5th ed. Philadelphia, WB Saunders, 1982.)

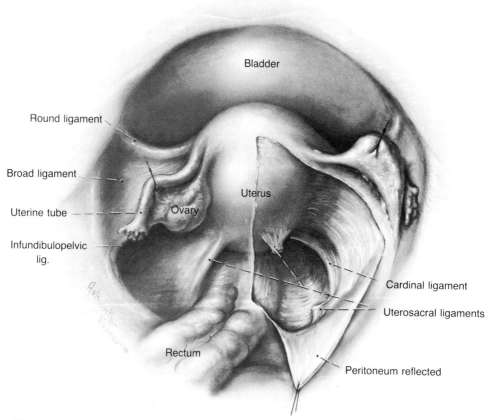

Figure 21–3. The uterus and ligaments as viewed from above. The peritoneum has been reflected back to show the cardinal ligament. (From Jacob S, Francone C, Lossow WJ: Structure and Function in Man, 5th ed. Philadelphia, WB Saunders, 1982.)

mature ovum to the uterus for fertilization. Each tube is about 4 inches long and ½ inch wide. The tube is suspended by a portion of the broad ligament of the uterus called the *mesosalpinx*. That portion of the tube that communicates with the uterus is called the *isthmus*. The central portion of the tube, which curves around the ovary, is the *ampulla*. The *infundibulum* is the funnel-shaped end portion that receives the ovum from the ovary. Small multiple projections called *fimbriae* vibrate slowly and help capture the egg at the infundibulum. The egg is then transported along the inner passageway of the tube by peristalsis and with the aid of cilia, which line the inner surface of each fallopian tube.

External Genitalia and Associated Structures

The external genital structures of the female (Fig. 21–4) are collectively called the *vulva*. These structures include the mons pubis, labia majora, labia minora, clitoris, vestibular glands, and hymen.

Mons Pubis

The mons pubis is an elevated portion of fatty tissue that lies directly over the symphysis pubis, the pubic bone. This protective area is covered by hair and lies in close proximity to the labia majora.

Labia Majora

The labia majora are bisectional folds of adipose tissue that extend from the mons pubis toward the anterior portion of the vulva. They encircle the vestibule of the external genitalia.

Labia Minora

The labia minora are also bisectional and lie directly beneath the labia majora. These folds of tissue are delicate and are attached anteriorly by the frenulum. Anteriorly, they meet just in front of the clitoris and form the prepuce (hood) of that structure.

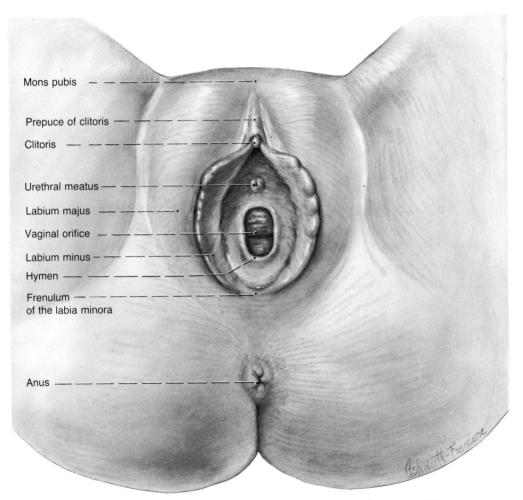

Figure 21–4. Female external genitalia. (From Jacob S, Francone C, Lossow WJ: Structure and Function in Man, 5th ed. Philadelphia, WB Saunders, 1982.)

Clitoris

The clitoris is a highly vascular and sensitive organ that lies at the anterior end of the labia minora. This organ is protected by the folds of the labia and is homologous to the penis in the male.

Vestibular Glands

The vestibular glands, so called because they lie within the vestibule of the external genitalia, include Skene's glands (paraurethral glands) and Bartholin's glands. Skene's glands are two small paired glands that lie beneath the floor of the urethra. These glands are the rudimentary homologue of the prostate gland in the male. Bartholin's glands lie on both sides of the vestibule and secrete mucus during coitus. These glands are homologous to the bulbourethral glands in the male.

Hymen

The hymen is a thin vascular fold of tissue that attaches around the entrance of the vagina. In the young female, the membrane is usually but not always intact, and its orifice may vary from pinpoint size to several centimeters. The membrane is generally broken during coitus and then remains as a notched tissue, which may be further reduced during childbearing.

INDICATIONS FOR OBSTETRIC AND GYNECOLOGIC SURGERY

To have a more complete understanding of gynecologic and obstetric surgery, the technologist should become familiar with terms and complications that are frequently encountered in the patient's history and physical report.

Obstetric Complications

Before birth, the fetus may abort because of disease or injury to the mother or fetus. Most abortions require that the patient have a dilatation and curettage. A *missed abortion* is a condition in which the product of conception (fetus) is nonliving and is retained in the uterus for over 2 months. An *incomplete abortion* is one in which only part of the products of conception have aborted. An *imminent abortion* is one in which the patient is about to abort. This may be indicated by uterine bleeding.

Just before or during childbirth, the patient and fetus may suffer from complications that require an emergency cesarean section. *Dystocia* is a term associated with painful and difficult labor. During *placenta previa*, the placenta is abnormally implanted in the lower uterine segment and may completely cover the os cervix. In *abruptio placentae*, the placenta is prematurely separated from the wall of the uterus. If the mother's pelvis is too small to accommodate the head of the fetus, the complication is termed *cephalopelvic disproportion*. The

manner in which the fetus is presented (positioned in relation to the cervix) may also necessitate emergency surgery. In a *breech* presentation, the buttocks are presented; in a *transverse* presentation, the fetus is presented crosswise; in a *footling*, the feet are presented; and in a *vertex*, the upper back of the head is presented. If the fetal heart tones diminish or are completely absent, cesarean section may be performed immediately. The absence of fetal heart tones often indicates that the umbilical cord has twisted on itself or is otherwise obstructed, thus preventing blood flow to the fetus.

Gynecologic Complications

Functional or metabolic complications may be indications for surgery. In *metrorrhagia*, the patient suffers from active uterine bleeding at times other than during menstruation. *Amenorrhea* indicates the absence of menstruation. This condition may be caused by disease or physiologic imbalance but can also be caused by emotional upset. Painful or difficult menstruation is termed *dysmenorrhea*. *Menometrorrhagia* is excessive bleeding that occurs both during menstruation and at irregular intervals. *Menorrhagia* is excessive bleeding during menstruation. The surgeon may perform a dilatation and curettage to determine the causes of the above conditions.

ABDOMINAL PROCEDURES

During abdominal procedures, the right-handed surgeon stands at the patient's left side. This provides the best access to the pelvis. The technologist should stand to the patient's right, unless otherwise directed.

Abdominal Hysterectomy

Definition

This is surgical removal of the uterus through an abdominal incision. Hysterectomy is performed for a variety of diseases. The most common indications are benign fibromas (leiomyomas), endometriosis, and cancer.

Highlights

1. The abdomen is entered.
2. The uterus is partially mobilized.
3. The bladder is separated from the uterus.
4. The uterus is removed.
5. The bladder is reattached.
6. The wound is closed.

Description

The patient is placed in the supine position. After a routine abdominal and vaginal prep, a Foley catheter is inserted for continuous urinary drainage. Even though

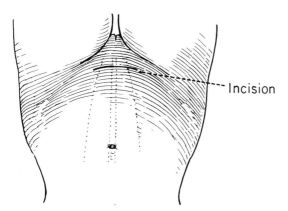

Figure 21–5. Abdominal hysterectomy. The Pfannenstiel incision. (From Parsons L, Ulfelder H: Atlas of Pelvic Operations, 2nd ed. Philadelphia, WB Saunders, 1968.)

a lower midline incision can be used for a hysterectomy, the *Pfannenstiel* ("bikini") incision will be discussed here because many gynecologic procedures, including the abdominal hysterectomy, are performed through this incision. The location of the incision is illustrated in Figure 21–5. After incising the skin, the surgeon deepens the incision through the subcutaneous tissue with the deep knife or cautery pencil. The next layer, the fascia, is nicked with the knife and incised with curved Mayo scissors (Fig. 21–6). The surgeon then grasps one edge of the fascial margin with two or more Kocher clamps. Using blunt dissection, the surgeon separates the fascia from the underlying muscle.

This procedure is repeated on the lower fascial margin (Fig. 21–7). The surgeon divides the muscle layer manually. The peritoneum is then nicked with the knife, and the incision is lengthened with Metzenbaum scissors. A self-retaining O'Sullivan-O'Connor or Balfour retractor is placed in the wound. The surgeon packs the bowel away from the uterus with moist lap sponges. The technologist must have stick sponges available throughout the procedure. These may be placed on the field while the surgeon packs the bowel.

During the first portion of the procedure, the surgeon isolates the uterus by severing it from the uterine liga-

ments and adnexa (ovaries and fallopian tubes). Beginning with the round ligaments, the surgeon double-clamps sections of ligament, divides the tissue between the clamps, and ligates the sections with suture ligatures. This process is repeated many times until the surgeon has gone deep into the pelvis, dividing sections of ligament on each side of the uterus. Various types of clamps are used to grasp the ligaments. Most surgeons have a preference for a particular set of clamps, which should appear on the surgeon's preference card. Most commonly used are Heaney, Ochsner, Kocher, and O'Hanlon clamps. The technologist should have at least 10 such clamps of the surgeon's choice available on the Mayo stand.

Absorbable suture is almost always used to ligate the ligaments. If chromic catgut is used, the technologist should allow enough time during the set-up to prepare it, since at least 24 strands will be needed to complete the mobilization of the uterus. The suture is mounted on heavy, tapered Mayo needles or similar needles. To divide the ligaments, the surgeon uses curved Mayo scissors or a scalpel. If the patient is very large, long instruments should be available.

As described earlier, the surgeon mobilizes the uterus to the level of the bladder. At this level the bladder is continuous with the uterus, both organs being attached by a peritoneal covering. Using Metzenbaum scissors and long tissue forceps, the surgeon separates the two structures by dissecting the peritoneal covering away from the bladder (Fig. 21–8). This is called the *bladder flap* and will be reattached (reperitonealized) later. Once the bladder has been separated from the uterus, mobilization is continued, as previously described.

At the level of the cervix, long Allis or Kocher clamps are placed around the edge of the cervix, and it is divided from the vagina. The surgeon uses long scissors (such as Mayo scissors) or the long knife to divide the tissue. This maneuver completely frees the uterus, which is passed to the technologist as a specimen. All instruments that have come in contact with the cervix or vagina must be treated as contaminated and discarded into a basin that can be passed off to the circulator.

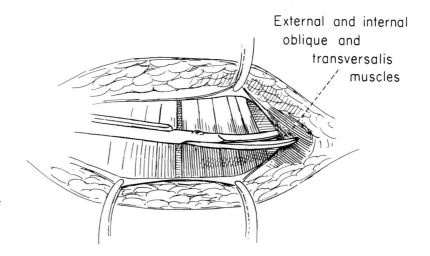

Figure 21–6. Abdominal hysterectomy. Separation of fascia from muscle with heavy curved scissors. (From Parsons L, Ulfelder H: Atlas of Pelvic Operations, 2nd ed. Philadelphia, WB Saunders, 1968.)

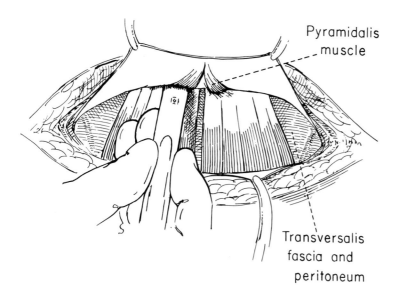

Pyramidalis muscle

Transversalis fascia and peritoneum

Figure 21–7. Abdominal hysterectomy. The fascia is incised with heavy curved scissors. (From Parsons L, Ulfelder H: Atlas of Pelvic Operations, 2nd ed. Philadelphia, WB Saunders, 1968.)

To close the wound, the surgeon begins by suturing the vagina (vaginal vault) where it has been separated from the cervix (Fig. 21–9). Absorbable suture of the same type as that used on the uterine ligaments is commonly used to close the vaginal vault. After closure of the vagina, the bladder flap must be reperitonealized. This is done with chromic catgut or Dexon swaged to a fine needle. Size 2-0 or 3-0 suture is commonly used (Fig. 21–10).

To close the abdomen, the surgeon grasps the edges of the peritoneum with several Mayo clamps. The peritoneum is closed with a running suture of 0 chromic catgut or Dexon swaged to a taper needle. The muscle tissue may be loosely approximated with three or four sutures of 4-0 chromic catgut. The fascia is closed with a wide variety of sutures, absorbable or nonabsorbable. Size 0 or 2-0 suture is most commonly used. The subcutaneous tissue is usually approximated with plain catgut or Dexon suture, size 3-0, mounted on tapered

needles. The skin is closed using the surgeon's suture preference.

Salpingo-oophorectomy

Definition

This is removal of one or both of the fallopian tubes and ovaries. The procedure may be performed in con-

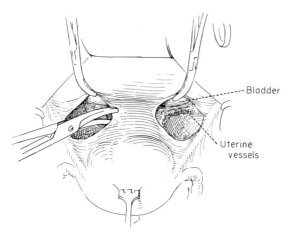

Bladder

Uterine vessels

Figure 21–8. Abdominal hysterectomy. Separation of the bladder from the uterus. (From Parsons L, Ulfelder H: Atlas of Pelvic Operations, 2nd ed. Philadelphia, WB Saunders, 1968.)

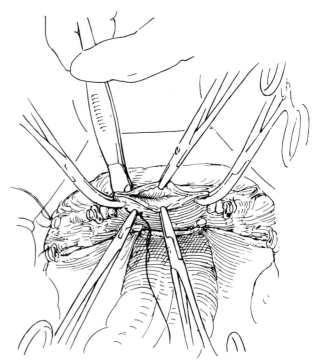

Figure 21–9. Abdominal hysterectomy. Closure of the vaginal vault after the uterus has been removed. (From Parsons L, Ulfelder H: Atlas of Pelvic Operations, 2nd ed. Philadelphia, WB Saunders, 1968.)

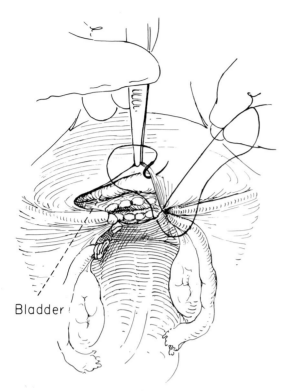

Figure 21–10. Abdominal hysterectomy. Reperitonealization of the bladder flap. (From Parsons L, Ulfelder H: Atlas of Pelvic Operations, 2nd ed. Philadelphia, WB Saunders, 1968.)

junction with a hysterectomy or as a separate procedure to treat conditions such as endometriosis or an abscess of the tube and ovary.

Highlights

1. The abdomen is entered.
2. The uterus is retracted.
3. The ovarian vessels are ligated.
4. The ovary and tube are mobilized.
5. The ovary and tube are removed.
6. The raw surface is reperitonealized.
7. The wound is closed.

Description

The patient is placed in the supine position and prepped and draped for an abdominal incision.

The abdomen is entered through a lower paramedian, median, or Pfannenstiel incision, depending on the size of the patient and the known condition of the tubes and ovaries. (If both tubes and ovaries are to be removed, a lower midline incision is used.)

The surgeon first examines the tubes and ovaries to determine the nature of the disease. The assistant retracts the uterus (unless it has been previously removed) with a tenaculum or uterine elevator. To begin the procedure, the surgeon grasps the tube with one or two Babcock clamps. Two Mayo or uterine clamps are then placed across the ovarian vessels. The tissue is divided between the clamps with the knife or dissecting scissors.

A suture ligature of chromic catgut or Dexon, size 0, is then used to ligate the ovarian vessel (Fig. 21–11).

This procedure is repeated along the edge of the ovarian and uterine ligaments until the tube and ovary are attached only by the uterus itself. Two uterine clamps are then placed across the fallopian tube where it emerges from the uterus. The tube is severed between the clamps and a suture ligature is placed over the tubal stump.

The raw surfaces on the uterine ligaments left by the dissection are reperitonealized with a running suture of size 0 or 2-0 chromic catgut swaged to a tapered needle (Fig. 21–12). The wound is then closed in routine fashion.

Salpingectomy for Ruptured Ectopic Pregnancy

Definition

This is removal of a ruptured fallopian tube and ectopic fetus. An ectopic pregnancy occurs when the fetus lodges in an area other than the uterine cavity. If the fetus lodges in the fallopian tube, it soon becomes too large for the tube and causes it to rupture.

Highlights

1. The abdomen is entered.
2. Large blood clots are evacuated.
3. The fallopian tube is mobilized and removed.
4. The wound is closed.

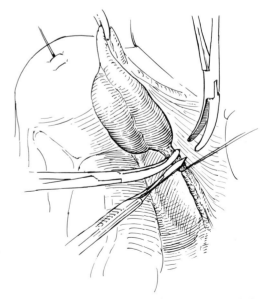

Figure 21–11. Salpingo-oophorectomy. Ligation of the ovarian vessels. (From Parsons L, Ulfelder H: Atlas of Pelvic Operations, 2nd ed. Philadelphia, WB Saunders, 1968.)

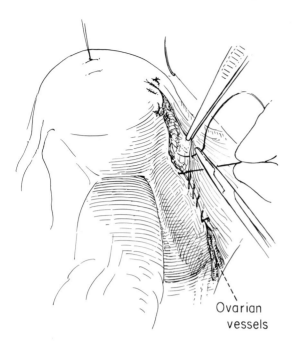

Ovarian
vessels

Figure 21–12. Salpingo-oophorectomy. Closure of the raw surface on the uterine ligaments. (From Parsons L, Ulfelder H: Atlas of Pelvic Operations, 2nd ed. Philadelphia, WB Saunders, 1968.)

Description

This procedure is similar to the salpingo-oophorectomy previously described. It differs primarily in that a ruptured ectopic pregnancy often necessitates emergency surgery. If bleeding vessels are not occluded quickly, the patient may die of loss of blood.

The patient is placed in the supine position, prepped, and draped, for a lower midline incision. Suction must be immediately available as soon as the abdomen is entered. If there is significant hemorrhage, the technologist should detach the suction tip from the suction tubing. This creates a larger opening so that clots can be evacuated quickly. A large basin should also be available to receive blood clots. The bleeding vessels are clamped immediately.

To begin the procedure, the surgeon places two Mayo or Kelly clamps across the tissue that lies between the ovary and fallopian tube (Fig. 21–13). This tissue is divided and a suture ligature of chromic catgut or Dexon, size 0, on a tapered needle is placed through the tissue (Fig. 21–14). Mobilization continues in the same manner up to the uterine border. A final suture ligature is placed across the tube where it joins the uterus (Fig. 21–15). The tube is then divided from the uterus with the knife or scissors and passed to the technologist as a specimen (Fig. 21–16).

The raw surfaces of tissue are sewn together with interrupted sutures of size 0 or 2-0 chromic catgut, as shown in Figure 21–17. The wound is irrigated with warm saline solution to remove any remaining blood clots and is closed in routine fashion.

Tubal Ligation: Pomeroy and Irving Techniques

Definition

This is ligation of the fallopian tubes for elective sterilization. The Irving technique ensures that the two severed ends of the tube will not rejoin. The Pomeroy

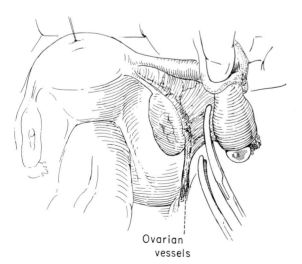

Ovarian
vessels

Figure 21–13. Ectopic pregnancy. Clamps placed between ovary and fallopian tube. (From Parsons L, Ulfelder H: Atlas of Pelvic Operations, 2nd ed. Philadelphia, WB Saunders, 1968.)

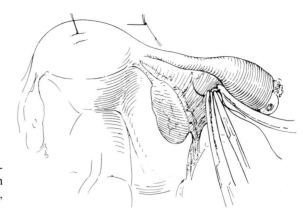

Figure 21–14. Salpingectomy. The tissue between the ovary and fallopian tube has been divided and is ligated with a suture ligature. (From Parsons L, Ulfelder H: Atlas of Pelvic Operations, 2nd ed. Philadelphia, WB Saunders, 1968.)

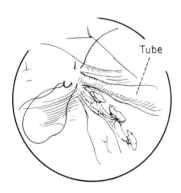

Figure 21–15. Salpingectomy. Final suture ligature through the fallopian tube where it joins the uterus. (From Parsons L, Ulfelder H: Atlas of Pelvic Operations, 2nd ed. Philadelphia, WB Saunders, 1968.)

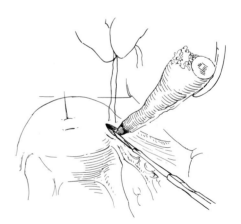

Figure 21–16. Salpingectomy. Division of the fallopian tube from the uterus. (From Parsons L, Ulfelder H: Atlas of Pelvic Operations, 2nd ed. Philadelphia, WB Saunders, 1968.)

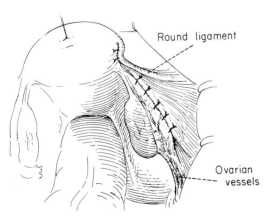

Figure 21–17. Salpingectomy. The raw surface on the uterine ligaments is closed with interrupted sutures. (From Parsons L, Ulfelder H: Atlas of Pelvic Operations, 2nd ed. Philadelphia, WB Saunders, 1968.)

method is faster but carries the risk that the ends of the tube may recommunicate at a later date. Tubal ligation is often performed on the postpartum patient a few hours after delivery.

Highlights

Pomeroy Technique

1. The abdomen is entered.
2. The fallopian tube is grasped and ligated.
3. The wound is closed.

Irving Technique

1. The abdomen is entered.
2. The fallopian tube is clamped, ligated, and divided.
3. The proximal end of the tube is buried in the serosa of the uterus.
4. The wound is closed.

Description

The surgeon enters the abdomen through a short lower midline or Pfannenstiel incision. The assistant retracts the abdominal wall with a medium Richardson retractor. Using a Babcock clamp, the surgeon grasps the fallopian tube and brings it into the wound site. The full length of the tube is examined to be certain that the round ligament has not been grasped unintentionally. (Their appearances are similar at the proximal end.)

Pomeroy Technique

The surgeon places a single tie of size 0 or 2-0 chromic catgut or Dexon around the looped tube while the assistant retracts it (Fig. 21–18). The loop is then severed and passed to the technologist as a specimen. The technologist must keep the right and left specimens separate, because they must be identified by the side from which they came. The severed tube is replaced in

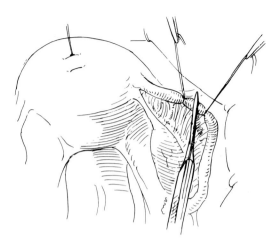

Figure 21–19. Irving technique of tubal ligation. The tube is ligated in two places and a section between the ligatures removed. (From Parsons L, Ulfelder H: Atlas of Pelvic Operations, 2nd ed. Philadelphia, WB Saunders, 1968.)

the abdominal cavity. The opposite tube is ligated and severed in the same way.

Irving Technique

The assistant elevates the tube with a Babcock clamp while the surgeon ligates it in two places using size 0 or 2-0 chromic catgut. The suture ends on the proximal side are left long. The surgeon then removes a section of tube between the ties (Fig. 21–19). A small incision is made in the serosal layer of the uterus with the knife (Fig. 21–20). A fine taper needle is threaded with the long proximal suture end. The surgeon then grasps the cut end of the tube with plain tissue forceps, places it inside the pocket made in the uterus, and secures it with one or two sutures (Fig. 21–21). The other end of the tube may be sewn within the broad ligament of the uterus (Fig. 21–22). The same procedure is performed on the opposite tube (Fig. 21–23). The wound is closed in routine fashion.

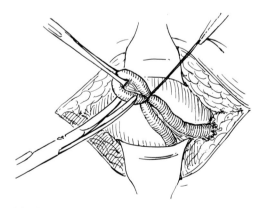

Figure 21–18. Pomeroy technique of tubal ligation. A loop of fallopian tube is ligated and removed. (From Parsons L, Ulfelder H: Atlas of Pelvic Operations, 2nd ed. Philadelphia, WB Saunders, 1968.)

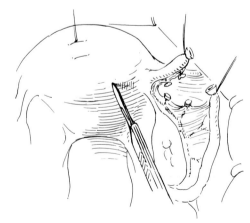

Figure 21–20. Tubal ligation. A small incision is made in the uterine serosa. (From Parsons L, Ulfelder H: Atlas of Pelvic Operations, 2nd ed. Philadelphia, WB Saunders, 1968.)

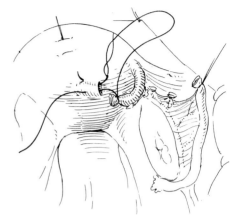

Figure 21–21. Tubal ligation. The severed end of the fallopian tube is sutured into the pocket in the serosa. (From Parsons L, Ulfelder H: Atlas of Pelvic Operations, 2nd ed. Philadelphia, WB Saunders, 1968.)

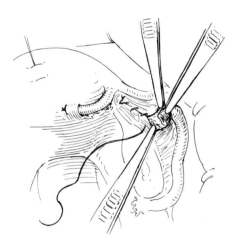

Figure 21–22. Tubal ligation. The distal end of the severed fallopian tube is buried within the broad ligament. (From Parsons L, Ulfelder H: Atlas of Pelvic Operations, 2nd ed. Philadelphia, WB Saunders, 1968.)

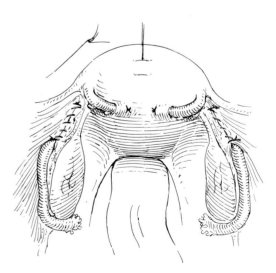

Figure 21–23. Tubal ligation. The procedure is repeated on the opposite tube. (From Parsons L, Ulfelder H: Atlas of Pelvic Operations, 2nd ed. Philadelphia, WB Saunders, 1968.)

Excision of Ovarian Cyst

Definition

This is removal of a cyst from the surface of the ovary. Ovarian cysts (Fig. 21–24) are usually benign but are removed when they cause pain, amenorrhea, or abnormal uterine bleeding. If a large cyst ruptures in the abdomen, serious bleeding could result. The so-called chocolate cyst is caused by endometriosis and is named for the thick brown fluid it contains. This fluid is actually an accumulation of old blood from cystic bleeding of the lining of the endometrioid tissue.

Highlights

1. The abdomen is entered.
2. The cyst is incised at its base and removed.
3. The ovary is oversewn.
4. The abdomen is closed.

Description

The patient is placed in the supine position and prepped and draped for an abdominal incision.

The surgeon enters the abdomen through a lower midline, paramedian, or Pfannenstiel incision. The fallopian tube is grasped with a Babcock clamp. The assistant then elevates the ovary. If the cyst can be "shelled out," as a nut from its shell, the surgeon makes a small incision at its base (Fig. 21–25).

Using blunt dissection, the surgeon separates the cyst from the ovary (Fig. 21–26). If the cyst is firmly attached to the ovary the surgeon may place two Kelly or Mayo clamps across the base of the cyst, incise between the clamps, and ligate the base with chromic catgut or Dexon. Once the cyst is removed, the surgeon oversews the ovary in the area where the cyst adhered to it. Chromic catgut, size 3-0, swaged to a fine needle is used to suture the ovary (Fig. 21–27). The reconstructed ovary is shown in Figure 21–28. The wound is closed in routine fashion.

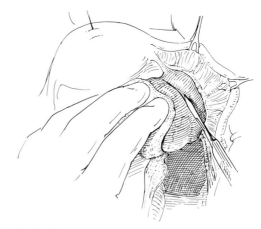

Figure 21–25. Removal of ovarian cyst. The surgeon makes a small incision at the base of the cyst. (From Parsons L, Ulfelder H: Atlas of Pelvic Operations, 2nd ed. Philadelphia, WB Saunders, 1968.)

Cesarean Section

Definition

This is the surgical delivery of an infant through the abdominal and uterine wall. Among other reasons, this procedure is commonly performed in the event of previous cesarean section, abruptio placentae, placenta previa, or cephalopelvis disproportion. The procedure is often performed as an emergency.

Highlights

1. The pelvis and uterus are entered.
2. The head of the infant is delivered and the infant's airways are cleared.
3. The infant's body is delivered.
4. The placenta is removed.
5. The uterus is closed.
6. The abdomen is closed.

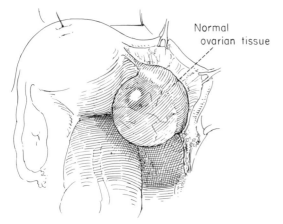

Figure 21–24. Ovarian cyst. (From Parsons L, Ulfelder H: Atlas of Pelvic Operations, 2nd ed. Philadelphia, WB Saunders, 1968.)

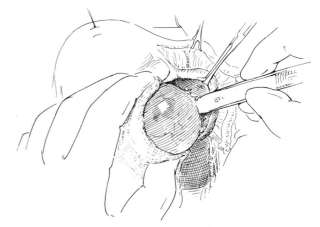

Figure 21–26. Removal of ovarian cyst. The surgeon separates the cyst from the ovary using blunt dissection. (From Parsons L, Ulfelder H: Atlas of Pelvic Operations, 2nd ed. Philadelphia, WB Saunders, 1968.)

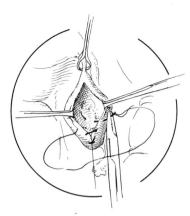

Figure 21–27. Removal of ovarian cyst. The raw surface on the ovary is oversewn. (From Parsons L, Ulfelder H: Atlas of Pelvic Operations, 2nd ed. Philadelphia, WB Saunders, 1968.)

Description

In preparation for cesarean section, a warmed mobile crib equipped with suction and infant resuscitative equipment is brought into the surgery suite. A second team consisting of a nurse and pediatrician is available to care for the infant immediately after delivery.

The patient is placed in the supine position. In the event of extreme emergency, a general anesthetic may be employed. In this case the skin prep and draping take place *before* induction so that the infant will receive as little anesthetic as possible across the placental barrier. If the procedure is not an emergency, a spinal anesthetic is commonly used.

The surgeon enters the abdomen through a lower midline or Pfannenstiel incision. The tissues of the abdomen are divided in standard fashion. The peritoneal covering of the bladder is incised as for a hysterectomy; this exposes the distended uterus. As soon as the uterus is exposed, the technologist must be ready with dry lap sponges, a bulb syringe, and suction. The suction tip is

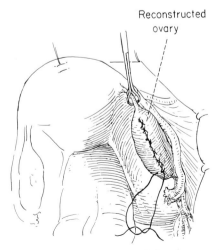

Reconstructed
ovary

Figure 21–28. Reconstructed ovary following ovarian cystectomy. (From Parsons L, Ulfelder H: Atlas of Pelvic Operations, 2nd ed. Philadelphia, WB Saunders, 1968.)

detached from the suction tubing so that amniotic fluid can be quickly evacuated from the field.

To enter the uterus, the assistant retracts the bladder downward with the bladder blade of a Balfour retractor or other similar retractor. The surgeon nicks the uterus with the deep knife and extends the incision with bandage scissors, whose blunt tips prevent injury to the fetus. As soon as the uterus is entered, *suction must be immediately available.* The technologist may be required to remove the bladder retractor at this time. Simultaneously, the assistant pushes firmly on the patient's upper abdomen while the surgeon grasps the infant's head and rotates it upward. The head is then delivered from the wound. The infant's airways are immediately suctioned with the bulb syringe. The surgeon delivers the infant's body from the wound and places it up on the mother's abdomen. Two Mayo clamps are then placed across the umbilical cord and it is divided with bandage scissors. Cord blood samples may be taken at this time. The technologist should have available a small basin or blood sample tube into which the surgeon can milk blood from the cord. The blood should be passed off to the circulator as soon as possible.

The infant is handed over to the circulator or pediatrician and placed in the previously warmed crib. The infant is then revived and oxygen or emergency drugs are given, as needed. If the mother has been given a spinal anesthetic, the infant is taken to the head of the table so that she can see it. It is then customary for the nurse to take the infant to the father, who is usually waiting anxiously outside the operating room. If the infant cannot be revived or if there appears to be a serious congenital defect, the anesthesiologist may sedate the patient heavily as soon as the abnormalities are discovered, so as not to upset her during surgery. In either case, the infant is taken to the nursery for observation.

As the infant is handed over to the circulator or pediatrician, attention must again be directed toward the surgical patient because much blood can be lost in a short time due to oozing from the severed uterine wall. Before closing the uterus, the surgeon removes the placenta from the uterus with his or her hand. The technologist should have a large basin on the field to receive the placenta. The surgeon then grasps the edges of the uterine incision with six to eight clamps; the type of clamp used depends on the surgeon's preference. Some surgeons use sponge forceps while others may use Duval lung-grasping clamps or Collin tongue clamps.

The uterine incision is closed with a two-layered running suture of size 0 chromic catgut, Vicryl, or Dexon swaged to a tapered needle. After the uterus is closed, the bladder flap is reperitonealized with a running suture of size 2-0 or 3-0 absorbable suture swaged to a fine tapered needle. The wound is then closed in routine fashion.

VAGINAL PROCEDURES

During vaginal procedures, with the patient in the lithotomy position, the surgeon usually operates while seated. The technologist should stand at the surgeon's right.

Dilatation and Curettage

Definition

This is dilatation of the os cervix and curetting of endometrial tissue. This procedure is performed to obtain tissue for microscopic examination or to halt uterine bleeding. The operation may also be performed to terminate pregnancy or to remove tissue following an incomplete or missed abortion. Placenta retained from a normal vaginal delivery is also removed by dilatation and curettage.

Highlights

1. The cervix is dilated.
2. The uterus is sounded for depth.
3. The endometrium is curetted.

Description

With the patient in the lithotomy position, the surgeon inserts a weighted speculum into the vaginal outlet and grasps the cervix with a tenaculum (Fig. 21–29). To determine the depth and direction of the uterine cavity and to prevent perforation during the procedure, a graduated sound is carefully introduced into the cervix (Fig. 21–30).

Using Hagar or Hanks uterine dilators, the surgeon

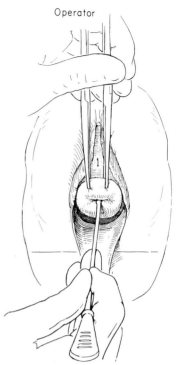

Figure 21–30. Dilatation and curettage. The uterus is sounded to measure its depth to prevent its perforation during dilatation and curettage. (From Parsons L, Ulfelder H: Atlas of Pelvic Operations, 2nd ed. Philadelphia, WB Saunders, 1968.)

slowly dilates the cervix (Fig. 21–31). As soon as the cervix is sufficiently dilated the surgeon places a sponge or Telfa strip over the speculum. The uterus is then gently curetted, allowing the specimen to collect on the Telfa or sponge (Fig. 21–32). The technologist should have several types of curettes available; these may be smooth, sharp, or serrated. The specimen is passed to the technologist, and the speculum is removed. The perineum is dressed with a perineal pad.

Conization of the Cervix

Definition

This is excision of a cone of tissue from the cervix. The procedure is performed to remove a cancerous lesion from the cervix or to obtain tissue for biopsy. If the procedure is performed in conjunction with a dilatation and curettage, the latter precedes the conization.

Highlights

1. Two suture ligatures are placed in the cervix.
2. The cone of tissue is excised.

Description

In preparation for a conization of the cervix, the routine vaginal prep may be omitted or limited to the application of antiseptic paint solution to the cervix and

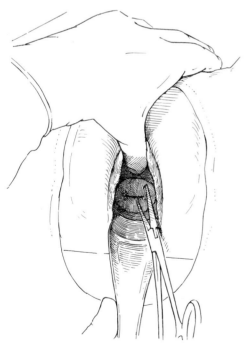

Figure 21–29. Dilatation and curettage. The surgeon grasps the cervix with a uterine tenaculum. (From Parsons L, Ulfelder H: Atlas of Pelvic Operations, 2nd ed. Philadelphia, WB Saunders, 1968.)

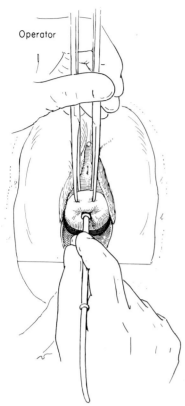

Figure 21–31. Dilatation and curettage. The surgeon dilates the cervix using cervical dilators in graduated sizes. (From Parsons L, Ulfelder H: Atlas of Pelvic Operations, 2nd ed. Philadelphia, WB Saunders, 1968.)

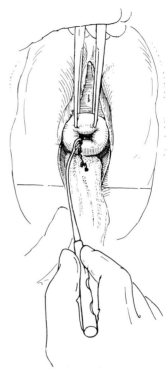

Figure 21–32. Dilatation and curettage. Uterine curettings are collected on a sponge or strip of Telfa. (From Parsons L, Ulfelder H: Atlas of Pelvic Operations, 2nd ed. Philadelphia, WB Saunders, 1968.)

vaginal vault. This is to prevent cancer cells from dislodging and spreading the disease.

With the patient in the lithotomy position, the surgeon inserts a weighted speculum into the vaginal outlet. Some surgeons apply a solution of iodine (Lugol's solution) to the cervix before starting the procedure. Healthy tissue will be stained by the solution while cancerous tissue will not.

The surgeon grasps the cervix with a tenaculum. Two suture ligatures of chromic catgut, size 0, mounted on a stout tapered needle, are then placed across the cervix. One suture is placed on each side of the os cervix. The ends are left long and are tagged (Fig. 21–33). Using a No. 11 or double-edged angled Beaver blade, the surgeon incises the cervix in a conical shape (Fig. 21–34). The cone is then removed and passed to the technologist (Fig. 21–35). The long suture ends are then cut. If the cervix continues to bleed in spite of the ligatures, the surgeon may place additional ligatures or a hemostatic agent over the oozing tissue.

Therapeutic Abortion

Definition

This is termination of pregnancy by removing the fetus from the uterus through the vagina. A technologist may refuse to participate in therapeutic abortions if the procedure contradicts his or her religious, ethical, or moral beliefs.

Highlights

1. The uterus is sounded and the cervix is dilated.
2. A curettage is performed.
3. The uterine contents are aspirated mechanically by a special suction apparatus.

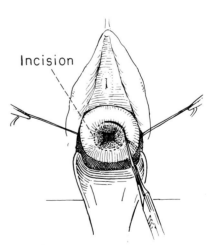

Figure 21–33. Conization of the cervix. The surgeon places two suture ligatures around the os cervix. (From Parsons L, Ulfelder H: Atlas of Pelvic Operations, 2nd ed. Philadelphia, WB Saunders, 1968.)

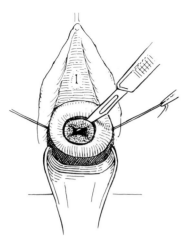

Figure 21–34. Conization of the cervix. The cervix is incised. (From Parsons L, Ulfelder H: Atlas of Pelvic Operations, 2nd ed. Philadelphia, WB Saunders, 1968.)

Description

This procedure involves the use of a special vacuum device that evacuates the contents of the uterus (Fig. 21–36). A routine dilatation and curettage is performed, as previously described. Sterile suction tubing and a suction tip are given to the technologist or surgeon. One end of the suction tubing is passed to the circulator, who then attaches it to the vacuum device. The vacuum is activated by the circulator, and the uterus is suctioned clean. The technologist must retrieve the specimen from the suction bottle at the close of the procedure. The vagina is dressed with a perineal pad.

Excision of Cystic Bartholin's Gland

Definition

The Bartholin gland, which secretes mucus, is a common site of cyst formation. These cysts often become infected, and, in such cases, surgical removal of the

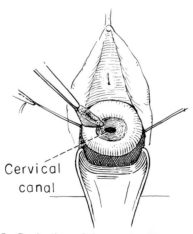

Figure 21–35. Conization of the cervix. The cone is removed and passed to the technologist as a specimen. (From Parsons L, Ulfelder H: Atlas of Pelvic Operations, 2nd ed. Philadelphia, WB Saunders, 1968.)

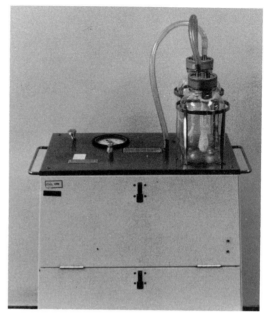

Figure 21–36. Suction apparatus used for therapeutic abortion.

cystic gland may be indicated. Fenestration (creating a "window" in the gland) with preservation of normal function is often performed as well.

Highlights

1. The cyst is excised.
2. The wound is closed.

Description

With the patient in the lithotomy position, the surgeon makes a small incision at the perimeter of the cyst with a No. 15 knife blade (Fig. 21–37). The incision is carried into the bed of the cyst with Metzenbaum scissors (Fig.

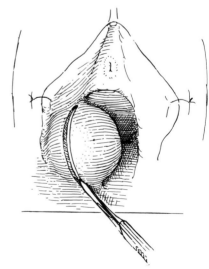

Figure 21–37. Excision of Bartholin's gland cyst. A small incision is made at the base of the cyst. (From Parsons L, Ulfelder H: Atlas of Pelvic Operations, 2nd ed. Philadelphia, WB Saunders, 1968.)

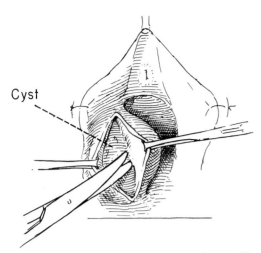

Figure 21–38. Removal of Bartholin's gland cyst. Sharp dissection of the cyst. (From Parsons L, Ulfelder H: Atlas of Pelvic Operations, 2nd ed. Philadelphia, WB Saunders, 1968.)

21–38). The surgeon may grasp the edge of the cyst with several Allis clamps. With the use of both sharp and blunt dissection, the cyst is mobilized. Small bleeders may be clamped with curved mosquito or Kelly hemostats and cauterized or ligated with fine catgut suture.

When the cyst has been removed completely, the surgeon closes the empty space left by the cyst with interrupted sutures of catgut, size 3-0, on a small taper needle (Fig. 21–39). A small length of Penrose drain may be placed in the wound (Fig. 21–40).

Repair of Vesicovaginal Fistula

Definition

This is excision of a fistula occurring between the bladder and vagina. The fistula allows urine to escape

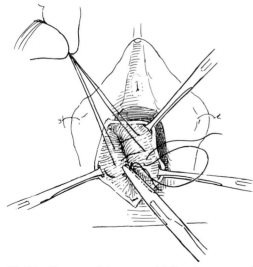

Figure 21–39. Closure of the wound following removal of the cystic Bartholin's gland. (From Parsons L, Ulfelder H: Atlas of Pelvic Operations, 2nd ed. Philadelphia, WB Saunders, 1968.)

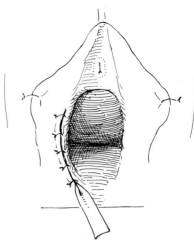

Figure 21–40. Removal of cystic Bartholin's gland. Completed closure. Note small Penrose drain at the end of the incision. (From Parsons L, Ulfelder H: Atlas of Pelvic Operations, 2nd ed. Philadelphia, WB Saunders, 1968.)

through the vagina, thereby causing pain and incontinence.

Highlights

1. The fistula is excised.
2. The defect in the bladder is closed.
3. The wound is closed.

Description

With the patient in the lithotomy position, the surgeon places a vaginal retractor to expose the fistula (Fig. 21–41). A malleable probe is placed in the fistula. The surgeon then makes a circular incision around the fistula with a No. 15 knife blade (Fig. 21–42) and carries the dissection further with Metzenbaum scissors (Fig. 21–43). The anterior vaginal mucosa is incised to expose the bladder wall (Fig. 21–44). The assistant grasps the

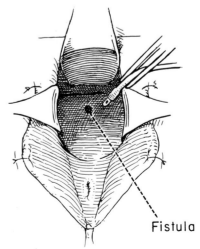

Figure 21–41. Vesicovaginal fistula. (From Parsons L, Ulfelder H: Atlas of Pelvic Operations, 2nd ed. Philadelphia, WB Saunders, 1968.)

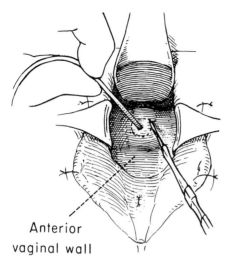

Figure 21–42. Repair of vesicovaginal fistula. A small probe is placed in the fistula and an incision made around it. (From Parsons L, Ulfelder H: Atlas of Pelvic Operations, 2nd ed. Philadelphia, WB Saunders, 1968.)

edges of the vaginal mucosa with several Allis clamps. The surgeon then sews the edges of the bladder wall with several interrupted sutures of Dexon or chromic catgut, size 3-0.

The cut edges of the vaginal mucosa are approximated with interrupted chromic catgut sutures, size 0 or 2-0 (Fig. 21–45). A Foley catheter may be inserted into the bladder at the close of the procedure.

Repair of Rectovaginal Fistula

Definition

This is repair of a fistula between the rectum and vagina. The fistula allows the passage of fecal material

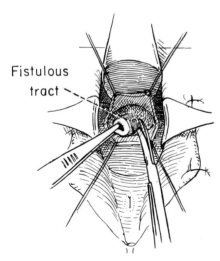

Figure 21–43. Repair of vesicovaginal fistula. The fistula is further dissected with Metzenbaum scissors. (From Parsons L, Ulfelder H: Atlas of Pelvic Operations, 2nd ed. Philadelphia, WB Saunders, 1968.)

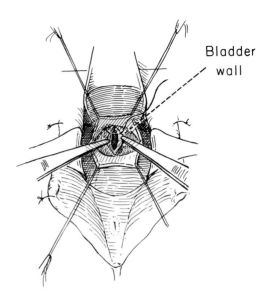

Figure 21–44. Repair of vesicovaginal fistula. The surgeon incises the anterior vaginal mucosa to expose the bladder wall. (From Parsons L, Ulfelder H: Atlas of Pelvic Operations, 2nd ed. Philadelphia, WB Saunders, 1968.)

into the vagina, thereby causing inflammation and infection.

Highlights

1. The fistula is excised.
2. The defect is sutured.
3. The perineal floor is strengthened with sutures.
4. The wound is closed.

Description

With the patient in the lithotomy position, the surgeon examines the fistula. A malleable probe may be inserted

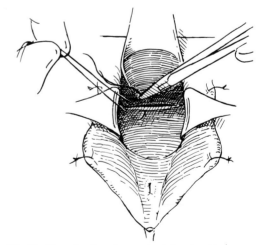

Figure 21–45. Repair of vesicovaginal fistula. The vaginal wall is approximated with absorbable sutures. (From Parsons L, Ulfelder H: Atlas of Pelvic Operations, 2nd ed. Philadelphia, WB Saunders, 1968.)

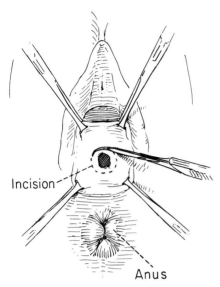

Figure 21–46. Rectovaginal fistula. The surgeon makes a circular incision around the fistula. (From Parsons L, Ulfelder H: Atlas of Pelvic Operations, 2nd ed. Philadelphia, WB Saunders, 1968.)

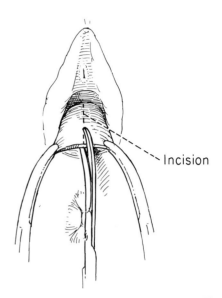

Figure 21–48. Repair of rectovaginal fistula. The surgeon incises the vaginal wall to expose the rectum. (From Parsons L, Ulfelder H: Atlas of Pelvic Operations, 2nd ed. Philadelphia, WB Saunders, 1968.)

into the fistula to determine its depth. Grasping the posterior wall of the vagina with Allis clamps, the assistant offers traction across the fistula. The surgeon then makes a circular incision around the fistula with a No. 15 knife blade (Fig. 21–46). The edge of the fistula is grasped with toothed tissue forceps and the incision is deepened with Metzenbaum scissors (Fig. 21–47).

The vaginal wall is then incised with the scissors (Fig. 21–48), thus exposing the wall of the rectum. The surgeon excises the edges of the fistula (Fig. 21–49). The defect is then closed with a pursestring suture. To strengthen the perineal floor, the surgeon approximates the levator muscles, which lie on either side of the rectum (Fig. 21–50). The vaginal mucosa is then ap-

proximated with an interrupted layer of chromic catgut sutures, size 0 or 2-0 (Fig. 21–51). A Foley catheter may be inserted at the close of the procedure.

Repair of Cystocele and Rectocele (Anterior and Posterior Repair)

Definition

This is surgical repair of a bulging of the bladder (cystocele) and rectum (rectocele), where there is weakened vaginal mucosa. These two conditions can occur together or independently. Anterior repair is indicated

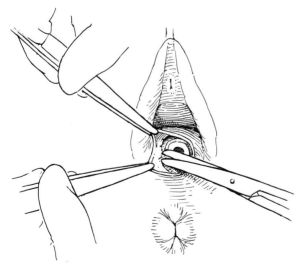

Figure 21–47. Repair of rectovaginal fistula. The circular incision is deepened. (From Parsons L, Ulfelder H: Atlas of Pelvic Operations, 2nd ed. Philadelphia, WB Saunders, 1968.)

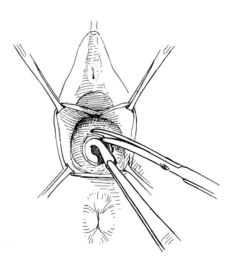

Figure 21–49. Repair of rectovaginal fistula. The fistula is excised at the rectum. (From Parsons L, Ulfelder H: Atlas of Pelvic Operations, 2nd ed. Philadelphia, WB Saunders, 1968.)

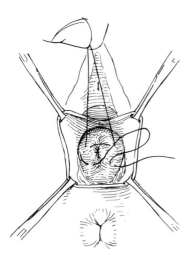

Figure 21–50. Repair of the rectovaginal fistula. To strengthen the perineal floor, the surgeon approximates the levator muscles that lie on either side of the rectum. (From Parsons L, Ulfelder H: Atlas of Pelvic Operations, 2nd ed. Philadelphia, WB Saunders, 1968.)

for cystocele and posterior repair for rectocele. Both of these conditions are usually the result of childbirth.

Highlights

Anterior Repair

1. The anterior vaginal wall is incised.
2. The incised edges are grasped with Allis clamps.
3. A plane of tissue is formed in the vaginal wall up to the bladder.
4. The bladder fascia is sutured.
5. The vaginal wall is reconstructed, and the excess mucosa is excised.

Posterior Repair

1. An incision is made in the posterior vaginal wall.
2. The incision is deepened to the rectum.

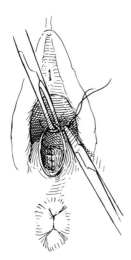

Figure 21–51. Repair of rectovaginal fistula. The vaginal wall is approximated with absorbable sutures. (From Parsons L, Ulfelder H: Atlas of Pelvic Operations, 2nd ed. Philadelphia, WB Saunders, 1968.)

3. Sutures are placed through the levator muscles.
4. The excess mucosa is excised, and the posterior vaginal wall is reconstructed.

Description

Before the procedure begins, the circulator inserts a Foley catheter. With the patient in the lithotomy position, the surgeon inserts a weighted speculum into the vaginal outlet. The cervix is grasped with a tenaculum and brought forward. Using a No. 10 knife blade or Mayo scissors, the surgeon makes an incision in the anterior vaginal wall (Fig. 21–52A). The edges of the incision are grasped with several Allis clamps, and the assistant retracts the edges in a fan shape. The surgeon deepens the incision with sharp and blunt dissection. Curved Mayo scissors, knife, and sponges are used to advance the incision through the vaginal wall and into the fascia that lies behind it (Fig. 21–52B through E). The assistant may be required to retract the bladder upward with a lateral (Sims) retractor during the dissection. As the surgeon deepens the tissue flaps, additional Allis clamps are placed on the edges of the tissue.

When the surgeon reaches the bladder neck, several sutures of size 0 chromic catgut are placed through the fascia, thus tightening the tissue. These sutures prevent the bladder from bulging (Fig. 21–52F through H). The excess vaginal mucosa is then excised, and the vaginal walls are approximated with sutures of size 0 chromic catgut (Fig. 21–52I).

To begin the posterior repair, the surgeon places two Allis clamps on each side of the vaginal outlet on the posterior side. The assistant offers traction with the clamps while the surgeon makes a transverse incision in the mucosa (Fig. 21–53A). The incision is deepened with curved Mayo or Metzenbaum scissors to the level of the rectum (Fig. 21–53B through D). To prevent the rectum from bulging, the surgeon brings the levator muscles together with interrupted sutures of size 2-0 chromic catgut (Fig. 21–53E). The excess vaginal mucosa is excised and the vaginal wall is reconstructed with interrupted sutures of size 2-0 chromic catgut swaged to a small needle (Fig. 21–53F). The surgeon usually inserts a Foley catheter at the close of the procedure and dresses the vagina with packing impregnated with an antibiotic cream.

Simple Vulvectomy

Definition

This is excision of the vulva (labia and clitoris) as treatment for cancer of the vulva. The procedure is indicated for small lesions of the vulva when no known lymph node metastasis has occurred.

Highlights

1. An elliptical incision is made around the labia.
2. A second incision is made around the vagina and urethral orifice.
3. The vulva is removed en bloc.

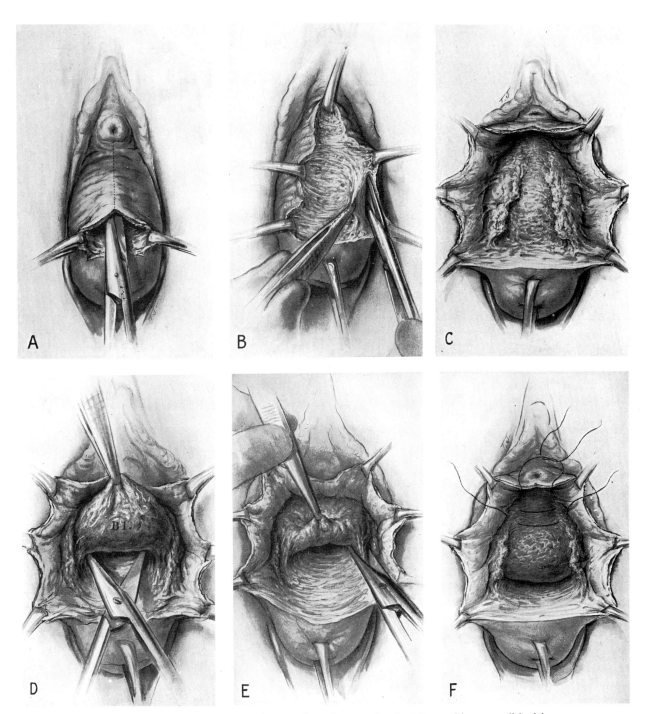

Figure 21–52. Anterior repair of cystocele and rectocele. *A.* After making a small incision in the anterior vaginal wall, the surgeon lengthens it with Mayo scissors. *B* through *E.* As the incision is advanced, more Allis clamps are added and the bladder is pushed upward.

Illustration continued on following page

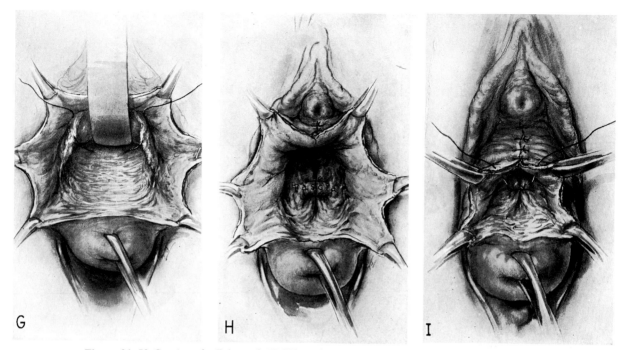

Figure 21–52 *Continued.* *F* through *H*. When the surgeon reaches the bladder neck, several sutures are placed across it to prevent it from bulging forward. *I.* After removing the excess vaginal tissue, the walls are closed. (From Jacob S, Francone C, Lossow WJ: Structure and Function in Man, 5th ed. Philadelphia, WB Saunders, 1982.)

4. The perineal floor is strengthened with sutures.
5. The wound is closed.

Description

With the patient in the lithotomy position, the surgeon incises the skin around the labia (Fig. 21–54). A second incision is made around the vagina and urethral orifice. The surgeon places many Allis clamps on the skin edges, and the assistant offers traction by pulling the clamps upward. The surgeon then deepens the incision with the knife, Metzenbaum scissors, and cautery pencil (Fig. 21–55). Large bleeding vessels are controlled with Kelly hemostats and ligated with chromic catgut or Dexon sutures, size 3-0. The vulva is removed en bloc when mobilization is complete (Fig. 21–56).

To strengthen the perineal floor, the surgeon sutures the levator muscles together. To gain access to these muscles, the surgeon incises the posterior vaginal mucosa (Fig. 21–57). The muscles are then sutured together with interrupted sutures of size 2-0 chromic catgut (Fig. 21–58).

To begin wound closure, the flap of vaginal mucosa is replaced. Using interrupted silk sutures, size 3-0 or 4-0, on a fine cutting needle, the surgeon approximates the skin to the vaginal outlet and to the incised tissue edges around the urethral orifice (Fig. 21–59). The completed reconstruction with a Foley catheter in place is shown in Figure 21–60.

Radical Vulvectomy

Definition

This is radical excision of the vulva and groin tissue. The procedure is performed in an attempt to cure cancer of the vulva. Because the disease metastasizes very early in its course, the lymph chain that drains the vulva is excised through groin incisions.

Highlights

1. The skin is incised as for simple vulvectomy.
2. The block of tissue is removed.
3. Both groins are entered, and the lymph nodes are removed.
4. The wound is closed.

Description

This procedure follows the same techniques as those used for a simple vulvectomy. A major difference between the two procedures is the removal of lymph nodes from both groins, which necessitates three separate incisions.

With the patient in the lithotomy position, the surgeon performs a simple vulvectomy. One or both groins are then incised and the lymph nodes are removed by sharp dissection. Bleeders are clamped and ligated with silk or Dexon sutures. At the completion of the groin dissection, the tissues are closed in layers.

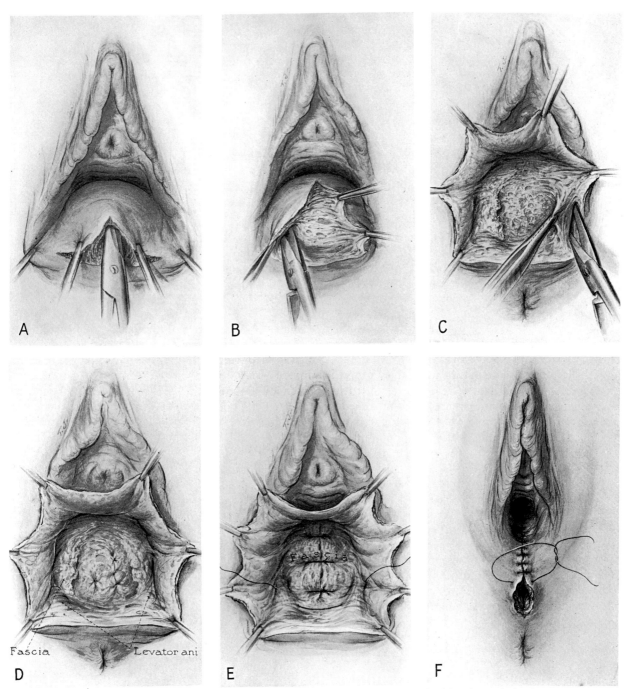

Figure 21–53. Posterior repair of cystocele and rectocele. *A.* An incision is made in the posterior mucosa. *B* through *D.* The incision is deepened by sharp and blunt dissection. *E.* The bulging rectocele is bound by sutures of chromic catgut or absorbable synthetic material. *F.* After the vaginal flaps are trimmed, they are approximated. (From Jacob S, Francone C, Lossow WJ: Structure and Function in Man, 5th ed. Philadelphia, WB Saunders, 1982.)

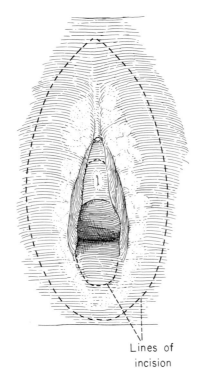

Figure 21–54. Simple vulvectomy. Area to be incised. (From Parsons L, Ulfelder H: Atlas of Pelvic Operations, 2nd ed. Philadelphia, WB Saunders, 1968.)

Wound closure may require a skin graft (see Chapter 29), depending on the amount of skin that remains after the dissection. Hemovac drains are used to evacuate blood and serum fluid from the wound postoperatively.

Vaginal Hysterectomy

Definition

This is surgical removal of the uterus through the vagina. The indications for vaginal hysterectomy are the same as those for an abdominal hysterectomy. Although a vaginal approach is technically difficult, it is less traumatic for the patient because the abdominal wall remains intact.

Highlights

1. The cervix is incised to gain access to the uterine ligaments.
2. The uterus is partially mobilized.
3. The peritoneal covering of the bladder is dissected free.
4. The uterus is completely mobilized and removed.
5. The bladder is reperitonealized.
6. The peritoneum is closed.
7. The vaginal vault is closed.

Description

A major portion of the operation for vaginal hysterectomy is the serial clamping, division, and ligation of

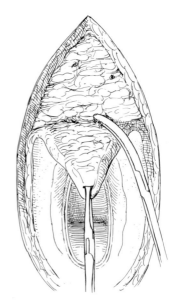

Figure 21–55. Vulvectomy. The surgeon deepens the incision with Metzenbaum scissors. (From Parsons L, Ulfelder H: Atlas of Pelvic Operations, 2nd ed. Philadelphia, WB Saunders, 1968.)

ligaments and vessels of the uterus, as for an abdominal hysterectomy. The surgeon may use Heaney, Kocher, Ochsner, or O'Hanlon clamps to secure the uterine segments before their division from the uterus.

With the patient in the lithotomy position, the surgeon grasps the cervix with a uterine tenaculum. Using the knife or curved Mayo scissors, the surgeon makes a circular incision around the cervix (Fig. 21–61). This exposes the first set of ligaments, which are double-clamped, divided, and ligated with suture ligatures of

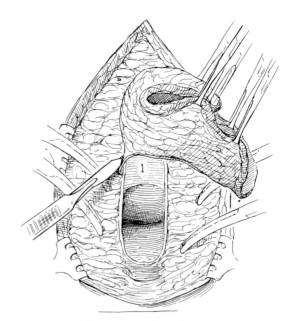

Figure 21–56. Vulvectomy. The vulva is removed en bloc. (From Parsons L, Ulfelder H: Atlas of Pelvic Operations, 2nd ed. Philadelphia, WB Saunders, 1968.)

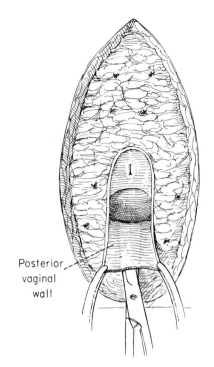

Posterior
vaginal
wall

Figure 21–57. Vulvectomy. The surgeon incises the posterior vaginal wall to gain access to the levator muscles. These will be sutured together to strengthen the perineal floor. (From Parsons L, Ulfelder H: Atlas of Pelvic Operations, 2nd ed. Philadelphia, WB Saunders, 1968.)

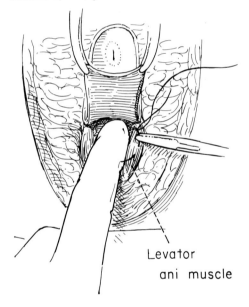

Levator
ani muscle

Figure 21–58. Vulvectomy. The levator muscles are approximated. (From Parsons L, Ulfelder H: Atlas of Pelvic Operations, 2nd ed. Philadelphia, WB Saunders, 1968.)

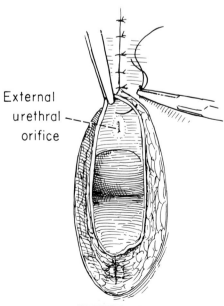

External
urethral
orifice

Figure 21–59. Vulvectomy. The vaginal wall is approximated to the skin. (From Parsons L, Ulfelder H: Atlas of Pelvic Operations, 2nd ed. Philadelphia, WB Saunders, 1968.)

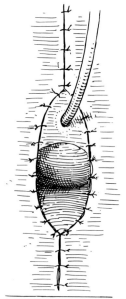

Figure 21–60. Vulvectomy. Completed closure. (From Parsons L, Ulfelder H: Atlas of Pelvic Operations, 2nd ed. Philadelphia, WB Saunders, 1968.)

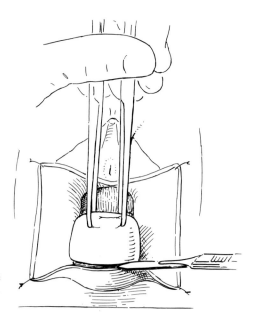

Figure 21–61. Vaginal hysterectomy. The cervix is incised to expose the uterine ligaments. (From Parsons L, Ulfelder H: Atlas of Pelvic Operations, 2nd ed. Philadelphia, WB Saunders, 1968.)

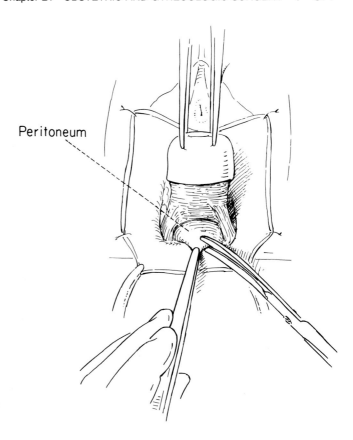

Peritoneum

Figure 21–62. Vaginal hysterectomy. The posterior peritoneum is incised. (From Parsons L, Ulfelder H: Atlas of Pelvic Operations, 2nd ed. Philadelphia, WB Saunders, 1968.)

size 0 chromic catgut mounted or swaged to a heavy tapered needle.

The surgeon picks up the posterior peritoneum with toothed tissue forceps and incises it with the knife or scissors (Fig. 21–62). With the peritoneal cavity open, the peritoneal attachment to the bladder is detached from the uterus with Metzenbaum scissors. The technologist must have long tissue forceps and long dissecting scissors available as the mobilization is carried deeper into the pelvis. The assistant may retract the bladder upward with a Sims or Heaney retractor.

Mobilization of the uterus continues until the uterus is completely free. It is then removed and delivered to the technologist as a specimen. When the uterus is removed, the peritoneal cavity is exposed. Before closing the peritoneum, the surgeon reperitonealizes the bladder with a running suture of size 2-0 chromic catgut swaged to a fine tapered needle. The peritoneum is then closed with a running chromic catgut suture, size 0 or 2-0. The wound is dressed with a perineal pad.

Shirodkar Procedure

Definition

This is the application of a strip of synthetic material to the internal os cervix to prevent premature dilatation and subsequent spontaneous abortion. The procedure is performed on the patient who has a history of spontaneous abortion in the first trimester of pregnancy.

Highlights

1. The cervix is incised.
2. Synthetic tape is placed around the internal os.
3. The cervix is closed.

Description

The patient is placed in the lithotomy position, prepped, and draped as for a dilatation and curettage. The surgeon places a weighted speculum in the vagina and grasps the cervix with a tenaculum. The anterior cervix is then incised, and the incision is extended to the posterior vaginal wall. A 0.5-cm Mersilene or Dacron tape is then passed around the internal os and tied. The incision is closed with absorbable sutures (chromic catgut, Dexon, or Vicryl), size 0 or 2-0.

Bibliography

Crooks L: Operating Room Techniques for the Surgical Team. Boston, Little, Brown & Co, 1979.

Gardner E, Gray D, O'Rahilly R: Anatomy: A Regional Study of Human Structure, 4th ed. Philadelphia, WB Saunders, 1984.

McVay C: Surgical Anatomy, 6th ed. Philadelphia, WB Saunders, 1984.

Moore CML: Realities in Childbearing, 2nd ed. Philadelphia, WB Saunders, 1983.

Purtilo R: Health Professional/Patient Interaction, 4th ed. Philadelphia, WB Saunders, 1990.

Sabiston DC Jr (ed): Davis-Christopher Textbook of Surgery, 14th ed. Philadelphia, WB Saunders, 1991.

Walter JB: An Introduction to the Principles of Disease, 3rd ed. Philadelphia, WB Saunders, 1992.

Urogenital Surgery

Urogenital surgery involves procedures of the male and female urinary systems and the male reproductive structures. Urinary procedures are classified as *open* or *closed*. An open procedure is performed when the focal point of the surgery is exposed through an incision, while closed procedures are performed through cystoscopy (direct visualization of structures by means of the fiberoptic cystoscope inserted into the urethra and bladder). The patient is placed in the lateral position for operations involving the kidney and ureter. The supine position is preferred for procedures on the bladder and reproductive structures. Closed procedures are performed with the patient in the lithotomy position. Closed procedures of the urinary system are performed more commonly than open procedures.

SURGICAL ANATOMY

Internal Organs of the Urinary System

Kidneys

The kidneys (Fig. 22–1) are paired organs that lie behind the parietal peritoneum between the level of the twelfth thoracic vertebra and the third lumbar vertebra. The kidney is bean shaped and weighs approximately 150 g.

Each kidney is covered by three separate tissue layers that protect it from injury and also help hold it in place. The outer layer, or *renal fascia*, anchors the kidney. The next layer, called the *perirenal fat,* is an adipose layer that surrounds the kidney and helps to protect it

from injury. The innermost layer, or true *capsule* (sometimes called *Gerota's capsule*), is a smooth fibrous tissue closely adherent to the organ.

From the *hilum,* the notched portion of the kidney, emerge the renal vein and artery, which supply and remove blood from the organ. Also at the hilum, an enlarged portion of the ureter joins the kidney; this structure is called the *renal pelvis*.

The inner structure of the kidney (Fig. 22–2) consists of several tissue layers within which lies the complex filtering system that rids the blood of impurities. The outer layer is called the *cortex*. The *medulla*, or middle layer, consists of 8 to 12 large collecting areas called the *renal pyramids*. The pyramids extend out away from the renal pelvis and the area where the ureter joins the kidney. The cavities of the kidney into which the pyramids converge are called the *calyces* (singular—calyx). The microscopic filtering system of the kidney lies within the bounds of the cortex and the medulla. This filtering system is composed of many single units called *nephrons* (Fig. 22–3).

Adrenal Glands

Above each kidney, but adherent to them, is the *adrenal,* or *suprarenal,* gland. This gland is enclosed by tough connective tissue and consists of a cortex and medulla. The adrenal gland is important in the production of norepinephrine and epinephrine, which act to stimulate or slow down heart rate, the activities of the gastrointestinal system, and certain portions of the respiratory system.

Ureter

The *ureter* emerges from the renal pelvis where filtered urine is shunted away from the kidney and out of

378

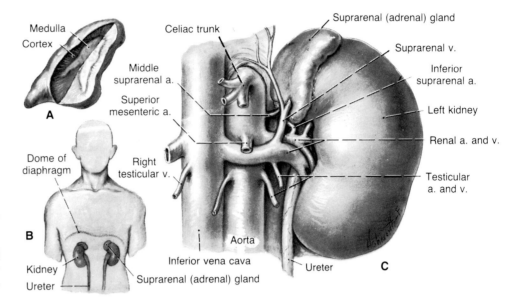

Figure 22–1. The kidneys. *A.* Adrenal (suprarenal) gland. *B.* Anatomic position of the kidneys. *C.* Gross structure. (From Jacob S, Francone C, Lossow WJ: Structure and Function in Man, 5th ed. Philadelphia, WB Saunders, 1982.)

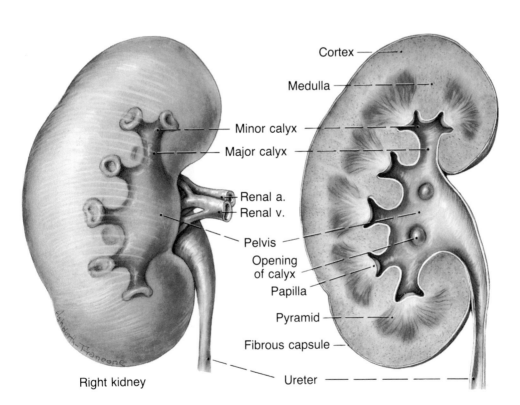

Figure 22–2. Internal structure of the kidney showing layers, calyces, renal pelvis, and ureter. (From Jacob S, Francone C, Lossow WJ: Structure and Function in Man, 5th ed. Philadelphia, WB Saunders, 1982.)

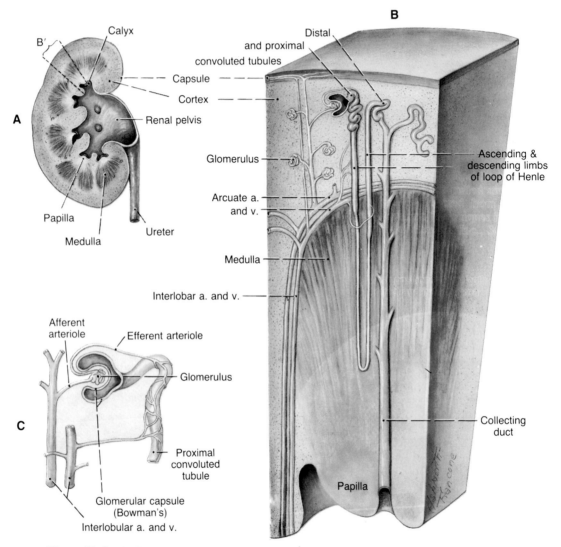

Figure 22–3. *A.* Sagittal section of kidney showing gross structure. *B.* The nephron and its relationship to the medulla and cortex. *C.* Magnified view of nephron. (From Jacob S, Francone C, Lossow WJ: Structure and Function in Man, 5th ed. Philadelphia, WB Saunders, 1982.)

the body. The ureters lead directly to the urinary bladder, which lies below. Each ureter is about 30 cm long and about 5 mm in diameter. Because of its small dimension, the ureter is often a site for lodged kidney stones. The ureter is a three-layered tube, including an outer fibrous layer, a middle mucous membrane layer, and an inner muscular layer. Urine is moved down the ureter by the peristaltic action of the muscular layer.

Urinary Bladder

The urinary bladder (Fig. 22–4) lies behind the symphysis pubis in the pelvic cavity. In the female, this hollow organ is separated from the rectum by the vagina and uterus. In the male, the seminal vesicles separate the bladder from the rectum.

The wall of the bladder is composed of four tissue layers. The outermost layer is a thin tissue called the *serosa.* Next is the *muscular layer,* the *submucosa,* and finally the inner *mucosa.*

At the base or neck of the bladder (the lowest portion) lies an area known as the *trigone.* This is a triangular area whose points correspond with the junction of both ureters and the *urethra.* Urination is accomplished by a complex series of nervous impulses that are finally transmitted to the trigonal area where a sphincter contracts or relaxes to allow the retention or escape of urine.

Urethra

As previously mentioned, the urethra emerges from the bladder at the trigone. The female urethra is quite short, whereas the male homologue is considerably longer. Its function is to convey urine from the urinary bladder to the outside of the body.

The *male urethra* is divided into several distinct portions. The *prostatic urethra,* or uppermost portion, is approximately 3 cm long and begins at the bladder neck. The *membranous urethra,* the shortest portion, is about 2 cm long. The *cavernis urethra,* or penile portion, is approximately 15 cm long and lies within the spongiosum layer of the penis.

The *female urethra* is about 4 cm long and follows a direct course from the bladder to the external *meatus,* or urethral opening. Because of its short length and proximity to the anus, the female urethra is often the site of infection owing to contamination by intestinal bacteria.

External Reproductive Organs of the Male

Scrotum and Testicles

The *scrotum* is a pouch that lies at the base of the penis. It is an extension of the abdominal wall that houses and protects the testicles—the male reproductive organs. The scrotum is divided into two subpouches by a septum, with one testicle resting in each pouch. The wall of the scrotum contains a subcutaneous tissue of smooth muscle fibers called the *dartos layer.* When the ambient temperature is unsuitable for maximum sperm protection, the dartos layer causes the scrotum to tighten or pull upward (in the case of a cold ambient surrounding) or to relax and hang farther away from the body (in the case of warm ambient temperatures).

Each *testicle* (Fig. 22–5) is suspended in the scrotum by the *epididymis.* The epididymis is a convoluted duct that secretes *seminal fluid,* the medium that gives the sperm mobility to travel along the reproductive tract of the male. Each testicle manufactures testosterone, the male hormone, and also serves as the housing for the production of sperm. Within the testicles are complicated ductal systems connected to the epididymis.

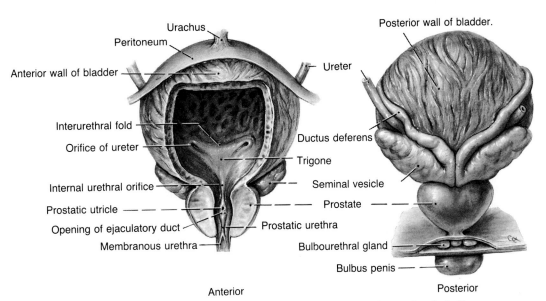

Figure 22–4. Internal and external views of the urinary bladder. (From Jacob S, Francone C, Lossow WJ: Structure and Function in Man, 5th ed. Philadelphia, WB Saunders, 1982.)

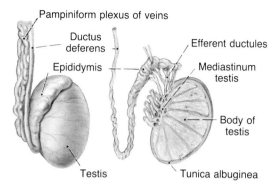

Figure 22–5. The testicle. (From Jacob S, Francone C, Lossow WJ: Structure and Function in Man, 5th ed. Philadelphia, WB Saunders, 1982.)

Penis

The penis (Fig. 22–6*A*), or male copulatory organ, is a highly vascular structure that is flaccid except during sexual stimulation, when it becomes engorged with blood and becomes rigid. It lies just in front of the scrotum and is suspended at the pubic arch by fascial tissue. The penis is composed of several columns of tissue. Two dorsal columns called the *corpora cavernosa*

are spongy vascular tissue that make up the greatest portion of the organ. The two columns are separated by a septum but are bound together by a fibrous sheath. A third tissue column that runs ventrally is the *corpus spongiosum*. Within this section lies the penile portion of the urethra. A slightly enlarged distal end of the corpus spongiosum forms the *glans penis,* which is normally covered by a skin fold called the *prepuce,* or *foreskin*. At the tip of the glans penis lies the *urethral orifice*.

Internal Reproductive Organs of the Male

The internal reproductive organs of the male (Fig. 22–6*B*) include the prostate, bulbourethral glands, vas deferens, seminal vesicles, and ejaculatory duct.

Prostate

The prostate gland is a musculoglandular structure approximately the size of a chestnut. It is conical and lies with its base in close proximity to the bladder. The prostate surrounds the prostatic portion of the urethra

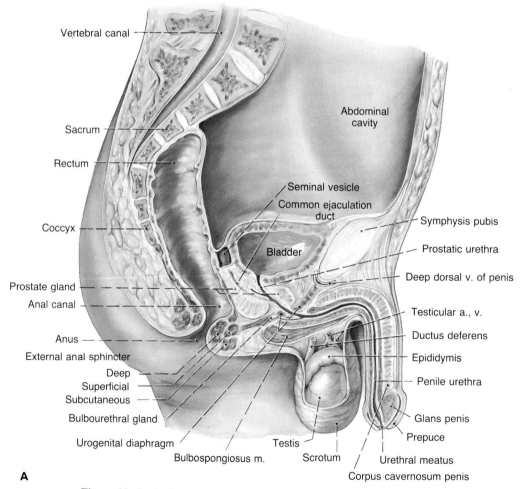

Figure 22–6. *A.* Sectioned view of bladder, prostate gland, and penis.

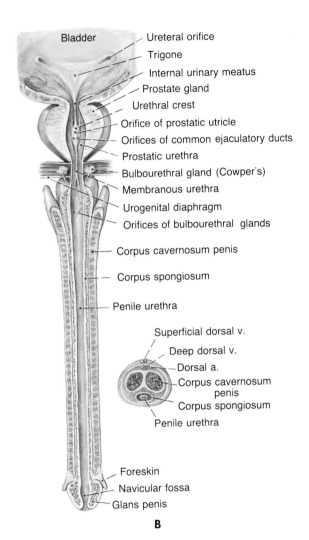

Bladder
Ureteral orifice
Trigone
Internal urinary meatus
Prostate gland
Urethral crest
Orifice of prostatic utricle
Orifices of common ejaculatory ducts
Prostatic urethra
Bulbourethral gland (Cowper's)
Membranous urethra
Urogenital diaphragm
Orifices of bulbourethral glands
Corpus cavernosum penis
Corpus spongiosum
Penile urethra
Superficial dorsal v.
Deep dorsal v.
Dorsal a.
Corpus cavernosum penis
Corpus spongiosum
Penile urethra
Foreskin
Navicular fossa
Glans penis

B

Figure 22–6 *Continued. B.* Section of male internal reproductive organs. (From Jacob S, Francone C, Lossow WJ: Structure and Function in Man, 5th ed. Philadelphia, WB Saunders, 1982.)

and secretes an alkaline fluid that is part of the liquid needed to nourish and give mobility to sperm. The gland is divided into six main lobes: anterior, posterior, middle, subcervical, right lateral, and left lateral.

The prostate gland is covered by a fibrous tissue called the *capsule.* Behind the prostatic capsule lies a sheath called the *true prostatic capsule* that separates the gland and seminal vesicles from the rectum.

Bulbourethral Glands

The bulbourethral glands (also called Cowper's glands) are paired glands that lie just below the prostate. They are about the size of a pea and rest on each side of the urethra. These glands secrete mucus, a portion of the fluid that makes up semen.

Vas Deferens

The vas deferens (also called the ductus deferens or seminal duct) is a portion of the path that the seminal

fluid travels. It is a continuation of the epididymis and begins along the back or posterior edge of a testicle, traverses the inguinal canal, and enters the abdomen. As the vas deferens enters the abdomen through the *inguinal canal* and *internal ring,* it is encompassed by the *spermatic cord.* This cord contains not only the vas deferens but also blood vessels and lymphatics. The vas deferens continues across the bladder and ureter where it meets the opening of the *seminal vesicle* and forms the *ejaculatory duct.*

Seminal Vesicles

The seminal vesicles are two pouches that lie behind the bladder at its base and actually represent a tube curved back on itself. Each seminal vesicle secretes a large portion of the total seminal fluid. The lower end of each vesicle joins its corresponding vas deferens to form the ejaculatory duct.

Ejaculatory Duct

As previously discussed, the ejaculatory duct is formed by the joining of the vas deferens and the duct or lower end of the seminal vesicle. This duct travels through the base of the prostate gland where it then enters the prostatic urethra.

OPEN PROCEDURES

Instrumentation for open procedures is similar to that used for general surgery. Right-angled, Allis, and Babcock clamps are needed for most procedures. The use of special prostatic retractors, stone-grasping forceps, and kidney pedicle clamps may also be required. Since the approach to most urinary structures often crosses muscle tissue, which is highly vascular, the technologist should have an ample supply of lap sponges and hemostatic clamps available. Sponge dissectors and stick sponges are needed for nearly all of the procedures. Chromic catgut and synthetic absorbable sutures (Dexon or Vicryl) are used when the surgeon is suturing in and around the tissues of the urinary tract, since nonabsorbable sutures can cause the formation of stones (calculi).

Simple Nephrectomy

Definition

This is surgical removal of a kidney. Severe infection that results in widespread damage to the kidney, cancer, severe trauma, and tuberculosis are all indications for a nephrectomy.

Highlights

1. The flank is entered.
2. The kidney and ureter are mobilized.
3. The renal artery and vein are divided.

4. The ureter is divided.
5. The wound is closed.

Description

The kidney is most often approached from a flank incision (Fig. 22–7). The patient is placed in the lateral position with the affected side up. Drapes are placed as for an abdominal incision, with the fenestration over the flank.

To begin the surgery, a curved incision is made across the flank by the surgeon. Fascia and muscle tissue are divided with dissecting scissors and cautery. Occasionally a rib must be sacrificed to gain access to the retroperitoneal space in which the kidney lies. If a rib is to be taken, the technologist should have periosteal

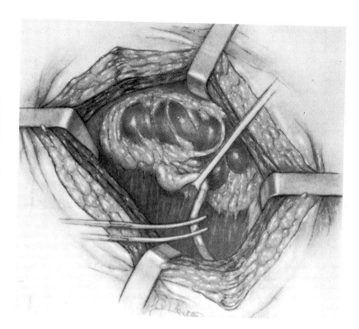

Figure 22–8. Simple nephrectomy. Ligation of the ureter. (From Harrison JH et al: Campbell's Urology, 4th ed. Philadelphia, WB Saunders, 1978.)

elevators and rib shears available. Once the surgeon has divided the tissues of the flank, the rib is stripped of periosteum and its attaching ligaments. The rib is then divided with shears. The divided rib is passed to the technologist, who retains it as a specimen. If the incision is far enough toward the head of the patient, the peritoneum or pleura may also be incised. A Balfour retractor is placed in the wound.

To mobilize the kidney, the surgeon must first free it from Gerota's capsule (the fascia that encompasses the kidney). Using a knife, the surgeon incises the capsule and extends the incision with Metzenbaum scissors. Blunt dissection is then used to separate the kidney from the capsule and surrounding fatty tissue. Once the kidney is separated from the capsule, the surgeon identifies and frees the ureter from its attachments by sharp dissection. The technologist should have a narrow Penrose drain available to sling around the ureter. The assistant can then use the drain to retract the ureter.

Using right-angled clamps, the surgeon dissects the renal artery and vein free. The vessels may be clamped individually or together. When they are divided individually, the surgeon uses two right-angled clamps to occlude the vessels. They are ligated with size 0 silk suture mounted on a passer and divided with Metzenbaum scissors. When divided together, kidney pedicle clamps are placed across the kidney pedicle. The surgeon then divides between the clamps and ligates the pedicle with heavy silk suture, size 0.

The surgeon next places two clamps across the ureter and divides it (Fig. 22–8). The distal end of the ureter is ligated with a suture ligature of size 0 or 2-0 chromic catgut swaged to a taper needle. Thus freed, the kidney is then passed to the technologist as a specimen.

The wound is closed in separate layers. The peritoneum, if it has been incised, is closed with a running

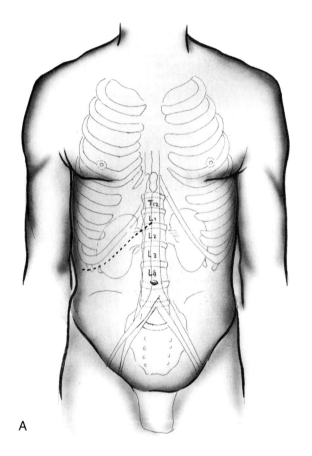

A

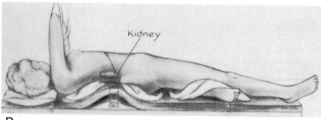

B

Figure 22–7. A. Subcostal incision for anterior approach. B. Flank incision. This is a common approach to the kidney and ureters. (From Harrison JH, et al: Campbell's Urology, 4th ed. Philadelphia, WB Saunders, 1978.)

suture of size 0 chromic catgut. Muscle layers are closed with the surgeon's preferred suture; a variety of materials are used to close the muscle. The fascia is usually closed with Dexon or a synthetic suture, size 2-0. Subcutaneous tissue is closed with size 3-0 absorbable suture. Skin is closed according to the surgeon's preference for suture or skin staples.

Nephrostomy

Definition

This is the establishment of a drain in the renal pelvis for temporary urinary diversion to the outside of the body. When a ureter becomes obstructed because of infection, injury, or other cause, the renal pelvis becomes distended with urine, a condition called *hydronephrosis*. By placing a drain in the renal pelvis, the condition is relieved until the obstruction can be removed.

Highlights

1. The retroperitoneal space is entered.
2. The renal pelvis is identified.
3. A tunnel is formed in the kidney.
4. The drain is inserted.
5. The wound is closed.

Description

The patient is placed in the lateral position. The surgeon gains access to the retroperitoneal space using a flank incision. Gerota's fascia at the lower pole of the kidney is incised with the deep knife. The surgeon then identifies the ureter, which is isolated with Metzenbaum scissors. A small Penrose drain is slung around the ureter for retraction.

Using blunt dissection, the surgeon exposes the renal pelvis. A small incision is then made into the pelvis. The technologist should have small hemostatic forceps, such as Kelly, Crile, or Randall stone forceps, available for the surgeon to tunnel through the kidney. The surgeon pushes the forceps through the kidney to create a passageway for the catheter (Fig. 22-9A). The technologist should have several different sizes of nephrostomy tubes available at this time. After the surgeon tunnels through the kidney, the catheter is grasped with the clamp and pulled back through the previously made tunnel (Fig. 22-9B and C). The winged tip of the catheter is now drawn back into the renal pelvis (Fig. 22-9D).

To close the incision made in the kidney, the surgeon places several sutures of size 4-0 chromic catgut swaged to a fine taper needle. The end of the catheter is brought out of the abdominal wall through a stab wound made near the incision. A large Penrose drain is placed near the kidney, and the wound is cleaned in routine fashion, as previously described. The nephrostomy tube is secured to the skin with heavy silk sutures, size 0.

Kidney Transplantation

Definition

This is the transplant of a kidney from a living donor or cadaver. Kidney transplant is performed on an otherwise healthy patient who suffers from renal failure. Ideally, the donor should be a close family member such as a twin, parent, or sibling. Two surgical teams work

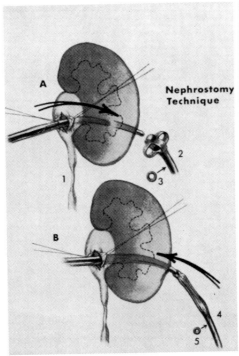
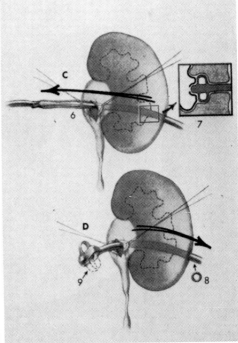

Figure 22–9. *A.* Nephrostomy. The surgeon creates a tunnel in the kidney with a blunt clamp. *B* and *C.* The surgeon grasps the catheter and withdraws it into the kidney. *D.* The winged tip of the catheter is drawn into the renal pelvis. (From Harrison JH, et al: Campbell's Urology, 4th ed. Philadelphia, WB Saunders, 1978.)

simultaneously so that the time that elapses between the recipient's nephrectomy and the implantation of the donor's kidney is as short as possible. The following is a *basic* description of a transplant. More detailed techniques should be learned in actual training.

Highlights

1. A nephrectomy is performed on the donor.
2. The donor kidney is placed in the recipient's iliac fossa.
3. Arterial and venous anastomoses are performed.
4. The donor ureter is implanted in the bladder.
5. The wound is closed.

Description

After a routine prep and draping, a nephrectomy is performed on the donor. Careful attention is given to preserving the renal vein, artery, and ureter. Before applying clamps to the renal vessels, the patient is given a heparinized saline injection to prevent coagulation.

Once the kidney has been removed, it must be kept cold before its transfer to the recipient. This is accomplished by using a cold electrolyte solution, which is infused into the kidney through an intravenous catheter and sterile intravenous tubing. The kidney is placed in a basin of cold saline solution, and the catheter is inserted into the renal artery. The electrolyte solution is then allowed to drip into the artery, thus reducing its temperature and flushing the donor's blood from the kidney. The kidney is flushed for 4 to 5 minutes.

The kidney is brought to the recipient team by the donor's surgeon. The surgeon of the recipient team makes a long inguinal incision. The incision is carried down to the iliac fossa by blunt and sharp dissection. The kidney will be placed in the patient's iliac fossa to avoid peritonitis, in case of postoperative infection (Fig. 22–10). The surgeon identifies the external iliac vein and hypogastric artery. Anastomoses are then performed between the renal artery and hypogastric artery and between the renal vein and external iliac vein. The anastomoses are performed with size 4-0 or 5-0 nonabsorbable vascular suture (Tevdek, Ti-Cron, or Prolene). Before the anastomoses, the patient is given a systemic dose of heparin.

The surgeon then implants the donor ureter in the bladder. The bladder is grasped with two or more Allis clamps and then incised. A separate incision is made to accommodate the ureter. The surgeon sutures the ureter through the first incision, using size 3-0 or 4-0 chromic catgut or Dexon. A Penrose drain is implanted near the bladder wall. The first incision is closed in three layers with size 2-0 or 3-0 chromic catgut or Dexon. This completes the procedure, and the wound is closed in layers, as for an inguinal hernia.

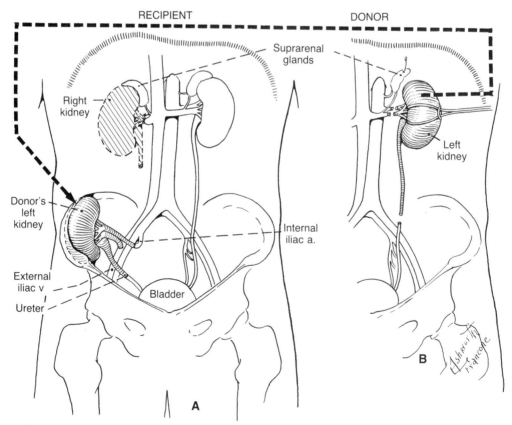

Figure 22–10. *A.* Kidney transplanted to right pelvis. *B.* Donor kidney. (From Jacob S, Francone C, Lossow WJ: Structure and Function in Man, 5th ed. Philadelphia, WB Saunders, 1982.)

Pyelolithotomy

Definition

This is surgical removal of calculi (stones) from the renal pelvis. A large stone that fills the renal pelvis can completely obstruct the flow of urine.

Highlights

1. The retroperitoneal space is entered.
2. The renal pelvis is incised.
3. The stone is removed.
4. The renal pelvis is closed.
5. The wound is closed.

Description

With the patient in the lateral position, the surgeon enters the retroperitoneal space through a flank incision as for a simple nephrectomy. The surgeon mobilizes the ureter with both blunt and sharp dissection. A small Penrose drain is slung around the ureter both for traction and to prevent a stone from migrating down the ureter during the procedure.

Before incising the renal pelvis, the surgeon may place two or three traction sutures of size 3-0 chromic catgut on either side of the incision site. The kidney is then incised with the knife (Fig. 22–11). The stone is lifted out with tissue forceps and is passed to the technologist as a specimen.

After the stone has been removed, the surgeon passes a ureteral catheter down the ureter and into the bladder to make sure that no stones have migrated down the ureter.

The incision in the renal pelvis may be closed with interrupted sutures of chromic catgut, size 4-0 or 5-0, swaged on a fine taper needle. The wound is irrigated with warm saline solution. The technologist should have one or two large Penrose drains available, which are placed near the renal pelvis. The wound is then closed in routine fashion.

Ileal Conduit

Definition

This is implantation of the ureters into a divided segment of the ileum and the creation of an ileostomy to provide urinary diversion. There are many different types of urinary diversion procedures that use a segment of bowel to replace the bladder. The ileal conduit is a common procedure performed for malignancy of the bladder, severe stricture of the distal ureter, or other conditions that require urinary diversion.

Highlights

1. A portion of the colon and ileum are mobilized.
2. The ureters are divided.
3. The ileum is divided.
4. The proximal end of the ileal segment is closed.

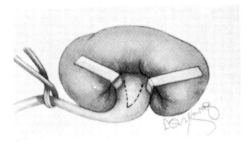

Figure 22–11. Pyelolithotomy. V-shaped incision in the renal pelvis. (From Harrison JH, et al: Campbell's Urology, 4th ed. Philadelphia, WB Saunders, 1978.)

5. An end-to-end anastomosis of the ileum is performed.
6. The ureters are implanted into the ileum.
7. An ileostomy is performed.
8. The wound is closed.

Description

Many of the techniques used in this procedure have been discussed in Chapter 21. In preparation for the procedure, the technologist should have gastrointestinal and long instruments available.

The patient is placed in the supine position, prepped, and draped for an upper midline incision. To begin the procedure, the surgeon enters the abdomen and retroperitoneal cavity. A Balfour retractor is placed in the wound. A portion of the large intestine and adjoining ileum are mobilized, as for a bowel resection.

Four intestinal clamps, such as Allen-Kocher clamps, are placed across a segment of the ileum, two at each end (Fig. 22–12A). The surgeon then divides the ileum in both places, cutting between the sets of clamps with the knife or cautery pencil. The proximal end of the ileum is closed with double layers of chromic catgut sutures, size 3-0, swaged to a fine taper needle. A third layer of size 4-0 silk sutures may be placed over the anastomosis (Fig. 22–12B). The surgeon then performs an end-to-end anastomosis of the severed ileum to restore its continuity (Fig. 22–12C).

After identifying the ureters, the surgeon divides them and performs an end-to-side anastomosis between the ureters and the isolated segment of ileum (Fig. 22–12D). The anastomosis is performed with interrupted sutures of 4-0 chromic catgut.

To perform the ileostomy, the surgeon first incises the skin over the area of the proposed stoma, taking a small disk of tissue from the abdominal wall. The open end of the ileal segment is then brought through the hole and everted (Fig. 22–12E). The surgeon sutures the everted ileal segment to the skin using size 3-0 interrupted Dexon sutures swaged to a fine cutting needle. The wound is then irrigated with warm saline solution and closed in routine fashion.

Related Procedures

Ureterosigmoidostomy
Ureteroenterocutaneous diversion

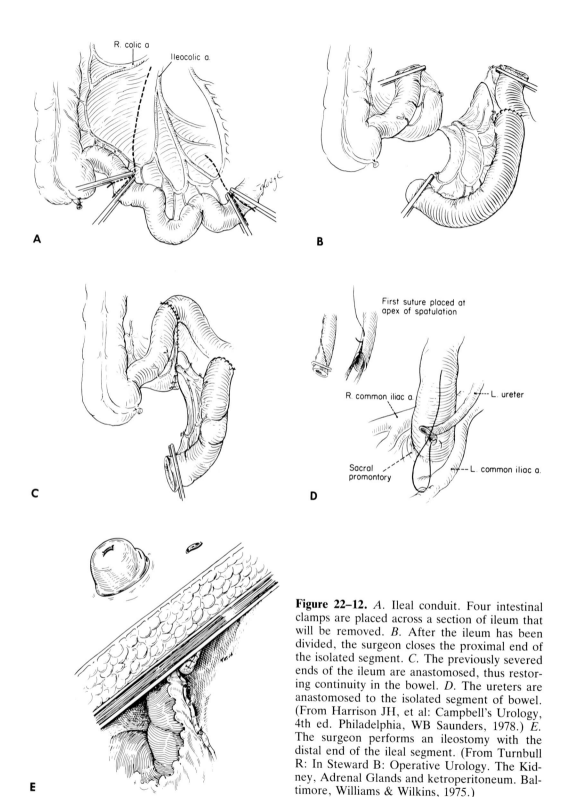

Figure 22–12. *A.* Ileal conduit. Four intestinal clamps are placed across a section of ileum that will be removed. *B.* After the ileum has been divided, the surgeon closes the proximal end of the isolated segment. *C.* The previously severed ends of the ileum are anastomosed, thus restoring continuity in the bowel. *D.* The ureters are anastomosed to the isolated segment of bowel. (From Harrison JH, et al: Campbell's Urology, 4th ed. Philadelphia, WB Saunders, 1978.) *E.* The surgeon performs an ileostomy with the distal end of the ileal segment. (From Turnbull R: In Steward B: Operative Urology. The Kidney, Adrenal Glands and ketroperitoneum. Baltimore, Williams & Wilkins, 1975.)

Sigmoid conduit diversion
Ureterojejunal cutaneous diversion

Ureterolithotomy

Definition

This is surgical removal of a stone from the ureter.

Highlights

1. The retroperitoneal space is entered.
2. The ureter is incised.
3. The stone is removed.
4. The wound is closed.

Description

Depending on the location of the stone in the ureter, the surgeon may choose one of several incisions to gain access to the ureter (Fig. 22–13). For the midline and inguinal approaches, the patient is placed in the supine position. The lateral position is used for a flank approach. Once the surgeon has entered the retroperitoneal space, the location of the stone is identified by manual examination. Metzenbaum scissors are used to dissect the ureter free. A small Penrose drain is placed around the ureter above the area of the stone to prevent its migration into the renal pelvis. The surgeon may place a Babcock clamp across the ureter below the stone to prevent it from moving downward.

Using a No. 15 knife blade, the surgeon makes a small incision over the stone. The stone is removed with fine tissue forceps.

The ureteral incision may, in some instances, be closed with interrupted chromic catgut sutures, size 4-0 or 5-0. Some surgeons prefer to leave the ureteral incision open and allow it to close spontaneously.

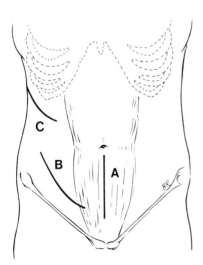

Figure 22–13. Surgical approaches to the ureters: A, lower midline incision; B, inguinal approach; C, flank incision. (From Harrison JH, et al: Campbell's Urology, 4th ed. Philadelphia, WB Saunders, 1978.)

Related Procedures

Ureterectomy
Ureteroureterostomy

Suprapubic Cystostomy

Definition

This is the placement of a suprapubic catheter into the bladder for drainage. A suprapubic catheter is used when a urethral catheter is undesirable, such as in the event of a urethral stricture. A suprapubic catheter is more comfortable for the patient than a urethral catheter and may be used when urinary diversion is required for a long period of time.

Highlights

1. The space of Retzius is entered.
2. The bladder is incised.
3. The catheter is positioned in the bladder.
4. The bladder is closed.
5. The wound is closed.

Description

The patient is placed in the supine position, prepped, and draped for a suprapubic incision. This area lies just above the pubic symphysis. The incision passes through the skin, fatty subcutaneous layer, fascia, and muscle fibers. The peritoneal cavity is *not* entered, since the area lying between the bladder and the symphysis pubis (the space of Retzius, which is the operative site) is bounded superiorly (at the top) by the abdominal peritoneum. Because the muscle fibers are quite vascular and contain many large veins, the technologist should have an ample supply of lap sponges available. The incision is made with the knife and carried through to the bladder with the cautery pencil or dissecting scissors.

The surgeon places two Allis clamps on the bladder wall and makes a small incision between the clamps. A pursestring suture is then placed around the bladder incision, and the catheter is threaded into the bladder. Malecot or Pezzer catheters are commonly used. The pursestring suture is tied snugly around the catheter, and the bladder incision is closed with interrupted sutures of size 0 or 2-0 chromic catgut swaged to a taper needle. The suprapubic incision is then closed in layers.

An alternative method of suprapubic cystostomy involves the use of a Silastic catheter that is placed in the bladder through a stab wound made in the skin over and through the bladder wall. A Cystocath catheter (made by Dow Corning Wright, Arlington, TN) is commonly used. To insert the catheter, the surgeon makes a small stab incision using a No. 11 knife blade. The Cystocath kit comes complete with a trocar and cannula that are thrust through the stab incision. The trocar is then removed and the catheter inserted through the cannula. The surgeon removes the cannula and places a special Silastic disk over the catheter and glues it to the patient's skin with surgical adhesive. The wound is neither sutured nor dressed.

Vesicourethral Suspension (Marshall-Marchetti-Krantz Procedure)

Definition

This is suspension of the bladder neck and urethra to the cartilage of the pubic symphysis to treat urinary stress incontinence in the female. The patient with urinary stress incontinence experiences urine leakage while straining in such activities as coughing, laughing, or bending.

Highlights

1. The space of Retzius is entered.
2. The bladder neck and urethra are sutured to the symphysis.
3. The wound is closed.

Description

Before the procedure begins, the circulator places a Foley catheter in the patient's bladder. The patient is placed in the supine position, prepped, and draped for a suprapubic incision. The technologist should have long instruments available, including long needle holders and long Allis clamps.

After entering the space of Retzius, the surgeon begins the procedure by placing his or her hand over the bladder to retract it upward. This exposes the urethra (Fig. 22–14A). The surgeon may grasp the bladder neck with several long Allis clamps. Several interrupted sutures of Dexon or Dacron, size 2-0, mounted on a small, stout, tapered needle, are then placed through the tissue surrounding the urethra (Fig. 22–14B). The needle is passed through the cartilage attached to the symphysis. Several of these sutures are placed in succession. The sutures are left long. The assistant is then required to place a finger in the vagina to release the pressure on the sutures while the surgeon ties them in place. Following this maneuver, the technologist must, of course, reglove the assistant. This completes the procedure. A large Penrose drain is placed in the space of Retzius, and the wound is closed in routine fashion.

Suprapubic Prostatectomy

Definition

This is removal of the prostate gland through an incision in the bladder. Approximately 90% of all prostatectomies are performed transurethrally, while a suprapubic or retropubic approach is the next most commonly used technique. (The transurethral approach is discussed later in this chapter.) Prostatectomy is performed to treat cancer of the prostate and for benign hypertrophy (enlargement) of the prostate, which occurs in the geriatric patient and causes urinary obstruction.

Highlights

1. The space of Retzius is entered.
2. The bladder is incised.
3. The prostatic mucosa is incised.
4. The prostate is removed.
5. A suprapubic catheter is inserted.
6. The bladder is closed.
7. The wound is closed.

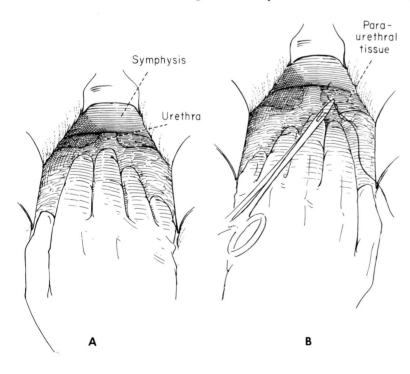

Figure 22–14. *A.* Vesicourethral suspension. After entering the pelvis, the surgeon gains access to the ureter by placing his hand over the bladder to retract it upward. *B.* The surgeon suspends the bladder neck by placing several sutures through the tissue surrounding the urethra and attaching them to the cartilage of the symphysis. (From Parsons L, Ulfelder H: Atlas of Pelvic Operations, 2nd ed. Philadelphia, WB Saunders, 1968.)

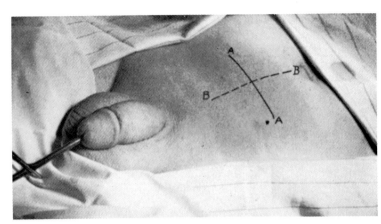

Figure 22–15. Surgical approaches for suprapubic prostatectomy. The surgeon may make a transverse (A) or longitudinal (B) incision over the pelvis. (From Harrison JH, et al: Campbell's Urology, 4th ed. Philadelphia, WB Saunders, 1978.)

Description

The patient is placed in the supine position, and shoulder braces are attached to the operating table so that the patient can be tipped into a severe Trendelenburg position. The patient is prepped and draped for a suprapubic incision.

The surgeon makes a transverse or longitudinal incision above the pubis (Fig. 22–15). After access is gained to the space of Retzius, a Balfour retractor may be placed in the wound. As for any suprapubic procedure, the technologist can expect a very bloody field and should have an ample supply of lap sponges, hemostats, and suction available. Stick sponges are used frequently during the procedure.

Before opening the bladder, the surgeon places two traction sutures of size 0 chromic catgut on either side of the incision site. The bladder may be grasped with Allis clamps and pulled up by the assistant. The surgeon then makes a short incision in the bladder, using a No. 10 or No. 15 knife blade mounted on a No. 7 knife handle. The technologist should have suction available as soon as the bladder is incised to drain its contents (Fig. 22–16). After draining the bladder, the surgeon places a bladder retractor (Judd) or Deaver retractor in the bladder wound. The surgeon incises the prostatic mucosa with the No. 15 knife blade or cautery pencil. The bladder retractors are then removed.

Using his or her fingers, the surgeon *enucleates* (removes cleanly without trauma to the tissue) the diseased prostate from its fossa (cavity) (Fig. 22–17). The prostate is passed to the technologist as a specimen.

The surgeon replaces the bladder retractor and examines the prostatic fossa for bleeding vessels. Many surgeons prefer to pack the fossa with a sponge for a few minutes to maintain hemostasis. Large bleeding vessels are ligated with suture ligatures of chromic catgut, size 0 or 2-0. Oozing surfaces are covered with a hemostatic agent, such as Surgicel or Avitene. A Foley catheter with a size 30-mL balloon is then inserted by the surgeon with the balloon at the bladder neck. Most surgeons prefer to drain the bladder through a suprapubic catheter, which is inserted at this time. A Malecot or Pezzer catheter is placed in the wound and brought out through a small stab incision near the suprapubic incision (Fig. 22–18). The bladder is then closed with

two layers of size 0 or 2-0 chromic catgut; the sutures may be interrupted or running. Before closing the wound, a large Penrose drain is placed in the space of Retzius. The wound is then closed in routine fashion.

Retropubic Prostatectomy

Definition

This is surgical removal of the prostate gland. Unlike a suprapubic prostatectomy, the bladder is not entered. The indications for retropubic prostatectomy are the same as for suprapubic prostatectomy. The choice of approach is based on the surgeon's preference or familiarity with one of the procedures.

Highlights

1. The space of Retzius is entered.
2. The prostatic capsule is incised.
3. The prostate is removed.
4. The prostatic capsule is closed.
5. The wound is closed.

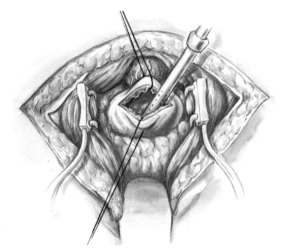

Figure 22–16. Suprapubic prostatectomy. The bladder is incised to gain access to the prostate. Note traction sutures on each side of the incision. (From Harrison JH, et al: Campbell's Urology, 4th ed. Philadelphia, WB Saunders, 1978.)

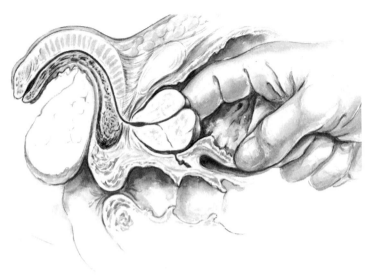

Figure 22–17. Suprapubic prostatectomy. The surgeon bluntly dissects the prostate from the fossa. (From Harrison JH, et al: Campbell's Urology, 4th ed. Philadelphia, WB Saunders, 1978.)

Description

The patient is placed in the supine position, prepped, and draped for a suprapubic incision. The surgeon enters the space of Retzius as previously described, through a low transverse incision. A Balfour retractor is placed in the wound.

Before incising the prostatic capsule, the surgeon may place two traction sutures of size 0 chromic catgut through the capsule (Fig. 22–19A). The sutures should be swaged to a taper needle. Using the deep knife, the surgeon incises the capsule and extends the incision with Metzenbaum scissors or the cautery pencil. The gland is then dissected free with sharp and blunt dissection and passed to the technologist as a specimen (Fig. 22–19B).

The surgeon packs the fossa with sponges to control bleeding; the sponges are left in place for several minutes. The technologist should have a hemostatic agent (Surgicel or Avitene) of the surgeon's preference available. This is placed in the fossa to control oozing from small vessels. Large bleeding vessels are ligated with suture ligatures of size 0 or 2-0 chromic catgut.

Before the wound is closed, the surgeon places a Foley catheter with a 30-mL balloon in the patient's bladder. A large Penrose drain is placed in the space of Retzius, and the wound is then closed in routine fashion.

Circumcision

Definition

This is surgical removal of the prepuce (foreskin). Circumcision is commonly performed on the male infant at birth. However, the uncircumcised adult may experience difficulty in retracting the prepuce from the glans of the penis because of a stricture in the prepuce (Fig. 22–20A). This condition (phimosis) is surgically treated by circumcision. The condition of paraphimosis (the

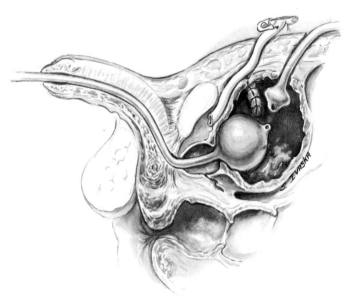

Figure 22–18. Suprapubic prostatectomy. At the completion of the procedure, a Malecot catheter is inserted in the wound and brought out through a stab wound made near the incision. (From Harrison JH, et al: Campbell's Urology, 4th ed. Philadelphia, WB Saunders, 1978.)

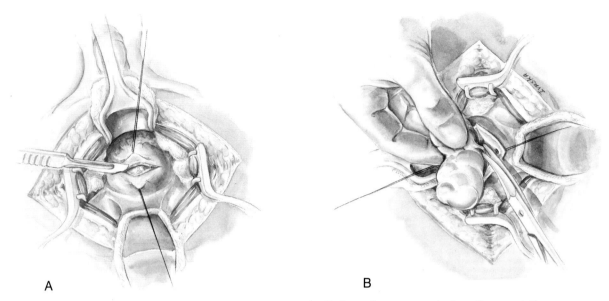

Figure 22–19. *A.* Retropubic prostatectomy. Before the surgeon incises the prostatic capsule, he or she places two traction sutures through the capsule. *B.* The prostate is dissected from its capsule with Metzenbaum scissors. (From Harrison JH, et al: Campbell's Urology, 4th ed. Philadelphia, WB Saunders, 1978.)

inability of the foreskin to fall forward over the glans) is also treated by circumcision.

If the procedure is performed for religious purposes on the Jewish male, all *female* surgical team members may be barred from the operating room suite during the procedure.

Highlights

1. The prepuce is grasped with straight hemostats.
2. The prepuce is incised and removed.
3. The wound is closed.

Description

With the patient in the supine position, the surgeon places several straight Kelly or Crile hemostats on the edge of the prepuce. Using fine dissecting scissors, a longitudinal incision is then made through the prepuce. A circular incision through the prepuce is made similarly (Fig. 22–20B). The surgeon passes the excised prepuce to the technologist as a specimen. Small bleeders are controlled with the cautery pencil. The surgeon then approximates the skin edges with interrupted sutures of size 4-0 or 5-0 chromic catgut or Dexon swaged to a fine

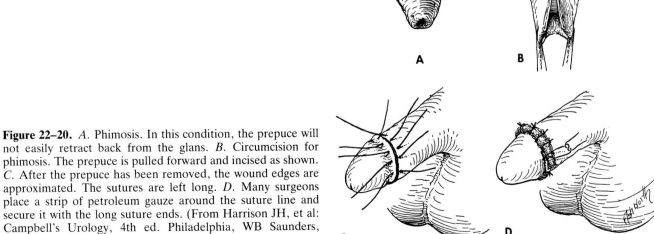

Figure 22–20. *A.* Phimosis. In this condition, the prepuce will not easily retract back from the glans. *B.* Circumcision for phimosis. The prepuce is pulled forward and incised as shown. *C.* After the prepuce has been removed, the wound edges are approximated. The sutures are left long. *D.* Many surgeons place a strip of petroleum gauze around the suture line and secure it with the long suture ends. (From Harrison JH, et al: Campbell's Urology, 4th ed. Philadelphia, WB Saunders, 1978.)

cutting needle (Fig. 22–20C). The skin is not approximated in the very young infant. The technologist should have a strip of nonadherent gauze (Xeroform or Adaptic) available, since some surgeons tie the previously placed sutures around the gauze (Fig. 22–20D) as a dressing. No other dressings are necessary.

Repair of Hypospadias

Definition

This is surgical correction of a urethral meatus, found abnormally on the undersurface of the penis. Hypospadias is a congenital defect that interferes with normal urination and fertilization of the female. It is often associated with abnormal curvature of the penis caused by stricture of its fibrous tissue, a condition known as *chordee*.

Highlights

1. The chordee is released.
2. A flap of skin is taken from the penis.
3. The flap is fashioned into a tube.
4. The tube is sutured to the distal urethra.
5. The skin is approximated.

Description

With the patient in the lithotomy position, the surgeon makes an incision into the penis to the level of the strictured fascia. The fascia is then excised. The surgeon creates a flap in the prepuce and brings the penis through the flap. Sutures of interrupted Dexon are then used to approximate the skin (Fig. 22–21). The technique for hypospadias repair is illustrated and described in Figure 22–22.

Insertion of Penile Implant

Definition

This is the insertion of a rigid or semirigid implant (Fig. 22–23) into the body of the penis in cases of organic impotence. Diseases such as Peyronie's disease, multiple sclerosis, or atherosclerosis of the iliac artery may cause impotence. Radical pelvic surgery may also cause this condition. The insertion of a prosthesis allows the patient to resume normal sexual activity. Patients are carefully screened for the procedure, and the patient's wife may also be consulted.

Highlights

1. An appropriate prosthesis is chosen.
2. A small incision is made at the base of the penis.
3. Each corpus cavernosum is incised and dilated.
4. The prosthesis is inserted.
5. The wound is closed.

Description

Before beginning the procedure, the surgeon usually indicates which size prosthesis is to be used. The prosthesis should be handled with utmost care. Do not allow the prosthesis to come in contact with linen towels, because small lint particles could adhere to it. If the prosthesis is the inflatable type, no sharp objects should come in contact with it. A complete discussion on handling Silastic prosthetic materials is presented in Chapter 29.

The patient is placed in the lithotomy position, and the penile-scrotal area is prepped. The inguinal area should also be prepped as for a hernia repair.

The surgeon makes a small incision at the base of the penis and uses cautery to control small bleeding vessels. The corpus cavernosum (spongy portion) of the penis is then identified on each side. At this time, the surgeon may insert a Foley catheter to aid in the identification of the urethra during the rest of the procedure. Using Hagar dilators and/or a Pean clamp, the surgeon dilates each corpus cavernosum to allow passage of the prosthesis. The prosthesis is then inserted. If the prosthesis includes an inflation pump, it is placed into the scrotum. The pump reservoir is placed inside the internal ring. The pump is then tested for function and integrity. The wound is closed with interrupted sutures of 2-0 or 3-0 Dexon and dressed with compression-type dressing.

Simple Orchiectomy

Definition

This is surgical removal of one or both testicles. It is indicated for malignancy of the testicles or prostate gland. When the testicle has suffered *torsion* (twisting of the testicle around the vas deferens) and its blood supply is interrupted, the testicle may become gangrenous. Orchiectomy is performed in this instance. A testicle may also be removed to treat chronic infection.

Highlights

1. The scrotum is incised.
2. The vas deferens and vessels are divided and ligated.
3. The testicle is removed.
4. The wound is closed.

Description

The patient is placed in the supine position, prepped, and draped for a scrotal incision. The surgeon incises the scrotum over the testicle and delivers it from the wound. Small bleeding vessels are cauterized or clamped with mosquito hemostats and ligated with size 4-0 chromic catgut or Dexon sutures.

The surgeon then places two Mayo clamps across the vas deferens and vessels. The tissue is ligated with the knife or dissecting scissors. The testicle, now released,

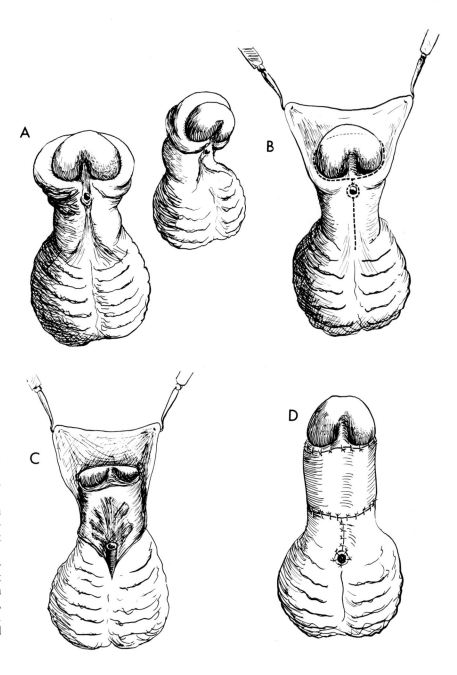

Figure 22–21. Release of chordee. *A.* Condition of hypospadias with chordee. *B.* Dotted lines indicate area of incision. Prepuce is retracted forward with skin hooks. *C.* Once the skin is incised, the surgeon releases the chordee by incising the strictured fascia. The prepuce is then brought over the glans in a buttonhole fashion. *D.* The skin is approximated with fine interrupted sutures, thus covering the defect left from the release of chordee. (From Schwartz SI, et al: Principles of Surgery, 2nd ed. New York, McGraw-Hill, 1974. Used with the permission of McGraw-Hill Book Company.)

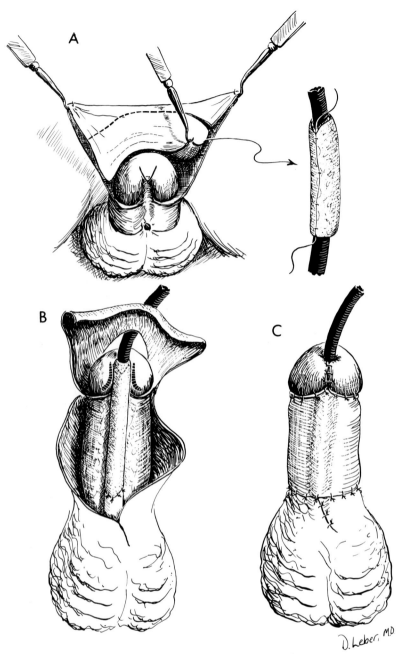

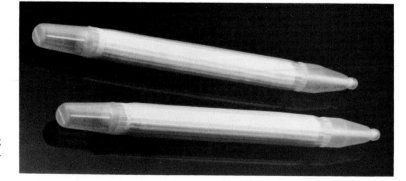

Figure 22–22. Repair of hypospadias. *A.* The surgeon excises the inner surface of the prepuce and wraps the graft around a catheter. The edges of the graft are approximated with fine sutures. (If the patient has already been circumcised, the graft may be taken from the skin of the inner arm.) *B.* After incising the penis as shown, the surgeon sutures the graft to the distal urethra. *C.* The skin is approximated with fine interrupted sutures. (From Schwartz SI, et al: Principles of Surgery, 2nd ed. New York, McGraw-Hill, 1974. Used with the permission of McGraw-Hill Book Company.)

Figure 22–23. AMS 600, Dynaflex, and 700 Ultrex Plus penile prostheses. (Courtesy of American Medical Systems, Inc., Minnetonka, MN.)

is passed to the technologist as a specimen. The vas and its vessels are then ligated with heavy chromic catgut or Dexon, size 0 or 1.

Before closing the wound, the surgeon may place a testicular prosthesis in the scrotum. Silastic prostheses are available in different sizes. It may be placed loose in the scrotal sac or the surgeon may suture the prosthesis to the scrotal wall. A small Penrose drain is placed in the scrotum, which is then closed in layers with size 4-0 Dexon or chromic catgut swaged to a fine cutting needle. The scrotum is then dressed with gauze dressing and a scrotal support.

Orchidopexy

Definition

This is surgical correction of an undescended testicle. During normal fetal life, the testicles are retained within the abdomen. Occasionally one or both testicles fail to descend into the scrotum. Orchidopexy is the attachment of the previously undescended testicle to the scrotal wall. This procedure is usually performed on the child before he is of school age.

Highlights

1. The inguinal area is incised.
2. The testicle is located and mobilized.
3. A tunnel is made through the inguinal region into the scrotum.
4. The testicle is brought through the tunnel and sutured in place.
5. The wounds are closed.

Description

The patient is placed in the supine position, prepped, and draped, with the inguinal and groin area on the affected side exposed. Using a No. 10 knife blade the surgeon makes an incision over the area of the external ring, as for a hernia repair. The incision is deepened with Metzenbaum scissors and cautery pencil on a very low setting. Small bleeding vessels are cauterized or clamped with mosquito hemostats and ligated with fine surgical catgut or Dexon ties. The surgeon dissects the spermatic cord free using both sharp and blunt dissection. A small hemostat is then placed at the tip of the testicle.

To create a tunnel for the testicle, the surgeon may use a finger or a blunt clamp, such as a Mayo clamp or sponge forceps (Fig. 22–24). The instrument or finger is pushed forcibly through the groin and into the scrotum. The testicle is then brought through the tunnel. The scrotum is incised to expose the scrotal septum and several sutures of size 3-0 or 4-0 Dexon mounted on a fine cutting needle are placed through the septum and testicle, thus securing it in place (Fig. 22–25). Rather than attaching the testicle to the scrotum, some surgeons attach a rubber band to a suture placed in the testicle and tape the rubber band to the thigh. However, it has been found that this device does not afford enough

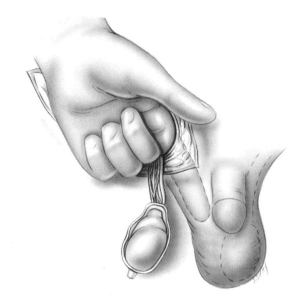

Figure 22–24. Orchidopexy for an undescended testicle. To create a passageway for the testicle, the surgeon pushes his or her finger forcibly through the groin and into the scrotum. (From Harrison JH, et al: Campbell's Urology, 4th ed. Philadelphia, WB Saunders, 1978.)

traction on the testicle because of the active movements of a normal child.

The scrotal incision is closed with interrupted sutures of size 4-0 Dexon or chromic catgut swaged to a fine cutting needle. The inguinal incision is closed in layers with fine catgut or Dexon. A subcuticular suture is usually used on skin if the child is very young.

Vasectomy

Definition

This is surgical removal of a small portion of the vas deferens performed as an elective sterilization proce-

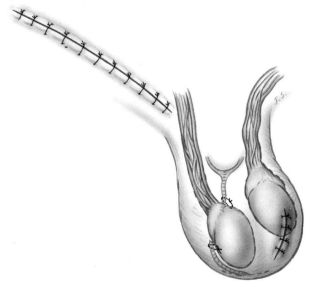

Figure 22–25. Orchidopexy. The testicle is secured to the scrotal wall with several sutures.

dure. It can be easily done under a local anesthetic and is often performed in the outpatient department of the hospital.

Highlights

1. The scrotum is incised.
2. The vas deferens is resected.
3. The scrotum is closed.

Description

With the patient in the supine position, the surgeon makes a small incision in the scrotum with a No. 10 or No. 15 knife blade. The surgeon grasps the vas with an Allis clamp and separates it from surrounding tissue with a hemostat or dissecting scissors (Fig. 22–26). The vas is then grasped with two Kelly clamps, and a small section of vas lying between the clamps is removed. The cut ends are cauterized. The surgeon may choose to bury the severed ends within the scrotal fascia with one or two sutures of fine chromic catgut or Dexon size 3-0 (Fig. 22–27). The procedure is repeated on the opposite vas.

The incisions are closed in layers with interrupted sutures of size 3-0 or 4-0 Dexon on a fine cutting needle (Fig. 22–28).

Hydrocelectomy

Definition

This is the surgical removal of a fluid-filled sac located around the testicle in the scrotum. A hydrocele is caused by trauma, infection, irritation, or tumor within the scrotum. A hydrocele is often seen in conjunction with an inguinal hernia.

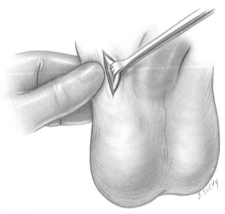

Figure 22–26. Vasectomy. After incising the scrotum, the surgeon grasps the vas with an Allis clamp and separates it from surrounding tissue with dissecting scissors. (From Harrison JH, et al: Campbell's Urology, 4th ed. Philadelphia, WB Saunders, 1978.)

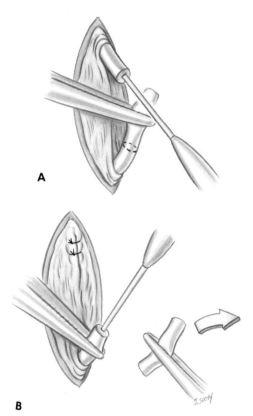

Figure 22–27. Vasectomy. *A.* After severing the vas, the surgeon cauterizes the ends. *B.* The severed ends may be buried within the scrotal fascia and sutured in place. (From Harrison JH, et al: Campbell's Urology, 4th ed. Philadelphia, WB Saunders, 1978.)

Highlights

1. The scrotum is incised.
2. The sac is removed.
3. The scrotum is closed.

Description

The patient is placed in the supine position, prepped, and draped for a scrotal incision. The surgeon makes a

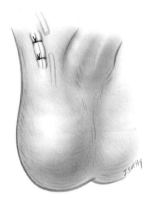

Figure 22–28. Vasectomy. The scrotal incision is closed with interrupted sutures. (From Harrison JH, et al: Campbell's Urology, 4th ed. Philadelphia, WB Saunders, 1978.)

small incision over the sac (Fig. 22–29). The cautery pencil is used to coagulate small bleeding vessels. The surgeon delivers the hydrocele through the incision and makes a small hole in the sac with the knife, cautery pencil, or dissecting scissors. The technologist should have suction available as soon as the sac is punctured to aspirate the liquid and prevent the drapes from becoming saturated. The surgeon then excises the sac and passes it to the technologist as a specimen (Fig. 22–30).

The surgeon checks the wound for small bleeding vessels, inserts a small Penrose drain, and closes the scrotum in layers with interrupted sutures of 3-0 Dexon on a fine cutting needle. The scrotum is then dressed with bulky gauze and a scrotal support.

CLOSED PROCEDURES: CYSTOSCOPY

The surgeon can perform a variety of procedures on the urethra, bladder, ureters, and prostate gland through the use of the fiberoptic cystoscope inserted into the bladder. Most modern hospitals are equipped with a special "cysto" room that is equipped with overhead x-ray equipment, a cystoscopy table specially designed to receive x-ray cassettes, and a storage area for supplies and instruments. Some "cysto" rooms are also equipped with wall units for anesthetic gas, oxygen, and suction. A typical "cysto" room is shown in Figure 22–31.

Special Equipment

Catheters

Urinary catheters (Fig. 22–32) are used for a variety of purposes, both in and out of surgery. These include (1) short-term urinary drainage, (2) long-term urinary drainage, (3) hemostasis, (4) evacuation of blood clots or blood, (5) diagnosis, and (6) maintenance of continuity of the urethra. Most hospitals maintain a supply

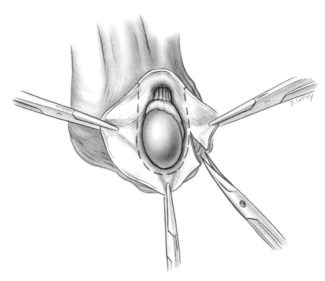

Figure 22–30. Hydrocelectomy. After incising the sac, the surgeon dissects it free and passes it to the technologist as a specimen. (From Harrison JH, et al: Campbell's Urology, 4th ed. Philadelphia, WB Saunders, 1978.)

of sterile catheters packaged by the manufacturer and designed for one-time use only. These are made of flexible nonirritating materials, such as latex rubber, Teflon-coated rubber, and plastic.

The lumen or bore of the catheter is measured in French sizes and ranges from 10 to 26 F. The most common sizes are those that range from size 16 to 18. Retention catheters also have a retention balloon size that is measured in cubic centimeters.

Urethral Catheters

Straight. The straight catheters are usually made of rubber and do not have a retention balloon. The most commonly used straight catheters are the Robinson and the Wishard catheters. The Robinson catheter, also called a utility or Red Robinson catheter, has one or two holes at the end. The Wishard catheters have just one hole at the end. These types of catheters are used for catheterization for diagnostic purposes. Examples of their use include checking residual urine and injecting contrast media for cystography. The utility catheter may also be used to simply drain the bladder before a surgical procedure.

Foley. The Foley catheter is the most commonly used retention catheter and has a variety of uses. The catheter remains in place in the bladder by means of an inflatable balloon located at the end of the catheter, which prevents it from sliding back out of the bladder. This type of catheter is available in sizes 8 through 30 F, and the retention balloon may be from 5 to 30 cc depending on the specific use of the catheter. The smaller balloon is used for simple retention, whereas the larger retention balloon is used for providing hemostasis postoperatively. The balloon is inflated with air or sterile water and should be tested before it is inserted to ensure its integrity. The larger balloons may also be intentionally

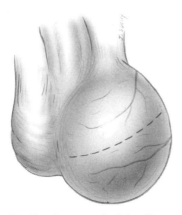

Figure 22–29. Hydrocelectomy. Incision line over hydrocele. (From Harrison JH, et al: Campbell's Urology, 4th ed. Philadelphia, WB Saunders, 1978.)

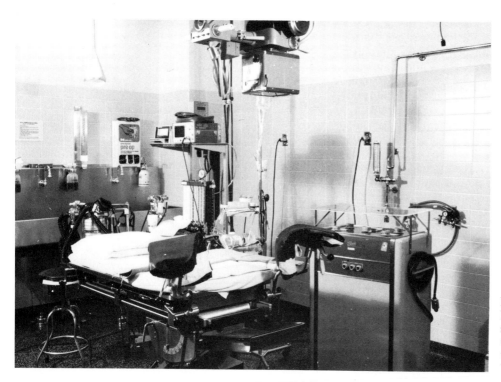

Figure 22–31. Cystoscopy room. Note overhead x-ray unit and special cystoscopy table. (From Greene LF, Segura JW: Transurethral Surgery. Philadelphia, WB Saunders, 1979.)

overinflated up to 120 cc for greater hemostatic efficiency.

Phillips. The Phillips catheter is straight but differs from the utility catheter in that one end has a screw tip designed to accept a filiform (small catheter used to locate a true passage through the urethra in case of stricture or the presence of a small passage). The filiform is of a much smaller diameter than the catheter and is easily manipulated in the urethra.

Coudé. The Coudé catheter can be straight or may be a Foley retention type. This type of catheter has a firm rubber tip or beak commonly used to facilitate its passage through a false urethral passage or beyond anatomic prominences in the urethra.

Gibbon. The Gibbon catheter is a long, thin catheter used mainly for long-term drainage of the bladder. A major disadvantage of the Gibbon catheter is that it has no device for self-retention and must be taped to the patient's thigh.

Ureteral Catheters

Ureteral catheters are used chiefly for retrograde pyelography (injection of contrast media into the kidney for diagnostic studies) and for the collection of urinary specimens directly from the kidney. Ureteral catheters are available in a variety of sizes and tip configurations (see Fig. 22–32). When these catheters are used for continuous urine collection and attached to collection bags, an adapter must be attached to the end of each catheter.

Irrigation and Evacuation

During cystoscopic examination and transurethral resection, it is necessary for the bladder to be distended.

This is done with the use of continuous irrigation. The irrigating fluid must not be an electrolyte because an electrolyte, such as a normal saline solution, will cause the dissipation of electricity when the electrosurgical unit is in use. Water must never be used during resection procedures because the irrigating solution is absorbed into the venous system during these procedures, and water will cause hemolysis (breakdown of red blood cells). Commonly used irrigation fluids are a sorbitol-mannitol combination of 1.5% glycine. Neither of these conducts electricity nor is harmful in case it should be absorbed by the body during resection procedures. All solutions should be stored at not more than 65°C. Temperatures greater than this tend to deteriorate the solutions. Solutions should not be used except at body temperature. Bladder spasm or hypothermia may occur when cold irrigation solutions are used.

Irrigation solutions are commercially prepared and are available in plastic bottles or pouches that are suspended above the operating table. During lengthy procedures, the bottles are piggybacked or connected to a Y tube that allows the circulator to change one bottle while another is in use (Fig. 22–33). (*Note:* It is important that empty bottles be replaced *immediately* during cystoscopic procedures.) Irrigation bottles should be hung 2½ to 3 feet above the cystoscopy table to maintain the correct amount of pressure within the bladder.

The fluid is evacuated from the bladder by the surgeon (by simply rotating a stopcock on the cystoscope), or the cystoscope may be equipped with a suction attachment.

Cystoscopy Table

The cystoscopy table differs from the standard operating table in that it is designed to maintain the patient

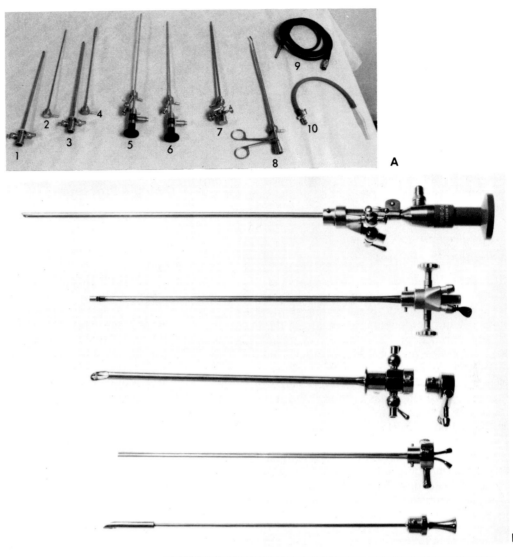

A

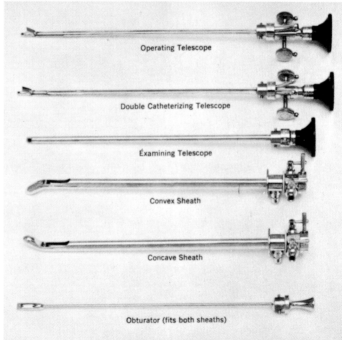

Operating Telescope

Double Catheterizing Telescope

Examining Telescope

Convex Sheath

Concave Sheath

Obturator (fits both sheaths)

B

C

Figure 22–34. *A.* Various types of cystoscopy instruments: 1 through 4, examination sheaths and obturators; 5, 6, telescopes; 7, catheter deflector; 8, biopsy forceps; 9, fiberoptic light cable; 10, irrigation tube. *B.* Greene cystoscope—utilizes fiberoptic lighting and ACMI microlens. *C.* Brown-Buerger cystoscope. By permission from American Cystoscope Makers. (*B* and *C* from Greene LF, Segura JW: Transurethral Surgery. Philadelphia, WB Saunders, 1979. *C* Courtesy of American Cystoscope Makers, Stamford, CT)

in intensity. The cable may attach to the telescope or the sheath, depending on the type of cystoscope in use. (See Chapter 20 for a more complete discussion of the fiberoptic light source and cable.)

Duties of the Cystoscopic Assistant

The circulating technologist who assists in cystoscopic and transurethral resection procedures is responsible for setting up the instrument table and all other equipment. The assistant dons sterile gloves to set up the instruments and other sterile supplies. The urologist does not require a scrubbed assistant so, after setting up the supplies, the assistant removes his or her gloves and functions as a circulator during the case.

Positioning the Patient

It is the technologist's duty to assist in positioning the patient on the cystoscopy table. The cystoscopy stirrups are a more modified (lower) version of those used commonly in open procedures involving the lower genital and perianal area. However, many patients who arrive for cystoscopic procedures suffer from hip deformities, including ankylosis or total hip fusion. In these cases, the cystoscopy stirrups are replaced with standard right-angled stirrups such as those used in gynecologic procedures. Extreme care must be taken when positioning the patient. The technologist must be particularly careful not to overextend the fixed joints in the patient with a hip deformity. The hip can usually be flexed but not necessarily abducted. The patient's chart should be checked before positioning the patient, and, if a hip deformity is present, the surgeon may assist and direct the safe positioning. All bony prominences must be padded properly. The proper positioning of the cystoscopy patient with a severe hip deformity is shown in Figure 22–35.

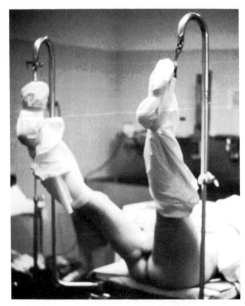

Figure 22–35. Proper positioning for patient with severe hip deformity. (From Greene LF, Segura JW: Transurethral Surgery. Philadelphia, WB Saunders, 1979.)

Electrosurgical Grounding and Settings

During cystoscopic procedures, the electrosurgical unit may be in frequent use, particularly during resection procedures. The grounding plate may be placed on the patient's thigh or waist. It must be placed over a fleshy area and never over a bony prominence. The electrosurgical unit should be placed on the lowest setting, which is increased gradually as directed by the urologist. (See Chapter 13 for a more complete discussion of the electrosurgical unit and precautions in its use.)

During a Procedure

During a cystoscopic procedure, the technologist has the following responsibilities:

1. Remain in the room at all times, unless otherwise directed by the urologist.
2. Connect the nonsterile ends of the power cables or suction tubing.
3. Open sterile supplies for the urologist, as needed.
4. Replace irrigation bottles as they empty. Note the number of bottles used.
5. Receive any specimens from the urologist and label them properly.
6. Monitor the patient's vital signs every 15 minutes, in case the procedure is done with the use of a local anesthetic.

Following a Procedure

Following a cystoscopic procedure, the technologist has the following responsibilities:

1. Assist in transferring the patient from the cystoscopy table to the stretcher, and accompany the urologist and/or anesthesiologist to the post-anesthesia care unit.
2. Transfer any tissue or fluid specimens to the designated area and record them in the specimen log.
3. Put away nonsterile supplies used during the procedure.
4. Transfer soiled equipment to the workroom and carry out terminal sterilization or decontamination on the equipment properly (see Chapters 6 and 7). In some operating rooms the cystoscopic equipment is washed and decontaminated in the cystoscopy room itself. If the instruments are to be decontaminated in a liquid chemical, they should be removed from the liquid promptly after a certain time, as specified by the manufacturer. Oversoaking can damage delicate instruments.

Diagnostic Procedures

The following are some common cystoscopic procedures used for diagnosis. They vary somewhat according to the surgeon or according to the specific equipment available.

Cystoscopy

During a simple cystoscopy, the urologist inserts the cystoscope into the bladder and examines it while it is distended. In addition to viewing the urethra, bladder neck, and bladder, the surgeon may take biopsy specimens of the inner mucosa or may obtain urine specimens from each separate kidney. The urine specimens are obtained with ureteral catheters and a catheter deflector. The urologist may also insert radiopaque dye into the kidney through the catheter and obtain radiographs of the flow of dye through the kidney and ureter. This is called a retrograde pyelogram. Biopsy tissue is taken with the biopsy forceps or with the brush biopsy instrument (Fig. 22–36).

Cystometrography

During cystometrography, the urologist instills irrigation fluid into the patient's bladder to measure the bladder's response to pressure and its capacity for fluid. The results of this procedure are shown on a cystometrogram.

Needle Biopsy of the Prostate

A needle biopsy is performed to obtain tissue from the prostate gland. The needle is inserted through the perineum and into the lobes of the prostate gland. The tissue obtained through the needle is passed to the technologist as a specimen and is later examined for malignancy. The tissue can be removed from the biopsy needle with a hypodermic needle.

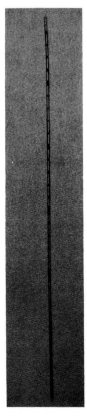

Figure 22–36. Brush biopsy instrument. (Courtesy of Vance Products.)

Surgical Procedures

Transurethral Resection

Transurethral resection means removing tissue piecemeal by inserting specialty cutting and coagulating instruments through the urethra, thereby gaining access to the tissue. Transurethral resection of the prostate (TURP) and transurethral resection of the bladder (TURB) are two common procedures that are approached in this manner.

The *resectoscope* (Fig. 22–37) is the instrument used to cut and coagulate tissue during transurethral resection. It consists of a telescope, cutting electrode (often called a "loop"), working element, sheath, and obturator. The resectoscope uses electric current generated by the electrosurgical unit to remove tissue piece by piece. Ball or curette-shaped electrodes are also used for hemostasis during the procedure.

There are several different types of working elements that vary according to the way in which the cutting electrode operates. Some require the surgeon to use both hands to operate the electrode, whereas others require only one hand. The elements that need two hands use a rack-and-pinion gear; these include the McCarthy type. The elements that require only one hand use a spring device; these include the Nesbit, Baumrucker, and Iglesias types. The Iglesias type also uses continuous irrigation and suction of fluid; this permits the urologist to work uninterrupted.

During TURP, the surgeon removes the prostate gland while leaving the prostatic capsule intact (Fig. 22–38). As the urologist excises bits of tissue with the cutting electrodes, the tissue collects within the bladder, along with the irrigation fluid. To remove the tissue, the fluid empties into an evacuator such as the Ellik evacuator (Fig. 22–39). The urologist then empties the tissue and solution from the evacuator over the wire mesh plate that extends from the operating table where the technologist can later retrieve and retain the tissue pieces as specimens. The McCarthy evacuator shown in Figure 22–40 may also be used to withdraw bits of prostatic tissue from within the bladder.

During TURB, the surgeon removes a bladder tumor as for transurethral resection of the prostate. Instruments used for a TURB are illustrated in Figure 22–37. The tumor or tumors are removed piecemeal with the resectoscope, and the specimens are evacuated with the McCarthy or Ellik evacuator.

Urethral Dilatation

Urethral dilatation is performed to release a stricture resulting from inflammation due to disease or trauma. Congenital strictures are very rare. Strictures are released with graduated dilators called sounds (Fig. 22–41), with filiforms (Fig. 22–42), or with the use of a urethrotome (special cutting device designed to release a stricture that does not respond to dilatation).

Text continued on page 411

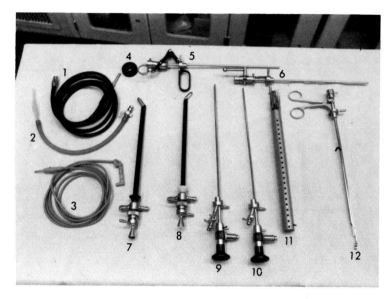

Figure 22–37. Resectoscope and accessories: 1, fiberoptic light cable; 2, irrigation tubing; 3, electrosurgical power cable; 4, protective eyepiece; 5, 6, working elements; 7, 8, resectoscope sheaths with obturators; 9, 10, telescopes; 11, resectoscope loops; 12, biopsy forceps.

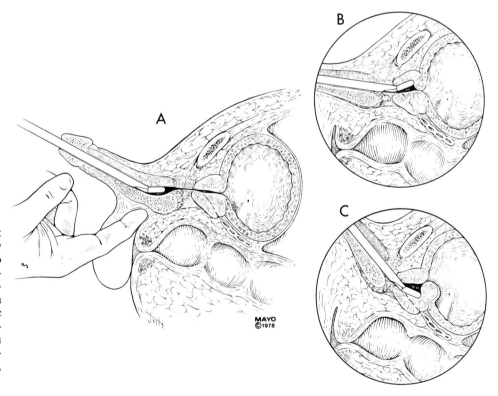

Figure 22–38. The urologist gains access to the prostate by inserting the resectoscope into the urethra. Insertion of the rectoscope in the presence of obstruction in the bulbous urethra *(A)*, at the anterior prostatic commissure *(B)*, and by an enlarged median lobe *(C)*. (From Greene LF, Segura JW: Transurethral Surgery. Philadelphia, WB Saunders, 1979.)

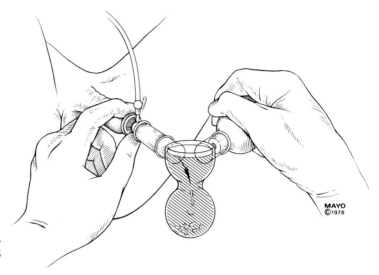

Figure 22–39. Ellik evacuator. (From Greene LF, Segura JW: Transurethral Surgery. Philadelphia, WB Saunders, 1979.)

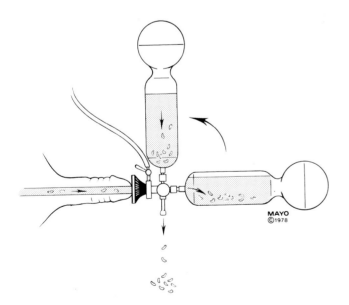

Figure 22–40. McCarthy evacuator. (From Greene LF, Segura JW: Transurethral Surgery. Philadelphia, WB Saunders, 1979.)

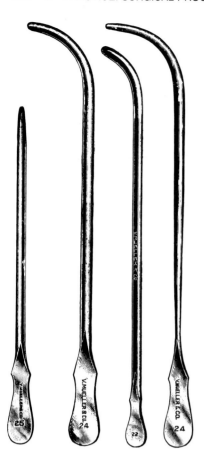

Figure 22–41. Urethral sounds. (Courtesy of V. Mueller Co.)

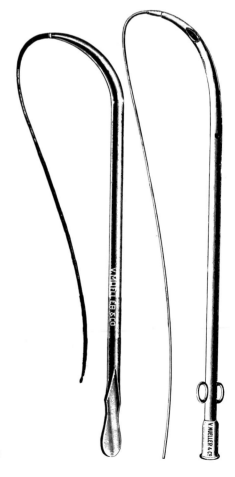

Figure 22–42. Urethral sounds and filiforms. (Courtesy of V. Mueller Co.)

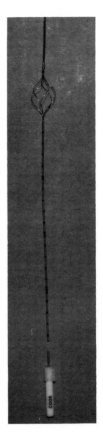

Figure 22–43. Cook helical stone dislodger. (Courtesy of Vance Products.)

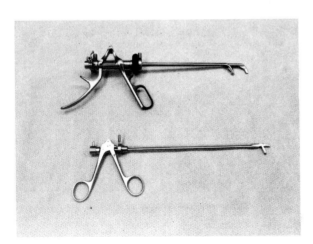

Figure 22–44. Lithotrites. Used for crushing urinary stones within the bladder.

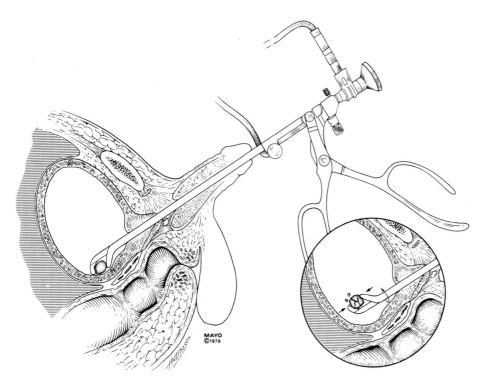

Figure 22–45. The urinary stone is grasped with the lithotrite and fragmented in the center of the bladder. (From Greene LF, Segura JW: Transurethral Surgery. Philadelphia, WB Saunders, 1979.)

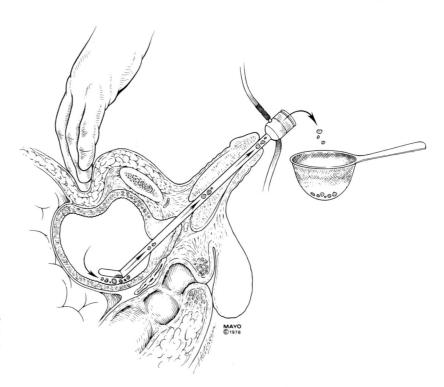

Figure 22–46. The crushed urinary stone is evacuated and must be retained as a specimen. (From Greene LF, Segura JW: Transurethral Surgery. Philadelphia, WB Saunders, 1979.)

Stone Manipulation and Litholapaxy

Calculi (stones) occurring in the urethra, bladder, and ureters may be successfully removed by the use of a *stone basket* (Fig. 22–43) or *lithotrite* (Fig. 22–44). Stone baskets are used to retrieve a small stone lodged in the ureter. The urologist retracts the basket into the catheter and then inserts it into the affected ureter. The basket is then opened, and the stone is "captured" with the basket. The urologist then retracts the basket again, encapsulating or crushing the stone within the lumen of the catheter.

The lithotrite is used to grasp and crush large stones occurring in the bladder. The calculous material is then evacuated with irrigation solution and an evacuator, such as the Ellik evacuator. This technique is illustrated in Figures 22–45 and 22–46.

Bibliography

Crawford D, Borden TA: Genitourinary Cancer Surgery. Philadelphia, Lea & Febiger, 1977.

Finney RP: New hinged silicone penile implant. J Urol 118:568, 1977.

Furlow WL: Inflatable penile prosthesis: Mayo Clinic experience with 175 patients. Urology 13:166, 1979.

Gardner E, Gray D, O'Rahilly R: Anatomy: A Regional Study of Human Structure, 5th ed. Philadelphia, WB Saunders, 1986.

Greene LF, Segura W (eds): Transurethral Surgery. Philadelphia, WB Saunders, 1979.

Jacob S, Francone C, Lossow WJ: Structure and Function in Man, 5th ed. Philadelphia, WB Saunders, 1982.

McVay C: Surgical Anatomy, 6th ed. Philadelphia, WB Saunders, 1984.

Roen P: Atlas of Urological Procedures. Norwalk, CT, Appleton-Century-Crofts, 1967.

Tannenbaum M: Urologic Pathology: The Prostate. Philadelphia, Lea & Febiger, 1977.

Walsh PC, Retik AB, Stamey TA, Vaughan ED: Campbell's Urology, 5th ed. Philadelphia, WB Saunders, 1993.

Orthopedic Surgery

Orthopedic surgery is performed to correct a fracture, replace diseased bone, correct a congenital defect, and treat injury or disease of the soft connective tissues, such as ligaments and tendons. Orthopedic procedures change very frequently as new techniques and equipment are developed. Because of the rapid changes in orthopedic technology, in this chapter the focus is on the basic techniques of surgery, equipment, and anatomic exposure of the skeletal system. Some procedures that demonstrate common techniques are described pictorially.

SURGICAL ANATOMY

The Skeleton

The human skeleton (Figs. 23–1 and 23–2) contains 206 bones. These bones are divided into groups according to their location in the body. The *axial* skeleton contains the bones of the head, neck, and trunk. The *appendicular* skeleton contains the bones of the limbs. Table 23–1 is a list of the bones of the body.

Classification of Bones

Bones are further classified according to their shape.

Long bones are those whose length is greater than their width or circumference. This group includes the clavicle, humerus, radius, ulna, femur, tibia, and fibula. Also included are the bones of the fingers and toes: the metacarpals, metatarsals, and phalanges. Each long bone has geographic landmarks. The *shaft* of the long bone is called the *diaphysis*. The ends of the bone are called the *epiphyses*.

Short bones are those whose dimensions are approximately equal all around. Included in this group are the numerous small bones of the hands and feet.

Sesamoid bones are sometimes called "floating" bones and are those that occur mainly in the hands and feet. They are actually a type of short bone but are embedded in the joint capsules or tendons. The patella (knee cap) is an example of a sesamoid bone.

Flat bones are usually curved, thin, and flat. These bones serve to protect soft body parts or as attachments for wide muscles. Included in this group are the ribs, pelvic bones, scapula, and many skull bones.

Irregular bones are those bones that do not actually fit into any of the other groups. These bones are peculiar in shape, although many closely resemble the short and flat bones. Included in this group are the vertebrae, ossicles of the ear, and some of the skull bones.

Bone Tissue Types and Membranes

There are two types of bone tissue. *Cancellous bone* (also called spongy bone) is not actually soft but contains many small open spaces, which make it appear soft. *Compact bone* is, as its name implies, very dense with few open spaces. The shaft of long bones (Fig. 23–3) is compact. Within the shaft is a space called the *medullary canal*. The medullary canal contains red or yellow marrow. Marrow is also contained in the small spaces of the cancellous bones. *Red marrow* is highly vascular and functions as the site of red and white blood cell formation. *Yellow marrow* consists mainly of fat cells and is found primarily in the shaft of the long bones.

The *periosteum* is a tough fibrous tissue that covers bones except at their ends or articular surfaces (those that form a joint). The periosteum has two layers: an

412

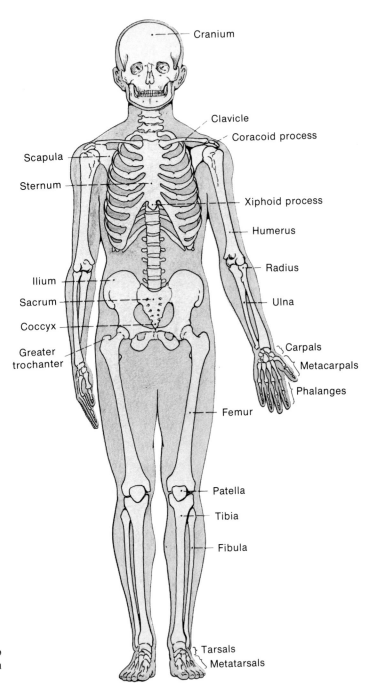

Figure 23–1. Anterior view of the skeleton. (From Jacob S, Francone C, Lossow WJ: Structure and Function in Man, 5th ed. Philadelphia, WB Saunders, 1982.)

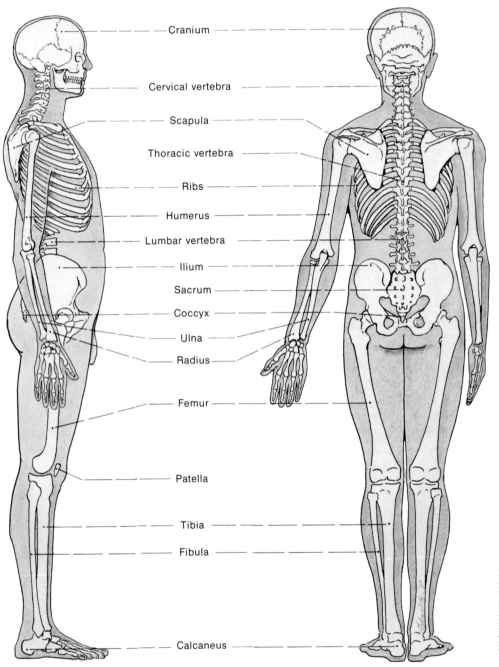

Figure 23–2. Lateral and posterior views of the skeleton. (From Jacob S, Francone C, Lossow WJ: Structure and Function in Man, 5th ed. Philadelphia, WB Saunders, 1982.)

Table 23–1. BONES

Bone	Number	Location
Skull	28 bones	
Cranium	8 bones	
Occipital	1	Posterior cranial floor and walls
Parietal	2	Forms the greater part of the superolateral aspect and roof of the skull between frontal and occipital bones
Frontal	1	Forms forehead, most of orbital roof, and anterior cranial floor
Temporal	2	Inferior lateral aspect and base of the skull, housing middle and inner ear structures
Sphenoid	1	Midanterior base of the skull; forms part of floor and side of orbit
Ethmoid	1	Between nasal bones and sphenoid, forming part of anterior cranial floor, medial wall of orbits, part of nasal septum, and roof
Face	14 bones	
Nasal	2	Upper bridge of nose
Maxillary	2	Upper jaw
Zygomataic (malar)	2	Prominence of cheeks and part of the lateral wall and floor of the orbits
Mandible	1	Lower jaw
Lacrimal	2	Anteromedial wall of the orbit
Palatine	2	Posterior nasal cavity between maxillae and the pterygoid processes of sphenoid
Vomer	1	Posterior nasal cavity, forming a portion of the nasal septum
Inferior nasal conchae (inferior turbinates)	2	Lateral wall of nasal cavity
Auditory Ossicles	6 bones	
Malleus (hammer)	2	Small bones in inner ear in temporal bone, connecting the tympanic membrane to the inner ear and functioning in sound transmission
Incus (anvil)	2	
Stapes (stirrup)	2	
Hyoid	1 bone	Horseshoe-shaped, suspended from styloid process of temporal bone
Trunk	51 bones	
Vertebrae	26 bones	
Cervical	7	Neck
Thoracic	12	Thorax
Lumbar	5	Between thorax and pelvis
Sacrum	1 (5 fused)	Pelvis—fixed, or false, vertebrae
Coccyx	1 (4 fused)	Terminal vertebrae in pelvis—fixed, or false, vertebrae
Ribs	24	True ribs—upper seven pairs fastened to sternum by costal cartilages; false ribs—lower five pairs; eighth, ninth, and tenth pairs attached indirectly to the seventh rib by costal cartilages; last two pairs do not attach and are called floating ribs
Sternum	1	Flat, narrow bone situated in median line anteriorly in chest
Upper Extremity	64 bones	
Clavicle	2	Together, clavicles and scapulae form the shoulder girdle; the clavicle articulates with the sternum
Scapula	2	
Humerus	2	Long bone of upper arm
Ulna	2	The ulna is the longest bone of forearm, on medial side of radius
Radius	2	Lateral to ulna shorter than ulna, but styloid process is larger
Carpals	16	Two rows of bones composing the wrist
Scaphoid		
Lunate		
Triangular		
Pisiform		
Capitate		
Hamate		
Trapezium		
Trapezoid		
Metacarpals	10	Long bones of the palm of the hand
Phalanges	28	Three in each finger and two in each thumb
Lower Extremity	62 bones	
Pelvic	2	Fusion of ilium, ischium, and pubis
Femur (thigh bone)	2	Longest bone in body
Patella	2	Kneecap; located in quadriceps femoris tendon; a sesamoid bone
Tibia	2	Shin bone; anteromedial side of the leg
Fibula	2	Lateral to tibia
Tarsals	14	Form heel, ankle (with distal tibia and fibula), and proximal part of the foot
Calcaneus		
Talus		
Navicular		
Cuboid		
First cuneiform (medial)		
Second cuneiform (intermediate)		
Third cuneiform (lateral)		
Metatarsals	10	Long bone of the foot
Phalanges	28	Three in each lesser toe and two in each great toe

From Jacob S, Francone C, Lossow WJ: Structure and Function in Man, 5th ed. Philadelphia, WB Saunders, 1982.

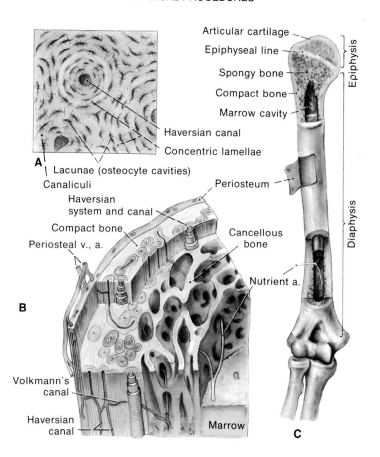

Figure 23–3. Cross section of a long bone showing internal and external structures. *A.* Relation of osteocytes to the Haversian system. *B.* Haversian system and lamellae. *C.* Structure of the long bone. (From Jacob S, Francone C, Lossow WJ: Structure and Function in Man, 5th ed. Philadelphia, WB Saunders, 1982.)

outer layer, which is dense and vascular, and an inner layer, which is much more loose and contains growing bone cells (osteoblasts).

The *endosteum* is a fine membrane that lines all compact bone cavities.

Bone Landmarks

Bones have certain landmarks, which are irregularities or markings that serve various functions and are named separately according to their shape and function. Some of these markings may serve as attachments for muscle or tendon, whereas others are passageways for nerves or blood vessels. Whenever we discuss skeletal anatomy, we often refer to these landmarks to make the exact location of the discussion more clear.

Crest: a ridge of bone (e.g., iliac crest)
Spine: a more or less sharp, narrow projection (e.g., spinous process)
Condyle: a knuckle-shaped portion of bone, generally found in association with a joint
Process: a projection of bone (e.g., coracoid process)
Tubercle: a small rounded projection (e.g., deltoid tubercle)
Tuberosity: a large rounded projection (e.g., ischial tuberosity)
Foramen: a rounded orifice in bone (e.g., olfactory foramen). A foramen is the bony passageway for blood vessels or nerves.
Sinus: a cavity within a bone (e.g., nasal sinus)
Sulcus: a groove in a bone

The Bones of the Body

The major bones of the body are illustrated in Figures 23–4 through 23–12.

The Muscular System

Muscles are responsible for the majority of movement in the human body. Some muscles may move an entire limb, whereas others are responsible for the movement of fluid or for a heartbeat. There are three major muscle types in the human body:

Striated: under voluntary control, such as those used to move an arm or leg
Smooth: activated *involuntarily*, that is, we have no direct ability to cause their contraction
Cardiac: the muscles of the heart; also involuntary but represent a separate group because they are different in structure and mechanism from smooth muscle tissue.

Striated Muscle

Striated muscle, also commonly called *skeletal muscle*, is composed of fibers that are bound together by sheaths of protective tissue. The fibers exist both on a microscopic level and also grossly. Each group of fibers and its associated sheath is bound together to form one muscle. Beginning with the smallest fiber and ending

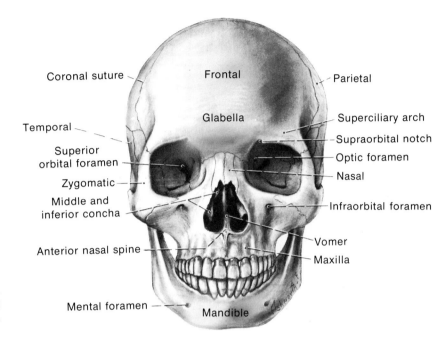

Figure 23–4. Frontal view of the skull. (From Jacob S, Francone C, Lossow WJ: Structure and Function in Man, 5th ed. Philadelphia, WB Saunders, 1982.)

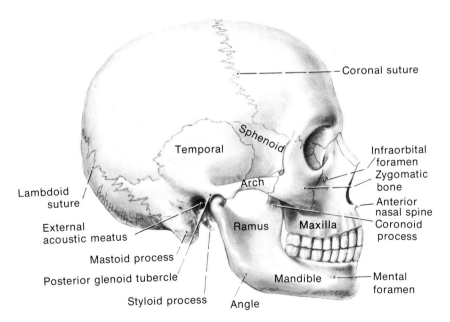

Figure 23–5. Right side of the skull. (From Jacob S, Francone C, Lossow WJ: Structure and Function in Man, 5th ed. Philadelphia, WB Saunders, 1982.)

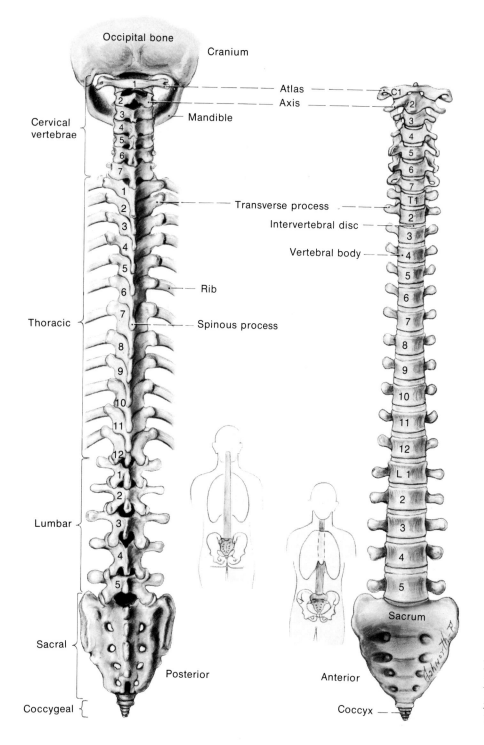

Occipital bone

Cranium

Atlas

Axis

C1

Mandible

Cervical vertebrae

Transverse process

Intervertebral disc

Vertebral body

Rib

Spinous process

Thoracic

Lumbar

Sacral

Posterior

Anterior

Sacrum

Coccygeal

Coccyx

Figure 23–6. The vertebral column. (From Jacob S, Francone C, Lossow WJ: Structure and Function in Man, 5th ed. Philadelphia, WB Saunders, 1982.)

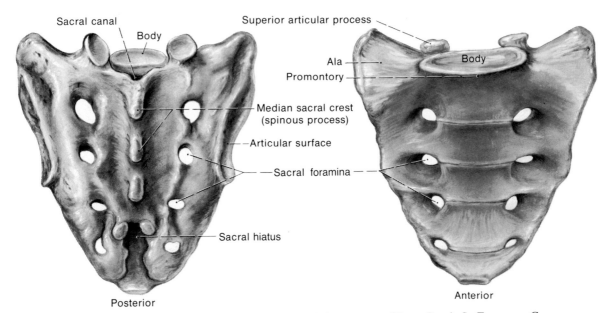

Figure 23–7. Posterior and anterior views of the sacrum. (From Jacob S, Francone C, Lossow WJ: Structure and Function in Man, 5th ed. Philadelphia, WB Saunders, 1982.)

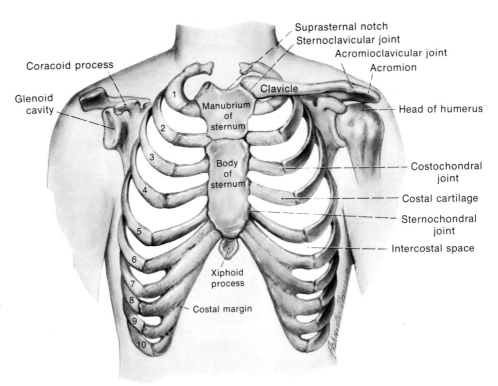

Figure 23–8. Anterior view of the rib cage. (From Jacob S, Francone C, Lossow WJ: Structure and Function in Man, 5th ed. Philadelphia, WB Saunders, 1982.)

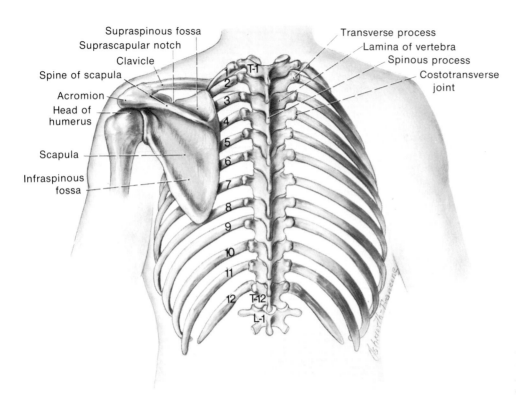

Figure 23–9. Posterior view of rib cage and scapula. (From Jacob S, Francone C, Lossow WJ: Structure and Function in Man, 5th ed. Philadelphia, WB Saunders, 1982.)

with the largest group of fibers, each is discussed as follows.

Myofibrils are the smallest contractile units of striated muscle tissue. These fibers are microscopic and appear as parallel structures. The myofibrils are bound together in groups, and, in turn, these groups form a larger fiber called the *fasciculi.*

Fasciculi (singular, fasciculus) are many groups of myofibrils that form one of many strands in the muscle. The fasciculi are each covered individually by a strong sheath called the *perimysium.* Many bound fasciculi form one section of muscle. Each section of muscle is then covered by the *epimysium*—a tough connective tissue that separates one muscle section from another. Other connective tissues with which we are more familiar then surround whole muscle groups; these include *fascia* and also *fatty (adipose) tissue.*

Smooth Muscle

Smooth muscle tissue is also called *involuntary muscle,* because under normal circumstances we have no control over its function. These muscles are found in the respiratory, digestive, and urinary tracts and also in other structures such as the iris and blood vessels. When found in structures such as the bladder and intestine, smooth muscle contains two layers—one outside, longitudinal layer and another inner, circular layer. When the muscles contract, they actually diminish the diameter and length of the structure of which they are a part, thus moving the contents along the structure.

Cardiac Muscle

As the name implies, cardiac muscle is the muscle of the heart. Like voluntary muscle, cardiac muscle is striated, but these muscles are involuntary. Cardiac muscle is responsible for the sustained contractions of the heart and for the movement of blood in and out of that organ. This mechanism, and also the rate of contraction, occurs through a complex series of impulses by the autonomic nervous system.

The Articular System

The articular system or joint system includes those areas of the body where two bones meet and where movement occurs because of this. The degree of movement may be small, such as in the ossicles of the ear, or large, such as in the hip joint.

Classification of Joints

Joints are classified according to the *degree of movement* they allow and also by the *shape* of the articulating surfaces (union of the bones themselves; Fig. 23–13). The first classification includes the following:

Synarthroses: immovable joint (e.g., union of the major skull bones)
Amphiarthroses: slightly moveable (e.g., the vertebra)
Diarthroses: freely moveable (e.g., the hip)

The diarthroses include most of the joints of the body. These joints are also called *synovial joints,* because the

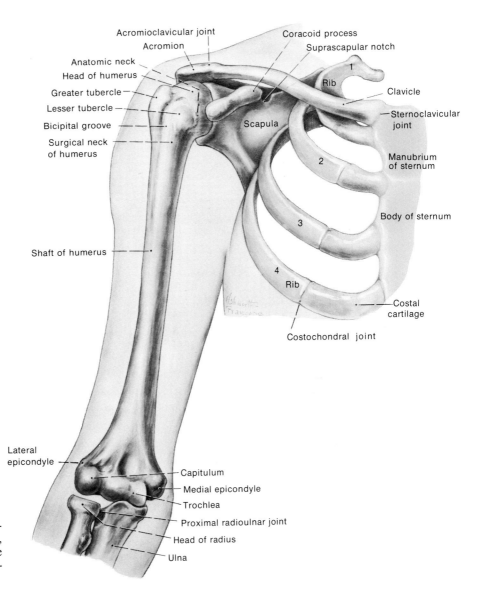

Figure 23–10. Right scapula, humerus, and rib cage. (From Jacob S, Francone C, Lossow WJ: Structure and Function in Man, 5th ed. Philadelphia, WB Saunders, 1982.)

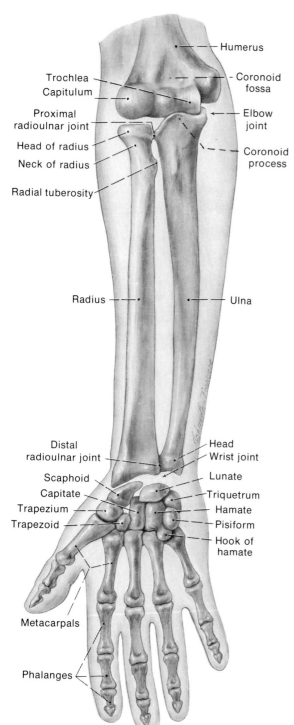

Figure 23–11. Anterior view of bones of the forearm and hand. (From Jacob S, Francone C, Lossow WJ: Structure and Function in Man, 5th ed. Philadelphia, WB Saunders, 1982.)

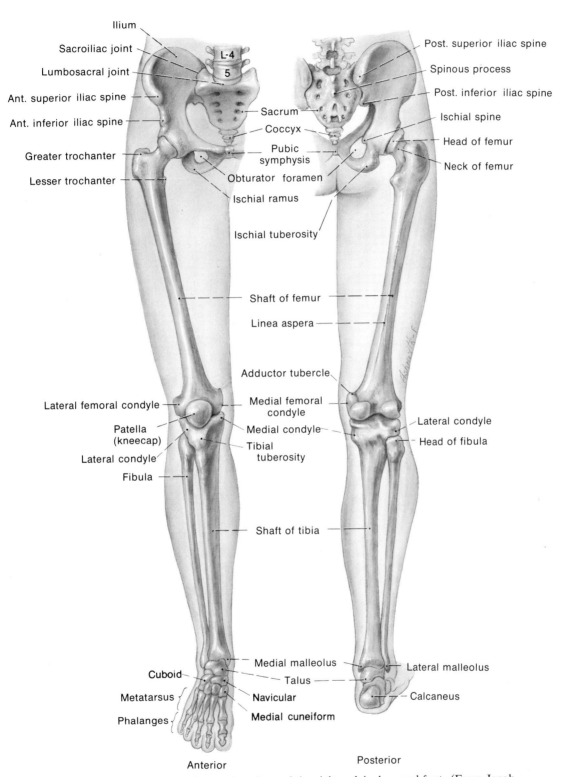

Anterior

Posterior

Figure 23–12. Anterior and posterior views of the right pelvis, leg, and foot. (From Jacob S, Francone C, Lossow WJ: Structure and Function in Man, 5th ed. Philadelphia, WB Saunders, 1982.)

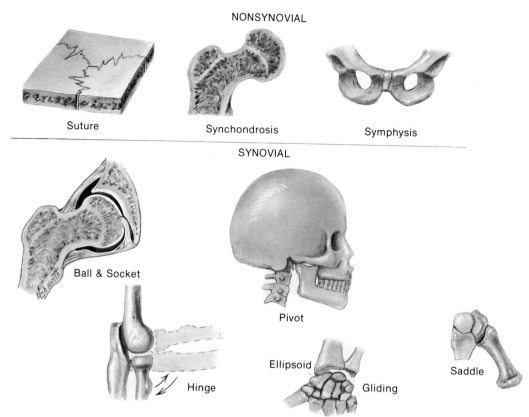

Figure 23–13. Classification of joints: nonsynovial, including suture, synchondrosis, and symphysis; and synovial including ball and socket, pivot, hinge, ellipsoid, gliding, and saddle. (From Jacob S, Francone C, Lossow WJ: Structure and Function in Man, 5th ed. Philadelphia, WB Saunders, 1982.)

joint capsule contains a fluid called *synovia,* or *synovial fluid.* The role of synovial fluid is discussed in more detail in the next section.

Types of Synovial Joints

The synovial joints are further classified according to the shape of the articular surfaces, which in turn governs the types of movement they allow. These types are as follows:

Ball and socket: This joint allows the greatest freedom of movement. One articular surface is ball shaped, whereas the other is a concave plate (socket). The ball portion slides freely across the plate portion, allowing rotation as well as lateral movement (e.g., the hip joint).

Pivot joint: This joint consists of a *process* and a *fossa.* The pivot joint allows rotation only (e.g., the atlas and axis of the neck).

Hinge joint: One articular surface is concave, whereas the other is convex. This type of joint allows only extension and flexion (e.g., the elbow).

Gliding joint: The articular surfaces are usually curved, allowing one to slide over the other (e.g., the vertebral inferior processes).

Saddle joint: This is similar to the ellipsoid joint but freer. One surface is concave in one direction and convex in the other. The opposite articular surface

is the reverse—convex in one direction and concave in the other. This joint occurs between the carpus and the first metacarpal, which joins the thumb.

Joint Structure

Synovial Joint

The *synovial joint* (Fig. 23–14) consists of the articulating bone ends and the connective tissues that surround and bind them. Surrounding the joint is a tough fibrous tissue called the *joint capsule.* The joint capsule is lined with a membrane called the *synovial membrane.* This membrane produces a thick clear fluid, *synovial fluid,* which lubricates and nourishes the joint. Each bone surface within the joint is covered with *cartilage,* a strong smooth tissue that, combined with the lubricating effect of the synovial fluid, aids in the smooth gliding of one bone surface over the other.

Ligaments are the strong fibrous bands of tissue that join bones together and limit or help facilitate their motion. In addition, where a muscle is joined to a bone, an intermediary tissue—the *tendon*—forms the actual attachment.

Nonsynovial Joints

Joints that do not have a capsule include the *sutures* (such as those joints that connect the bones of the skull), *synchondroses* (temporary joints that occur during growth), *symphyses* (joints whose bones are connected by a disk of cartilage), and *syndesmoses* (those bones joined by ligaments).

FRACTURES

Complications that arise from fractured bones include hemorrhage, edema, and soft tissue injury. Frequently, the displaced bone ends cause tendon and muscle tissue to be pulled, twisted, or bruised. Nerves, blood vessels, or organs that lie adjacent to the fracture site may be injured during the trauma, or the displaced bones themselves can cause further injury. During clinical evaluation of the orthopedic patient, extensive examination may be necessary to discover these additional injuries. Orthopedic repair is often performed on an emergency basis to prevent subsequent injury.

Classification of Fractures

Fractures (Fig. 23–15) are classified by the extent and type of injury to the bone and surrounding tissues. These classifications are clinically significant because some fracture sites are contaminated and present the risk of infection:

1. A *simple fracture* is one in which there is a single fracture line.

2. A *comminuted fracture* consists of multiple bone fragments and fracture lines. The force needed to produce this type of injury usually results in soft tissue damage and may require extensive repair of both soft tissue and bone. Depending on the site of injury, bone fragments may be approximated with steel wires, pins, or screws. Soft tissue repair may require the reattachment of ligaments with sutures, staples, or screws. Tendon repair is performed with fine sutures.

3. An *open* or *compound fracture* is one in which the bone fragments protrude through the skin. This type of fracture is considered an emergency because of the immediate risk of infection. Débridement (see Chapter 11) is usually performed as part of the surgical procedure to repair the fracture. Debris such as metal fragments, paint, wood, glass, or devitalized tissue is removed during the débridement. Because the wound is contaminated, this type of fracture requires special management. It is undesirable to use any internal fixation device at the fracture site, because it would be rejected in the presence of infection. Repair of soft tissues resulting from the original trauma must sometimes be deferred. The fracture may be stabilized by an internal device placed some distance from the wound site, and traction can be employed during healing. Very often the wound is left open to facilitate drainage and allow further débridement. After the risk of infection has passed, the wound may be closed or skin grafts employed as needed.

4. A *greenstick fracture* occurs in children, whose bones are resilient and covered with a durable, tough periosteum. Because of this resiliency, children's bones may "bend" rather than break. When this occurs, the concave side of the fracture surface is compressed and the convex side is pulled apart. Thus, the bone appears angled but is not broken. If the fracture extends through the epiphyseal plate (growth center of the bone), future bone growth may be disturbed. If the break lies completely within the epiphysis, and there is no displacement into metaphysis, normal bone growth can be anticipated.

5. A *pathologic fracture* is one caused by disease such as metastatic carcinoma. The fracture most often occurs at the tumor site, where the bone is weak. Osteoporosis, which is the softening and weakening of bone tissue occurring in the elderly patient, may also give rise to a pathologic fracture.

6. An *impacted fracture* is one caused by violent impact along the longitudinal axis of a bone. This occurs at the junction between the metaphysis and diaphysis, where the cortex is quite thin. The diaphysis is usually

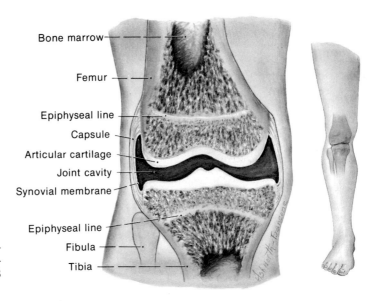

Bone marrow
Femur
Epiphyseal line
Capsule
Articular cartilage
Joint cavity
Synovial membrane
Epiphyseal line
Fibula
Tibia

Figure 23–14. A synovial joint (the knee) showing components. (From Jacob S, Francone C, Lossow WJ: Structure and Function in Man, 5th ed. Philadelphia, WB Saunders, 1982.)

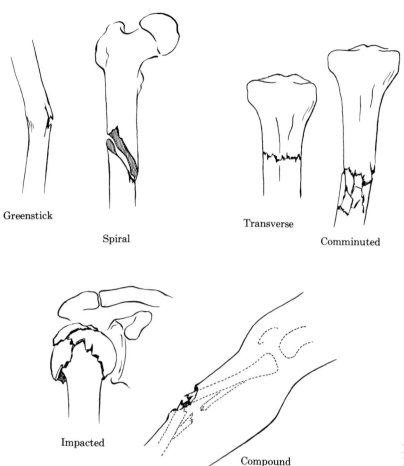

Greenstick

Spiral

Transverse

Comminuted

Impacted

Compound

Figure 23–15. Common types of fractures. (From Dorland's Illustrated Medical Dictionary, 27th ed. Philadelphia, WB Saunders, 1988.)

forced into the metaphysis, tightly wedging the two fragments together.

7. A *spiral fracture* is caused by the twisting or torquing of a bone. In this type of fracture, the bone is twisted apart into two fragments.

Fracture Management

Reduction

Reduction is the physical approximation of the fracture ends so that healing can begin. Reduction can occur *externally*, by manipulation of the bone from the outside of the body, or *internally*, when the bone ends themselves are handled, manipulated, and brought together during surgical intervention. External manipulation is possible only when the orthopedist can overcome the force of the spasms that occur in the muscles that bridge the fracture site. When the fracture occurs in areas such as the proximal humerus or femur, these spasms are often too strong for manual reduction. In these cases, prolonged pull on the fractured bones is necessary. This can be accomplished through *traction* (Fig. 23–16). A transverse pin or rod is placed through the limb, and continuous weight is applied to the end. This draws the fractured bones together.

When a fracture cannot be reduced by external manipulation or traction, surgery is necessary. This is called *open reduction*.

Some fractures require removal of bone fragments or complete replacement of the bone with a prosthesis. Fractures of the radial or femoral head, which result in painful irregular surfaces between the two joint components, often require this type of surgery.

Some types of fractures are stable and require no reduction. Even though surgical intervention may not be necessary for their reduction, these fractures may be seen in the operating room because of the need for general anesthesia.

Immobilization

Reduction is the *internal* or *external* means of *stabilizing* the broken bones in their correct anatomic position while healing occurs.

Casts (External Stabilization)

When a cast is applied, it must immobilize the joints above and below the fracture site. Plaster of Paris is available in individual rolls or strips (called *splints*). Before applying the cast, the limb is wrapped with

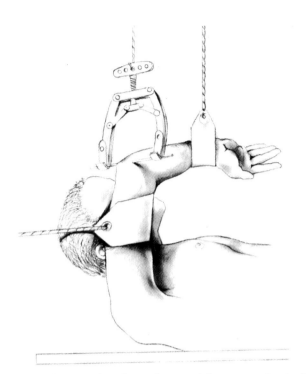

Figure 23–16. Traction for a fractured humerus. A pin is inserted through the bone and suspended by weights and pulleys. (From Schwartz SI, et al: Principles of Surgery, 2nd ed. New York, McGraw-Hill, 1974. Used with the permission of McGraw-Hill Book Company.)

expandable webbing and further protected with a layer of soft compressed cotton (called *Webril*). This is followed by a layer of thick, soft, cotton sheeting. It is critical that all layers of padding be free of wrinkles to prevent pinching or deformation of the skin. The casting splints are then dipped in *cold* water and applied along the long axis of the bone. Cold water must be used because when the plaster begins to dry it gives off heat. Additional heat caused by hot water could cause a burn.

Following application of the splints, rolled plaster bandages are moistened and wrapped around the limb. Should swelling occur at the fracture site, prominent blood vessels can be compressed and the limb's circulatory function can become compromised. Therefore, the tip of the limb must be cleaned of all plaster and the patient monitored for signs of circulatory disruption. If this occurs, there will be increasing pain in the limb, progressing to numbness, and the skin will turn cyanotic and cold. Different types of casts are shown in Figure 23–17.

Traction (External Stabilization)

Traction may also be used to stabilize a limb until casting is possible.

Orthopedic Implants (Internal Stabilization)

Orthopedic implants are applied across, over, or through a fracture *during surgery* to hold the bone fragments together. These implants may be left in the body or removed at a later date. Examples include plates, pins, screw, rods, or staples. There are many types of implants available, and new ones are constantly being developed. The techniques used to place some common types of implants are discussed later in this chapter.

Summary

Fractures require *reduction* (approximation of bone fragments) and *immobilization* (stabilization of the bone fragments while healing takes place). In surgery, immobilization is called *fixation*. When a procedure is *closed*, the bone fragments are not surgically exposed. An *open* procedure is one in which the bones are surgically exposed.

Closed Reduction With External Fixation

In this type of procedure, the bone ends are reduced externally (without surgery), by manipulation. The fractured bone is then immobilized or *fixated* by external means such as a plaster cast or traction.

Open Reduction With External Fixation

In this procedure, open surgery is performed because the fractured bone is reduced *internally*, through an incision. The bones are then held in approximation with an external device—one that is applied outside the body, such as a cast.

Closed Reduction With Internal Fixation

In this procedure, the bone ends are approximated (reduced) externally and then held in place by an internally placed device such as a rod or pin. This type of procedure requires surgical intervention because the stabilizing (fixation) appliance must be inserted. However, instead of making an incision to insert the fixating device, the device is pushed or drilled through the skin and then into the bone fragments.

Open Reduction With Internal Fixation

This procedure requires both the internal manipulation of the bone fragments and the application of a stabilizing or fixating device within the surgical wound. It is this type of reduction that is done most frequently in the operating room and the one that requires the most complex surgical intervention. The various types of fixation devices used in open reduction are discussed in this chapter.

ORTHOPEDIC EQUIPMENT AND SUPPLIES

There are numerous types of appliances and tools used in orthopedic surgery for the reduction and fixation of fractures, and each employs a slightly different tech-

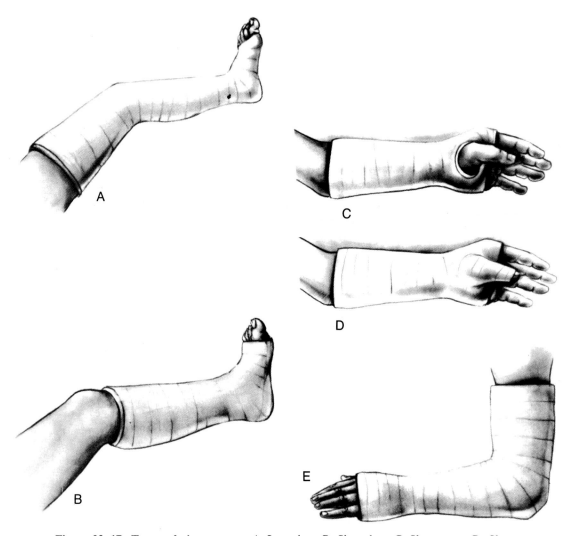

Figure 23–17. Types of plaster casts. *A.* Long leg. *B.* Short leg. *C.* Short arm. *D.* Short arm with thumb immobilized. *E.* Long arm. (From Schwartz SI et al: Principles of Surgery, 2nd ed. New York, McGraw-Hill, 1974. Used with the permission of McGraw-Hill Book Company.)

nique. These appliances and tools are distributed by individual manufacturers and require instruction by the manufacturer's representatives. Individual orthopedic surgeons frequently use a specific technique based on their own personal preference or education. Because of the wide variation in technique, instrument sets and specific fixation devices presented in this chapter are grouped according to anatomic location. These appliances and tools represent those most commonly used for basic orthopedic procedures.

Special Equipment

Power Equipment

Power-driven equipment is often used in orthopedic surgery. Drills, saws, reamers, and screwdrivers are commonly driven by compressed nitrogen. All surgery personnel should be familiar with the proper handling, storage, and use of hoses, tanks, and regulators used in the operating room. The nitrogen source in most operating rooms is located away from the surgical department and piped into ceiling-mounted fixtures. When these fixtures are not available, nitrogen must be brought into surgery in tanks. The nitrogen tank is fitted with a regulator and valve. The proper use of these fittings during surgery is illustrated in Figure 23–18. All personnel must become familiar with these fittings because any gas cylinder represents a significant hazard in the event of leaks or breakage. A cylinder carrier should always be used when handling tanks, and the tank must

be securely locked into the carrier before transportation. Tanks should be stored in a designated location away from heat sources, where they are secured and prevented from falling over.

Whenever power-driven saws, reamers, or other cutting instruments are in use, the scrub assistant should lightly irrigate the area at the instrument's cutting edge with saline solution. This reduces friction and prevents the tissue from drying out and heating up. Using a rubber rather than a glass bulb syringe prevents shattering of the syringe tip, in the event it is caught in the instrument's cutting edge.

Pneumatic Tourniquet

The pneumatic tourniquet is used during most orthopedic procedures. All personnel should become familiar with the proper application and handling of the tourniquet and oxygen source. A complete discussion of this equipment is presented in Chapter 13.

Methyl Methacrylate Cement

Methyl methacrylate cement is used to hold many types of metal or synthetic prostheses in place, such as during total joint replacement. It is the responsibility of the scrub assistant to mix this chemical. Because the fumes from methyl methacrylate are toxic to the respiratory system, closed mixing units (Fig. 23–19) must be used whenever the cement is prepared. These units are equipped with a suction outlet that vents the fumes away from the sterile field. In addition, a second set of gloves

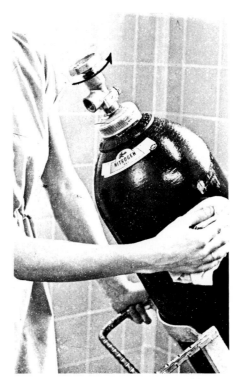

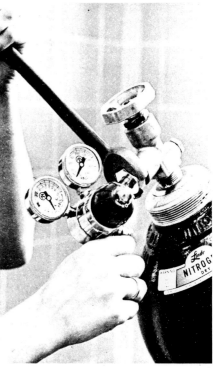

Figure 23–18. Proper handling of the nitrogen tank and regulator. (Courtesy of Zimmer, Inc., Warsaw, IN.)

Illustration continued on following page

1. Wipe off cylinder and carrier; open tank valve (counter-clockwise: see arrows) very slowly and allow only enough gas to escape to blow out possible debris.

2. Attach regulator by hand and secure with 1⅛" wrench. Ensure that regulator is turned completely off by turning green knob counterclockwise until it stops.

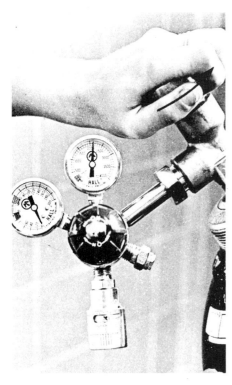

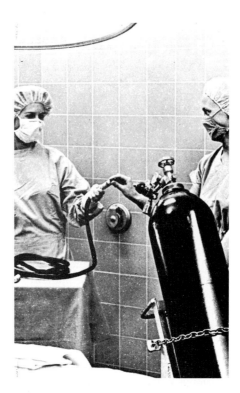

3. Slowly turn tank valve fully open. Tank pressure should read 2000 to 2500 PSI on right-hand gauge when full. Listen for air leaks.

4. Circulating nurse takes the connector end of the instrument from the scrub nurse.

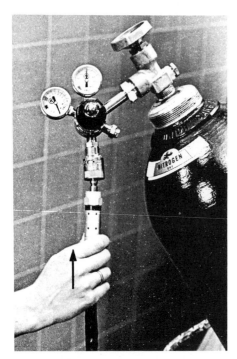

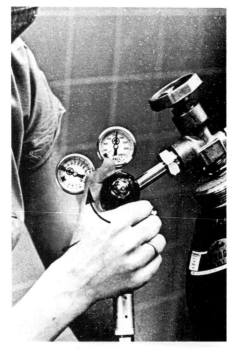

5. Connector end of instrument is thrust into the regulator outlet. Be sure tank valve is fully opened.

6. Turn the green knob "ON" (clockwise: see arrows) and set pressure on left-hand regulator gauge according to needs of instruments and surgeon. NOTE: Pressure settings must be made with instrument running, or too low an operating pressure will result.

Figure 23–18 *Continued.*

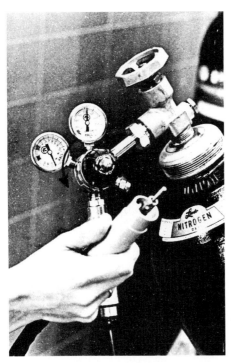

7. When finished, turn tank off. Actuate instrument to bleed off air in tubing and gauge. Regulator gauge should read zero. Turn off regulator by turning green knob counterclockwise until it stops.

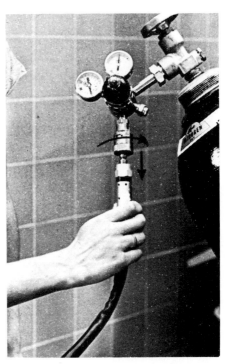

8. Turn connector on regulator (clockwise: see arrows) holding instrument diffuser to prevent diffuser from falling.

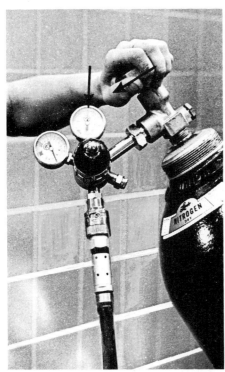

9. If pressure remaining in tank is 500 PSI or more, return to storage. CAUTION: Replace if cylinder pressure gauge shows less than 500 PSI.

Figure 23–18 *Continued.*

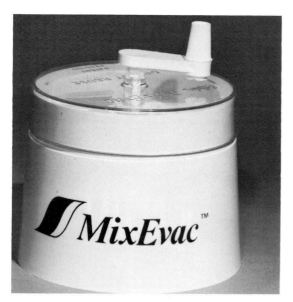

Figure 23–19. Closed mixing unit for methylmethacrylate. (Courtesy of the Stryker Corporation, Kalamazoo, MI.)

should be worn while the cement is in use to prevent skin irritation.

Methyl methacrylate is formed from two components, one a liquid and the other a powder. The powder is placed in the mixing unit, and the liquid is poured over it. At least 4 minutes of continuous mixing is required to prepare the cement (mixing time varies with humidity and temperature). When the cement takes on a doughy consistency and no longer adheres to the gloved hand, it is ready for use.

Orthopedic Table

The orthopedic table (also called a fracture table) is used during repair of hip fractures. Extreme caution must be observed when positioning the anesthetized patient on this table to prevent injury to soft tissues adjacent to the fracture site and to prominent blood vessels and nerves. A complete discussion of this equipment is given in Chapter 10.

Surgical Armboard

The surgical armboard is an extension placed on the operating table to provide a large sterile surface during surgical procedures of the hand, wrist, and arm. The table in use is shown in Figure 23–20.

Orthopedic Instruments

Orthopedic instruments are classified according to their use. Listed here are those commonly used.

Cutdown or Soft Tissue Instruments

To gain access to the fracture or operate on soft tissue injuries, the surgeon uses a cutdown or soft tissue set of instruments (Fig. 23–21). This instrument tray includes the following:

Scalpel handles
Tissue forceps
Metzenbaum scissors
Mayo scissors
Suture scissors
Needle holders
Mosquito clamps
Kelly clamps
Kocher clamps
Towel clamps
Allis clamps
Mayo clamps

In addition to these instruments, a plastic surgery tray including fine skin hooks, Senn retractors, plastic surgery scissors, tissue forceps, and micro needle holders may be used for repair of tendons, fascia, and nerves of the hand, wrist, and forearm.

Internal Fixation Devices—Implants

Internal fixation devices (Fig. 23–22) are surgical steel or steel alloy appliances used to stabilize the fracture during healing. Each type of device is implanted with a particular tool.

Pins and bolts are inserted across two small bone fragments such as those of the hand, ankle, or wrist. They may also provide an attachment for traction. They are inserted with a *drill or driver.*

Nails are used to span the longitudinal axis of the neck of the trochanter to stabilize a fracture in that location. They may also be driven into the medullary canal to span two fracture ends. Nails are driven with a *driver* or *impactor.*

Plates are spanned across the surface of two large bone fragments such as in a fracture of the femur. These are held in place with *screws.* Some plates are a combination nail and plate assembly. The nail portion is driven into the trochanteric neck, and the plate is then secured with individual screws.

Staples are used to reconnect soft tissue portions of a joint such as during ligament repair of the knee. Staples are available in various sizes and weights. They are driven with a *staple driver.*

Intermedullary rods are driven into the predrilled medullary canal to span two fracture ends. These rods are implanted with a *driver.*

Screws are placed across the fracture ends of small bones such as those of the ankle. They are also used to attach a plate to bone or to attach some soft tissues to bone. Screws are implanted with a surgical *screwdriver.*

Care of Orthopedic Implants

Metal implants are extremely expensive. Once an implant has been scratched, bent, or dented, it cannot be used. Scratches on the surface of an implant deepen once the implant has been placed in the body. This can cause the implant to weaken and may lead to its failure. Hence, all surgical personnel should follow these basic guidelines to prevent implant damage:

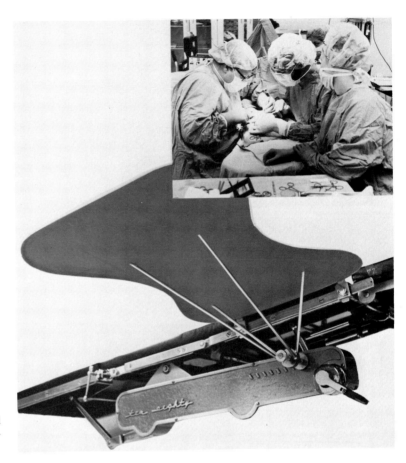

Figure 23–20. Surgical hand table used during hand or wrist surgery. (Courtesy of the Stryker Corporation, Kalamazoo, MI.)

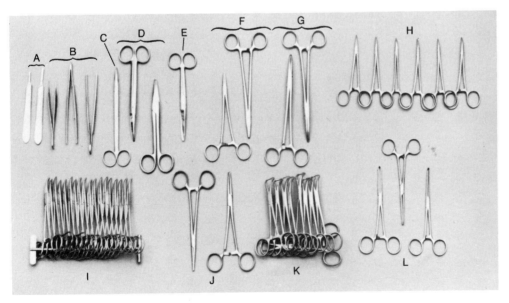

Figure 23–21. Cutdown instruments. *A.* Scalpel handles. *B.* Toothed and plain tissue forceps. *C.* Metzenbaum scissors. *D.* Mayo scissors. *E.* Suture scissors. *F.* Needle holders. *G.* Mayo clamps. *H.* Mosquito clamps. *I.* Kelly clamps. *J.* Kocher clamps. *K.* Towel clamps. *L.* Allis clamps.

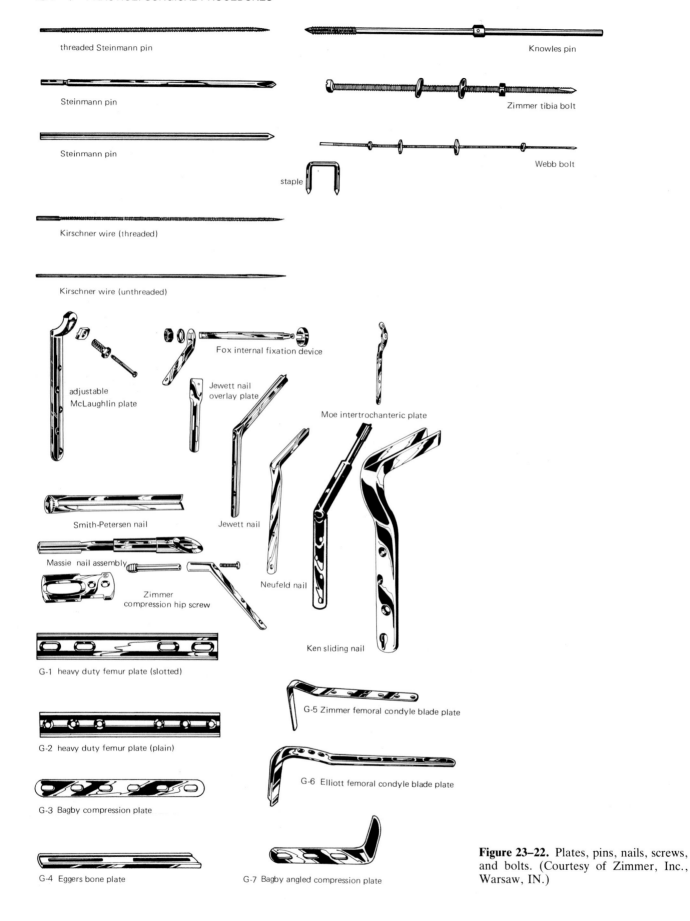

threaded Steinmann pin

Steinmann pin

Steinmann pin

Kirschner wire (threaded)

Kirschner wire (unthreaded)

Knowles pin

Zimmer tibia bolt

Webb bolt

staple

adjustable McLaughlin plate

Fox internal fixation device

Jewett nail overlay plate

Moe intertrochanteric plate

Smith-Petersen nail

Jewett nail

Massie nail assembly

Zimmer compression hip screw

Neufeld nail

Ken sliding nail

G-1 heavy duty femur plate (slotted)

G-2 heavy duty femur plate (plain)

G-3 Bagby compression plate

G-4 Eggers bone plate

G-5 Zimmer femoral condyle blade plate

G-6 Elliott femoral condyle blade plate

G-7 Bagby angled compression plate

Figure 23–22. Plates, pins, nails, screws, and bolts. (Courtesy of Zimmer, Inc., Warsaw, IN.)

1. When implants are stored or prepared for sterilization, they should not be allowed to contact each other or any metal surface.

2. Implants should be handled as little as possible.

3. Implants should never be intentionally bent.

4. If the implant is driven by force, an appropriate driver with a Teflon head must be used.

5. Different metals should not be mixed within an implant because they may react chemically with each other and weaken both components. If an implant such as a plate requires screws for fixation, the screws should be of the same metal as the plate and, preferably, should be obtained from the same manufacturer.

6. When an implant requires "sizing" (templates of the implant inserted for size), the implants themselves must never be used.

Impactors, Drivers, Extractors, Screwdrivers

These instruments (Fig. 23–23) are used to place or remove surgical implants. Impactors and drivers are placed over the head or fixed to the end of the implant, which may then be driven with a mallet. This prevents the mallet from contacting the fixation device and scratching, nicking, or denting it. Extractors are designed to fit over the head of the fixation device for its removal. The screwdriver may be manually operated or power driven.

Cutting Instruments

Rasps (Fig. 23–24) are used to smooth the surface of bone or to evacuate the medullary canal so that a stemmed prosthesis can be inserted.

Reamers (Fig. 23–25) are used to form a hollow area in the bone. Reamers may be bell shaped, such as those used in creating a space in the acetabulum for a prosthesis, or they may be long and narrow, such as those used to create a hole to accommodate a large nail.

Knives (Fig. 23–26) are used to cut heavy connective tissue such as cartilage. Orthopedic knives may be one unit (no detachable blade), or they may require the insertion of a single-use blade. When blades are inserted in orthopedic knives, an instrument must be used to grasp the blade. The hand should never be used to insert the blade.

Elevators (Fig. 23–27) are used to lift the periosteum from the surface of the bone and to perform fine dissection during tendon and ligament repair.

Rongeurs (Fig. 23–28) are used to cut bone. These are *double action* (two hinges) or *single action* (single hinge). The rongeur removes bone in small bites, which the scrub assistant must retain as specimens. When the surgeon uses a ronguer, he may offer the tip toward the scrub assistant who then removes the bits of bone with a moist sponge.

Saws are used to cut through fine bone. These are power driven and available in two types. The *recipro-*

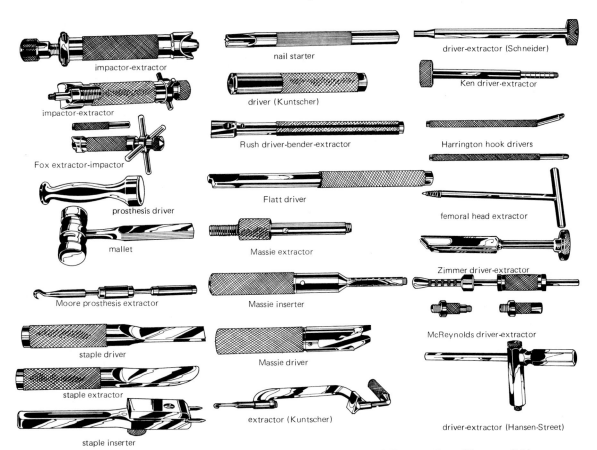

Figure 23–23. Impactors, drivers, and extractors. (Courtesy of Zimmer, Inc., Warsaw, IN.)

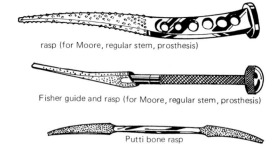

rasp (for Moore, regular stem, prosthesis)

Fisher guide and rasp (for Moore, regular stem, prosthesis)

Putti bone rasp

Figure 23–24. Rasps. (Courtesy of Zimmer, Inc., Warsaw, IN.)

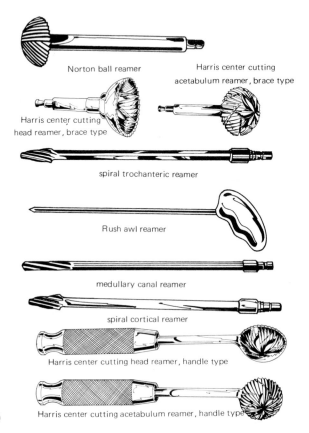

Norton ball reamer

Harris center cutting
acetabulum reamer, brace type

Harris center cutting
head reamer, brace type

spiral trochanteric reamer

Rush awl reamer

medullary canal reamer

spiral cortical reamer

Harris center cutting head reamer, handle type

Harris center cutting acetabulum reamer, handle type

Figure 23–25. Reamers. (Courtesy of Zimmer, Inc., Warsaw, IN.)

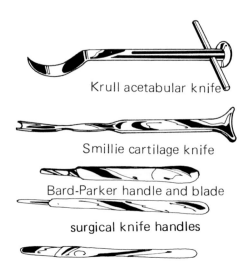

Krull acetabular knife

Smillie cartilage knife

Bard-Parker handle and blade

surgical knife handles

Beaver blade handle with chondroplasty blade

Figure 23–26. Orthopedic knives. (Courtesy of Zimmer, Inc., Warsaw, IN.)

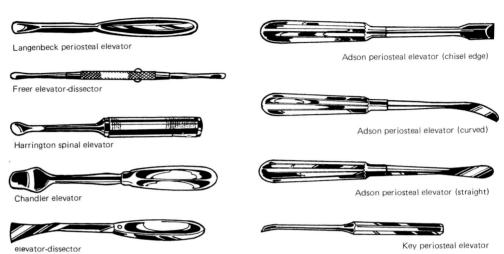

Figure 23–27. Elevators. (Courtesy of Zimmer, Inc., Warsaw, IN.)

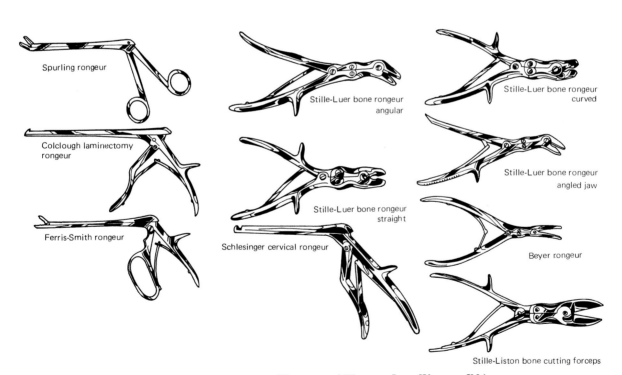

Figure 23–28. Rongeurs. (Courtesy of Zimmer, Inc., Warsaw, IN.)

cating saw blade vibrates in and out. The *oscillating* saw blade vibrates back and forth. These are used to remove small spurs or to smooth the surface of a bone. Both types of orthopedic saws are shown in Figure 23–29.

Osteotomes, curettes, and *gouges* (Fig. 23–30) are used to trim bone or to remove bone to be used as an autologous graft. The osteotome creates a sliver of bone that can be used as a graft and leaves a flattened surface. The curette is used to spoon out bits of bone from a curved area. The gouge creates a grooved surface on the bone. These instruments are heavy and sharp and should be handled carefully. Their cutting edges should be protected.

Drills (Fig. 23–31) may be hand or power operated and are used in conjunction with a *drill bit.* These are small, graduated pins that have a spiral cutting edge. A drill bit is used to drill a hole to accept a screw or pin. Drill bits are kept in a rack that protects their sharp edges and allows easy access.

Measuring devices (Fig. 23–32) are used during implant procedures. Two commonly used measuring devices are the *caliper* and the *depth gauge.* The caliper is used to measure the width of a ball joint head such as the femoral or humeral head, in preparation for a prosthetic implant. The depth gauge is used to measure the depth of the hole made by a drill bit to determine what length of screw is needed.

Retractors and bone clamps (Fig. 23–33) are used to hold a bone or to retract soft tissue away from the wound site. Some orthopedic clamps, such as the meniscus clamp, have sharp teeth within their jaws to grasp heavy tissue. Bone clamps are available in large, heavy sizes, such as the Lane clamp, or they may be delicate, such as the Lewin clamp.

SURGICAL EXPOSURE AND PROCEDURES

Arthroscopic Surgery

In addition to their valuable use as diagnostic tools, arthroscopic equipment and instruments allow the orthopedic surgeon to perform a wide variety of procedures.

Knee
  Synovial biopsy
  Removal of loose bodies
  Resection of plicae (obstructive synovial folds)
  Patellar shaving
  Synovectomy
  Meniscus repair
  Anterior and posterior cruciate ligament repair
Shoulder
  Removal of loose bodies
  Lysis of adhesions
  Synovial biopsy
  Bursectomy
  Stabilization of dislocation
  Biceps tendon and rotator cuff repair
  Impingement syndrome
Elbow
  Extraction of loose bodies
  Débridement of osteochondritis dissecans
  Partial synovectomy in rheumatoid disease
  Débridement and lysis of adhesions
Ankle
  Removal of loose bodies
  Biopsy
  Lateral ligament reconstruction

The advantages of arthroscopic surgery over open procedures include the following:

- Minimal tissue trauma
- Decreased postoperative infection
- Preservation of joint mobility
- Decreased postoperative pain
- Early postoperative recovery
- Decreased hospital stay

Arthroscopic Equipment

Arthroscope

The arthroscope (Fig. 23–34) is a lensed, fiberoptic telescope that is inserted into a joint space. Surgery is performed through the arthroscope with specialized instruments. Care and handling of the arthroscope is the same as that for the *laparoscope.* A complete discussion

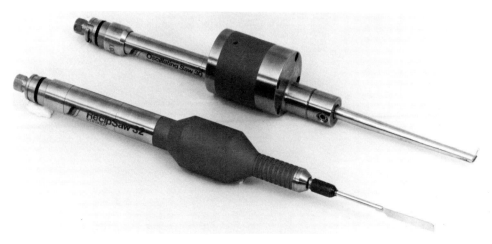

Figure 23–29. Special bone saws—the reciprocating saw and the oscillating saw. (Courtesy of the Stryker Corporation.)

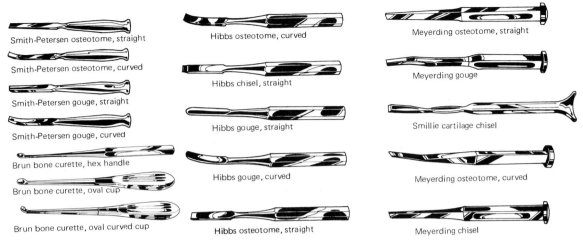

Figure 23–30. Osteotomes, curettes, chisels, and gouges. (Courtesy of Zimmer, Inc., Warsaw, IN.)

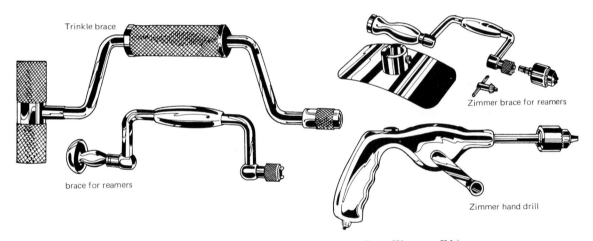

Figure 23–31. Drills. (Courtesy of Zimmer, Inc., Warsaw, IN.)

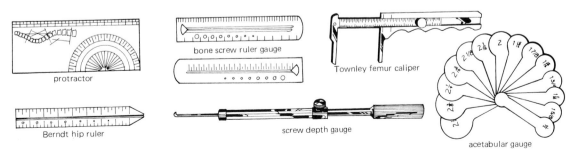

Figure 23–32. Measuring devices. (Courtesy of Zimmer, Inc., Warsaw, IN.)

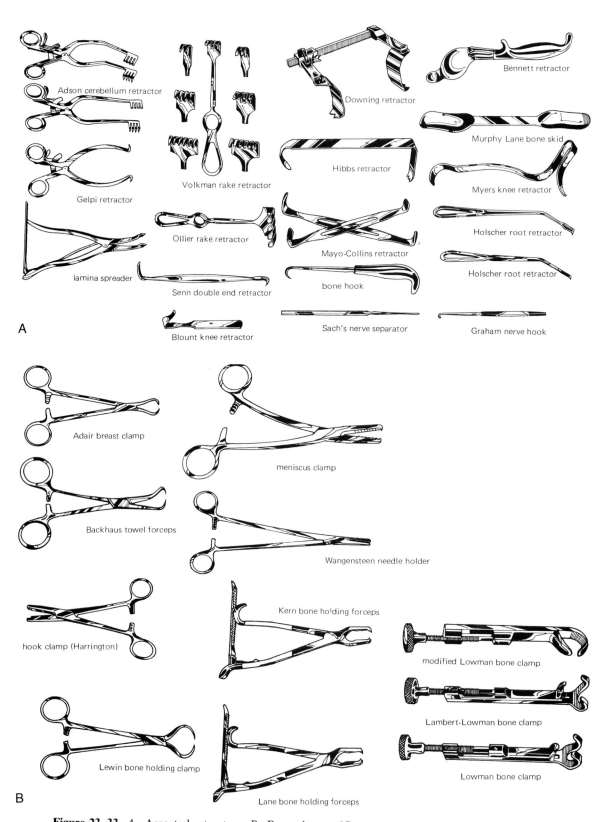

Figure 23–33. *A.* Assorted retractors. *B.* Bone clamps. (Courtesy of Zimmer, Inc., Warsaw, IN.)

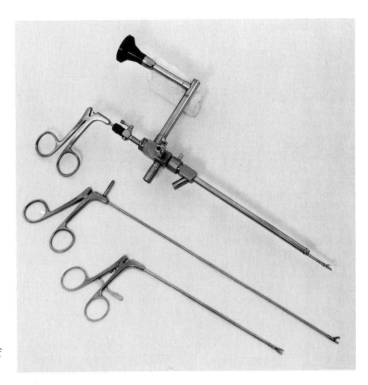

Figure 23–34. Arthroscope and accessories. (Courtesy of the Stryker Corporation.)

of endoscopic principles and techniques is presented in Chapter 20.

Video Camera System

A complete discussion of the video camera system is provided in Chapter 20. The surgeon may use this system or operate by direct visualization through the arthroscope.

Visualization and Exposure Equipment

Equipment and instruments used to distend the joint space and expose the internal structures are similar to those used during laparoscopic procedures. Whereas in laparoscopy the abdomen is filled with carbon dioxide gas to distend its walls, in arthroscopy normal saline or lactated Ringer's solution is used to fill the joint cavity. This distends the joint space and allows the surgeon to view its internal structures. The solution is pumped into the joint through a Veress needle, which is connected to the solution by a length of tubing. The solution is drained from the joint space through an additional portal near the operative site. Once the joint space is distended, trocars and sleeves are inserted to allow passage of the arthroscope and instruments.

A pneumatic tourniquet (see Chapter 13) may be used to prevent blood from entering the operative area.

Instrumentation

Instruments used during arthroscopic surgery include forceps, scissors, biopsy and grasping clamps, meniscus instruments, meniscus suture needles, anterior cruciate ligament reconstruction instruments, and arthroscopic orthopedic tools such as saws, curettes, rongeurs, and knives. Additional specialty equipment such as instruments used to take autologous grafts for ligament repair are also used. All arthroscopic instruments are delicate and should be handled with care to prevent damage to their tips.

Because all arthroscopic procedures have the potential to become open procedures, a basic orthopedic instrument tray should be included in all set-ups.

Patient Position, Prepping, and Draping

The patient positions used during arthroscopic surgery are similiar to those employed in open techniques. During *knee* procedures, the patient lies in supine position and the operative leg is prepped from thigh to ankle. Rolled towels or sterile blankets may be placed under the knee to support it. These may be removed during the course of surgery to allow the surgeon to rotate the leg and gain better exposure of the joint space. The leg is prepped and draped from mid thigh to ankle or foot.

For procedures on the *shoulder,* the patient is placed in the lateral position, with the operative arm suspended in an overhead traction device. Before surgery, the surgeon adjusts the abduction angle and flexion of the arm to facilitate exposure. The surgeon operates from behind the patient during the procedure. The arm is prepped from the wrist to the axilla.

During procedures on the *ankle,* the patient is placed in supine position with the operative leg flexed at the knee, or a sandbag may be placed under the hip on the operative side. The leg is prepped and draped from knee to ankle.

Open Procedures: Exposure and Description

Clavicle

The clavicle is a frequent site of injury because it is relatively unprotected by soft tissue. Fractures may be treated by open or closed reduction. Surgical exposure of the clavicle is shown in Figure 23–35. Two types of repair are commonly employed: screw fixation (Fig. 23–36) and fixation with a Steinmann pin (Fig. 23–37).

Shoulder

Recurrent dislocation of the shoulder is most often the result of injury that weakens the soft tissues encompassing the shoulder joint and causes the soft tissues to detach from the joint. The surgical exposure of the shoulder is shown in Figure 23–38. Of the more than 100 procedures used to repair the shoulder, two are commonly employed. The Bankart and Putti-Platt procedures are similar and involve the reattachment of the soft tissues to their proper anatomic location. To accomplish this, the surgeon drills several holes in the edge of the glenoid. The joint capsule is then incised, and a portion of the soft tissue is sutured to the glenoid by passing the sutures through the drill holes. The remaining portion of the capsule is then overlapped and sutured in place. This technique and the necessary instrumentation are illustrated in Figure 23–39.

Forearm

Transverse fractures of the forearm are a common result of injury to the arm by a direct blow or fall. Many heal satisfactorily by closed reduction and application of a plaster cast. With more complex fractures, open reduction may be necessary. The surgical exposure of the forearm is shown in Figure 23–40. When internal fixation is employed the bone fragments are fused with an intermedullary rod or pin (Figs. 23–41 through 23–43). Combinations of plates and rods are also employed.

Wrist and Hand

Wrist

The wrist is commonly injured when the patient suffers a fall and attempts to break the fall by extending the arms and hands forward. Most fractures of the wrist can be treated by closed reduction and application of a plaster cast. Open reduction and internal fixation are performed with small pins, screws, or plates. The surgical exposure of the wrist is shown in Figure 23–44.

Hand

The hand is subject to disease of the tendons and ligaments and to injury from industrial or other types of accidents. A special hand table (see Fig. 23–20) is used during hand surgery.

Two common surgically treatable diseases of the hand are Dupuytren's contracture and carpal tunnel syn-

drome. Dupuytren's contracture is a disease that causes the palmar fascia to constrict. The fingers bend in toward the patient's palm, and it becomes impossible for the patient to extend them. Surgical treatment is aimed toward releasing the fascia by sharp dissection (Fig. 23–45).

Carpal tunnel syndrome is a condition resulting in pressure on the median nerve as it passes through the carpal tunnel. The pressure may be due to an increased thickening of the synovium, injury, or structural anomaly. Surgical treatment of the disease involves release of the stricture by sharp dissection (Fig. 23–46).

Injury of the hand is given serious consideration by the surgeon, since unsuccessful treatment may seriously affect the patient's livelihood or life-style. Fracture of the finger may be treated by closed reduction and external fixation with a splint or may require internal fixation with a small Steinmann pin or wire (Kirschner wire).

Tendon injuries (Fig. 23–47) are commonly repaired with fine sutures. The technique used in tendon repair is shown in Figure 23–48. The extensive pulley system in the hand sometimes makes repair and rehabilitation of these injuries difficult.

Fractures and dislocations of the fingers (Fig. 23–49) may be repaired with fine wires or pins or with screws and usually heal without complications.

Hip

The femur and acetabulum are commonly referred to in medicine as the hip. Surgical exposure of the hip is shown in Figure 23–50. Fractures of the femoral neck, trochanter, and femoral head are commonly seen in the elderly patient who sustains a fall. Pathologic fractures are also indications for surgical repair of the hip. Fractures of the femoral neck and trochanter may be treated by the insertion of nails, pins, or rods that are inserted across the fracture to bind the fragments together. If the femoral head is damaged, the surgeon may choose to remove it and insert a prosthesis. Total hip replacement (replacement of both the femoral head and acetabulum) may be indicated when degenerative disease or injury involves both of these structures. There are many different types of procedures for total hip replacement. Basic instruments for hip procedures are common to most of these procedures. More specific instrumentation for a given type of hip replacement should be presented to the operating room staff by the manufacturer's representative.

Fractures of the femoral shaft are treated with rods, pins, or plates. Compression plates that reduce the fracture mechanically are commonly employed.

Common procedures of the hip and femoral shaft and their associated instruments are shown in Figures 23–51 through 23–58.

Knee

The knee is a relatively weak structure that carries a great deal of stress and weight. Injury to the knee during athletic sport is common. The ligaments and menisci are

Text continued on page 458

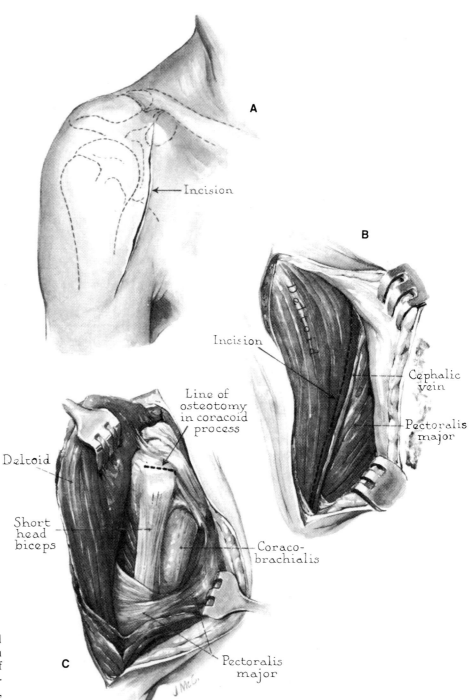

Figure 23–35. *A* through *C*. Surgical exposure of the clavicle. (From Banks SW, Laufman H: An Atlas of Surgical Exposures of the Extremities. Philadelphia, WB Saunders, 1953.)

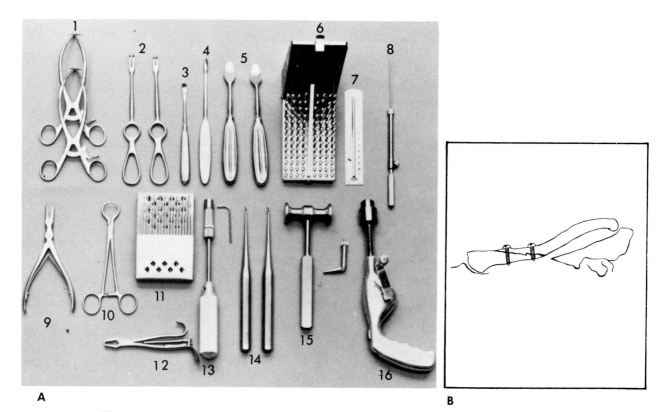

Figure 23–36. *A*. Screw fixation of the clavicle. 1, Gelpi retractors; 2, rake retractors; 3, Adson periosteal elevator; 4, Langenbeck periosteal elevator; 5, Chandler elevators; 6, Woodruff screws; 7, ruler; 8, depth gauge; 9, Beyer rongeur; 10, Lewin bone clamp; 11, drill bits; 12, Kern bone clamp; 13, screwdriver; 14, curettes; 15, mallet; 16, hand drill and key. *B*. Indication—transverse fracture of the clavicle. (Courtesy of Zimmer Inc., Warsaw, IN.)

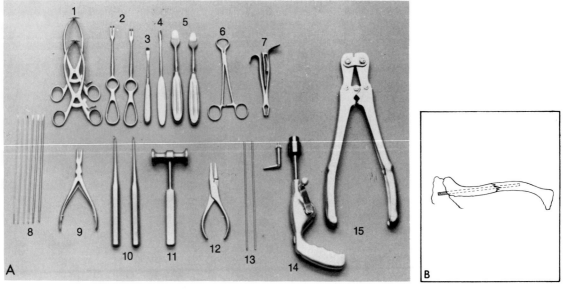

Figure 23–37. *A*. Steinmann pin fixation of the clavicle. 1, Gelpi retractors; 2, rake retractors; 3, Adson periosteal elevator; 4, Langenbeck periosteal elevator; 5, Chandler elevators; 6, Lewin bone clamp; 7, Kern bone clamp; 8, assorted Steinmann pins; 9, Beyer rongeur; 10, curettes; 11, mallet; 12, needle-nosed pliers; 13, clavicle pins; 14, hand drill and key; 15, pin cutter. *B*. Indication—transverse fracture of the clavicle. (Courtesy of Zimmer Inc., Warsaw, IN.)

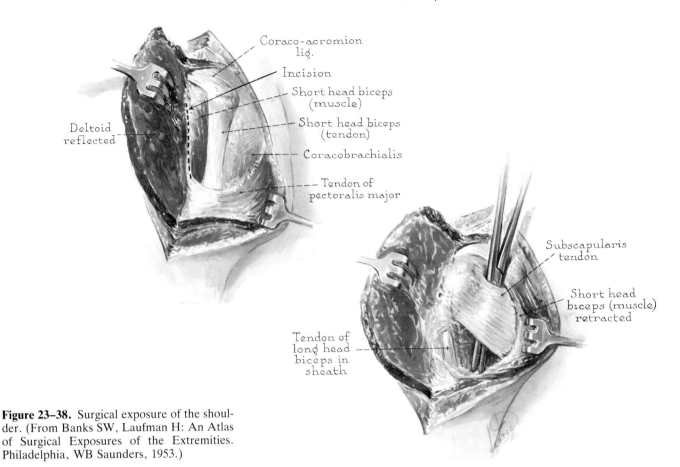

Figure 23–38. Surgical exposure of the shoulder. (From Banks SW, Laufman H: An Atlas of Surgical Exposures of the Extremities. Philadelphia, WB Saunders, 1953.)

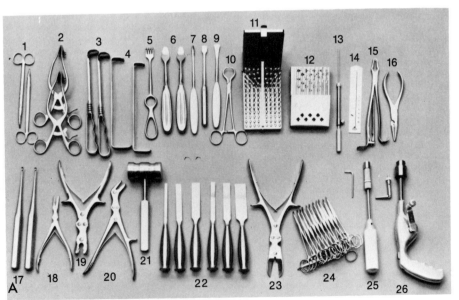

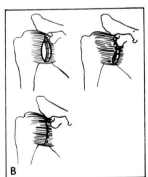

Figure 23–39. A. Bankart or Putti-Platt instrumentation. 1, Metzenbaum scissors; 2, Weitlaner retractors; 3, Richardson retractors; 4, U.S. retractors; 5, rake retractor; 6, Chandler elevators; 7, Langenbeck periosteal elevator; 8, Key periosteal elevator; 9, Langenbeck periosteal elevator; 10, Lewin bone clamp; 11, Woodruff screws; 12, drill bits; 13, depth gauge; 14, ruler; 15, Kern bone clamp; 16, needle-nosed pliers; 17, curettes; 18, Beyer rongeur; 19, Stille-Luer rongeur; 20, Stille-Luer rongeur; 21, mallet; 22, osteotomes; 23, bone cutter; 24, Kelly hemostats; 25, screwdriver; 26, hand drill and key. B. Indication—recurrent shoulder dislocation. (Courtesy of Zimmer Inc., Warsaw, IN.)

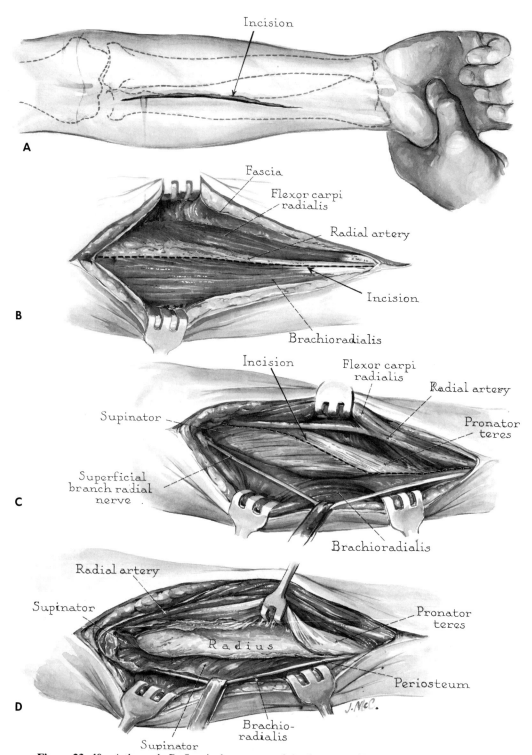

Figure 23–40. *A* through *D*. Surgical exposure of the forearm. (From Banks SW, Laufman H: An Atlas of Surgical Exposures of the Extremities. Philadelphia, WB Saunders, 1953.)

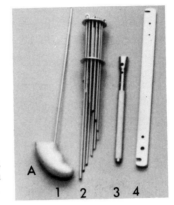

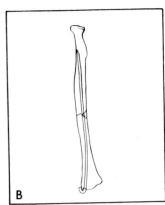

Figure 23–41. *A.* Rush rod instruments. 1, Rush awl reamer; 2, Rush rods in rack; 3, Rush driver-bender-extractor; 4, Rush bender. *B.* Indication—transverse fracture of the radius. (Courtesy of Zimmer Inc., Warsaw, IN.)

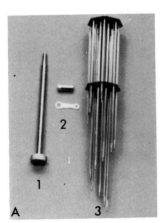

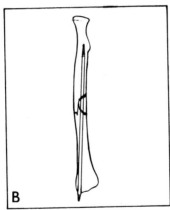

Figure 23–42. *A.* 1, Schneider driver-extractor; 2, cap and anchor plate; 3, Schneider nails. *B.* Indication—transverse fracture of the radius. (Courtesy of Zimmer Inc., Warsaw, IN.)

Figure 23–43. *A.* 1, Steinmann pins; 2, large pin cutter. *B.* Indication—transverse fractures of both the radius and ulna. (Courtesy of Zimmer Inc., Warsaw, IN.)

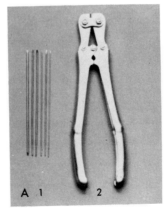

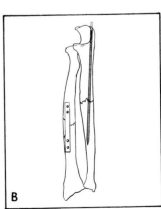

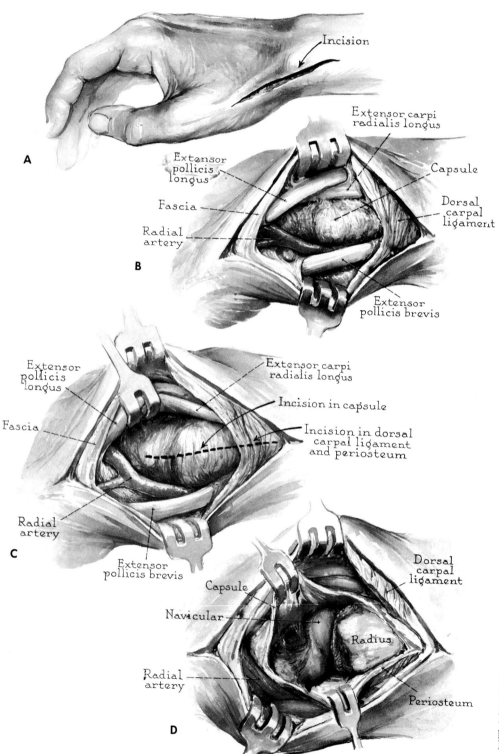

Figure 23–44. *A* through *D*. Surgical exposure of the wrist. (From Banks SW, Laufman H: An Atlas of Surgical Exposures of the Extremities. Philadelphia, WB Saunders, 1953.)

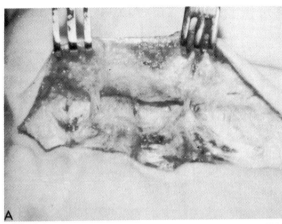

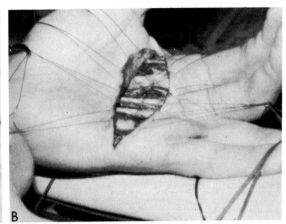

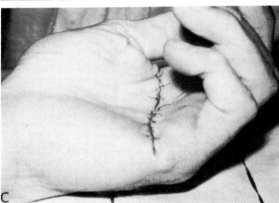

Figure 23–45. Surgical treatment of Dupuytren's contracture. *A.* Exposure of the constructed palmar fascia. (From Converse JM (ed): Reconstructive Plastic Surgery, 2nd ed. Philadelphia, WB Saunders, 1977.) *B.* Once the fascia has been released, transfixion sutures are employed to approximate the skin flaps. *C.* Skin closure. (*B* and *C* from Hueston JT: Dupuytren's contracture: selection for surgery. Br J Hosp Med 13:361, 1974.)

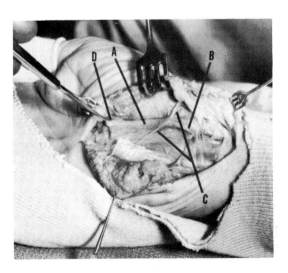

Figure 23–46. Release of carpal tunnel stricture. Carpal ligament is retracted. A, atrophy; B, pseudoneuroma of median nerve; C, Cutaneous nerve branches; D, motor nerve branch. (From Converse JM (ed): Reconstructive Plastic Surgery, 2nd ed. Philadelphia, WB Saunders, 1977.)

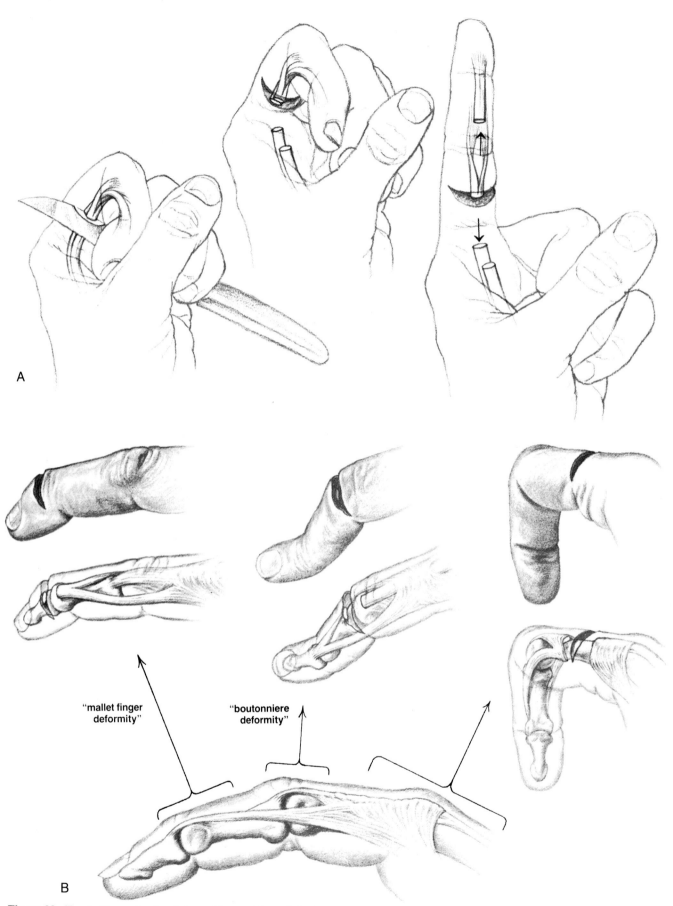

A

"mallet finger
deformity"

"boutonniere
deformity"

B

Figure 23–47. *A.* Flexor tendon injury. The position of the hand and fingers at the time of injury is particularly important since the level of tendon laceration may be quite distal to the skin laceration if the fingers were acutely flexed during injury. *B.* Extensor tendon injury and resultant deformity. (Courtesy of Ethicon, Inc., Somerville, NJ.)

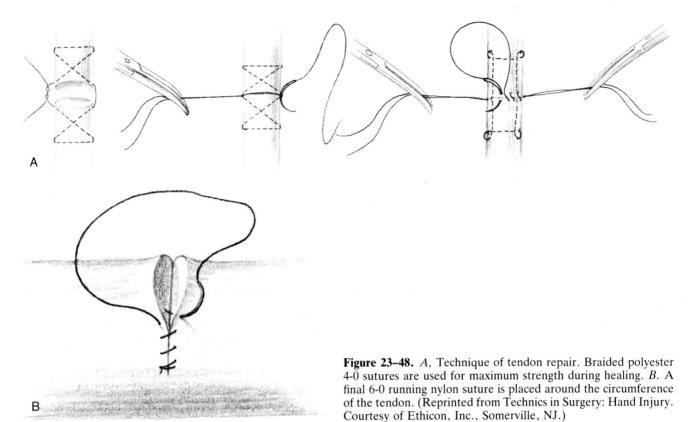

Figure 23–48. *A,* Technique of tendon repair. Braided polyester 4-0 sutures are used for maximum strength during healing. *B.* A final 6-0 running nylon suture is placed around the circumference of the tendon. (Reprinted from Technics in Surgery: Hand Injury. Courtesy of Ethicon, Inc., Somerville, NJ.)

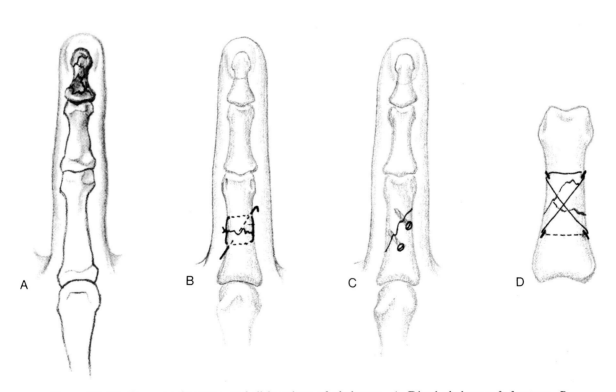

Figure 23–49. Common fractures and dislocations of phalanges. *A.* Distal phalanx tuft fracture. *B* through *D.* Use of fixation in phalangeal fracture. (Courtesy of Ethicon, Inc., Somerville, NJ.)

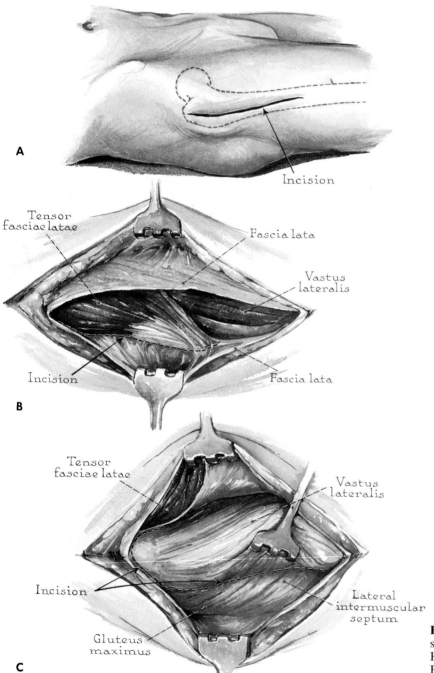

A

Incision

Tensor
fasciae latae

Fascia lata

Vastus
lateralis

Incision

Fascia lata

B

Tensor
fasciae latae

Vastus
lateralis

Incision

Lateral
intermuscular
septum

Gluteus
maximus

C

Figure 23–50. *A* through *C.* Surgical exposure of the hip. (From Banks SW, Laufman H: An Atlas of Surgical Exposures of the Extremities. Philadelphia, WB Saunders, 1953.)

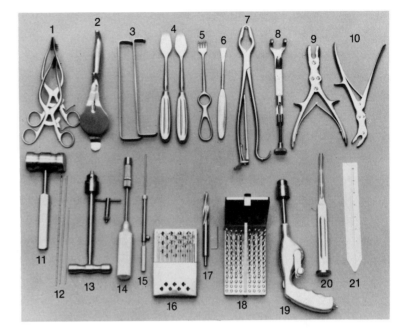

Figure 23–51. Basic instrumentation for hip nailing. 1, Weitlaner retractors; 2, Bennett retractor; 3, U.S. retractors; 4, Chandler elevators; 5, rake retractor; 6, Langenbeck periosteal elevator; 7, Lane bone clamp; 8, Lowman bone clamp; 9, Stille-Luer rongeur; 10, Stille-Luer rongeur; 11, mallet; 12, calibrated guide wire; 13, hand chuck and key; 14, screwdriver; 15, depth gauge; 16, drill bits; 17, cortical drill; 18, screws; 19, hand drill; 20, gouge; 21, ruler. (Courtesy of Zimmer Inc., Warsaw, IN.)

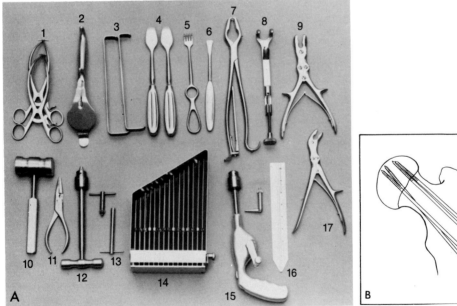

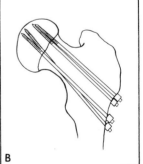

Figure 23–52. *A.* Instrumentation for Knowles pins. 1, Gelpi retractors; 2, Bennett retractor; 3, U.S. retractors; 4, Chandler elevators; 5, small rake retractor; 6, periosteal elevator; 7, Lane bone clamp; 8, Lowman bone clamp; 9, Stille rongeur; 10, mallet; 11, needle-nosed pliers; 12, hand chuck and key; 13, cannulated wrench; 14, set of Knowles pins; 15, hand drill and key; 16, ruler; 17, angled Stille rongeur. *B.* Indication—fracture of the femoral neck. (Courtesy of Zimmer Inc., Warsaw, IN.)

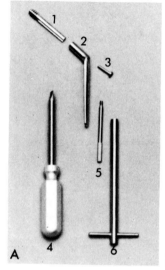

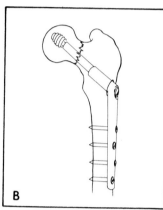

Figure 23–53. *A.* Compression screw. 1, Compression lag screw; 2, compression tube and nail; 3, compression set screw; 4, screwdriver; 5, plate, tube guide; 6, compression inserter-extractor; *B.* Indication—fracture of the femoral neck. (Courtesy of Zimmer Inc., Warsaw, IN.)

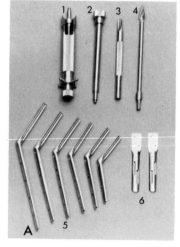

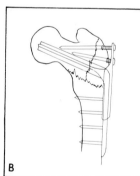

Figure 23–54. *A.* Jewett nail. 1, Impactor-extractor; 2, Jewett driver; 3, nail starter; 4, spiral cortical reamer; 5, set of Jewett nails; 6, overlay plates. *B.* Indication—fracture of the femoral neck. (Courtesy of Zimmer Inc., Warsaw, IN.)

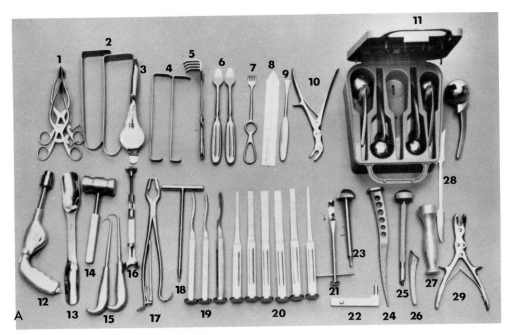

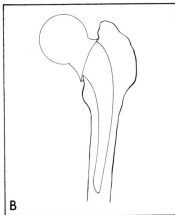

Figure 23–55. *A.* Thompson femoral head prosthesis instrumentation. 1, Weitlaner retractors; 2, Hibbs retractors; 3, Bennett retractor; 4, U.S. retractors; 5, Israel retractor; 6, Chandler elevators; 7, rake retractor; 8, ruler; 9, Langenbeck periosteal elevator; 10, Stille-Luer rongeur; 11, Thompson prostheses; 12, hand drill; 13, bone skid; 14, mallet; 15, bone hooks; 16, Lowman bone clamp; 17, Lane bone clamp; 18, femoral head extractor; 19, gouges; 20, osteotomes; 21, acetabular knife; 22, caliper; 23, ball reamer; 24, rasp; 25, Fisher guide; 26, Fisher rasp; 27, prosthesis driver; 28, rasp; 29, Stille-Luer rongeur. *B.* Indication—injury or disease of the femoral head. (Courtesy of Zimmer Inc., Warsaw, IN.)

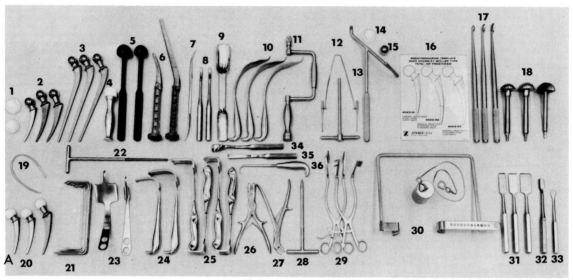

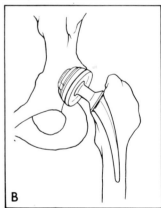

Figure 23–56. *A*. Muller-type total hip replacement. 1, Muller-type cups; 2, Muller-type total hip; 3, Muller-type total hip, extra long; 4, prosthesis driver; 5, acetabular gauges; 6, rasps; 7, Putti bone rasp; 8, Cobb gouges; 9, Murphy-Lane bone skid; 10, Cobra retractors; 11, brace; 12, pin retractor; 13, cup positioner; 14, replacement head; 15, replacement head; 16, prosthesis template; 17, curettes; 18, reamers; 19, medullary vent tubing; 20, provisional prosthesis; 21, Sofield retractors; 22, taper reamer; 23, Hohman retractors; 24, Meyerding retractors; 25, large rake retractors; 26, Stille rongeur; 27, angled Stille rongeur; 28, femoral head extractor; 29, Beckman retractors; 30, initial incision retractor; 31, Hibbs chisels; 32, gooseneck gouge; 33, periosteal elevator; 34, swan-neck gouge; 35, gouge; 36, bone hook. *B*. Indication—injury or disease of the acetabulum and femoral head. (Courtesy of Zimmer Inc., Warsaw, IN.)

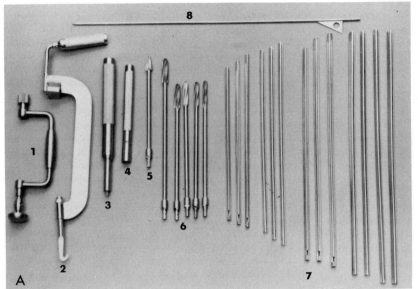
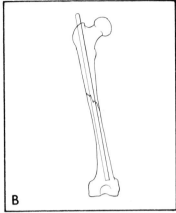

Figure 23–57. *A.* Küntscher nail. 1, Brace; 2, extractor; 3, nail set; 4, driver; 5, trochanteric reamer; 6, medullary canal reamers; 7, Küntscher nails; 8, femoral guide pin. *B.* Indication—transverse fracture of the femoral shaft. (Courtesy of Zimmer Inc., Warsaw, IN.)

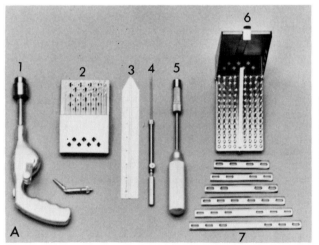
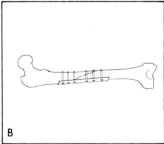

Figure 23–58. *A.* Instrumentation for heavy side plate. 1, Hand drill; 2, drill bits; 3, ruler; 4, depth gauge; 5, screwdriver; 6, screws; 7, femoral plates. *B.* Indication—oblique fracture of the femoral shaft. (Courtesy of Zimmer Inc., Warsaw, IN.)

particularly vulnerable to a "wrenching" type of injury. The torn meniscus is removed by sharp dissection. A torn ligament may be sutured in place or transferred to another location and attached with sutures or staples. Fracture of the patella may be caused by a direct blow or fall.

Total knee replacement is indicated when injury or disease has resulted in a nonfunctioning joint. There are many different types of partial and total knee replacement procedures, and, as with the total hip replacement techniques, the technologist should attend in-service lectures to become familiar with the total knee procedures practiced in his or her operating room.

Figure 23–59 shows the surgical exposure of the knee joint. Surgical procedures and instrumentation for operations on the knee are shown in Figures 23–60 through 23–63.

Tibia and Fibula

Fractures of the tibia and fibula are frequently caused by injury due to an accident (e.g., skiing, motorcycle,

Text continued on page 466

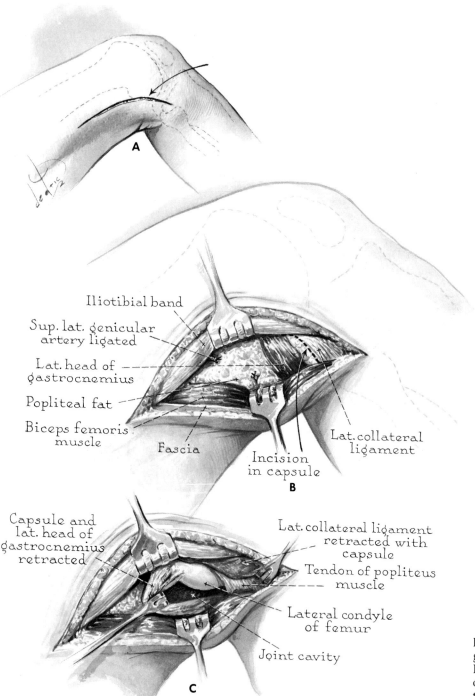

Figure 23–59. *A* through *C.* Surgical exposure of the knee. (From Banks SW, Laufman H: An Atlas of Surgical Exposures of the Extremities. Philadelphia, WB Saunders, 1953.)

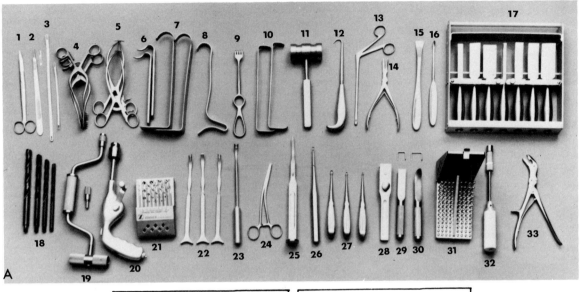

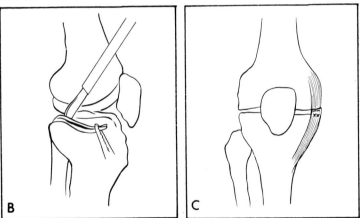

Figure 23–60. *A.* Instrumentation for meniscus and ligament. 1, Cartilage scissors; 2, No. 3 knife handle and No. 15 blade; 3, tendon passers; 4, Weitlaner retractors; 5, Gelpi retractors; 6, Blount knee retractors; 7, Hibbs retractors; 8, Myers knee retractor; 9, rake retractor; 10, U.S. retractors; 11, mallet; 12, bone hook; 13, Spurling rongeur; 14, Beyer rongeur; 15, elevator; 16, periosteal elevator; 17, osteotomes; 18, high-speed drills; 19, Trinkle brace and adapter; 20, hand drill; 21, drill bits; 22, Smillie cartilage knives; 23, Downing cartilage knife; 24, meniscus clamp; 25, gouge; 26, long curette; 27, short curettes; 28, staple inserter; 29, staple driver; 30, staple extractor; 31, screws; 32, screwdriver; 33, Stille-Luer rongeur. *B.* Indication—torn meniscus. *C.* Indication—repair of torn ligament. (Courtesy of Zimmer Inc., Warsaw, IN.)

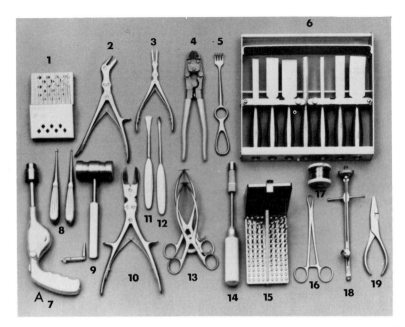
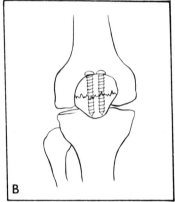

Figure 23–61. *A.* Instrumentation for repair of patella. 1, Drill bits; 2, Stille-Luer rongeur; 3, Beyer rongeur; 4, wire cutter; 5, rake retractor; 6, osteotomes; 7, hand drill and key; 8, curettes; 9, mallet; 10, Stille-Luer bone cutters; 11, periosteal elevator; 12, periosteal elevator; 13, Gelpi retractors; 14, screwdriver; 15, screws; 16, Adair breast clamp; 17, spool of wire; 18, Shifrin wire twister; 19, pliers. *B.* Indication—transverse fracture of the patella. (Courtesy of Zimmer Inc., Warsaw, IN.)

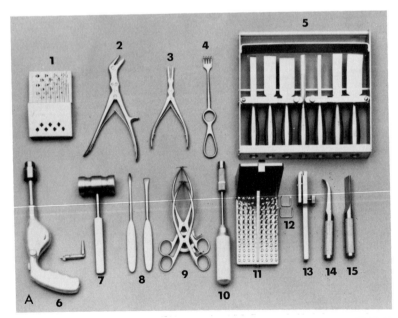
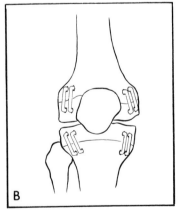

Figure 23–62. *A.* Instruments for epiphyseal stapling. 1, Drill bits; 2, Stille-Luer rongeur; 3, Beyer rongeur; 4, rake retractor; 5, osteotomes; 6, hand drill and key; 7, mallet; 8, periosteal elevators; 9, Gelpi retractors; 10, screwdriver; 11, screws; 12, staples; 13, staple inserter; 14, staple extractor; 15, staple driver. *B.* Indication—unequal growth of the legs. (Courtesy of Zimmer Inc., Warsaw, IN.)

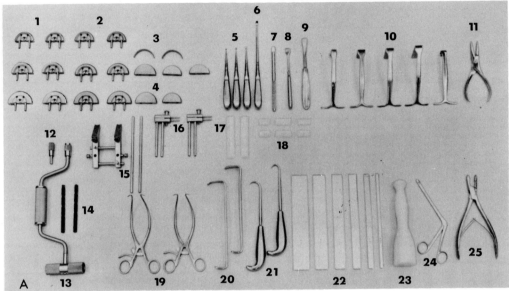

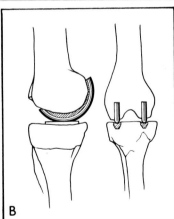

Figure 23–63. *A*. Instrumentation for polycentric-type total knee replacement. 1, Femoral components; 2, trial femoral components; 3, femoral condyle templates; 4, femoral drill guides; 5, straight curettes; 6, angled curette; 7, impactor; 8, rake retractor; 9, Cushing elevator; 10, Smillie retractors; 11, needle-nosed pliers; 12, adapter; 13, brace; 14, high-speed twist drills; 15, femoral positioning instruments; 16, tibial track holder; 17, tibial track template; 18, tibial components; 19, Gelpi retractors; 20, U.S. retractors; 21, bone hooks; 22, osteotomes; 23, mallet; 24, Spurling rongeur; 25, Adson rongeur; *B*. Indication—severe injury or degenerative disease of the knee joint. (Courtesy of Zimmer Inc., Warsaw, IN.)

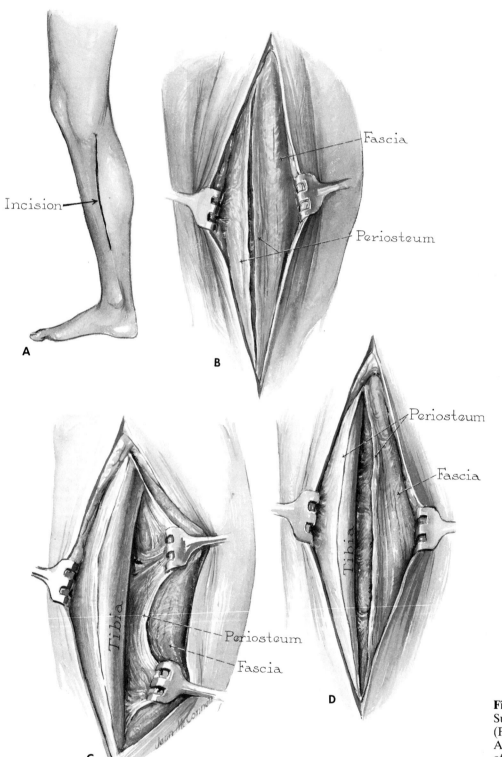

Figure 23–64. *A* through *D*. Surgical exposure of the tibia. (From Banks SW, Laufman H: An Atlas of Surgical Exposures of the Extremities. Philadelphia, WB Saunders, 1953.)

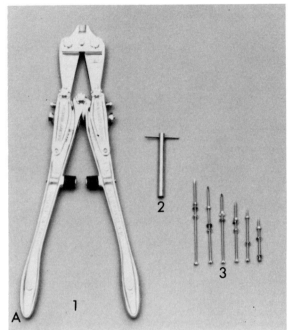
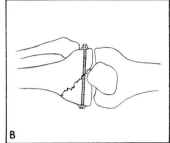

Figure 23–65. *A.* Bolt fixation of the tibia. 1, Pin cutter; 2, cannulated wrench; 3, tibia bolts. *B.* Indication—fracture of the tibia. (Courtesy of Zimmer Inc., Warsaw, IN.)

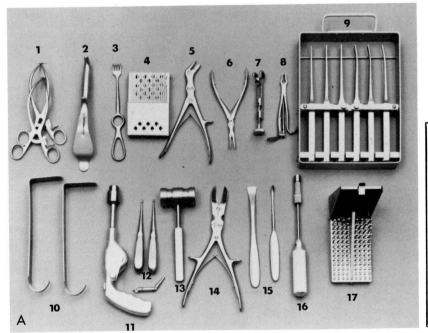
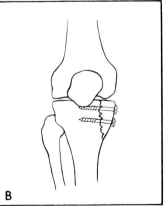

Figure 23–66. *A.* Screw fixation of the tibia. 1, Gelpi retractors; 2, Bennett retractor; 3, rake retractor; 4, drill bits; 5, Stille-Luer rongeur; 6, Beyer rongeur; 7, Lowman bone clamp; 8, Kern bone clamp; 9, osteotomes; 10, Hibbs retractors; 11, hand drill and key; 12, curettes; 13, mallet; 14, Stille-Luer bone cutter; 15, periosteal elevator; 16, screwdriver; 17, screws. *B.* Indication—fracture of the tibia. (Courtesy of Zimmer Inc., Warsaw, IN.)

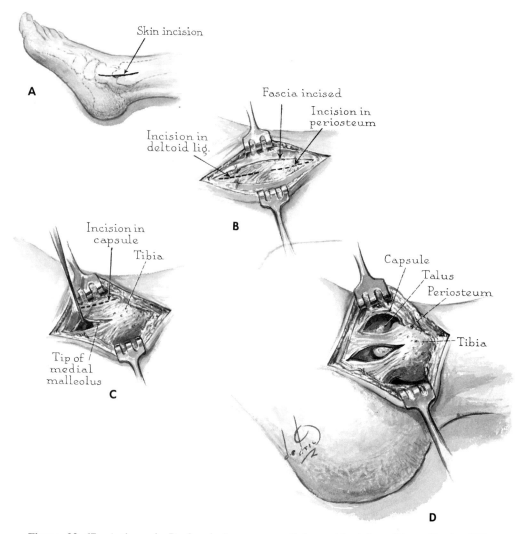

Figure 23–67. *A* through *D*. Surgical exposure of the ankle joint. (From Banks SW, Laufman H: An Atlas of Surgical Exposures of the Extremities. Philadelphia, WB Saunders, 1953.)

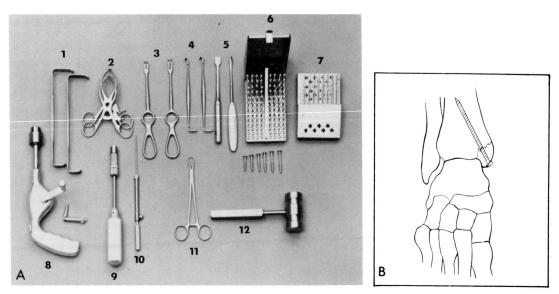

Figure 23–68. *A.* Screw fixation of the malleoli. 1, U.S. retractors; 2, Gelpi retractors; 3, two-prong rake retractors; 4, Senn retractors; 5, periosteal elevators; 6, screws; 7, drill bits; 8, hand drill and key; 9, screwdriver; 10, depth gauge; 11, Adair breast clamp; 12, mallet. *B.* Indication—fracture of the malleoli. (Courtesy of Zimmer Inc., Warsaw, IN.)

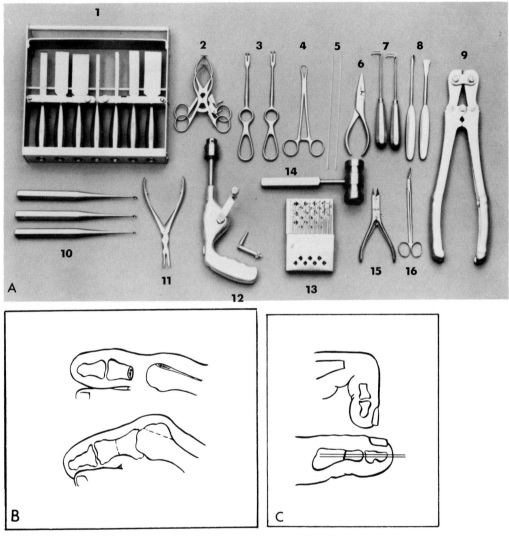

Figure 23–69. *A.* Toe and bunion instrumentation. 1, Osteotomes; 2, Gelpi retractors; 3, rake retractors; 4, Adair breast clamp; 5, Kirschner wires; 6, needle-nosed pliers; 7, hospital retractors; 8, periosteal elevators; 9, large pin cutter; 10, curettes; 11, Beyer rongeur; 12, hand drill and key; 13, drill bits; 14, mallet; 15, small bone cutters; 16, Dean scissors. *B.* Indication—bunion. *C.* Indication—hammertoe. (Courtesy of Zimmer Inc., Warsaw, IN.)

automobile). Although many of these fractures can be treated by closed reduction, others must be fixated with rods, nails, plates, or screws.

Figures 23–64 through 23–66 show the surgical exposure of the tibia and techniques of repair.

Ankle and Foot

Fracture and deformity of the foot may be due to injury or disease. When fracture of one of the ankle bones occurs, open reduction may be necessary. The bone fragments can be fixated with screws or pins. The diseased foot can be stabilized by a triple arthrodesis (binding of the subtalar, calcaneocuboid, and talonavicular joints with staples). Surgical exposure of the ankle is shown in Figure 23–67.

Various malformations of the toes and foot include bunions (excess tissue on the medial surface of the great toe) and hammertoe. Hammertoe deformity occurs when the toes are flexed (contracted). This painful condition causes the top of the toe to rub on the patient's shoe. The affected joint is resected and a small wire is inserted through the toe to hold it straight while healing occurs. When disease has caused the degeneration of the great toe joint, a Silastic prosthesis may be inserted to replace it.

Surgical procedures of the ankle and toe and their associated instrumentation are illustrated in Figures 23–68 and 23–69.

Bibliography

Banks SW, Laufman H: An Atlas of Surgical Exposures of the Extremities. Philadelphia, WB Saunders, 1973.

Boyes JH (ed): Bunnell's Surgery of the Hand, 5th ed. Philadelphia, JB Lippincott, 1970.

Chase RA: Atlas of Hand Surgery, vol 1. Philadelphia, WB Saunders, 1973.

Deyerle W, et al: Methylmethacrylate: uses and complications. AORN 29(4):696, 1979.

Dorland's Illustrated Medical Dictionary, 26th ed. Philadelphia, WB Saunders, 1981.

Drucker M: Arthroscopic Surgery of the knee joint. AORN 36(4):585, 1982.

Ethicon, Inc: Technics in Surgery: Hand Injury. Somerville, NJ, Ethicon, Inc.

Gardner E, Gray D, O'Rahilly R: Anatomy: A Regional Study of Human Structure, 4th ed. Philadelphia, WB Saunders, 1984.

Gartland J: Fundamentals of Orthopaedics, 3rd ed. Philadelphia, WB Saunders, 1979.

Jacob S, Francone C, Lossow WJ: Structure and Function in Man, 5th ed. Philadelphia, WB Saunders, 1982.

Laskin RS, Varrichio DM: Total Knee Replacement. AORN 36(4): 1982.

McVay C: Surgical Anatomy, 6th ed. Philadelphia, WB Saunders, 1984.

Turek S: Orthopaedics: Principles and Their Application. Philadelphia, JB Lippincott, 1967.

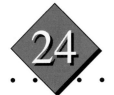

Cardiothoracic Surgery

The purpose of surgical intervention in the cardiothoracic system (the heart, associated great vessels, and pulmonary structures) varies according to the specific anatomy involved. The aim of cardiac surgery is to correct defects and improve the function of the heart. Abnormalities of the great vessels, particularly the aorta, are surgically corrected to improve the circulation of blood to the body. The aims of pulmonary surgery are to make a diagnosis by means of endoscopy and to treat diseased tissue by resection. The technologist should have a thorough knowledge of the anatomy involved in each specific procedure. He or she is encouraged to develop a solid background in general surgery to comprehend the surgical procedures presented in this chapter more fully.

SURGICAL ANATOMY

The Thoracic Cavity

The thoracic cavity is separated from the abdominal cavity by the diaphragm and contains the heart and its great vessels, the lungs and associated respiratory structures, the mediastinum, and a portion of the esophagus.

The Heart

The heart is a muscular organ that consists of four hollow spaces, or *chambers*. It lies between the two lungs within an enclosed cavity called the *mediastinum*. Most of the heart's mass lies to the left of the midline.

Enclosing the heart (Fig. 24–1) is a double-layered membrane called the *pericardium*. Between the inner

layer of the pericardium, the *visceral pericardium*, and the outer layer, the *parietal pericardium*, is a fluid called *pericardial fluid*, which lubricates the two tissue layers and prevents friction.

The walls of the heart contain three layers. The outer layer is called the *epicardium*, the middle layer is the *myocardium*, and the inner layer is the *endocardium*. Only the middle layer contains muscle tissue.

The four chambers of the heart are each divided by a *septum*, and each has a separate function. The upper chambers, the *atria* (singular *atrium*), are the receiving chambers. Blood is brought into the atria by veins and is then emptied into the lower chambers, the ventricles. The ventricles are the pumping chambers where blood is transferred back to various parts of the body. Because of the pumping function of the ventricles, their walls are much thicker than those of the atria. In Figure 24–2 the path of blood is shown as it flows from one chamber to another.

Blood flows from the atria to the ventricles and from the ventricles to the pulmonary artery and aorta by way of *valves* (see Fig. 24–2). The valves between the atria and ventricles (atrioventricular valves) each have a separate name. On the right side of the heart, the valve is the *tricuspid valve*. On the left side, the valve is called the *mitral* or *bicuspid valve*. When blood leaves the ventricles, it passes through the *semilunar valves*. These are named according to the vessel of destination—on the right side, it is the *pulmonary valve*, and, on the left side, it is the *aortic valve*.

The heart tissue itself is nourished by its own blood supply, which is separate from the blood that it pumps to the body. Two major arteries supply this need; these are the *coronary arteries*. The coronary arteries are smaller branches of the aorta. Blood is drained from the heart tissue by the *coronary veins*.

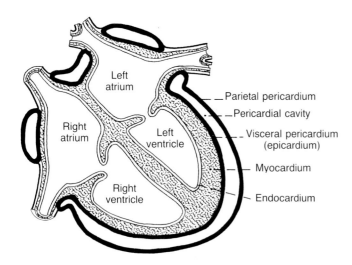

Left atrium

Right atrium

Left ventricle

Right ventricle

—Parietal pericardium

—Pericardial cavity

—Visceral pericardium (epicardium)

—Myocardium

—Endocardium

Figure 24–1. Schematic drawing of the heart showing tissue layers, spaces, and chambers. (From Jacob S, Francone C, Lossow WJ: Structure and Function in Man, 5th ed. Philadelphia, WB Saunders, 1982.)

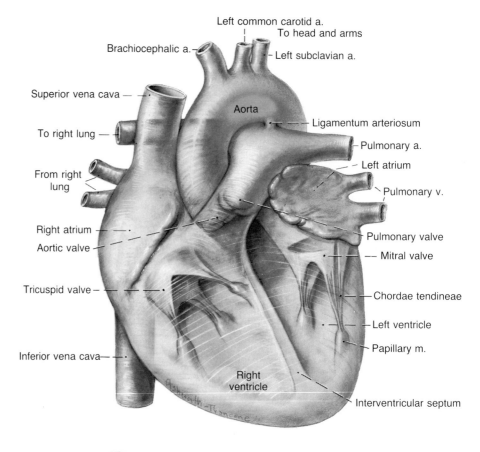

Left common carotid a.
To head and arms

Brachiocephalic a.

Left subclavian a.

Superior vena cava

Aorta

Ligamentum arteriosum

To right lung

Pulmonary a.

Left atrium

From right lung

Pulmonary v.

Right atrium

Pulmonary valve

Aortic valve

Mitral valve

Tricuspid valve

Chordae tendineae

Left ventricle

Papillary m.

Inferior vena cava

Right ventricle

Interventricular septum

Figure 24–2. Cutaway view of the heart showing position and types of valves. (From Jacob S, Francone C, Lossow WJ: Structure and Function in Man, 5th ed. Philadelphia, WB Saunders, 1982.)

VALVES

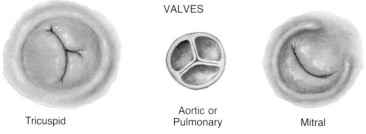

Tricuspid

Aortic or Pulmonary

Mitral

The *cardiac cycle* is divided into two distinct phases. The first phase is *systole* and occurs when the heart is contracting. *Diastole* is the relaxation phase. Venous blood enters the heart through the vena cava and fills the right atrium. From the right atrium, the blood is then shunted across the tricuspid valve into the right ventricle, where it then passes through the pulmonary valve into the pulmonary arteries. The blood is then carried along to the lungs, where it is oxygenated. From the lungs, the blood enters the left atrium through the pulmonary veins and then passes to the left ventricle through the mitral valve. During ventricular contraction, the blood passes through the aortic valve and enters the aorta. The aorta then carries the oxygenated blood to the rest of the body. Normal and abnormal flow of blood through the heart is shown in Figure 24–3.

Great Vessels of the Heart

The large vessels surrounding the heart (see Fig. 24–2) are an intrinsic part of cardiac circulation and are discussed in conjunction with the heart rather than with other vessels of the body.

The *vena cava* is divided into two sections: inferior and superior. The *inferior vena cava* brings blood into the heart from the legs and trunk. This blood is of course deoxygenated because at this level it has not passed through the cardiac cycle and hence the lungs, where it picks up oxygen. The *superior vena cava* brings blood into the heart from the head and arms. Both portions of the vena cava meet at the right atrium as previously discussed. The *pulmonary artery* exits from the right ventricle and branches into two portions: left and right. These arteries carry deoxygenated blood to the lungs. The four *pulmonary veins* bring blood back from the lungs and into the left atrium.

Oxygenated blood leaves the heart by way of the *aorta*. As the aorta crosses over the pulmonary artery, it is called the *aortic arch*. Three branches arise directly from the aortic arch and are the *innominate artery, left common carotid artery*, and *left subclavian artery*. These branches of the aorta carry blood to the upper portion of the body. The descending aorta, or lower portion of the aorta, carries oxygenated blood to the lower portion of the body.

The Lungs and Associated Respiratory Structures

In addition to the heart and its associated structures, the thoracic cavity also contains the lungs, a portion of the trachea, and the bronchi, all part of the respiratory system (Fig. 24–4).

The *trachea* is a tubular structure that conveys air from the outside atmosphere of the body to the lungs. Its proximal portion lies within the throat and neck area, but shortly after entering the thoracic cavity, it splits into two distinct tubes called the *primary bronchi*. This split occurs at the level of the fifth thoracic vertebra. The right bronchus is much shorter and larger in diameter than the left bronchus, and, because of this, it collects foreign bodies that enter the trachea. Both bronchi lie behind the pulmonary blood vessels, and the left bronchus is situated behind the aorta. The primary bronchi are further divided into *lobar bronchi*. There are three right and two left lobar bronchi. The lobar bronchi further divide into *tertiary* or *segmental bronchi*, which branch out into finer and finer tubules and terminate at the entrance of the lung into *terminal bronchioles*. The final branching results in the *respiratory bronchioles*. These respiratory bronchioles actually open into the alveolar ducts of the lungs.

The two *lungs* are situated in the mid-thoracic cavity and are bound by two *pleural cavities*. Each lung is separated by the mediastinum, which lies in the middle. The lungs are enveloped in a membrane called the *pleura*. The pleura is divided into two layers. The *visceral pleura* lies close to the lung and covers its surface. The *parietal pleura* lines the diaphragm and the inner surface of the chest cavity. The two layers of the pleura are separated by a fluid that acts as a lubricant and prevents friction caused by the layers.

The upper portion of the lung, called the *apex*, reaches just above the clavicle. Below the apex about one third the distance down is an area called the *hilum*. The bronchus, major blood vessels, and lymphatics leave and enter the lung in this area.

Each lung is divided into sections or *lobes*. The left lung contains only two lobes: the inferior and superior. The right lung is divided into the superior, inferior, and middle lobes. These lobes are separated by *fissures*.

The air pockets of the lung are called *alveoli*. These are coated with a protein-like substance that reduces the surface tension on the tissue and prevents the lung from collapsing entirely. The alveoli greatly increase the surface area of the lungs and allow a large amount of air and therefore oxygen to be taken in with each breath.

Inspiration, or the act of breathing in, is caused by the contraction of the diaphragm and intercostal muscles. As the diaphragm contracts, it elongates the thoracic cavity and causes the pressure within the lungs to lower. This forces air into the lungs. *Expiration*, or breathing out, occurs when the diaphragm and intercostal muscles relax. The alveoli contract, and air escapes out of the lungs. This allows the pressure between the outside atmosphere of the body and the lungs to equalize.

SPECIAL EQUIPMENT

Underwater Chest Drainage System

This is composed of a catheter (tube) and collection reservoir used to drain fluid and evacuate air postoperatively from the chest cavity. It is necessary to remove air and fluids from the chest cavity to prevent the lungs from collapsing. A disposable system called a *Pleur-Evac* is commonly used. The drainage system must always be kept below the level of the chest to ensure proper drainage and to prevent the introduction of the contents of the bottle into the chest cavity.

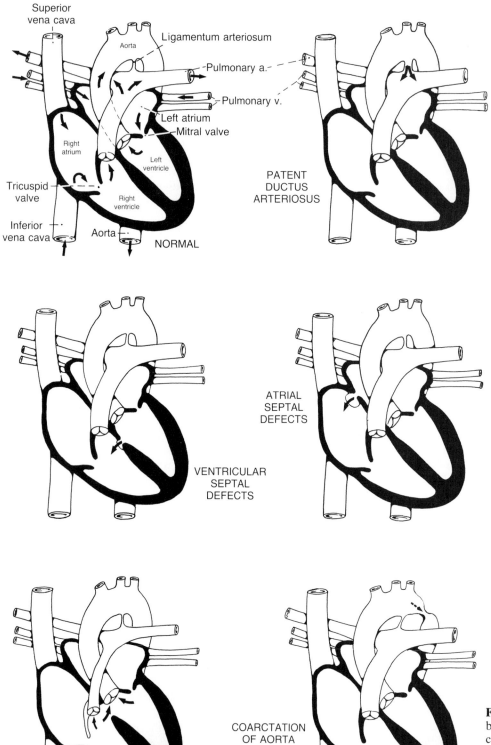

Figure 24–3. Normal flow of blood through the heart and some congenital defects that cause abnormal flow. (From Jacob S, Francone C, Lossow WJ: Structure and Function in Man, 5th ed. Philadelphia, WB Saunders, 1982.)

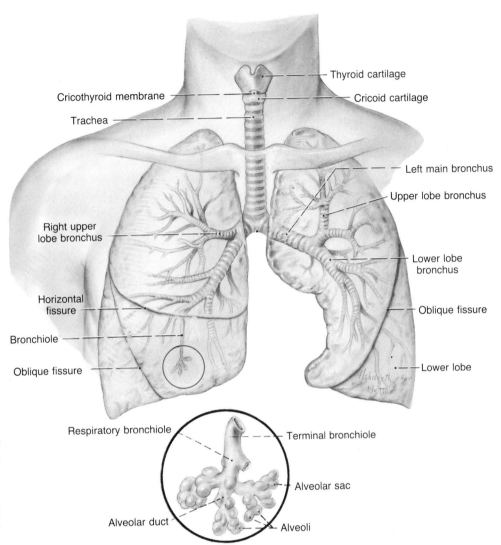

Figure 24–4. Lower portion of the respiratory anatomy. Enlarged inset shows terminal bronchi and alveolar ducts. (From Jacob S, Francone C, Lossow WJ: Structure and Function in Man, 5th ed. Philadelphia, WB Saunders, 1982.)

Prosthetic Grafts

Prosthetic grafts are used to replace a segment of an artery that has been surgically resected because of an abnormality such as a coarctation (stricture of a vessel) or an aneurysm (dilation of a vessel). There are many types of grafts that are available in assorted sizes. The technologist should be familiar with those used by the surgeons in his or her hospital. The two most common types of grafts are knitted and woven grafts. Knitted grafts are more porous and softer and allow the suture needle to pass through more easily. They are preferred for small artery anastomosis or when an artery is very friable. Woven grafts are used for large artery replacement because their tight weave prevents blood loss through the graft. This is advantageous whenever the patient has received a systemic dose of heparin. The surgeon may elect to pre-clot the graft before performing the anastomosis. To do this, the surgeon aspirates 30 to 50 mL of blood from the patient before the heparin is administered. The surgeon or the technologist then flushes the graft with the blood. The graft is usually placed in a small basin, where it is totally immersed in the blood. The blood clots and thus seals the spaces between the fibers of the graft.

Grafts may be made of Teflon or Dacron. They may be fashioned as a straight or bifurcated tube (a straight tube that divides into two equal tubes of smaller diameter). Straight and bifurcated grafts are shown in Figure 24–5.

To avoid waste and expense, only the appropriate size graft, as specified by the surgeon, should be opened for a particular procedure. The size, type, and serial number of the graft that is implanted must be recorded on the patient's operative record by the registered nurse circulator.

Patch Graft Materials

Made of Dacron or Teflon, patch grafts are used to strengthen a suture line or close a defect. Teflon felt material is often in the form of pledgets (tiny pieces of felt) that are used on the suture or along the suture line to reinforce the anastomosis. The technologist should place the pledgets on the end of a mosquito clamp for

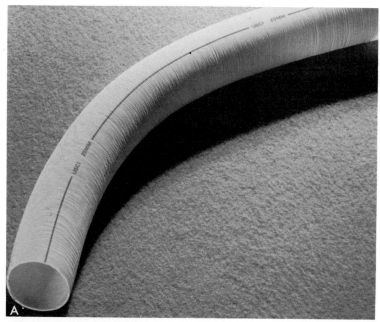

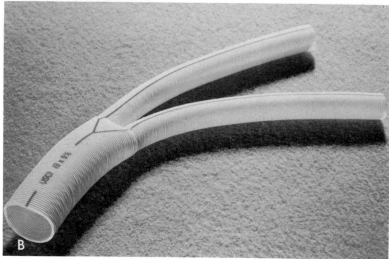

Figure 24–5. *A.* Straight tube graft. *B.* Bifurcated graft. (Courtesy of Bard Vascular Systems Division, Billerica, MA.)

easier handling. When a patch is to be used to close a defect, the surgeon cuts the patch to the desired size.

Segments of Rubber Tubing

Commonly called bolsters, segments of tubing are cut from a size 16 F Robinson catheter and are used to form tourniquets with the cannulation sutures to help hold the cannulae in place. They are also used when large vessels, such as the venae cavae, are to be occluded with an umbilical tape. A stylet, such as that from a Rummel tourniquet, is often used to snare the strands of suture or tape and bring them through the lumen of the tubing. The tubing may then be tightened against the cannula or vessel by pulling on the strands of the suture or the tape, thus forming a tourniquet. The tubing is held securely by placing a hemostat across its upper end.

Pacemaker

A pacemaker is used during some cardiac procedures. It is a device that is attached to an electrode for the purpose of stimulating the heart muscle, causing it to beat at a certain rate. This is referred to as *pacing* the heart. The batteries are external (temporary) or internal (permanent); the electrodes are either temporary or permanent. Temporary electrodes are implanted at the time of heart surgery. Permanent electrodes are of two types—endocardial (transvenous) or epicardial. The endocardial electrode is inserted into a vein and advanced into the right ventricle under fluoroscopy. The epicardial electrode is sutured directly to the heart, either on the atrium or ventricle or both.

The technologist should have a basic understanding of the purpose of pacemakers and should be able to identify their various components. The electrodes and battery are illustrated in Figure 24–6. The alligator cable (Fig. 24–7) is used to connect the electrode(s) to the external battery for pacing the heart temporarily. This cable may also be used as a fibrillator cable when it is connected to the fibrillator power source (Fig. 24–8). The heart is fibrillated when it is possible that air may be drawn into the heart and ejected into circulation by the beating action of the heart.

Defibrillator Paddles

Defibrillator paddles are required to convert fibrillation (ineffectual quivering of the heart) to normal sinus rhythm (normal beating of the heart). The paddles are kept readily available on the sterile field. When needed, such as during heart arrhythmia, the surgeon places the paddles on either side of the heart and instructs the circulating nurse to set the charge of electricity on the debrillator. The application of the electrical current to the heart shocks the cells of the heart, converting it back to normal rhythm. The paddles and debrillator are shown in Figure 24–9. When the defibrillator is in use, all personnel must stand clear of the patient to prevent their electrocution.

Diethrich Coronary Artery Set

This coronary artery set is composed of fine instruments, particularly scissors, that are used when operating on very small vessels, such as the coronary arteries (Fig. 24–10).

Prosthetic Valves

A full set of prosthetic valves, along with their respective sizers and holders, is required when valve replacement is performed. The technologist should be familiar with the types of valves and know how to handle each, along with their sizers and holders. These valves are very expensive and should be handled as little as possible. The type and identification number of the valve must be recorded on the patient's operative record by the circulator. Two commonly used valves are the St. Jude and Hancock porcine (pig) (Fig. 24–11).

Heart-Lung Machine

A heart-lung machine is used during surgical procedures of the heart and major blood vessels (pulmonary artery and aorta). It is described in the section on cardiopulmonary bypass in this chapter.

SPECIAL MEDICATIONS AND SOLUTIONS

Sodium Heparin

Sodium heparin is an anticoagulant that is administered before cannulation for cardiopulmonary bypass. It prevents clot formation while the patient is on the heart-lung machine. The drug dosage is calculated according to body weight and is referred to as a *systemic dose* because it circulates throughout all systems of the body.

Protamine Sulfate

This is a low-molecular-weight protein that, when combined with heparin, causes a loss of anticoagulant activity. (In other words, the clotting mechanism of the blood returns to normal.) Protamine sulfate is administered intravenously after bypass is completed and the cannulae are removed.

Cardioplegic Solution

This type of solution is used to stop the beating of the heart. It is prepared by a pharmacist and contains

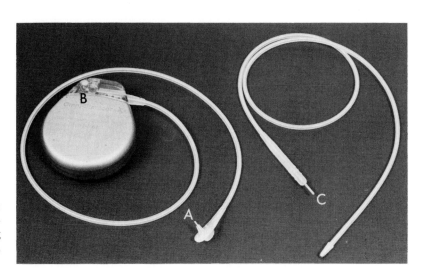

Figure 24–6. Epicardial pacing electrode (A) with internal pacemaker battery (B) and endocardial pacing electrode (C). (Courtesy of Long Beach Memorial Medical Center, Long Beach, CA.)

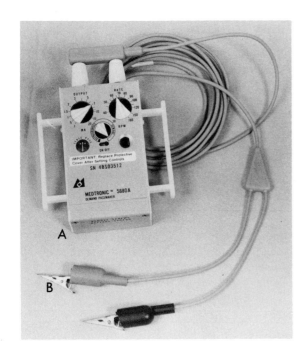

Figure 24–7. External pacemaker battery (A) with alligator pacing cable (B). (Courtesy of Long Beach Memorial Medical Center, Long Beach, CA.)

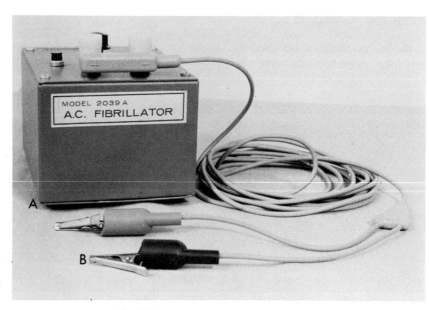

Figure 24–8. Fibrillator source (A) with alligator cable (B) used to fibrillate the heart. (Courtesy of Long Beach Memorial Medical Center, Long Beach, CA.)

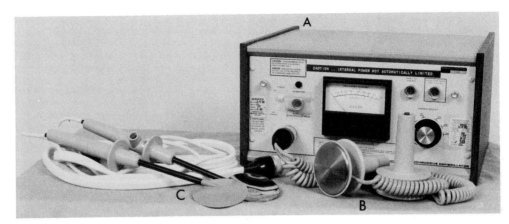

Figure 24–9. Defibrillator power source (A) with external (B) and internal (C) paddles. (Courtesy of Long Beach Memorial Medical Center, Long Beach, CA.)

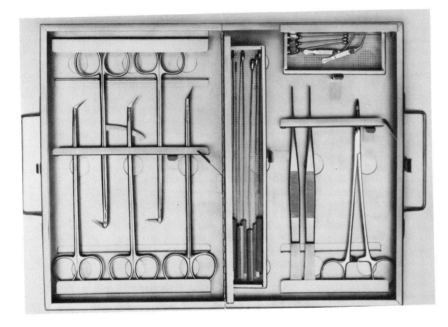

Figure 24–10. Diethrich coronary artery bypass instrument set. (Courtesy of Codman and Shurtleff, Inc., Randolph, MA.)

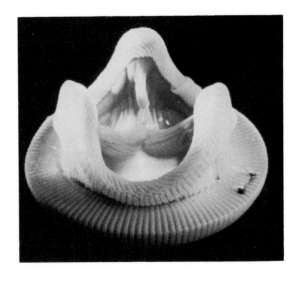

Figure 24–11. Hancock porcine valve. (Reprinted with permission of Medtronic, Inc., Minneapolis, MN.)

such ingredients as potassium chloride, lidocaine, dextrose, insulin, albumin, tromethamine, and Plasmanate. The exact type and amount of the ingredients vary according to hospital. The solution should be kept at 4°C for optimal results; it is administered intravenously.

Fixative Solution

A fixative solution hardens and preserves tissue, making it easier to examine. Two examples are Lugol's and Gey's solutions, which are used when a bronchoscopy is performed.

Other Drugs

A list of drugs used commonly in cardiothoracic surgery is presented in Table 24–1.

PULMONARY SURGERY

Bronchoscopy

Definition

This is the insertion of a lighted bronchoscope into the respiratory tree. The procedure allows direct visualization of the respiratory tree and lungs, extraction of tissue for pathologic examination, and detection of bacterial disease. It may also be performed to remove food or other foreign objects that the patient has aspirated.

Highlights

1. The bronchoscope is inserted into the respiratory canal.
2. The respiratory structures are examined.
3. A segment of tissue may be removed.
4. Secretions are collected from the bronchus.
5. The bronchoscope is withdrawn slowly.

Description

All necessary pieces of equipment and supplies are assembled and tested to make certain they are in good working order. Both the rigid and flexible bronchoscopes are used for a bronchoscopy. When the rigid bronchoscope is used, the technologist should know the age and weight of the patient so that the appropriate size scope and accessory items can be selected. The Jackson scope (8 mm × 40 cm) is the most common size used for the adult.

The following items may be necessary when a rigid scope is used, depending on the problem that is presented:

1. A fiberoptic cable or light carrier that fits both the scope and light source.
2. A right-angled telescopic lens for added light. (The technologist should dip the lens into warm normal saline solution just before insertion to prevent fogging.)
3. Biopsy cup forceps (angled and straight) to obtain a tissue specimen.
4. Grasping forceps to secure a foreign body.
5. Suction cannulae (rigid and flexible tips) used to remove secretions and the specimen. The technologist

Table 24–1. COMMONLY USED DRUGS IN CARDIOTHORACIC PROCEDURES

Name	Action
Absorbable gelatin sponge (Gelfoam)	Provides a good surface for and aids in clot formation
Aminophylline	Relaxes smooth muscle; stimulates the central nervous system; stimulates cardiac muscle to increase output
Atropine methylnitrate	Increases heart and respiratory rates
Bacitracin solution	Antibiotic effective against gram-positive organisms, the *Neisseria*, and some spirochetes
Betamethasone	Used to treat many inflammatory diseases because of its anti-inflammatory properties
Cefazolin sodium (Ancef, Kefzol)	Bacteriostatic and bactericidal antibiotic—blocks synthesis of the bacterial wall
Calcium chloride	Increases cardiac muscle and tone
Dobutamine (Dobutrex)	Increases myocardial contraction
Dopamine	Increases blood pressure by enhancing cardiac contractility
Epinephrine (adrenalin)	Raises blood pressure; increases force of the heartbeat
Furosemide (Lasix)	Potent diuretic; given to reduce circulatory overload
Heparin sodium	Prolongs the clotting time of blood in the treatment of thrombophlebitis, pulmonary embolism; used as an irrigant in cardiovascular surgery to prevent the formation of clots within the wound or vessels
Isoproterenol (Isuprel)	Increases myocardial contractility and conductivity of atrioventricular node
Levarterenol (noradrenaline)	A potent vasoconstrictor; raises blood pressure markedly with increased cardiac output
Lidocaine (Xylocaine)	Exerts antiarrhythmic effect by increasing the electrical stimulation threshold of the ventricles during diastole
Nitroglycerin	Relaxes smooth muscles; provides relief of angina pectoris
Oxidized cellulose (Oxycel)	Promotes coagulation at the wound site
Phentolamine (Regitine)	Reduces afterload
Potassium chloride	Promotes normal electrical activity of the cells by its electrolytic effect
Propranolol hydrochloride (Inderal)	Depresses pacemaker activity; allows the heart to beat at a slower rate and more effectively
Protamine sulfate	Causes a loss of anticoagulant activity; given to counteract the effects of heparin
Sodium bicarbonate	Raises the pH of the blood, especially during cardiac arrest
Sodium nitroprusside (Nipride)	Peripheral vasodilator; increases cardiac output

should be certain that the forceps and suction cannulae extend beyond the end of the scope; otherwise, they will be ineffective.

6. An eyepiece adapter used on the end of the scope to protect the eyes of the surgeon from contamination by the patient's secretions.

7. A specimen collection device, such as the Lukens collector, placed between the scope and the suction unit so that the specimen may be retrieved before it travels into the suction unit.

The set-up for a bronchoscopy using the rigid bronchoscope is shown in Figure 24–12.

A flexible bronchoscope, such as the Olympus, requires a slightly different set-up. The scope is often inserted through the endotracheal tube, thus allowing better control of the patient's ventilation during the procedure. The scope may also be introduced by way of the nasopharynx and then into the trachea. The flexibility of the scope enables the surgeon to manipulate the tip in many different directions so as to visualize a broad area and eliminate the need for the right-angled telescopic lens. A major disadvantage of this flexible scope is that it does not permit the surgeon to remove foreign objects and thick copious secretions through its lumen. The following items should be included when the flexible scope is used:

1. A fiberoptic cable that attaches to the scope and its light source.

2. Biopsy forceps to remove tissue.

3. A suction cannula that is specially constructed to fit through the lumen of the scope.

4. A stylet with a brush attached to the end, used to brush cells from the wall of the bronchi.

5. Glass slides onto which the specimen is placed.

6. A swivel adapter to be inserted on the end of the endotracheal tube through which the scope is inserted. The oxygen hose from the anesthesia machine is attached to the adapter. This adapter is used when a general anesthetic is given.

The set-up for a bronchoscopy using the flexible bronchoscope is shown in Figure 24–13.

A bronchoscopy may be performed using either a local or a general anesthetic. Local anesthesia is used for those patients who have a limited cardiac or respiratory reserve. General anesthesia is advantageous because the patient is asleep and totally relaxed. Pediatric patients require a general anesthetic because they are extremely apprehensive.

The anesthetized patient is placed in the supine position with the neck hyperextended to bring the respiratory canal into a straight line. This facilitates the insertion of the scope. Patients under local anesthesia usually sit upright in a chair during the procedure. The surgeon protects the patient's eyes with a towel and the teeth with gauze padding. The technologist applies lubricating jelly to the scope to facilitate its passage through the respiratory canal. Both the surgeon and the technologist must be gentle throughout the procedure to avoid tissue injury when the instruments are inserted into the respiratory canal.

The surgeon inserts the scope and examines the tissue in the bronchus. Suction is used to provide a clear view of the tissue. The technologist aids the surgeon by placing the suction tip or other instruments into the surgeon's hand, guiding the tip of the instrument into the lumen of the scope.

The specimen collection unit is held upright by the technologist throughout the procedure to prevent the specimen from escaping into the suction unit. To collect the specimen, the surgeon injects a fixative solution into the scope with a syringe. Cells are washed free from the bronchus and retrieved with the aid of the suction cannula.

If an actual piece of tissue is to be removed from the lining of the bronchus, the surgeon uses biopsy cup forceps. The technologist is responsible for removing the piece of tissue from the forceps. A hypodermic needle is useful in removing the tissue, which may then be placed on a piece of Telfa to prevent its loss.

When the flexible fiberoptic scope is used, the specimen is obtained on a brush or with the biopsy forceps. When the brush is used, the technologist smears the tissue from the brush onto a sterile glass slide and places the slide into a sterile container. When the biopsy forceps is used, the specimen is handled as described previously.

At the close of the procedure, before the scope is withdrawn, the surgeon suctions the patient free of all

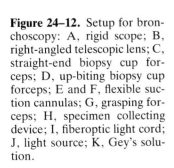

Figure 24–12. Setup for bronchoscopy: A, rigid scope; B, right-angled telescopic lens; C, straight-end biopsy cup forceps; D, up-biting biopsy cup forceps; E and F, flexible suction cannulas; G, grasping forceps; H, specimen collecting device; I, fiberoptic light cord; J, light source; K, Gey's solution.

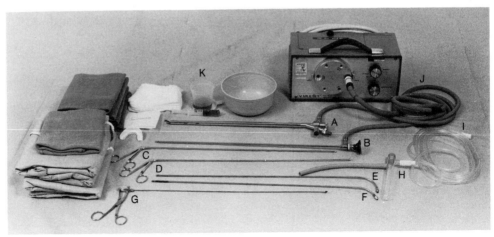

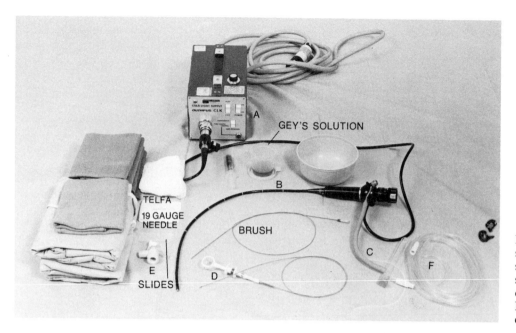

Figure 24–13. Bronchoscopy setup for flexible bronchoscope: A, light source; B, scope; C, specimen collecting device; D, grasping forceps; E, swivel adapter; F, suction cannula.

secretions and then withdraws the scope slowly. It is the technologist's responsibility to disconnect the specimen collection unit and take care that the specimen is not spilled. The circulator labels the specimen as "bronchial washings." All specimens are sent to the laboratory as soon as possible to prevent drying of the tissue cells, since this could alter the cells and cause a misdiagnosis.

Mediastinoscopy

Definition

This term refers to the insertion of a lighted instrument into the mediastinal space (located in the middle of the chest cavity between the heart and the two pleural cavities). The procedure is performed to look for evidence of abnormal pathology (particularly tumors) and to obtain tissue for examination. It is often performed as a final test to confirm a particular diagnosis, such as cancer.

Highlights

1. The mediastinal space is entered.
2. The mediastinoscope is introduced into the space.
3. The anatomy is visualized and identified.
4. Any suspect lymph nodes are removed for examination.
5. The wound is closed.

Description

A mediastinoscopy is both an endoscopic and a surgical procedure. The principles for assembling the endoscopic equipment are similar to those necessary for a bronchoscopy, but a mediastinoscopy is a *sterile* procedure because it involves a surgical incision. The set-up

and instruments used for a mediastinoscopy are illustrated in Figure 24–14. The set-up should include the mediastinoscope, light carrier and light source, grasping forceps, biopsy cup forceps, cautery/suction unit, and metal needle stylet.

The procedure is performed with the patient in the supine position under general anesthesia. The anesthesiologist positions the anesthesia machine next to the patient. The surgeon will perform the procedure standing at the patient's head. The patient's neck is hyperextended by a small rolled towel placed beneath the shoulders. This allows better access to and visualization of the structures that will be seen through the scope. The position of the patient and the scope is shown in Figure 24–15.

The surgeon makes an incision over the suprasternal notch using a No. 10 knife blade on a No. 3 knife handle. The incision is carried through the subcutaneous and muscle layers using Metzenbaum scissors and tissue forceps, and the fascial layer on the anterior surface of the trachea is identified. The surgeon ligates small veins by clamping them with mosquito clamps and tying them with a fine suture, such as 4-0 silk. Electrocautery may also be used to help achieve hemostasis. The surgeon uses blunt finger dissection to make a plane (flat open surface) between the tissues into the superior mediastinum. The scope is inserted into this plane.

The major arteries and veins lie in close proximity to the area being visualized and can be injured inadvertently. Good lighting and suctioning are therefore vital, and these are the responsibility of the technologist. The technologist must exercise care when handing instruments to avoid jarring the patient or surgeon while the scope or instruments are being used. Unexpected movements could lead to trauma of the surrounding vessels.

After the scope is in the proper position, the surgeon performs further dissection through the scope with small sponges mounted on grasping forceps. The surgeon

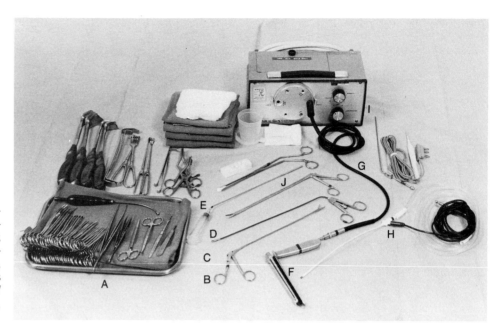

Figure 24–14. Setup for mediastinoscopy: A, soft tissue instruments; B, up-biting cup forceps; C, straight-end biopsy cup forceps; D, ligature clip applier; E, grasping forceps; F, Olympus scope; G, light cable; H, cautery/suction unit; I, light source; J, needle with metal stylet.

identifies the nodes or tissue to be biopsied. To confirm that this tissue is truly a node and *not* the wall of the pulmonary artery, a special needle attached to a metal stylet is used to pierce the tissue. The technologist attaches a syringe to the stylet before handing it to the surgeon, who then aspirates the contents of the tissue. If there is no evidence of blood return from the tissue being aspirated, the surgeon uses cup biopsy forceps to obtain a sample of the tissue for examination. The technologist removes the tissue from the forceps using a hypodermic needle. The specimen may be placed on a piece of Telfa for safekeeping until the entire specimen is obtained. The technologist then places the specimen

in a specimen cup and hands it to the circulator for proper labeling and handling.

The surgeon maintains hemostasis with electrocautery or a hemostatic agent, such as Gelfoam or Surgicel. A sponge count must be taken before the scope is removed to prevent having to reinsert the scope in case a small sponge is missing. The surgeon then closes the incision by reapproximating the subcutaneous tissue and skin with the suture of his or her choice.

Tracheotomy

Definition

This is the creation of a temporary or permanent opening into the trachea to allow air to enter the bronchi and lungs. A tracheotomy may be performed when an endotracheal tube (one entering through the mouth) is not tolerated by a conscious patient, when an airway must be maintained for more than 36 hours, or when endotracheal intubation is not advisable because of pharyngeal or laryngeal obstruction due to other causes. A tracheotomy may also be performed for long-term respiratory support or to assist in the removal of bronchial secretions for patients unable to do so themselves. The majority of tracheotomies are performed as emergencies; therefore, it is very important for the technologist to perform with speed and efficiency.

Tracheotomy tubes come in a variety of styles and sizes. The technologist should be familiar with the particular type preferred by the surgeon. The average size tubes for an adult range from a No. 5 to a No. 7. The tubes have three parts: the obturator, inner cannula, and primary tube with attached cuff. As soon as the technologist obtains the appropriate size tube, he or she inflates the cuff with 10 mL of air in a syringe to test for leakage. The cuff must remain airtight; otherwise,

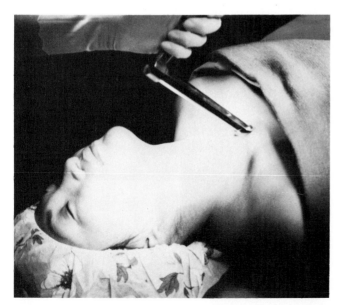

Figure 24–15. Position of patient during mediastinoscopy. (Courtesy of Long Beach Memorial Medical Center, Long Beach, CA.)

the tracheotomy tube will become dislodged from the trachea. The technologist replaces the inner cannula with the obturator to be used during insertion of the tube. A tracheotomy tube is shown in Figure 24–16.

Highlights

1. The skin and tissue overlying the trachea are incised.
2. The trachea is exposed and grasped with a hook.
3. The trachea is incised.
4. The tracheotomy tube is inserted.
5. The inner cannula is inserted.
6. The oxygen hose from the anesthesia machine is connected to the tracheotomy tube.
7. The tracheotomy tube is secured to the patient's neck.
8. Dressings are applied to the open wound.

Description

The patient is placed in the supine position with the neck hyperextended with a small sandbag or pillow placed beneath the shoulders. When the neck is fully extended, the trachea is brought forward and the spaces between the tracheal rings of cartilage are widened. Whenever feasible, this procedure is performed with the patient under local anesthesia.

Before the procedure is begun, the technologist should ask the surgeon what size tracheotomy tube he or she plans to insert. This tracheotomy tube must be available in the set-up before the trachea is incised, because as soon as the surgeon incises the trachea control over the patient's breathing (ventilation) is lost. Oxygen then escapes through the incision and fails to reach the lungs.

The surgeon makes either a transverse incision just above the sternal notch or a horizontal incision in the midline of the neck using the skin knife. The subcutaneous tissue and platysma muscle are divided with the deep knife, and the assistant retracts them with small rake (Senn) retractors. The surgeon divides the deeper tissue and muscle in the midline with Metzenbaum scissors and toothed Adson tissue forceps. Vessels in the line of dissection are clamped with mosquito hemostats and ligated with silk or catgut sutures. An electrocautery pencil may be used for hemostasis. The surgeon then retracts the deeper muscles with a U.S. Army, Green, or vein retractor. The assistant holds the retractor and exposes the trachea, taking special care to prevent trauma or laceration of the thyroid gland and accompanying vessels.

The surgeon grasps the trachea with a tracheal hook and incises it with a No. 11 or No. 15 knife blade. An Allis clamp is used to grasp the cut edge of tracheal tissue; the surgeon might insert a Trousseau dilator to expand the size of the opening. The technologist moistens the end of the tube with saline solution before handing it to the surgeon to facilitate insertion of the tube into the trachea. The surgeon then inserts the tracheotomy tube with the obturator in place. The tracheal hook and obturator are removed and the inner

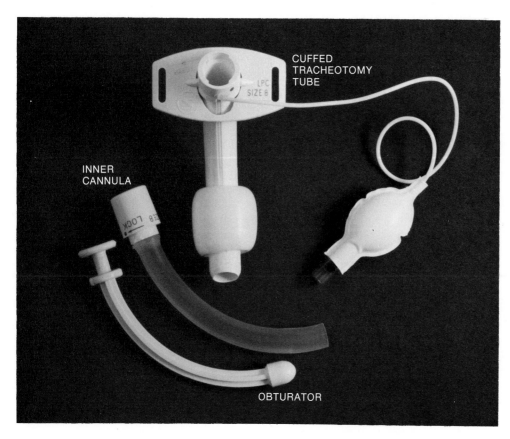

Figure 24–16. Tracheotomy tube. (Courtesy of Shiley Laboratories, Irvine, CA.)

cannula is then inserted and locked in place. The assistant or technologist should be prepared to suction the trachea and bronchus free of blood and mucus immediately by passing a suction catheter into the tracheotomy tube. A No. 14 or No. 16 Robinson catheter is commonly used. The anesthesiologist or circulator administers oxygen to the patient as soon as possible by connecting the oxygen hose from the anesthesia machine to the tracheotomy tube.

The surgeon secures the tube in place by tying cotton tapes around the patient's neck. (The tapes should be tied with the patient's head in a *normal* position rather than hyperextended. This prevents the tapes from being too loose, thus preventing the tube from dislodging.)

The wound is left open to allow drainage of secretions coughed up from the lungs. The technologist cuts a gauze dressing sponge so that it fits snugly around the tube. The dressing is applied beneath the tube. The technologist then rinses the obturator in saline solution to remove all blood and mucus. The obturator should be sent along with the patient in case the tube is dislodged and reinsertion is necessary.

Insertion of Chest Tube(s)

Definition

This is the insertion of one or more tubes into the pleural cavity to remove blood and air that accumulate following a thoracotomy, thus allowing the lung to expand. The use of chest tubes is indicated following any chest surgery (except total pneumonectomy) to prevent cardiac tamponade (inability of the heart to beat normally because of accumulated fluid or blood surrounding the heart).

Highlights

1. The chest wall is incised.
2. A tube-pulling clamp is inserted into the intercostal space.
3. The tube is positioned and secured to the skin.

Description

To insert a pleural tube, the surgeon makes an incision in the chest wall below the thoracotomy incision using the skin knife. (When a mediastinal tube is to be inserted, the skin is incised along the abdominal wall below the sternotomy incision. Mediastinal tubes do not require underwater seal drainage because the tube does not lie in the pleural cavity.) The surgeon then inserts a clamp, such as a long Péan, through the incision. The assistant inserts the tapered end of the tube into the jaws of the clamp and the surgeon withdraws the clamp with the tube through the tissue layers. The surgeon positions the tube so that all the tube's perforations lie inside the cavity. (The holes must be inside the cavity for the underwater seal drainage to be effective.) The tube is secured to the skin with silk sutures, size 0 or 2-

0. The tube is then connected to the Pleur-Evac drainage system.

At the completion of the surgical procedure, the connection between the tube and drainage system is taped securely by either the surgeon or circulator to avoid the possibility of disconnecting the tube and drainage system, which would allow air to enter the cavity. Otherwise, pneumothorax can occur.

Thoracotomy

Definition

This is a surgical incision into the thoracic cavity to provide access to the organs of the chest, particularly the lungs, heart, and aorta.

Highlights

Opening

1. The skin is incised.
2. The subcutaneous tissue and muscle layers are divided.
3. The intercostal space (space between two ribs) is entered.
4. The thoracic cavity is opened.

Closure

1. Sutures are placed around the two ribs that were separated.
2. The ribs are brought together with an approximator.
3. The subcutaneous tissue and muscle layers are approximated.
4. The skin is closed.

Description

Opening

The patient is placed in the lateral position. The surgeon incises the skin with the skin knife and divides the subcutaneous tissue and muscle layers with either a deep knife or an electrocautery pencil. The blood vessels severed in the incision may be cauterized or clamped with hemostatic forceps and tied with a free tie, such as size 2-0 chromic catgut or silk. The incision and division of the muscle layers is shown in Figure 24–17.

The surgeon inserts a Davidson scapular retractor beneath the shoulder muscles, elevates the scapula, and then inserts his or her hand beneath the scapula and counts the ribs. When the appropriate intercostal space for incision has been determined, the chest cavity is entered with the deep knife. The intercostal incision is extended with Metzenbaum scissors or the electrocautery pencil. Hemostasis of the periosteum is maintained by electrocautery.

If a rib is to be removed, the surgeon incises the periosteum along its anterior surface with the deep knife

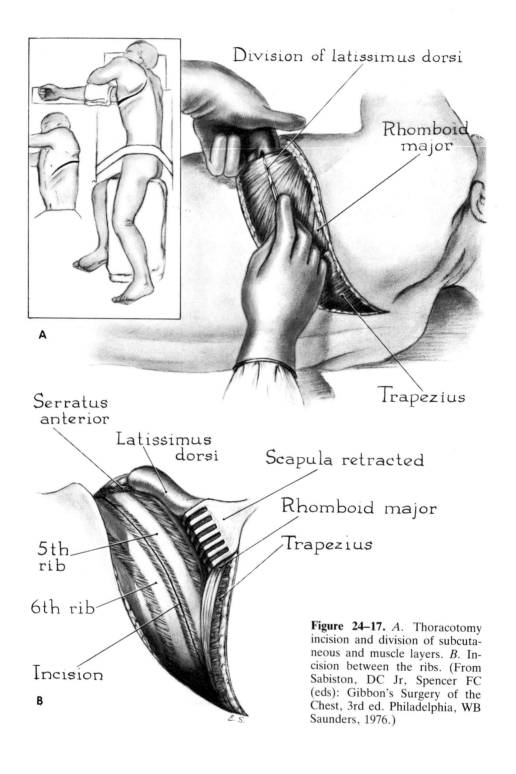

Figure 24–17. *A*. Thoracotomy incision and division of subcutaneous and muscle layers. *B*. Incision between the ribs. (From Sabiston, DC Jr, Spencer FC (eds): Gibbon's Surgery of the Chest, 3rd ed. Philadelphia, WB Saunders, 1976.)

or electrocautery pencil. A periosteal elevator or Alexander, Haight, or Doyen rib raspatory is used to strip the rib free from the periosteum. The periosteum is preserved because it contains blood vessels that nourish the bone, and the wound heals more quickly if there is good blood supply to all tissue layers. The surgeon cuts the rib free from its attachment to the spine and sternum with rib shears (usually Bethune rib shears). The entire rib is removed, as demonstrated in Figure 24–18. The surgeon then trims the sharp edges of the remaining rib stump using Sauerbruch rib shears. This prevents possible trauma to surrounding tissue by the sharply cut edges of the rib stump and guards against puncture of the surgeon's gloves during surgery.

The surgeon covers the edges of the wound with laparotomy sponges or sterile towels to protect the tissue from bruising caused by pressure from the retractor blades. The technologist provides the appropriate size retractor, which the surgeon then inserts between the ribs. The retractor is opened slowly to prevent rib fracture or tissue trauma. The chest cavity is now open.

Closure

After the specific surgical procedure has been completed and chest tubes have been inserted, the surgeon places pericostal sutures, such as No. 2 Dexon or No. 1 chromic catgut, around the two ribs and holds the ends of each suture with hemostatic forceps. Four to six sutures of this type are usually required. A rib approximator, such as the Bailey rib contractor, is used to bring the ribs together. The pericostal sutures are then tied securely while the approximater is in place (Fig. 24–19).

A running suture of size 0 chromic catgut or Dexon may be used to approximate the periosteum between the two ribs. The surgeon then reapproximates the various muscle layers individually with a running suture of size 0 chromic catgut or Dexon or interrupted nonabsorbable sutures, such as silk or Tevdek. The surgeon approximates the subcutaneous tissue in a similar fashion with a smaller size suture. The skin is then closed according to the surgeon's preference.

Lung Biopsy

Definition

This is the excision of a small piece of lung tissue for microscopic examination. The procedure is usually performed to establish a diagnosis in pulmonary disease.

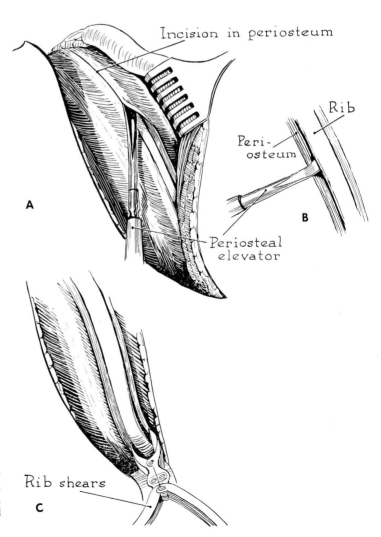

Figure 24–18. Technique for removal of a rib. *A.* Incision in periosteum. *B.* Periosteum stripped from rib with elevator. *C.* Rib cut with shear. (From Sabiston DC Jr, Spencer FC (eds): Gibbon's Surgery of the Chest, 3rd ed. Philadelphia, WB Saunders, 1976.)

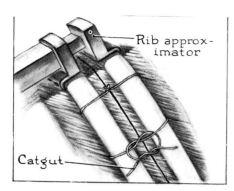

Figure 24–19. Technique for closure of chest cavity using rib approximator. (From Sabiston DC Jr, Spencer FC (eds): Gibbon's Surgery of the Chest, 3rd ed. Philadelphia, WB Saunders, 1976.)

Highlights

1. A thoracotomy is performed.
2. The lung tissue to be sampled is identified.
3. The lung tissue is divided, and the segment of lung to be sampled is removed.
4. The edges of the divided lung tissue are oversewn.
5. A chest tube is inserted, and the wound is closed.

Description

A thoracotomy is performed in standard fashion, as previously described. However, the incision required for a lung biopsy is usually smaller than that required for a standard thoracotomy.

After the surgeon opens the chest, the lung is examined and the segment to be removed for biopsy is identified. The surgeon may need to retract the lung with a moist laparotomy sponge to expose the segment of lung for biopsy. A Duval lung forceps is applied to stabilize the lung during excision of the segment. The assistant holds the lung forceps as the surgeon divides the lung tissue with a knife blade or surgical stapling instrument. (See Chapter 12 for a complete discussion of the use of the surgical stapling instrument.)

The surgeon removes the segment of lung tissue. The cut edges of the divided lung are then oversewn with a running suture, such as size 3-0 chromic catgut or Dexon. A lung biopsy is illustrated in Figure 24–20.

The surgeon inspects the suture line carefully for air leaks by filling the chest cavity with warm saline solution and then asking the anesthesiologist to inflate the lungs. The presence of bubbles in the solution indicates that air is leaking through the suture line. The surgeon or assistant aspirates the solution and the surgeon places additional sutures to occlude the areas of leakage. If air is allowed to leak into the pleural cavity, it will cause an increase in the intrapulmonic pressure, causing the lung to collapse. This condition is referred to as a *pneumothorax*. Pneumothorax is prevented by making certain that suture lines are airtight and by inserting chest tubes to drain the accumulated air and blood from the pleural cavity.

Once hemostasis is achieved, the surgeon inserts the chest tube(s) and closes the chest, as previously described.

Lobectomy

Definition

This is the surgical removal of a lobe of the lung that is diseased, most commonly due to carcinoma or infection.

Highlights

1. A thoracotomy is performed.
2. The diseased lobe is identified.
3. The veins and arteries supplying the lobe are dissected and ligated.
4. The bronchus is isolated, transected, and oversewn.
5. A lobe of the lung is removed.
6. The suture line is tested for leaks.
7. The bronchial stump is covered with pleura.
8. Chest tubes are inserted, and the chest is closed.

Description

A thoracotomy is performed with the affected side up, as previously described. The surgeon examines the entire lung and mediastinum closely to make certain there is no evidence of disease beyond that which had been originally diagnosed. The diseased lobe is identified and dissected free from the rest of the lung, using Metzenbaum scissors and smooth tissue forceps.

Long instruments may be needed, so the technologist should have them available. All sutures that are to be hand-tied should be on a passer, such as a Schnidt or right-angled clamp.

The surgeon isolates all major arteries and veins supplying the diseased lobe by sharp dissection with Metzenbaum scissors and smooth tissue forceps. Duval lung-grasping forceps may be used to retract the lung, thus providing exposure of the vessels and bronchus.

The vessels and bronchus may be encircled with an umbilical tape or heavy silk suture for retraction or control of the vessel. The technologist should wet the tape or silk before passing it to the surgeon to prevent it from cutting into the vessels.

The surgeon clamps the veins and arteries supplying blood to the diseased lobe with Schnidt clamps, transects them, and ties them with a suture such as size 2-0 silk.

The surgeon divides the bronchus with a scalpel. (Occasionally, a bronchus clamp may be applied before transection of the bronchus.) Once the bronchus is transected, the lobe of lung may be removed. Suctioning is very important while the bronchus is open to prevent any blood or fluid from draining into the opposite (nonaffected) lung. It may be necessary for the technologist to manage the suction while the surgeons are engaged in transecting and suturing the bronchus.

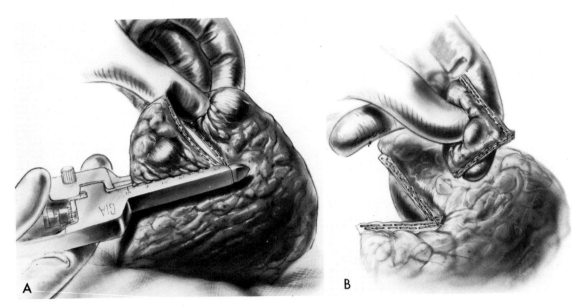

Figure 24–20. *A.* Technique of lung biopsy using suture stapling instrument. *B.* Specimen removed. (From Sabiston DC Jr, Spencer FC (eds): Gibbon's Surgery of the Chest, 3rd ed. Philadelphia, WB Saunders, 1976.)

The surgeon closes the open end of the remaining bronchus with interrupted sutures, such as size 3-0 Ti-Cron, or with a surgical stapling instrument, such as the Auto Suture Premium TA 55 (United States Surgical Corporation, Norwalk, CT). The open bronchus must be closed as quickly as possible to prevent the leakage of anesthetic gases into the atmosphere, spillage of blood into the remaining lung, and pneumothorax. Figure 24–21 illustrates the technique used for lobectomy.

After the surgeon closes the bronchus, the suture line is tested for air leaks in the same manner as described for a lung biopsy. The chest tube is inserted as previously described, and the wound is closed by the surgeon in routine fashion.

Pneumonectomy

Definition

This is the removal of a lung, commonly performed to treat lung cancer.

Highlights

1. A thoracotomy is performed.
2. The mediastinal pleura is incised.
3. The major vessels (bronchus, pulmonary artery, and superior and inferior pulmonary veins) are isolated.
4. The vagus, phrenic, and recurrent laryngeal nerves are identified.
5. Lymph nodes are dissected.
6. The pulmonary artery and veins are divided and ligated.
7. The bronchus is divided and closed.
8. The lung is removed, and the chest is closed.

Description

The surgeon performs a thoracotomy, as previously described. The entire lung and surrounding tissues are examined closely to evaluate the extent of the disease and to confirm the diagnosis. Adjacent lymph nodes may be biopsied and the specimen sent to the pathologist for a frozen section to determine whether there is metastasis from the cancerous lung.

Occasionally, the cancer may be so advanced that the surgeon considers it inoperable. In such a case, surgery is discontinued, chest tubes are inserted, and the chest is closed. The technologist should pay strict attention to the pathologist's verbal report so that he or she may anticipate the needs of the surgeon.

If surgery is to continue, the assistant retracts the lung to expose the mediastinal pleura using Deaver retractors, malleable retractors, or Duval lung forceps. The surgeon incises the mediastinal pleura using Metzenbaum scissors and smooth forceps. Blunt dissection is carried out with a sponge dissector along the edges of the parietal pleura.

The surgeon isolates the major structures connected to the lung (bronchus, pulmonary artery, and pulmonary veins) using sharp dissection with Metzenbaum scissors or blunt dissection with a sponge dissector. Adjacent to these structures are the vagus, recurrent laryngeal (left side only), and phrenic nerves. Because these nerves carry some very important functions, they must be preserved. The surgeon passes an umbilical tape or heavy silk suture mounted on a right-angled clamp around the nerves. The vessels may be encircled in the same way. To protect these structures from injury during the dissection of the surrounding tissue, the assistant retracts the vessels or nerves by pulling on the tape or silk.

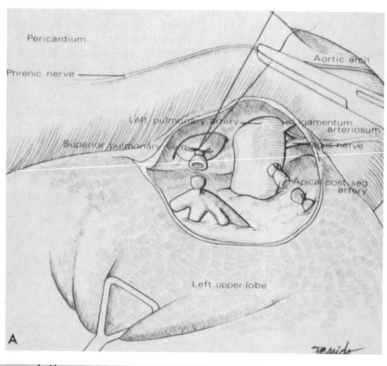

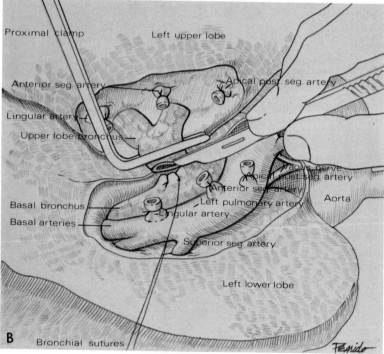

Figure 24–21. Lobectomy. *A.* The pulmonary artery and vein supplying the left upper lobe of lung are ligated and divided. *B.* Bronchus to left upper lobe is divided and sutured to left upper lobe.

The surgeon ligates the pulmonary artery with two sutures of size 0 silk mounted on a passer. The artery between the ligatures is divided with Metzenbaum scissors. The surgeon may oversew the cut edges of the artery with a fine suture, such as size 4-0 or 5-0 cardiovascular silk or Prolene for additional hemostasis. The superior and inferior veins are ligated and divided in a similar fashion. Ligation clips may be used for ligating smaller vessels.

The surgeon usually applies a bronchus clamp, such as a Sarot clamp, before the bronchus is divided with the deep knife. The lung is then removed from the chest cavity. The surgeon quickly closes the open end of the bronchus using interrupted sutures, such as size 3-0 Ti-Cron. The technologist may need to manage the suction while the surgeons are suturing the bronchus. Every precaution must be taken to preserve the remaining lung and to keep it free from contamination because the patient cannot tolerate any further loss of lung tissue. After the surgeon closes the bronchus, he or she tests for air leaks, as previously described for a lung biopsy. Lymph nodes that are diseased or those that look suspect are removed along with the lung specimen.

The surgeon examines the mediastinal pleura for bleeding vessels, which are treated with suture ligatures or electrocautery. The upper mediastinal pleura is closed with a chromic catgut or Dexon suture. It is not necessary to insert chest tubes when the entire lung is removed because the threat of pneumothorax is eliminated. The surgeon closes the chest in standard fashion, as previously described.

THORACIC AORTA AND CARDIAC SURGERY

Closure of Patent Ductus Arteriosus

Definition

This is the closure of an unnatural communication between the pulmonary artery and the descending thoracic aorta. During fetal life, blood is pumped from the right ventricle into the systemic circulation by way of the ductus. The lungs are bypassed and remain unexpanded. At birth, the lungs expand and the ductus closes spontaneously. If the ductus fails to close, arterial blood recirculates through the lungs, causing an added burden on the lungs and heart. The heart becomes enlarged and may fail. The ductus is surgically closed to correct this defect, most commonly while the patient is still an infant.

Highlights

1. A thoracotomy is performed.
2. The mediastinal pleura is incised.
3. The ductus is isolated.
4. The ductus is closed.
5. The chest tube is inserted, and the chest is closed.

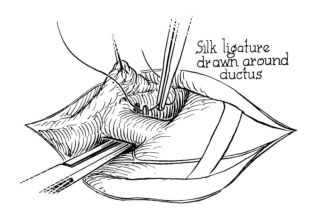

Figure 24–22. Closure of patent ductus arteriosus. Silk suture is drawn around ductus. (From Cooley DA, Hallman GL: Surgical Treatment of Congenital Heart Disease. Philadelphia, Lea & Febiger, 1966. Used with permission.)

Description

The surgeon performs a thoracotomy. A suture, such as size 3-0 silk, is placed through the edges of the pleura. The assistant applies a hemostat to the ends of the suture and then retracts the pleura. The surgeon carefully dissects between the aorta and pulmonary artery with Metzenbaum scissors to expose the ductus. A heavy silk suture mounted on a passer may be passed around the ductus (Fig. 24–22).

The surgeon continues the dissection until the ductus is totally isolated (Fig. 24–23). Straight or slightly angled vascular clamps are placed across the ductus, one close to the aorta and the other close to the pulmonary artery (Fig. 24–24). (In the newborn or a small infant, the surgeon simply ties the ductus with size 0 silk because the ductus is too small to allow placement of the vascular clamps. The infant is generally in critical condition and unable to tolerate the normal procedure.)

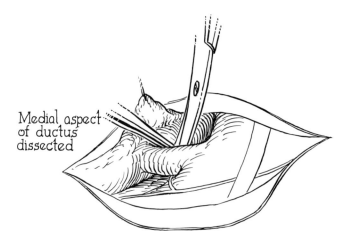

Figure 24–23. Closure of patent ductus arteriosus. Ductus is completely isolated. (From Cooley DA, Hallman GL: Surgical Treatment of Congenital Heart Disease. Philadelphia, Lea & Febiger, 1966. Used with permission.)

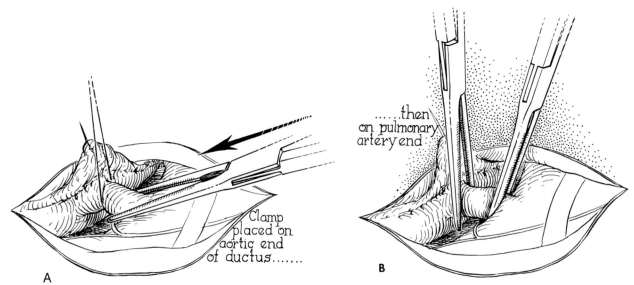

Figure 24–24. Closure of patent ductus arteriosus. Vascular clamps are placed across the ductus. *A.* Clamp placed on aortic end. *B.* Clamp placed on pulmonary artery end. (From Cooley DA, Hallman GL: Surgical Treatment of Congenital Heart Disease. Philadelphia, Lea & Febiger, 1966. Used with permission.)

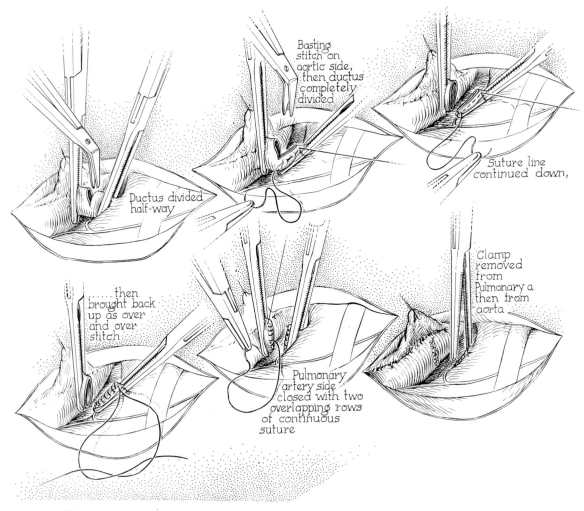

Figure 24–25. Technique of division of patent ductus arteriosus and oversewing of aortic and pulmonary side. (From Cooley DA, Hallman GL: Surgical Treatment of Congenital Heart Disease. Philadelphia, Lea & Febiger, 1966. Used with permission.)

The surgeon cuts halfway through the ductus using a knife blade or Potts scissors. A size 5-0 or 6-0 Prolene suture is used to begin closure of the ductus on the aortic side (Fig. 24–25). The surgeon then completes the cutting of the ductus and continues the suture to close the entire ductus on the aortic side. As soon as the aortic side of the ductus is securely sutured, the vascular clamp is slowly removed. Additional sutures are placed if there are any leaks. The end of the ductus closest to the pulmonary artery is sutured in the same manner.

A hemostatic agent, such as Surgicel, is often used to control bleeding along the suture line. The surgeon closes the mediastinal pleura with a continuous suture of size 3-0 or 4-0 silk or chromic catgut (Fig. 24–26). The surgeon inserts the appropriate size chest tube and closes the chest in standard fashion.

Correction of Coarctation of the Thoracic Aorta

Definition

This surgical procedure is performed to correct a congenital stenosis in the thoracic aorta, usually just below the origin of the left subclavian artery. This construction may obstruct the normal flow of blood through the thoracic aorta. The heart becomes enlarged owing to the added burden of trying to pump blood through the narrow lumen. The lower body may be underdeveloped as a result of the reduced blood flow.

Highlights

1. A thoracotomy is performed.
2. The mediastinal pleura is incised.
3. The aorta in the area of the coarctation is isolated.
4. The ligamentum arteriosum is ligated and divided.
5. The aorta is occluded proximal (above) and distal (below) to the coarctation.
6. The aorta is transected and reanastomosed.
7. The aorta is unclamped.
8. The wound is closed.

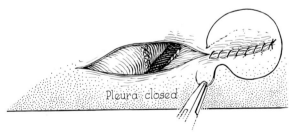

Figure 24–26. Closure of patent ductus arteriosus. The pleura is closed. (From Cooley DA, Hallman GL: Surgical Treatment of Congenital Heart Disease. Philadelphia, Lea & Febiger, 1966. Used with permission.)

Description

The surgeon performs a thoracotomy in standard fashion. A moist laparotomy sponge is placed over the lung, which is retracted by the assistant with a Deaver or malleable retractor. The surgeon uses Metzenbaum scissors and smooth forceps to incise the mediastinal pleura overlying the aorta. Atraumatic sutures of size 3-0 or 4-0 silk or Ti-Cron may be placed through the cut edges of the pleura to provide greater exposure of the aorta (Fig. 24–27). The surgeon then ligates the intercostal veins in the area of the coarctation by clamping them with Schmidt clamps and then dividing and ligating them with size 3-0 or 2-0 silk (Fig. 24–28). Metzenbaum scissors and forceps are used to dissect the aorta in the area of the coarctation.

The surgeon encircles the aorta with an umbilical tape or heavy silk tie mounted on a passer. The assistant secures the ends of the tape or silk in a hemostat and uses this to retract the aorta during the dissection.

The surgeon ligates the ductus to free the aorta and to prevent bleeding from the ductus if it is still patent. The surgeon encircles the ductus with size 0 silk sutures. The sutures are tied, and the ductus between the sutures is divided using a knife. Additional sutures of size 4-0 or 5-0 Prolene may be placed through the ends of the divided ductus.

The surgeon occludes the aorta proximal and distal to the coarctation with straight or angled vascular clamps. The arteries that supply the coarctated segment of the aorta are ligated, and bulldog clamps may be placed on any other vessels that lie between the coarctated segment and the occluding clamps (Fig. 24–29). The aorta above and below the coarctation is then transected with Metzenbaum scissors and the coarctated segment is removed (Fig. 24–30).

The surgeon performs the anastomosis between the two cut ends of the aorta using a continuous suture of size 3-0 or 4-0 Prolene for adults and size 5-0 or 6-0 Prolene for children. The anterior walls of the aorta in children may be anastomosed with interrupted sutures of Prolene rather than a continuous suture to allow the aorta to stretch while the child grows (Fig. 24–31).

When the cut ends of the aorta cannot be brought together easily, particularly in adults, a prosthetic tube graft may be used. The surgeon selects an appropriate size graft and completes the proximal anastomosis with a continuous nonabsorbable suture. A straight vascular clamp is placed across the graft and the proximal clamp is removed from the aorta to test for any leaks in the anastomosis. Additional sutures should be ready, as well as pledgets of Teflon felt.

The surgeon reapplies the vascular clamp to the aorta proximal to the anastomosis and removes the clamp from the graft. The graft is then cut to an appropriate length, and the distal anastomosis is completed. Before the suture is tied, the clamps on the aorta are temporarily released to flush out trapped air or blood clots in the graft.

The surgeon removes all clamps from the aorta and intercostal arteries. Blood flow to the lower body is thus

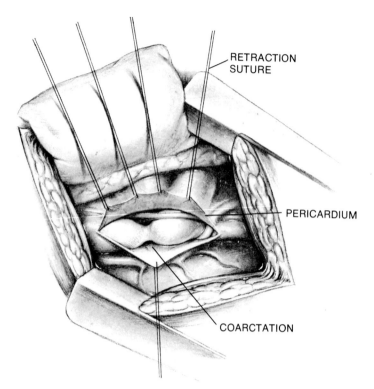

RETRACTION
SUTURE

PERICARDIUM

COARCTATION

Figure 24–27. Correction of coarctation of thoracic aorta. Pleura is incised and retracted to expose coarctation of aorta. (Courtesy of Ethicon, Inc., Somerville, NJ.)

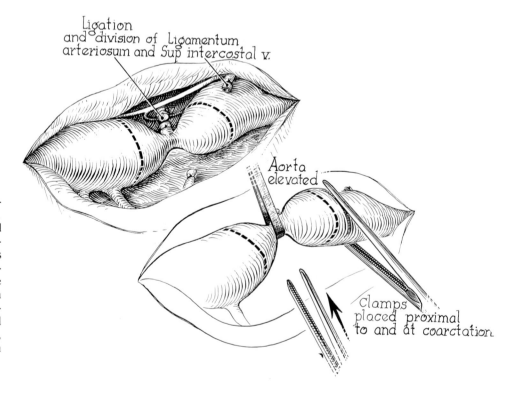

Ligation
and division of Ligamentum
arteriosum and Sup intercostal v.

Aorta
elevated

Clamps
placed proximal
to and at coarctation

Figure 24–28. Correction of coarctation of thoracic aorta. *A.* Intercostal vein is ligated and ligamentum arteriosum is divided. *B.* Umbilical tape is slung around aorta for retraction, and vascular clamps are placed across aorta. (From Cooley DA, Hallman GL: Surgical Treatment of Congenital Heart Disease. Philadelphia, Lea & Febiger, 1966. Used with permission.)

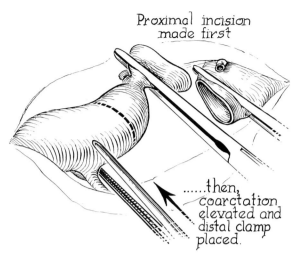

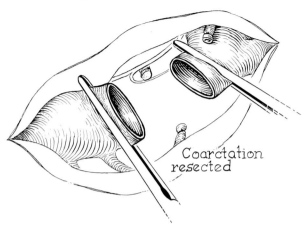

Figure 24–29. Correction of coarctation of thoracic aorta. Aorta is transected proximal and distal to coarctation. (From Cooley DA, Hallman GL: Surgical Treatment of Congenital Heart Disease. Philadelphia, Lea & Febiger, 1966. Used with permission.)

Figure 24–30. Correction of coarctation of thoracic aorta. Coarctation is resected. (From Cooley DA, Hallman GL: Surgical Treatment of Congenital Heart Disease. Philadelphia, Lea & Febiger, 1966. Used with permission.)

re-established. The surgeon inspects the anastomoses or leaks, and additional sutures may be placed or a topical hemostatic agent may be applied to control bleeding.

The surgeon closes the mediastinal pleura with size 3-0 or 4-0 silk or chromic catgut sutures (Fig. 24–32). An appropriate-sized chest tube is inserted, and the chest is closed in standard fashion.

Resection of Aneurysms of the Descending Thoracic Aorta

Definition

This is surgical removal of an aneurysmal segment of the descending aorta and the insertion of a prosthetic graft. An aneurysm is a widening or dilatation of the walls of the artery that may be caused by arteriosclerosis, infection, syphilis, trauma, or a congenital abnormality.

Aneurysms obstruct the normal flow of blood, leading to ischemia (a local and temporary anemia) of the organs and tissues that normally receive their blood supply from that particular artery. Aneurysms may rupture, resulting in severe blood loss and possible death.

The three major classes of aneurysms are saccular, fusiform, and dissecting (Fig. 24–33). A *saccular aneurysm* is created by the dilatation or ballooning out of a localized area in the artery. A *fusiform aneurysm* involves the entire circumference of the artery, causing it to become spindle shaped. *Dissecting aneurysms* occur when there is a tear in the intima (the inner layer of the vessel), allowing blood to flow between the layers of the vessel wall instead of through the normal channel. There are also three main types of dissecting aneurysms (Fig. 24–34).

Highlights

1. A thoracotomy is performed.
2. The aneurysm is located.

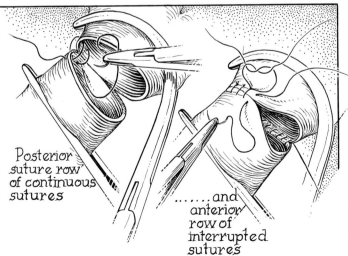

Figure 24–31. Correction of coarctation of thoracic aorta. Technique of anastomosing the proximal and distal ends of the aorta. (From Cooley DA, Hallman GL: Surgical Treatment of Congenital Heart Disease. Philadelphia, Lea & Febiger, 1966. Used with permission.)

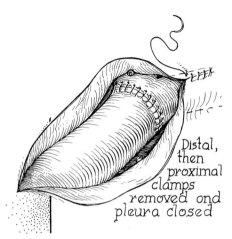

Distal, then proximal clamps removed and pleura closed

Figure 24–32. Correction of coarctation of thoracic aorta. The mediastinal pleura is closed. (From Cooley DA, Hallman GL: Surgical Treatment of Congenital Heart Disease. Philadelphia, Lea & Febiger, 1966. Used with permission.)

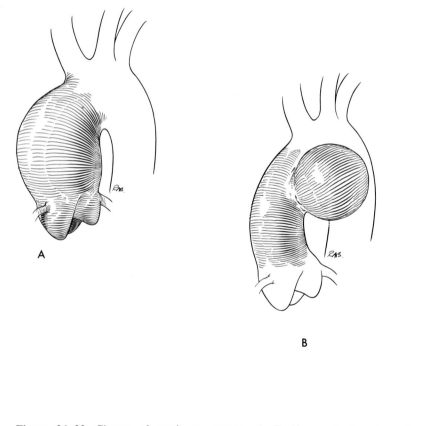

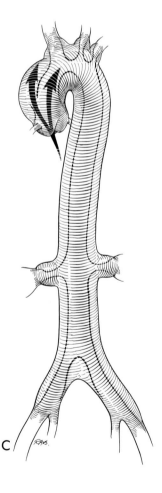

Figure 24–33. Classes of aortic aneurysms. *A.* Fusiform. *B.* Saccular. *C.* Dissecting (type I).

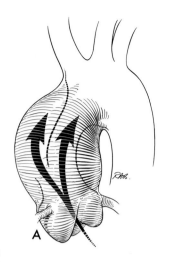
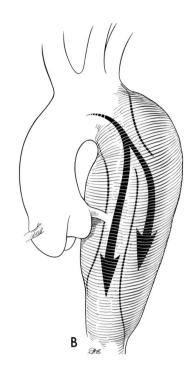

Figure 24–34. Types of dissecting aneurysms. In type I (Fig. 24–33C), dissection extends from aortic annulus to the aorta, well below the diaphragm. *A.* Type II. Dissection is localized to the ascending aorta. *B.* Type III. Dissection originates distal to the left subclavian artery and may continue below the diaphragm.

3. The mediastinal pleura is incised.

4. The aneurysm is freed from the surrounding tissue.

5. Partial cardiopulmonary bypass may be instituted, or a shunt may be inserted.

6. Vascular occluding clamps are applied to the aorta, and the aneurysm is resected.

7. The intercostal arteries are ligated.

8. A prosthetic graft is sutured in place.

9. The occluding clamps are removed from the aorta, and the graft is covered with any remaining aneurysmal tissue.

10. The mediastinal pleura is closed.

11. Chest tubes are inserted, and the chest is closed.

Description

The surgeon performs a thoracotomy in standard fashion. The surgeon may retract the edges of the pleura with sutures such as size 2-0 silk on an atraumatic needle to help expose the aneurysm. The intercostal veins that are in the line of the dissection are clamped and ligated.

The surgeon begins to dissect the aneurysm free from the surrounding tissue. The manner in which the dissection is continued depends on whether he or she uses an assist device (shunt or partial cardiopulmonary bypass) or resects the entire segment of aneurysmal aorta. Each of these three methods will be described.

Use of Shunt

The shunt is an artificial tube designed to prevent clot formation when blood flows through the tube. The Gott shunt, which is commonly used, is shown in Figure 24–35.

The surgeon isolates the aorta proximal and distal to the aneurysm using Metzenbaum scissors. The aorta may be encircled with an umbilical tape. A pursestring suture (3-0 Prolene or Ti-Cron) is then placed proximal to the aneurysm. The assistant places a bolster on the ends of the suture. The surgeon inserts one end of the shunt tubing into the aorta through a stab incision made within the pursestring suture. The technologist should control the end of the shunt to prevent it from flipping into the surgeon's face. The surgeon occludes the shunt with a tubing clamp. The assistant tightens the bolster against the shunt by pulling the pursestring suture taut, forming a tourniquet. The bolster is held secure with hemostatic forceps. The surgeon ties the bolster and shunt together with a heavy silk tie to keep the shunt in place. A pursestring suture is then placed distal to the aneurysm, and the other end of the shunt is inserted in the same manner. The tubing clamp is removed from the shunt.

The surgeon occludes the aorta proximal and distal to the aneurysm. The ends of the shunt remain outside the occluded segment of aorta to provide continuous blood flow to the lower body during the procedure. The surgeon then makes a longitudinal incision into the aneurysm with the knife and extends the incision with Metzenbaum scissors. The outer layer of the aneurysm is preserved and retracted with sutures of size 2-0 or 0 silk. The surgeon will later use this layer to cover the prosthetic graft to prevent the graft from adhering to the lung and to control bleeding.

The surgeon removes all debris and blood clots inside the aneurysm using suction and tissue forceps. The technologist should have a small basin available to collect the debris and clots. The surgeon ligates the intercostal vessels along the posterior wall of the aneurysm with sutures of silk or Ti-Cron. It may be difficult to identify the origin of these vessels; therefore, the surgeon rinses the area with warm saline solution and then looks for bleeding points, which usually indicate

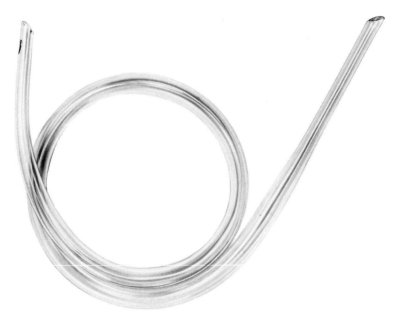

Figure 24–35. Gott shunt used to divert blood around the aneurysm during resection and repair. (Courtesy of Argyle, St. Louis, MO.)

an open vessel (Fig. 24–36). After the surgeon achieves hemostasis, he or she begins to anastomose the prosthetic graft to the aorta.

Partial Cardiopulmonary Bypass

Cannulation for partial cardiopulmonary bypass is performed in the same manner as described later in this chapter. It may be performed by the assistant while the surgeon performs the thoracotomy. If the aneurysm is ruptured, the surgeon may cannulate and begin bypass before performing the thoracotomy to prevent further blood loss and to restore blood flow to the lower body (Fig. 24–37).

In nonruptured cases, the surgeon isolates the aorta proximal and distal to the aneurysm using Metzenbaum scissors and then places vascular clamps across the aorta

to occlude the aneurysm. Partial cardiopulmonary bypass is used while the aorta is occluded. The surgeon continues the procedure in the same manner as described for the shunt.

Complete Resection

The surgeon performs the dissection along the entire circumference of the aneurysm using Metzenbaum scissors. All intercostal vessels involved in the aneurysm are ligated. The surgeon then places vascular clamps across the aorta, proximal and distal to the aneurysm. Speed is essential at this time because there is no blood flow to the lower body. The technologist must be very alert to the needs of the surgeon to prevent unnecessary loss of time when handing sutures and instruments. The surgeon transects the aorta immediately above and be-

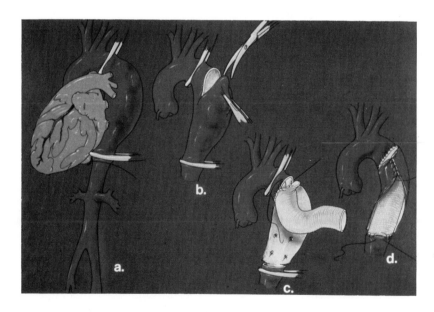

Figure 24–36. Technique of resection of descending thoracic aneurysm. *a.* Vascular clamps placed proximal and distal to aneurysm. *b.* Aneurysm incised and clot and debris removed. *c.* Intercostal vessels ligated and a graft anastomosed to distal and proximal aorta. *d.* Graft covered with remaining aneurysm sac and pleura.

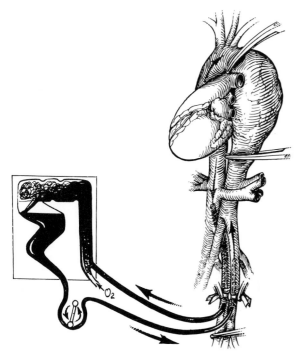

Figure 24–37. Femoral vein–femoral artery bypass with oxygenator used during resection of descending thoracic aneurysm. (From DeBakey ME: Thoracic aorta and great vessels. In Effler DB [ed]: Blades' Surgical Diseases of the Chest, 4th ed. St. Louis, CV Mosby, 1978.)

low the aneurysm and removes the transected segment. He or she then begins to anastomose the prosthetic graft to the aorta.

Anastomosing the Graft

The technique of anastomosing the graft to the aorta is the same for all three methods described above. The surgeon performs the proximal anastomosis with a continuous suture, such as size 3-0 or 4-0 Prolene or Ti-Cron. A straight vascular clamp is then placed across the graft while the proximal aortic clamp is temporarily released to test the suture line for leaks. The surgeon reapplies the aortic clamp, removes the clamp from the graft, and places any additional sutures needed to control leaks. Teflon felt pledgets may be placed under the sutures.

After the surgeon completes the proximal anastomosis, he or she cuts the graft to the appropriate length and completes the distal anastomosis. Before the surgeon ties the suture, the graft is flushed to clear it of clots and debris by temporarily releasing the clamp on the aorta. The suture is then tied and all clamps are removed, thus restoring blood flow to the lower body.

If partial cardiopulmonary bypass or a shunt has been used, it is discontinued at this stage of the procedure. The shunt is removed in a fashion similar to that for an atrial cannula.

The surgeon covers the graft with any remaining aneurysmal tissue using a running or interrupted suture,

such as size 3-0 or 2-0 chromic catgut. The mediastinal pleura is closed in a similar manner.

The chest tube is inserted in standard fashion, and the chest is closed as for a thoracotomy.

Median Sternotomy

Definition

This is an incision of the chest at the midline, through the sternum. The procedure provides access to the organs in the mediastinal cavity, particularly the heart. It is the most common incision used in open-heart surgery.

Highlights

Opening

1. The incision is made.
2. The xiphoid is divided.
3. The sternum is divided.
4. Hemostasis is achieved.
5. The retractor is inserted.
6. The pericardium is opened.

Closure

1. Wires are placed through the sternum.
2. The sternal edges are brought together.
3. The fascia and periosteum are reapproximated.
4. The subcutaneous tissue and skin are closed.

Description

Opening

The patient is placed in the supine position. The surgeon makes a midline incision with the skin knife from the level of the sternal notch to 2 to 3 inches below the xiphoid. The subcutaneous tissue and linea alba (fascial layer distal to the xiphoid) are divided with the deep knife or electrocautery pencil. The surgeon separates the underlying tissue from the sternal notch and xiphoid using finger dissection and divides the xiphoid in the center with curved Mayo scissors. A sternal saw blade or knife is then placed in the center of the divided xiphoid or the sternal notch, and the sternum is divided in half (Fig. 24–38A).

The assistant elevates the cut edges of the sternum using a U.S. Army retractor while the surgeon maintains hemostasis by applying bone wax to the marrow and cauterizing the periosteum and subcutaneous tissue layers. The surgeon covers the edges of the sternum with sterile towels or laparotomy sponges to protect the bone marrow from the blades of the retractor.

The surgeon slowly opens the retractor to expose the subcutaneous tissue. He or she divides it with Metzenbaum scissors and controls bleeding by ligating the vessels or using the electrocautery pencil.

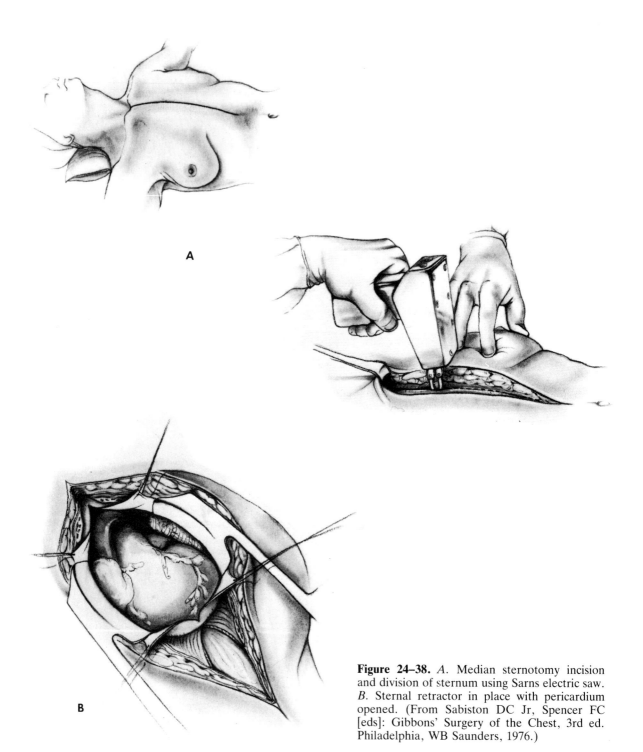

Figure 24–38. *A.* Median sternotomy incision and division of sternum using Sarns electric saw. *B.* Sternal retractor in place with pericardium opened. (From Sabiston DC Jr, Spencer FC [eds]: Gibbons' Surgery of the Chest, 3rd ed. Philadelphia, WB Saunders, 1976.)

The surgeon grasps the pericardium with smooth tissue forceps or a Schnidt clamp to elevate it and prevent injury to the heart, which lies just beneath. The pericardium is incised, and the incision is extended to expose the heart and ascending aorta. The surgeon may extend the incision laterally to expose the ventricles more completely.

The surgeon may place silk traction sutures through the edges of the pericardium (Fig. 24–38B) and encircle the ascending aorta with an umbilical tape. The heart and aorta are then cannulated for cardiopulmonary bypass.

Closure

After a particular procedure is performed, hemostasis is maintained and chest tubes are inserted. The surgeon places six to eight No. 5 wire sutures through each sternal edge. The technologist holds onto the free end of the wire until the assistant takes it so that it does not hit the surgeon's face.

The surgeon brings the sternal edges together by tightening the wires and then twisting each individual wire until it is snug against the sternum. The surgeon tightens the wire further with a wire twister and bends the ends over to bury them in the periosteum.

When the Wolvek sternal approximation fixation instruments are used, the ends of the wires are threaded through small metal plates instead of being twisted together. The ends of the wires are tightened and the wire is then locked in position by crimping the plate. The excess wires are cut and the sharp tips of the remaining wires are pushed into the periosteum with a wire twister (Fig. 24–39).

The surgeon reapproximates the fascial and periosteal layers with interrupted sutures, such as size 0 Tevdek or 2-0 braided silk, or a running suture of size 0 Prolene or chromic catgut. The subcutaneous tissue and skin are then closed in the surgeon's preferred manner.

Cardiopulmonary Bypass

Definition

Cardiopulmonary (heart-lung) bypass is the method used to divert blood away from the heart and lungs temporarily when surgery of the heart and major vessels is performed. A special heart-lung pump is used to collect the blood, oxygenate it, and return it to the body (Fig. 24–40). The pump tubing is connected to cannulae that are inserted into the vena cavae and ascending aorta through a median sternotomy incision. Occasionally, the femoral artery and femoral vein are used instead of the cavae and aorta.

Cardiopulmonary bypass may be either total or partial. Total bypass is achieved by tightening umbilical tapes around the vena cavae and cannulae. This forces all blood returning to the heart into the cannula, and thus to the pump. It also prevents air from entering the venous line and obstructing the flow of blood to the pump when the right side of the heart is opened. Total bypass is used for such procedures as valve replacements, repair of septal defects, and resection of ventricular and ascending aortic aneurysms. In partial bypass, blood can escape around the cannula and enter the heart. Partial bypass is adequate for procedures such as coronary artery bypass and resection of a thoracic aneurysm. It is also used to support a patient in emergency situations, such as a cardiac arrest or ruptured aneurysm. Partial cardiopulmonary bypass is illustrated in Figure 24–41.

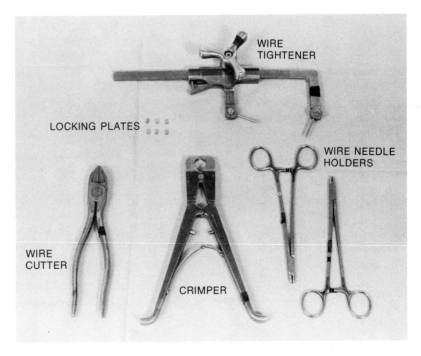

Figure 24–39. Wolvek sternal approximation fixation instrument used to approximate divided sternum. (Courtesy of Long Beach Memorial Medical Center, Long Beach, CA.)

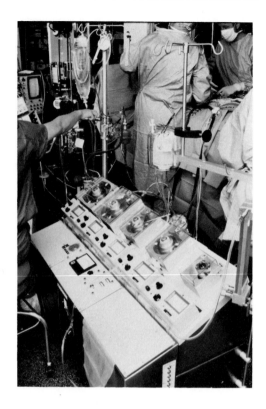

Figure 24–40. Heart-lung machine with tubing.

Figure 24–41. Partial cardiopulmonary bypass with cannulation of femoral artery and femoral vein. (From DeBakey ME, Diethrich EB: Ventricular assistive devices, present and future. In Burford TH, Ferguson TB (eds): Cardiovascular Surgery, Current Practice, vol 1, p 232. St. Louis, CV Mosby, 1969.)

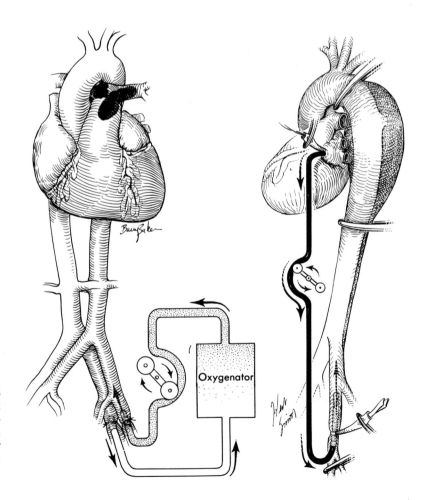

The tubing and oxygenator for the *heart-lung machine* are assembled and primed by the perfusionist (pump technician) before cannulation is performed. The technologist should be familiar with the basic functions and method of operation of the pump, the sizes of the pump lines, and how the lines connect to the patient. The technologist should also be familiar with the various types of *cannulae* and know where they are used in the body. The cannulae discussed here are shown in Figure 24–42. *Venous cannulae* are straight ended with multiple holes and are used to drain the blood from the body. The *aortic cannula* has an angled tip so that blood is directed toward the descending thoracic aorta. The *femoral cannula* is tapered to match the size of the artery and has a beveled end to allow for easier insertion. The femoral and aortic cannulae carry oxygenated (arterial) blood. The *coronary perfusion cannula* has a cuff near its tip to prevent the possibility of inserting the cannula too far, thus occluding a major branch of the artery. It is used to infuse cardioplegic solution directly into the heart. The *left ventricular sump catheter* is used to prevent injury to the heart muscle caused by distention when excess blood accumulates. The catheter drains the blood from the left ventricle when the aorta is occluded.

In both types of bypass, blood returns to the pump through the cannula, either by gravity drainage or by the pump roller head. Gravity drainage cannot be used if a chamber of the aorta is open because the venous line will fill with air and obstruct the flow of blood to the pump. When suction is used, it must be applied while the catheter is being inserted into the ventricle to prevent air from being drawn into the ventricle by the beating heart. Instead, the vacuum created by the pump draws the air away from the heart and down into the pump. The technologist must always watch for the presence of air in the heart or pump lines. Air must be removed immediately to prevent embolization to major body organs, particularly the brain and heart. The technologist should always have a *needle and syringe* readily available. A 10-mL syringe with a 19-gauge needle may be used for both adults and infants.

Highlights: Cannulation of the Superior and Inferior Venae Cavae

1. The right atrium is clamped.
2. A pursestring suture is placed in the occluded portion, and its ends are snared through a piece of tubing.
3. The atrium is opened, and its walls are held open.
4. The cannula is inserted, and all clamps are removed.
5. The cannula is introduced into the vena cava.
6. The suture is drawn tightly through the tubing, thus forming a tourniquet.
7. The cannula and tubing are tied together with a heavy silk suture.
8. The cannula is allowed to fill with blood and is then occluded with a tube-occluding clamp.
9. The cannulae are connected to the venous return line from the pump.

Description: Cannulation of the Superior and Inferior Venae Cavae

Shortly after heparin is administered to the patient by the anesthesiologist, the surgeon grasps the right atrial

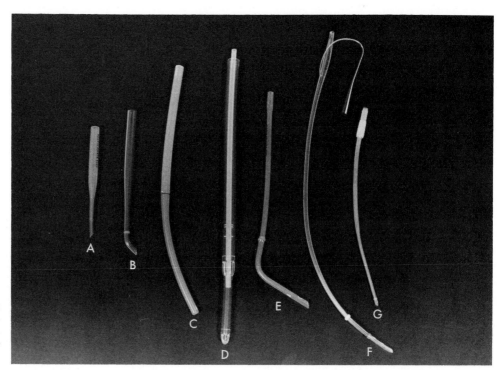

Figure 24–42. Types of cannulae for cardiopulmonary bypass. A, femoral artery; B, aorta; C, vena cava; D, atrium; E, left ventricle (right superior pulmonary vein approach); F, left ventricle (apex); G, coronary artery for direct perfusion.

appendage with Singley forceps and places a curved vascular clamp (Beck or Glover) across it. A pursestring suture, size 0 Ti-Cron or 3-0 Prolene, is placed through the occluded portion of the appendage. The assistant snares the ends of the suture through a piece of tubing and holds the ends with a hemostatic clamp.

The surgeon excises the tip of the appendage with Metzenbaum scissors and applies clamps (mosquito or Schnidt) to the two edges of the atrial wall. The assistant controls the vascular clamp and retracts one of the clamps on the atrial wall. The surgeon retracts the atrial wall with one hand as he or she inserts the cannula. The technologist should control the top end of the cannula to prevent it from hitting the surgeon's face. The assistant removes the vascular clamp and controls the suture to prevent bleeding from the atrium.

The surgeon introduces the cannula into the superior vena cava. (If only one cannula is used, it is left in the atrium.) The assistant forms a tourniquet by tightening the tubing against the suture and holding the end with a hemostatic clamp. The surgeon ties the cannula and tourniquet together with a heavy silk suture and then allows blood to fill the cannula by having the anesthesiologist inflate the lungs. The assistant places a tube-occluding clamp across the cannula.

The inferior vena cava is cannulated in a similar fashion. The major difference is that the cannula is inserted through the atrial wall instead of through the appendage. A knife blade and Potts scissors may be used to open the atrium. The cannulae are connected to the venous return line from the pump. The cannulation of the vena cava is shown in Figure 24–43.

Highlights: Cannulation of the Aorta

1. A pursestring suture is placed in the ascending aorta, and its ends are snared through a piece of tubing.
2. The aorta is incised.
3. The cannula is inserted and positioned.
4. The suture is tightened.
5. The cannula and tubing are tied together with a heavy silk suture.
6. The cannula is allowed to fill to evacuate all air.
7. A tube-occluding clamp is placed across the cannula.
8. The cannula is connected to the arterial perfusion line from the pump.

Description: Cannulation of the Aorta

The surgeon places a pursestring suture in the ascending aorta. The assistant snares the ends of the suture through a piece of tubing. A stab incision is made into the aorta, and the incision is dilated with an aortic dilator or Schnidt clamp. The surgeon controls bleeding by holding one finger over the hole as the cannula is inserted. The assistant controls the top end of the cannula, which is occluded by a tube-occluding clamp. The surgeon positions the cannula and the assistant tightens the suture, forming a tourniquet with the tubing. The surgeon ties the tourniquet to the cannula with

a heavy silk suture. He or she temporarily unclamps the cannula to allow it to fill with blood and evacuate the air. The cannula is then connected to the arterial perfusion line from the pump. The placement of the aortic cannula is shown in Figure 24–44.

Highlights: Cannulation of the Femoral Artery and Femoral Vein

1. An incision is made in the groin over the area of the femoral artery and vein.
2. The tissue layers are divided, and a self-retaining retractor is inserted.
3. The common femoral artery and its two major branches are isolated and encircled with umbilical tapes, and the ends of the tapes are snared through pieces of tubing.
4. The femoral vein is isolated in a similar fashion.
5. The artery is occluded with vascular clamps, and an arteriotomy is performed in the common femoral artery.
6. The cannula is inserted as the upper clamp is removed.
7. The cannula is allowed to fill with blood to evacuate all air and a tube-occluding clamp is applied across the cannula.
8. The cannula is connected to the perfusion line from the pump.
9. The femoral vein is cannulated in a similar fashion.

Description: Cannulation of the Femoral Artery and Femoral Vein

Cannulation of the femoral artery and vein are performed when partial bypass is needed to support the patient's circulation in emergency situations and during surgical resection of the descending thoracic aorta and the ascending aorta. The femoral artery is also cannulated any time the ascending aorta cannot be cannulated.

The surgeon makes an incision in the groin over the area of the vessels using the skin knife. The subcutaneous tissue and fascial layers are divided with Metzenbaum scissors. A self-retaining retractor (Gelpi or Weitlaner) is inserted to help expose the vessels. The surgeon isolates the common femoral artery and its two major branches (superficial and profunda) with Metzenbaum scissors. Each vessel is encircled with umbilical tapes secured in the jaw of a right-angled clamp. The assistant snares the ends of the tapes in pieces of tubing. The surgeon isolates the femoral vein in the same manner.

After heparin has been administered, the surgeon occludes the femoral artery with small angled vascular clamps (Glover or Cooley). An arteriotomy is performed in the occluded segment with a No. 11 knife and the incision is extended with Potts scissors. The surgeon may dilate the opening with a hemostatic clamp. He or she inserts the cannula as the assistant removes the upper vascular clamp. The assistant tightens the umbilical tape to hold the cannula in place. The surgeon ties a heavy silk suture around the tape and releases the

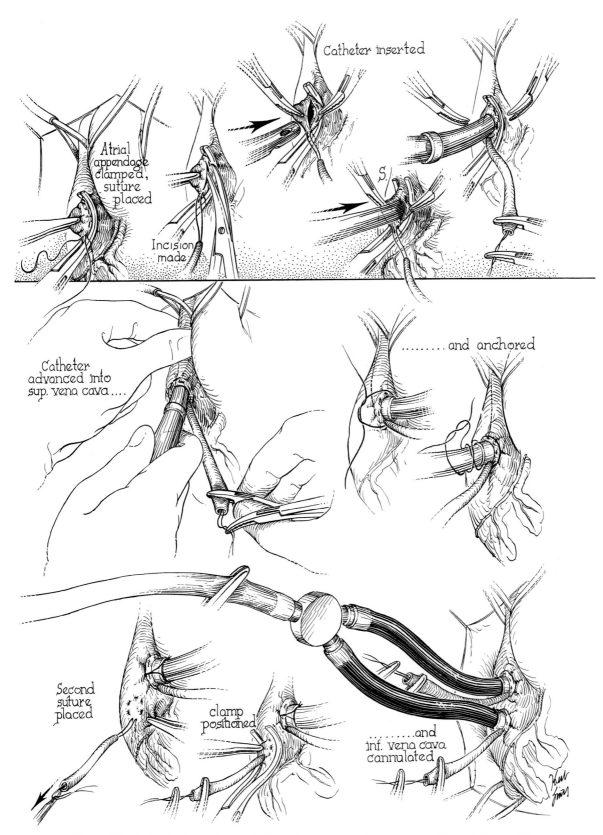

Figure 24–43. Technique of cannulation of vena cava. (From Cooley DA, Hallman GL: Surgical Treatment of Congenital Heart Disease. Philadelphia, Lea & Febiger, 1966. Used with permission.)

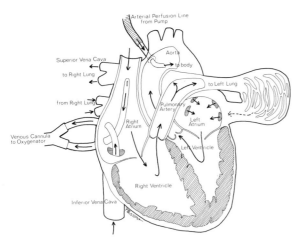

Arterial Perfusion Line from Pump
Aorta
Superior Vena Cava
to body
to Right Lung
to Left Lung
Pulmonary Artery
from Right Lung
Right Atrium
Left Atrium
Venous Cannula to Oxygenator
Left Ventricle
Right Ventricle
Inferior Vena Cava

Figure 24–44. Standard placement of cannula for cardiopulmonary bypass, showing flow of blood through heart to lungs and aorta during *partial* bypass.

tube-occluding clamp to allow blood to fill the cannula and evacuate air. The cannula is then connected to the arterial perfusion line. The cannulation of the femoral artery is described in Figure 24–45.

The surgeon cannulates the femoral vein in the same manner. The cannulae are secured to the patient's skin or to the drapes.

Highlights: Insertion of a Sump Catheter into the Apex of the Left Ventricle

1. The apex is elevated, and a pursestring suture is placed.
2. The ends of the suture are brought through a piece of tubing.
3. A stab incision is made in the ventricle, and the incision is dilated.
4. The catheter is inserted into the ventricle and held secure by tightening the suture with the tubing.
5. The catheter is tied to the tubing with a heavy silk suture.
6. The apex of the ventricle is lowered back to its normal position.

Description: Insertion of a Sump Catheter into the Apex of the Left Ventricle

As soon as bypass is instituted, the surgeon elevates the apex of the left ventricle with a laparotomy sponge. A pursestring suture is placed in the apex, and the assistant snares it through the tubing. The technologist connects the sump catheter to the pump line.

The surgeon makes a stab incision in the apex with a No. 11 knife blade and dilates the opening with a Schnidt clamp. He or she inserts the catheter, and the assistant secures it in place by forming a tourniquet with the suture and tubing. The surgeon ties the catheter and tourniquet together with a heavy silk suture and then lowers the apex to its normal position. The insertion of the sump catheter is shown in Figure 24–46.

Highlights: Insertion of a Sump Catheter into the Right Superior Pulmonary Vein

1. The right atrium is retracted to expose the right superior pulmonary vein.
2. A pursestring suture is placed in the vein.
3. A stab incision is made in the vein, and the incision is dilated.
4. The catheter is inserted and manipulated into the left atrium across the mitral valve and then into the left ventricle.
5. A tube-occluding clamp is placed across the cannula.
6. The tubing is tightened against the catheter and then tied to it.
7. The catheter is connected to the pump line.

Description: Insertion of a Sump Catheter in the Right Superior Pulmonary Vein

The assistant retracts the right atrium to expose the right superior pulmonary vein while the surgeon places the pursestring suture. The assistant brings the ends of the suture through a piece of tubing. The surgeon makes a stab incision into the vein with a No. 11 knife blade and dilates the incision with a Schnidt clamp. He or she inserts the catheter into the vein and then manipulates it into the left atrium, across the mitral valve, and into the left ventricle. The assistant forms a tourniquet with the suture and tubing and places a tube-occluding clamp across the catheter. The surgeon ties the catheter to the tourniquet with a heavy silk suture and then connects the catheter to the pump line.

Highlights: Decannulation of the Ventricle, Venae Cavae, and Aorta

1. A tube-occluding clamp is placed across the catheter or cannula.
2. The heavy silk tie and tubing from the suture are removed.
3. The catheter is withdrawn, and the suture is tied.

Description: Decannulation of the Left Ventricle, Venae Cavae, and Aorta

The left ventricular catheter is usually removed from the ventricle before bypass is discontinued. The catheter is occluded with a tube-occluding clamp, and the heavy silk suture and tourniquet are removed. The catheter is withdrawn, and the suture is tied securely to occlude the cannulation site.

The procedure for decannulation of the venae cavae and aorta is performed in a similar manner after bypass is discontinued.

Highlights: Decannulation of the Femoral Artery and Femoral Vein

1. The cannula is occluded.
2. The umbilical tape is released.

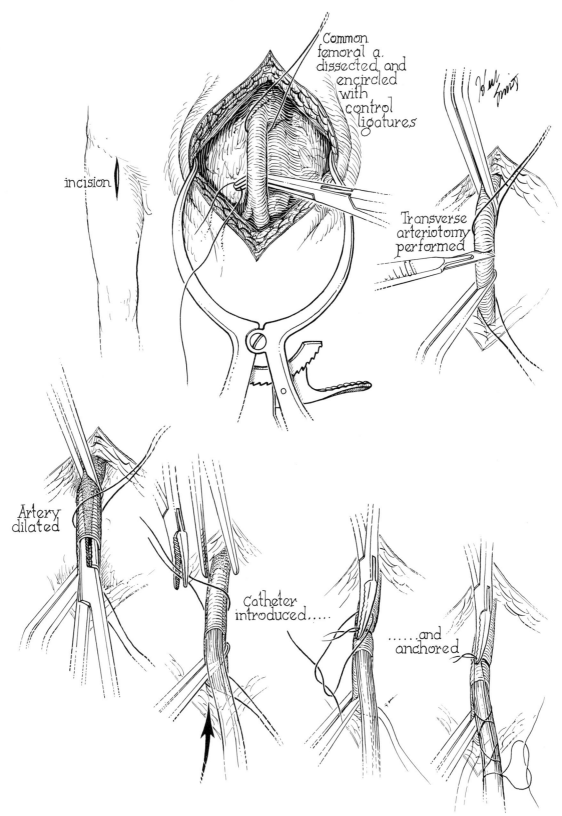

Figure 24–45. Technique for cannulation of femoral artery. (From Cooley DA, Hallman GL: Surgical Treatment of Congenital Heart Disease. Philadelphia, Lea & Febiger, 1966. Used with permission.)

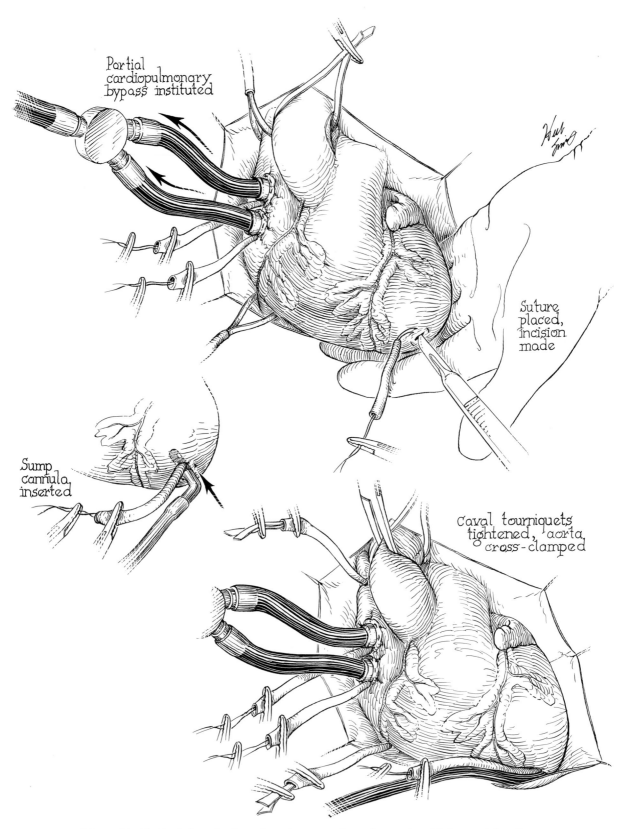

Figure 24–46. Technique for insertion of sump catheter into apex of left ventricle. (From Cooley DA, Hallman GL: Surgical Treatment of Congenital Heart Disease. Philadelphia, Lea & Febiger, 1966. Used with permission.)

3. The cannula is withdrawn, and the vein is occluded with a vascular clamp.

4. The venotomy is closed, and all clamps and tapes are removed.

5. The artery is decannulated in the same fashion.

Description: Decannulation of the Femoral Artery and Femoral Vein

At the conclusion of bypass, the surgeon occludes the femoral vein cannula. The assistant releases the cannula from the patient's skin or the drapes and also releases the umbilical tape from around the cannula and vein. The surgeon withdraws the cannula, and the assistant occludes the vein with a vascular clamp. The surgeon closes the venotomy with a running suture, such as size 6-0 or 5-0 Prolene. All clamps from the vein are removed, and then the artery is decannulated in the same manner.

Highlights: Coronary Artery Perfusion

This is the infusion of cardioplegic solution into the coronary arteries to preserve the cardiac muscle from damage when the aorta is occluded. The solution may be infused directly into the coronary artery or indirectly into the aortic root just above the aortic valve.

1. The ascending aorta is occluded and opened below the clamp.

2. The ostia (openings) of the coronary arteries are identified and then cannulated.

3. Solution of sufficient quantity to stop the heart is infused, and the cannulae are removed immediately after each infusion.

4. The aorta is closed when the surgery is completed.

Description: Coronary Artery Perfusion (Direct Method)

The surgeon occludes the ascending aorta and opens it below the clamp. The coronary ostia are located and the sizes of cannulae needed are determined. The technologist connects the appropriate size cannulae to the tubing. The surgeon gently inserts the cannulae into the ostia of the coronary arteries and holds them in position until the pump perfusionist or anesthesiologist completes the infusion of the cardioplegic solution. Enough solution is infused so that the heart stops. The technologist should keep the cannulae and tubing secure in a towel until they are needed for subsequent infusions of cardioplegic solution. The surgeon closes the aorta at the completion of the surgery.

Highlights: Coronary Artery Perfusion (Indirect Method)

1. The ascending aorta is occluded.

2. An indwelling catheter is inserted into the aortic root above the valve.

3. The catheter is connected to the tubing filled with cardioplegic solution.

4. Solution of sufficient quantity to stop the heart is infused.

5. The indwelling catheter is removed immediately before the aorta is unclamped.

6. The hole made by the catheter is oversewn.

Description: Coronary Artery Perfusion (Indirect Method)

The surgeon occludes the ascending aorta and inserts an indwelling catheter, such as a 14-gauge Angiocath, into the aorta below the clamp. The assistant connects the tubing from the cardioplegic solution to the catheter. The anesthesiologist or pump perfusionist infuses the solution into the aorta in sufficient quantity to stop the heart. The surgeon may secure the catheter to the aortic clamp with a heavy silk suture.

Cardioplegic solution is infused as often as necessary during the time the aorta is occluded, as directed by the surgeon. The surgeon withdraws the indwelling catheter and removes the clamp from the aorta. Air in the aorta escapes through the hole made by the catheter. The surgeon closes the hole with a suture, such as size 5-0 Prolene, as soon as all the air has been evacuated.

Implantation of a Pacemaker

Definition

This is the placement of pacemaker electrodes to the heart to correct bradycardia or heart block or to control arrhythmias. The *pulse generator* utilizes lithium to provide power for the pacemaker. Pacemaker implantation may be performed on a temporary basis such as during cardiac procedures, or the implantation may be permanent. Three approaches are employed for permanent implantation: transvenous, epicardial, and subxiphoid. The transvenous and subxiphoid procedures, which do not require a thoracotomy, are commonly performed with the patient under local anesthesia with monitored anesthesia care (see Chapter 9). When the transvenous approach is used, the electrodes are placed with the aid of fluoroscopy. A venotomy is performed and the electrode is advanced into the right atrium, through the tricuspid valve, and into the right ventricle, where it is placed in the right ventricular apex. The pulse generator is then placed within the superficial tissues of the chest wall.

The procedures for both permanent and temporary pacemaker implantation through a thoracotomy are more complex than the transvenous approach and are discussed below.

Highlights: Temporary Pacemaker

1. The electrode is sutured to the right ventricle or right atrium.

2. The free end of the electrode is brought through the skin and secured with a suture.

3. The electrode is connected to the alligator cable, which is attached to the pacemaker battery.

Description: Temporary Pacemaker

The surgeon usually sutures the electrode to the heart with size 0 Flexon steel after cardiopulmonary bypass is discontinued. The technologist should have the electrode open and loaded on the needle holder in case it is needed before bypass is discontinued. The assistant cuts the needle off the electrode after the surgeon places it through the myocardium. The surgeon then buries the tip of the electrode in the epicardium, using a mosquito clamp. The electrode may be secured with sutures of size 5-0 silk. The surgeon brings the opposite end of the electrode through the skin. The assistant secures the electrode to the skin with a suture of size 2-0 silk. The electrode is then connected to the alligator cable and pacemaker battery. The anesthesiologist or circulator can then pace the heart when necessary.

Highlights: Permanent Pacemaker

1. The chest is opened to expose the right ventricle.
2. Sutures are placed in the ventricle and into the electrode Silastic casing.
3. A small hole is made in the myocardium.
4. The coiled metal tip of the electrode is positioned in the hole.
5. The sutures are tied to secure the electrode.
6. The electrodes are tested and then connected to the permanent battery.
7. The battery is implanted in the abdominal wall.
8. The wound is closed.

Description: Permanent Pacemaker

The techniques for implanting the permanent pacemaker through a thoracotomy or a short transverse incision are the same. The surgeon makes a short transverse incision below the xiphoid and across the area of the diaphragm using the skin knife. The subcutaneous, fascial, and muscle layers are divided with the deep knife or electrocautery pencil. A self-retaining retractor, such as a small Finochietto or large Weitlaner retractor, is then inserted.

The surgeon exposes the right ventricle by opening the pericardium with the knife or Metzenbaum scissors. Size 2-0 silk sutures are placed on the edges of the pericardium so that the assistant can offer traction on the tissue. The surgeon then places several sutures of size 4-0 silk or Ti-Cron through the ventricle and into the electrode Silastic casing. The myocardium is incised with a No. 11 knife blade. The coiled metal tip of the electrode is placed in the incision, and the sutures are tied. Additional sutures may be needed to secure the electrode further (Fig. 24–47A).

To test the electrode, the surgeon connects it to an alligator cable attached to the external pacemaker battery. The circulator or anesthesiologist activates the battery. If the electrode functions normally, it is then connected to the permanent battery. The surgeon makes a pocket for the battery beneath the fascia of the abdomen using Metzenbaum scissors. He or she inserts the battery in the pocket and closes it with interrupted sutures of size 0 Ti-Cron or Tevdek. Dexon sutures are used to approximate the subcutaneous tissue, and the skin is closed with the surgeon's choice of suture.

Frequently, the screw-on epicardial lead is used instead of the type of lead that requires suturing. The technique of inserting this type of lead into the myocardium of the right ventricle is shown in Figure 24–47B.

Replacement of Pacemaker Battery

Definition

This is the replacement of a malfunctioning pacemaker battery with a new, functional one.

Highlights

1. The skin is incised over the area of the battery.
2. The tissue layers are divided to expose the battery and electrode(s).
3. The battery is removed from the tissue pocket.
4. The electrode is connected to an alligator cable.
5. The electrode is inserted into the new battery.
6. The new battery is inserted into the tissue pocket.
7. The wound is closed.

Description

The surgeon incises the skin over the area of the battery with the skin knife. The underlying tissue layers are then divided with the deep knife or Metzenbaum scissors to expose the electrode(s) and battery. The battery is removed from the tissue pocket and the electrode(s) is disconnected. The surgeon immediately connects the electrode(s) to the alligator cable so that the heart can be continually paced during the exchange of batteries. The electrodes are then connected to the new battery. The surgeon places the new battery into the tissue pocket. Interrupted sutures of size 3-0 Dexon are used to approximate the tissues over the battery. The skin is then closed with the surgeon's choice of suture.

Automatic Implantable Cardioverter Defibrillator

The automatic implantable cardioverter defibrillator (AICD) is an electronic, cardiac monitoring device that delivers defibrillatory shocks during ventricular fibrillation or ventricular tachycardia. The device consists of a generator, myocardial patches, and sensing electrodes.

The AICD may be implanted through a thoracotomy, subxiphoid, or median sternotomy incision. The sensing leads are placed in the right ventricle through a transvenous or epicardial approach. The ventricular patches are sutured to the epicardium, and the pulse generator is placed in the superficial tissues of the abdominal wall.

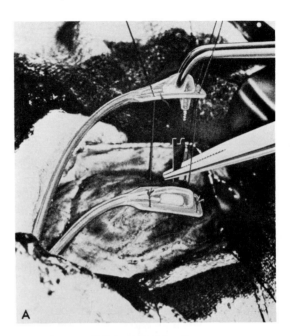

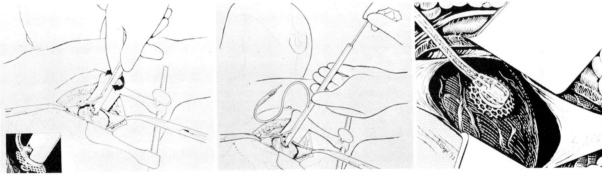

Figure 24–47. *A.* Technique of implanting epicardial lead. *B.* Technique of inserting screw-on epicardial leads. (Reprinted with permission of Medtronic, Inc., Minneapolis, MN.)

Coronary Artery Bypass

Definition

This is the bypass of an occluded segment of one or both coronary arteries, using an autogenous vein graft (a vein taken from elsewhere in the patient's body). The graft is anastomosed to the ascending aorta and the coronary artery to increase the blood supply to the heart muscle.

Highlights

1. A median sternotomy is performed.
2. A segment of autogenous vein is obtained from the leg.
3. The heart is cannulated for cardiopulmonary bypass.
4. The aorta is occluded and cardioplegic solution administered into the aortic root.
5. The coronary artery is isolated, opened, and anastomosed to the vein.

6. The aorta is unclamped.
7. The vein is anastomosed to the ascending aorta.
8. Cardiopulmonary bypass is discontinued, and decannulation is performed.
9. Chest tubes are inserted, and the wound is closed.

Description

The surgeon performs a median sternotomy in standard fashion and cannulates for cardiopulmonary bypass, as previously described. At the same time, the assistant removes a segment of vein (the greater saphenous) from the leg. There are two main approaches that may be used to remove the vein. The assistant may either begin at the groin and work toward the ankle, or he or she may begin at the ankle and work toward the groin. The vein from the lower leg is smaller and closer in size to the coronary artery than the vein taken from the groin area. The latter approach is most commonly used and is discussed here.

The technologist may be required to assist both the surgeon and the assistant, or a second technologist may assist in the vein removal. In the latter case, a separate set of instruments is usually required for the vein removal and the two teams work independently. This helps control possible contamination from the patient's legs and feet to the chest.

Description

Removal of Vein

The assistant begins the incision in the ankle area and extends it toward the knee. He or she incises the skin with the skin knife and extends the incision with either the skin knife or the Metzenbaum scissors. The subcutaneous tissue is divided with Metzenbaum scissors and smooth tissue forceps. The vein from the surrounding tissue is then mobilized, and all branches of the vein are ligated with fine silk sutures or small ligation clips. The vein as it is removed from the leg is shown in Figure 24–48.

When the assistant has isolated an adequate length of vein, he or she ligates both ends with size 2-0 silk suture. The upper and lower ends of the vein are noted so that its position can be reversed for anastomosis to the artery. (Veins have valves that allow blood to flow in one direction only. For blood to flow in the opposite direction, as in an artery, the vein must be reversed.) The assistant inserts a syringe adapter attached to a syringe filled with heparinized physiologic solution and flushes the solution to test for leaks. In case there are any leaks, they are repaired with fine vascular sutures. The assistant then places the vein in a basin filled with heparinized physiologic solution and passes it to the technologist, who places it on the instrument table until it is needed.

The assistant maintains hemostasis by clamping and tying bleeders or by using the electrocautery pencil. He or she then reapproximates the subcutaneous tissue with running sutures of size 3-0 absorbable suture. The skin is closed with the surgeon's choice of suture. The assis-

tant or technologist washes the leg free of blood and applies the dressing. The technologist may be required to hold the leg while the assistant wraps it in an Ace bandage; this is done to prevent the formation of a hematoma when the patient is heparinized. The surgeon then covers the legs with a sterile drape.

Coronary Artery Bypass

After cardiopulmonary bypass is instituted and the left ventricular sump catheter is inserted, the surgeon isolates the segment of coronary artery to which the vein will be anastomosed. This is done with a No. 64 Beaver blade, a No. 15 Bard-Parker blade, or Potts scissors. The surgeon then occludes the ascending aorta and inserts the indwelling catheter for infusion of cardioplegic solution, as previously described. Ice-cold physiologic solution is poured over the heart to lower its temperature and reduce its requirement for oxygen.

The surgeon opens the coronary artery with a No. 11 knife blade and extends the incision with Diethrich coronary scissors (Fig. 24–49). A Garrett dilator may be inserted into the lumen of the artery to assess its size (Fig. 24–50). The technologist places the vein on a saline solution–moistened towel and hands it to the surgeon, who makes a slit in the free end of the vein with Potts scissors. The vein is then sutured to the coronary artery with running or interrupted sutures, such as size 6-0 Prolene (Fig. 24–51). When the anastomosis is complete, the assistant inflates the vein with physiologic solution to test for leaks.

The surgeon performs all succeeding anastomoses to the coronary arteries in the same manner. At the completion of the anastomoses, the aorta is unclamped and the indwelling catheter is removed. A portion of the aorta is then occluded with a vascular clamp, such as the Lambert-Kay clamp (Fig. 24–52). A No. 11 knife blade and aortic punch (Fig. 24–53) are used to create

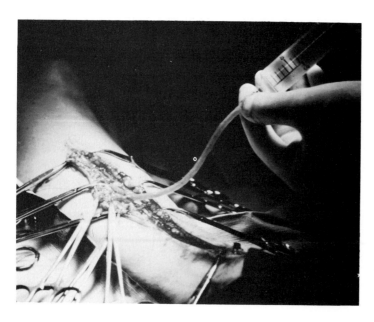

Figure 24–48. Technique of removal of saphenous vein from lower leg. Incision begins at ankle and extends to the knee.

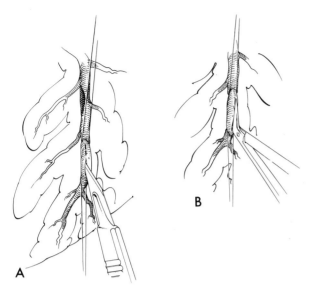

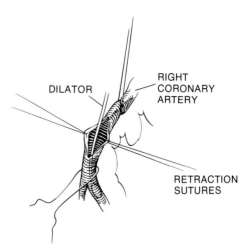

Figure 24–50. Insertion of dilator to assess size of lumen of coronary artery.

Figure 24–49. *A.* Arteriotomy performed with scalpel. *B.* Arteriotomy extended with Diethrich scissors.

a hole in the occluded portion. The surgeon inflates the vein to make certain it is not twisted and to determine the length needed to reach the aorta. He or she then cuts the vein to the appropriate length and makes a slit in the end with Potts scissors. The anastomosis is performed between the vein and the hole in the aorta (Fig. 24–54). The surgeon completes each of the anastomoses in the same manner and removes the clamp from the aorta. Air is evacuated from the vein grafts with a 25-

gauge needle (Fig. 24–55). The left ventricular sump catheter is then removed. The surgeon inspects each anastomosis for possible leaks; these are repaired before bypass is discontinued. The grafts are shown in functioning position in Figure 24–56.

Cardiopulmonary bypass is discontinued, and the surgeon removes the cannulae. A pacemaker electrode may be sutured to the heart, as described for implantation of a pacemaker.

Metal rings or radiopaque material may be placed around each vein graft on the aorta. These serve as

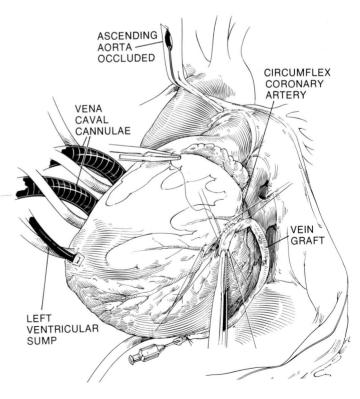

Figure 24–51. Technique of anastomosis of vein graft to coronary artery.

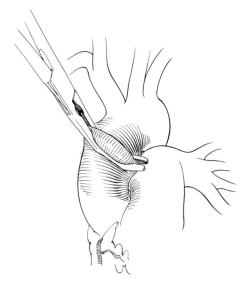

Figure 24–52. Ascending aorta partially occluded with vascular clamp.

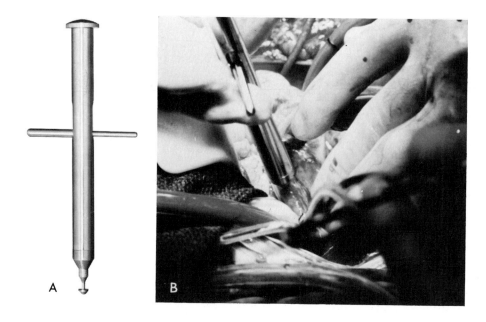

Figure 24–53. *A.* Aortic punch. *B.* Creation of hole in occluded segment of aorta. (*A,* courtesy of Scanlan, Inc., St. Paul, MN.)

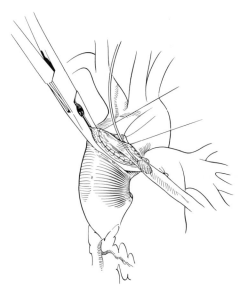

Figure 24–54. Vein graft is anastomosed to hole in ascending aorta. A dilator is passed to ensure a patent lumen.

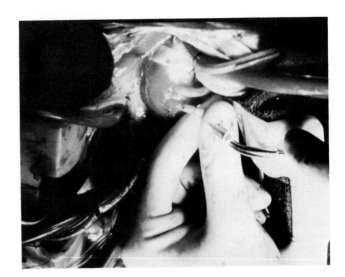

Figure 24–55. Technique for removal of air from vein grafts using a 25-gauge needle.

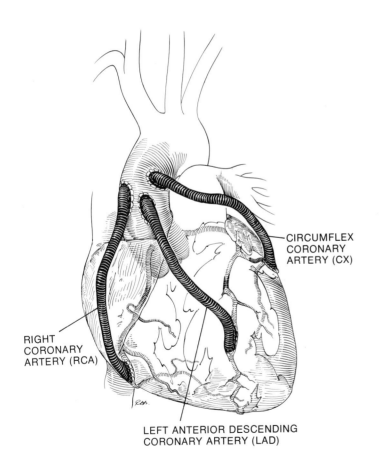

CIRCUMFLEX
CORONARY
ARTERY (CX)

RIGHT
CORONARY
ARTERY (RCA)

LEFT ANTERIOR DESCENDING
CORONARY ARTERY (LAD)

Figure 24–56. Illustration of vein grafts on completion of anastomosis and decannulation.

markers to assist in locating the vein grafts when cardiac catheterization is performed in the postoperative period. The surgeon inserts chest tubes and closes the median sternotomy, as previously described.

Some surgeons perform the proximal anastomoses first and then perform the distal anastomoses while the patient is on cardiopulmonary bypass. The technologist should be familiar with the particular method used by the surgeon.

Coronary Artery Angioplasty

Coronary artery angioplasty is performed to relieve stricture in the left coronary artery system caused by atherosclerotic plaque. This procedure is offered to patients who cannot tolerate a bypass grafting procedure.

Angioplasty is performed with the aid of fluoroscopy and may occur in the cardiac catheterization laboratory. To enlarge the coronary artery, the surgeon threads a balloon-tipped catheter into the artery through an incision in the femoral or brachial arteries. The balloon is then inflated. This forces the plaque against the arterial wall and enlarges the diameter of the lumen. During the procedure, Fluosol is administered to the patient through the catheter to maintain oxygenation to the myocardium.

In conjunction with balloon angioplasty, or as an alternative to the procedure, laser therapy may be used to vaporize the atherosclerotic plaque in the arterial wall.

Aortic Valve Replacement

Definition

This is the excision and replacement of the aortic valve with a prosthetic heart valve that permits blood to flow in only one direction. Common causes of valve insufficiency are rheumatic fever, subacute bacterial endocarditis, and congenital anomalies. When a valve becomes diseased, it loses its ability to close tightly and thus becomes inefficient. Blood then leaks back into the left ventricle instead of going through the aorta in normal fashion. Eventually, the left ventricle fails because of the added strain of trying to eject the excess blood out into the aorta.

The valve leaflets may also become stenotic because of calcification, which reduces the opening of the valve to a small slit. The ventricle is unable to pump a sufficient amount of blood through the stenotic valve, resulting in syncope (a temporary form of unconsciousness caused by lack of oxygen to the brain). Heart failure and sudden death commonly occur when the stenosis is severe.

Highlights

1. A median sternotomy is performed.
2. Cannulation for total cardiopulmonary bypass is

performed, and the left ventricular sump catheter is inserted.
3. The aorta is occluded distal to the valve.
4. An aortotomy (incision made in the aorta) is performed.
5. Direct coronary artery perfusion is performed.
6. The valve is excised.
7. The annulus (valve ring) is measured, and a prosthetic valve is inserted and sutured in place.
8. The aortotomy is closed.
9. Cardiopulmonary bypass is discontinued and decannulation is accomplished.
10. A temporary pacemaker electrode is sutured to the heart.
11. Chest tubes are inserted, and the wound is closed.

Description

The surgeon performs a median sternotomy in standard fashion. He or she performs cannulation for total cardiopulmonary bypass, and the left ventricular sump catheter is inserted, as previously described.

The ascending aorta is then occluded, and the aortotomy is performed using Metzenbaum scissors. The coronary arteries are perfused using the direct method, as described for cardiopulmonary bypass.

The surgeon excises the valve using the deep knife and Diethrich valve scissors (Fig. 24–57). The size of the annulus (remaining valve ring) is measured with the prosthetic valve sizer. The technologist obtains the correct size valve from the circulator. The surgeon places the commissure (area where the leaflets come together) sutures, and the assistants holds the ends of the sutures

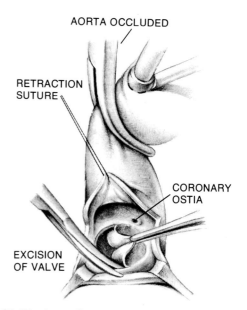

Figure 24–57. Ascending aorta occluded. Aortotomy performed and aortic wall retracted with a suture. The valve is excised with Diethrich valve scissors. (Courtesy of Ethicon, Inc., Somerville, NJ.)

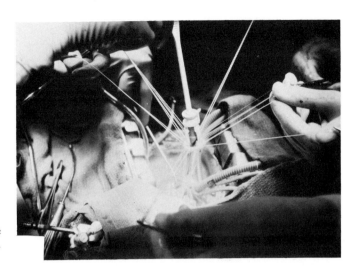

Figure 24–58. Technique of placing sutures through valve annulus and then through the prosthetic valve sewing ring. (Courtesy of Ethicon, Inc., Somerville, NJ.)

with straight mosquito clamps. The surgeon then places sutures around the entire annulus, alternating between blue and white sutures. The assistant places curved mosquito clamps on each suture to keep them separated. (A suture ring, such as the Crawford, may also be used to keep the sutures separated.)

After the surgeon places all sutures through the prosthetic valve sewing ring (Fig. 24–58), the valve is seated in position and all the sutures are tied (Fig. 24–59). The aortotomy is then closed with continuous sutures, such as size 3-0 Prolene; strips of Teflon felt may also be used along the suture line. Before removing the aortic occlusion clamp, the surgeon evacuates air from the left ventricle and aorta by allowing the heart to fill with blood and by aspirating it with a needle and syringe.

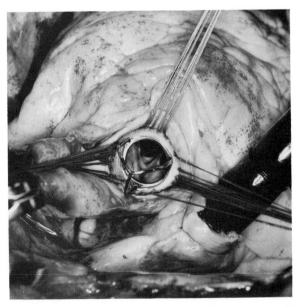

Figure 24–59. Prosthetic aortic valve seated in proper position and sutures tied. A ball valve is shown. The ball is often removed during insertion of the valve and then inserted after the valve is in place to allow air to escape from the left ventricle. (From Sabiston DC, Spencer FC (eds): Gibbons' Surgery of the Chest, 3rd ed. Philadelphia, WB Saunders, 1976.)

The left ventricular sump catheter is then removed, as previously described.

Cardiopulmonary bypass is discontinued and the surgeon removes the cannulae. A temporary pacemaker electrode may be sutured to the heart. Chest tubes are inserted, and the median sternotomy is closed in standard fashion.

Mitral Valve Replacement

Definition

This is the excision and replacement of the mitral valve with a prosthetic valve because of stenosis or insufficiency, most commonly caused by rheumatic heart disease. A malfunctioning valve causes the left atrium to become dilated and begin to fail. Surgery is performed to prevent or to treat heart failure.

Highlights

1. A median sternotomy is performed.
2. Cannulation for total cardiopulmonary bypass is performed.
3. The ascending aorta is occluded, and cardioplegic solution is infused through the aortic root into the coronary arteries.
4. A left atriotomy is performed and the mitral valve is excised.
5. A prosthetic valve is sutured in place.
6. The atriotomy is closed, and the aorta is unclamped.
7. Cardiopulmonary bypass is discontinued, and decannulation is accomplished.
8. Chest tubes are inserted and the wound is closed.

Description

Mitral Valve Replacement

The surgeon performs a median sternotomy and cannulates for total cardiopulmonary bypass. The ascending aorta is occluded and cardioplegic solution is infused through the aortic root into the coronary arteries.

The surgeon opens the left atrium with the deep knife and extends the incision with Metzenbaum scissors. He or she inserts a Cooley atrial retractor, which the assistant uses to expose the valve. The surgeon grasps the valve with a valve hook or long Allis clamp and excises the cusps, chordae tendineae, and papillary muscles with the Diethrich valve scissors or deep knife (Fig. 24–60). The annulus is then measured so that the technologist can obtain the correct size prosthetic valve from the circulating nurse. The surgeon places the sutures through the annulus and sewing ring of the prosthetic valve in a fashion similar to that described for aortic valve replacement. The surgeon then seats the valve in position and ties all sutures. The atriotomy is closed with running sutures of size 3-0 Prolene. Before tying the sutures, the surgeon temporarily releases the vena caval tourniquets and clamps the left ventricular sump to allow the heart to fill with blood. The blood is allowed to spill out of the heart to carry away any air bubbles. The surgeon then ties the sutures securely. The aortic clamp is removed, and the aorta is aspirated with a needle and syringe to further ensure that no air remains in the heart.

Cardiopulmonary bypass is discontinued and decannulation is done. A temporary pacemaker electrode may be sutured to the heart. Chest tubes are inserted, and the median sternotomy is closed in standard fashion.

Mitral Commissurotomy

Occasionally, a mitral commissurotomy (opening of the commissures that bring the cusps of the valve together) is performed rather than valve replacement to alleviate the stenosis. This procedure is carried out using cardiopulmonary bypass. The cusps are separated by incising between them with a knife blade or by breaking them apart with a mitral valve dilator, such as the Gerbode or Tubbs. The atrium is then closed, as described for mitral valve replacement.

Mitral Annuloplasty

An insufficient mitral valve is corrected by placing several sutures in the annulus to allow the valve leaflets to come together more efficiently. This procedure is preferred over the implantation of an artificial valve in the body because the presence of the foreign material requires that the patient receive anticoagulation therapy. The procedure is performed in a manner similar to that for mitral valve replacement.

Tricuspid Valve Replacement

In this procedure, the tricuspid valve is excised and replaced with a prosthetic valve through a right atriotomy in a manner similar to that used for mitral valve replacement.

Resection of an Aneurysm of the Ascending Aorta

Definition

This is the surgical removal of a segment of ascending aorta that is aneurysmal. The aneurysm may cause the aortic valve to become incompetent (leaflets fail to close properly).

Highlights

1. A median sternotomy is performed.
2. The femoral artery is isolated and cannulated.

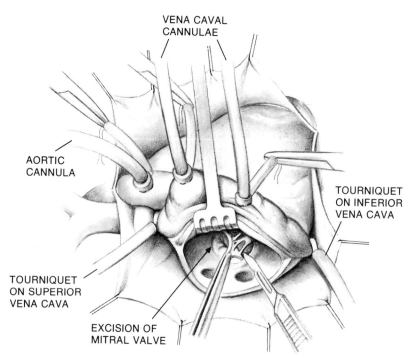

VENA CAVAL CANNULAE

AORTIC CANNULA

TOURNIQUET ON INFERIOR VENA CAVA

TOURNIQUET ON SUPERIOR VENA CAVA

EXCISION OF MITRAL VALVE

Figure 24–60. Mitral valve replacement. A retractor is inserted into the arteriotomy to expose the mitral valve. The valve is excised with the scalpel and Diethrich valve scissors. (Courtesy of Ethicon, Inc., Somerville, NJ.)

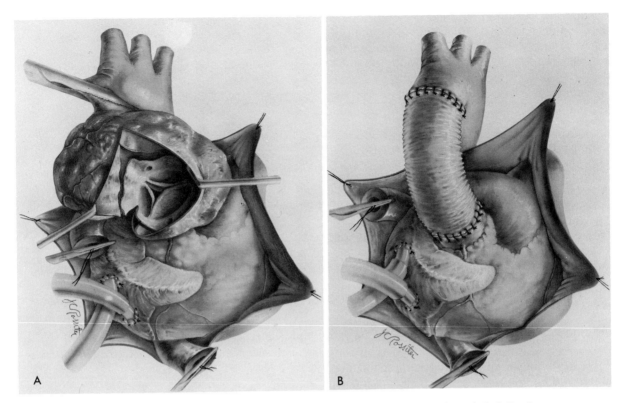

Figure 24–61. Resection of aortic aneurysm. *A.* The ascending aorta is occluded distal to the aneurysm. The aneurysm is incised and partially resected. The aortic valve and coronary ostia are clearly visible and normal. *B.* The aneurysm is resected and replaced with a woven prosthetic tube graft. The proximal and distal anastomoses are completed. (From Sabiston DC Jr, Spencer FC (eds): Gibbon's Surgery of the Chest, 3rd ed. Philadelphia, WB Saunders, 1976.)

3. The venae cavae are cannulated.

4. Total cardiopulmonary bypass is instituted, and a left ventricular sump catheter is inserted.

5. The aorta is occluded distal to the aneurysm, and the aneurysm is opened.

6. The coronary arteries are perfused directly.

7. A prosthetic graft is anastomosed to the proximal and distal aorta, and the aorta is unclamped.

8. Cardiopulmonary bypass is discontinued, and decannulation is performed.

9. Chest tubes are inserted, and the wound is closed.

Description

A median sternotomy is performed in standard fashion, and the femoral artery is isolated for cannulation, as described for a total cardiopulmonary bypass. After cannulation is completed and the left ventricular sump catheter is inserted, the surgeon occludes the aorta distal to the aneurysm. The aneurysm is opened with Metzenbaum scissors, and all clots and debris are removed (Fig. 24–61*A*). The coronary arteries are then cannulated, and the cardioplegic solution is administered.

The surgeon examines the aortic valve to determine the extent of its injury and to replace it, if necessary. The technologist should have valve instruments and sutures available on the set-up tray to avoid any delay.

The surgeon obtains the appropriate size graft from the technologist and performs the distal anastomosis

with a continuous suture, such as size 3-0 Prolene. When the anastomosis is completed, the surgeon occludes the graft with a vascular clamp and temporarily releases the aortic clamp to test the suture line. Additional sutures are placed as needed, along with Teflon felt pledgets to reinforce the suture line.

The surgeon cuts the graft to an appropriate length and performs the proximal anastomosis. Before tying the suture, he or she temporarily releases the aortic clamp to fill the graft and flush out all air and clots. The completion of the anastomoses with the graft in functioning position is illustrated in Figure 24–61*B*.

The surgeon removes the left ventricular sump catheter. After cardiopulmonary bypass is discontinued, decannulation is performed. The surgeon may cover the graft with aneurysmal tissue and pericardium. The assistant closes the groin incision while the surgeon inserts chest tubes and closes the median sternotomy in standard fashion.

Resection of Left Ventricular Aneurysm

Definition

This is the surgical correction of an aneurysm of the left ventricle, most commonly caused by a diminished blood supply from an occluded coronary artery. The tissue beyond the occlusion becomes necrotic, softens, and then dilates (Fig. 24–62). The aneurysm is surgically resected to reduce the incidence of embolization that occurs from clots forming inside the aneurysm and to prevent heart failure.

Highlights

1. A median sternotomy is performed.
2. Cannulation for cardiopulmonary bypass is carried out.
3. Total cardiopulmonary bypass is instituted.
4. A left ventriculotomy is performed, and the aneurysm is resected.
5. The ventricle is closed.
6. Decannulation is performed as soon as cardiopulmonary bypass is discontinued.
7. A temporary pacemaker electrode is sutured to the heart.
8. Chest tubes are inserted, and the wound is closed.

Description

The surgeon performs a median sternotomy in standard fashion. Cannulation for total cardiopulmonary bypass is accomplished.

The surgeon places a laparotomy sponge beneath the heart to elevate the left ventricle. The ventricle is incised

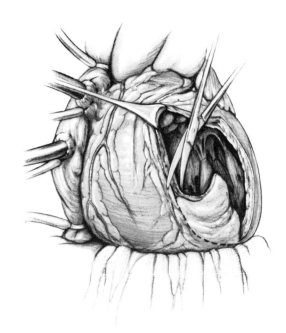

Figure 24–63. Resection of ventricular aneurysm. The left ventricular aneurysm is completely excised. (Courtesy of Ethicon, Inc., Somerville, NJ.)

with the deep knife, and the incision is extended with curved Mayo scissors. Allis clamps are applied to the edges of the aneurysm; these are held by the assistants. The surgeon inspects the intraventricular cavity to assess the mitral valve and to locate any clots; all clots are removed using forceps or suction. The technologist should wipe all instruments free of clots to prevent their escape into the bloodstream.

The surgeon may temporarily occlude the ascending aorta to prevent the escape of clots and to provide a drier field. The surgeon then excises the aneurysmal tissue with curved Mayo scissors and thumb forceps (Fig. 24–63). The edges of the ventricle are brought together with a running or interrupted suture, such as size 0 Prolene or Ti-Cron. The method of ventricular closure and size of needle vary with the size of the aneurysm and the surgeon's preference. The most common method of closure is to incorporate strips of Teflon felt or pledgets along with the sutures (Fig. 24–64). The surgeon then places a second or third row of sutures through the ventricular edges for a more secure closure.

The surgeon decompresses the ventricle using the sump catheter from the heart-lung machine to prevent distention of the intraventricular muscle as blood accumulates in the ventricle. Just before the final suture is tied, the surgeon removes the catheter, inserts a Schnidt clamp, and allows blood to spill out of the ventricle so that all air bubbles will be evacuated. The suture is then tied, and the apex of the ventricle is aspirated with a needle and syringe.

Cardiopulmonary bypass is discontinued and decannulation is accomplished, as previously described. A temporary pacemaker electrode is sutured to the heart in standard fashion. Hemostasis is maintained by placing additional sutures as needed or by applying a hemostatic

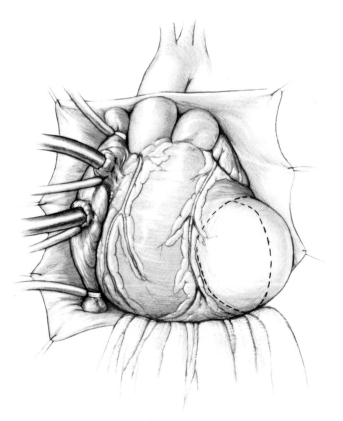

Figure 24–62. Resection of ventricular aneurysm. The pericardium is incised and retracted. The patient is on complete cardiopulmonary bypass with right atrial cannulation. The line of ventricular incision is shown. (Courtesy of Ethicon, Inc., Somerville, NJ.)

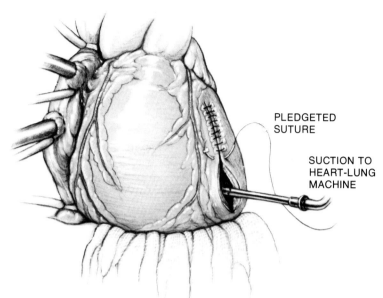

PLEDGETED
SUTURE

SUCTION TO
HEART-LUNG
MACHINE

Figure 24–64. Resection of ventricular aneurysm. The two edges of the ventricular wall are approximated with continuous or interrupted sutures using pledgets of Teflon felt. (Courtesy of Ethicon, Inc., Somerville, NJ.)

agent along the ventriculotomy. The surgeon inserts chest tube(s) and closes the median sternotomy in standard fashion.

Pulmonary Valvulotomy

Definition

This is the surgical correction of congenital pulmonary valve stenosis. The fused leaflets of the valve are surgically separated, thus allowing blood to flow from the right ventricle to the lungs. The procedure is most commonly performed on the pediatric patient. Thus, the following discussion includes the procedure for cardiopulmonary bypass as it is performed on the pediatric patient.

Highlights

1. A median sternotomy is performed, and the pericardium is opened.
2. The cannulae are inserted for cardiopulmonary bypass.
3. The venae cavae are encircled with umbilical tapes.
4. The pulmonary artery is opened, and the fused leaflets of the valve are separated.
5. The pulmonary artery is closed.
6. Cardiopulmonary bypass is discontinued, and decannulation is performed.
7. Chest tubes are inserted, and the wound is closed.

Description

The surgeon enters the chest through a median sternotomy. After a retractor is inserted, the pericardial sac is entered with a No. 15 knife blade and the incision is extended with Metzenbaum scissors downward to the diaphragm and upward to the innominate vein. The aorta and venae cavae are examined to determine the

sizes of cannulae needed. The technologist then obtains the cannulae from either the circulator or pump technician.

The surgeon encircles the ascending aorta with an umbilical tape and then places a size 4-0 Prolene or Ti-Cron pursestring suture. The assistant brings the ends of the suture through a bolster and holds the suture with a hemostat.

After heparin is administered to the patient by the anesthesiologist, the surgeon places a pediatric size vascular clamp, such as the Beck or Satinsky, across the right atrial appendage. A pursestring suture, size 3-0 Ti-Cron or Prolene, is then placed in the occluded portion of the appendage. The assistant brings the suture ends through a bolster and holds it with a hemostat. The surgeon excises the tip of the appendage with Metzenbaum scissors and applies mosquito clamps to the two edges of the cut atrium. Both the surgeon and assistant hold the atrium open with the mosquito clamps while the surgeon inserts the cannula. The assistant removes the occluding clamp from the appendage and tightens the pursestring suture to prevent bleeding. The surgeon introduces the cannula into the superior vena cava. The assistant holds it in position, forming a tourniquet by snugging the bolster down on the suture. The surgeon secures the cannula to the bolster with a heavy silk suture. He or she allows the cannula to fill with blood and then places a tube-occluding clamp across the cannula.

To cannulate the inferior vena cava, the surgeon applies the vascular clamp to the wall of the right atrium below the appendage. A pursestring suture is then placed.

The surgeon incises the occluded segment of the atrial wall with a No. 11 knife blade and extends the incision with Potts scissors. Mosquito clamps are applied, the cannula is inserted into the inferior vena cava, and it is secured as previously described. The two cannulae are then connected to the venous line from the pump.

The surgeon cannulates the aorta by first making a stab incision with a No. 11 knife blade within the pursestring suture. (The surgeon may apply a partially occluding vascular clamp in the aorta before making the incision.) The cannula is then inserted into the aorta and placed in proper position. The assistant tightens the pursestring suture, and the surgeon secures the cannula to the tubing.

The surgeon allows the cannula to fill with blood and then connects it to the arterial line from the pump. Air that remains in the tubing is evacuated by aspiration with a syringe. The surgeon removes all clamps from the cannulae and pump lines, and cardiopulmonary bypass is begun.

The surgeon encircles the venae cavae with umbilical tapes using a right-angled clamp. The assistant brings the ends of the tape through pieces of rubber tubing, tightens the tubing against the cavae to form a tourniquet, and holds the tubing in place with hemostatic clamps.

The surgeon opens the pulmonary artery just above the valve using Metzenbaum scissors. The aorta may be temporarily occluded to provide a drier field. The valve is examined, and then the fused leaflets are separated with Metzenbaum or Potts scissors (Fig. 24–65). The surgeon closes the pulmonary artery with a continuous suture, such as size 5-0 Prolene (Fig. 24–66).

Cardiopulmonary bypass is discontinued and decannulation is performed. Chest tubes are inserted.

The surgeon then places sutures through the sternum, on both sides. The type of suture varies with the size of the patient and the surgeon's preference. No. 4 wire sutures are commonly used for older children and No. 2 Mersilene or No. 1 wire is used for infants. The surgeon brings the two edges of the sternum together by tightening the wires or tying the sutures. The periosteal and fascial tissue layers are reapproximated with interrupted sutures of size 2-0 Tevdek or a running suture of size 3-0 chromic catgut or Dexon. The subcutaneous tissue is reapproximated with a running suture, such as size 4-0 Dexon, and the skin is closed with the surgeon's preferred suture material.

Closure of Atrial Septal Defect

Definition

This is the surgical correction of a congenital anomaly that involves defective formation of the interatrial sep-

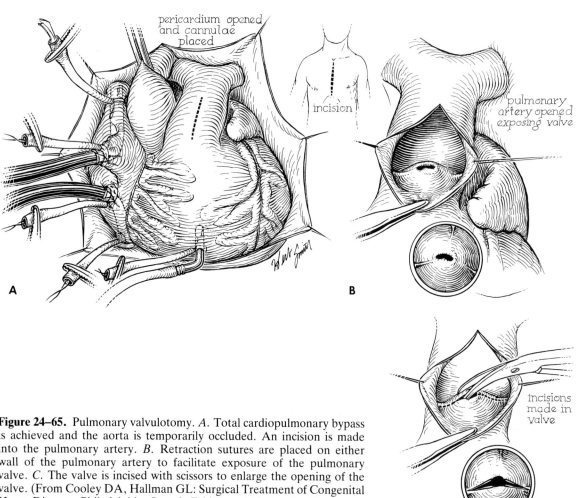

Figure 24–65. Pulmonary valvulotomy. *A.* Total cardiopulmonary bypass is achieved and the aorta is temporarily occluded. An incision is made into the pulmonary artery. *B.* Retraction sutures are placed on either wall of the pulmonary artery to facilitate exposure of the pulmonary valve. *C.* The valve is incised with scissors to enlarge the opening of the valve. (From Cooley DA, Hallman GL: Surgical Treatment of Congenital Heart Disease. Philadelphia, Lea & Febiger, 1966. Used with permission.)

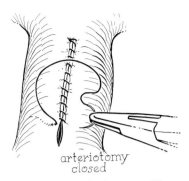

Figure 24–66. Pulmonary valvulotomy. The arteriotomy is closed with a continuous suture. (From Cooley DA, Hallman GL: Surgical Treatment of Congenital Heart Disease. Philadelphia, Lea & Febiger, 1966. Used with permission.)

tum. Blood from the left atrium flows across the defect into the right atrium, creating a left-to-right shunt. The added blood volume puts a strain on the right ventricle, causing it to hypertrophy (enlarge) and eventually to fail.

Atrial septal defects are usually closed surgically during childhood. However, some patients reach adulthood before developing symptoms that require surgical closure of the defect.

Highlights

1. A median sternotomy is performed.
2. Cannulation is performed for total cardiopulmonary bypass.
3. The aorta may be occluded.
4. A right atriotomy is performed, the defect is closed, and the atriotomy is closed.
5. Cardiopulmonary bypass is discontinued, and decannulation is accomplished.
6. Chest tubes are inserted, and the wound is closed.

Description

The surgeon performs a median sternotomy in standard fashion. He or she cannulates for cardiopulmonary bypass, as described previously.

The surgeon may fibrillate the heart and occlude the aorta before performing a right atriotomy. A retractor is then inserted, most commonly the Cooley for adults and a Richardson for pediatric patients. The assistant exposes the defect with the retractor as the surgeon examines the interatrial cavity for additional defects. The technologist should pay strict attention to the results of this examination, since additional supplies may be needed.

The surgeon may bring the edges of the defect together with a running suture (primary closure; Fig. 24–67). This does not require a prosthetic patch graft (see the section on special equipment in this chapter). For larger defects, a patch is usually required. The surgeon cuts the patch to the appropriate size and then places sutures, such as Prolene or Ethibond, through the edges of the patch and defect. The patch is secured in place

by tying all the sutures (Fig. 24–68). Before the last suture is tied, air is evacuated from the left side of the heart by allowing the heart to fill with blood. The surgeon then removes the aortic clamp, aspirates the aorta with a needle and syringe, and closes the atriotomy with running sutures, such as size 3-0 or 4-0 Prolene.

Cardiopulmonary bypass is discontinued and decannulation is done. Chest tubes are inserted, and the median sternotomy is closed in standard fashion.

Closure of Ventricular Septal Defect

Definition

This is the surgical closure of a defect or hole in the intraventricular septum, usually involving the use of a prosthetic patch. The higher pressure in the left ventricle causes blood to flow through the defect into the right ventricle. The increased volume of blood in the right ventricle creates a volume overload in the lungs and leads to congestive heart failure. Surgical closure of the defect is most commonly performed in the pediatric patient.

Highlights

1. A median sternotomy is performed.
2. Cannulation for total cardiopulmonary bypass is performed.
3. The aorta is occluded, and cardioplegic solution is infused into the coronary arteries.
4. A ventriculotomy is performed, and the defect is closed.
5. The aorta is unclamped, and the ventricle is closed.
6. Cardiopulmonary bypass is discontinued, and decannulation is performed.
7. A temporary pacemaker electrode is sutured to the heart.
8. Chest tubes are inserted, and the wound is closed.

Description

The surgeon performs a median sternotomy and cannulates for total cardiopulmonary bypass in the fashion used for the pediatric patient, as described for a pulmonary valvulotomy.

The surgeon occludes the aorta with a Cooley pediatric clamp and perfuses the coronary arteries, as described for a cardiopulmonary bypass. A right ventriculotomy is then performed with the deep knife and curved Mayo scissors (Fig. 24–69). The surgeon may place sutures, such as size 3-0 Prolene, through the edges of the ventricle. The assistant holds the ends of the sutures in hemostatic clamps and retracts them for better exposure of the defect.

The surgeon examines the septum for defects not previously determined. After the defect has been identified, the surgeon cuts a patch graft to the appropriate size and places the sutures through the edges of the patch and the defect (Fig. 24–70). Occasionally, pledgets

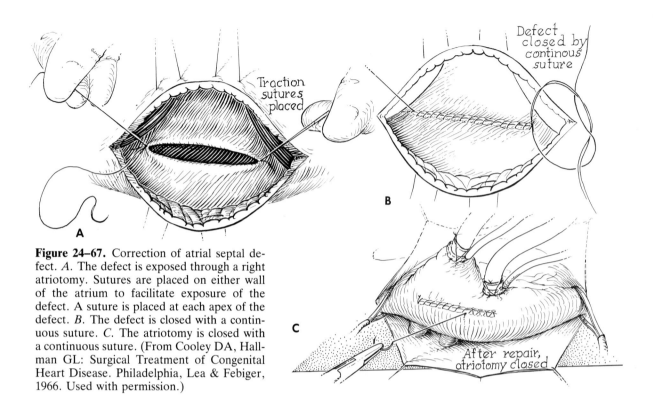

Figure 24–67. Correction of atrial septal defect. *A.* The defect is exposed through a right atriotomy. Sutures are placed on either wall of the atrium to facilitate exposure of the defect. A suture is placed at each apex of the defect. *B.* The defect is closed with a continuous suture. *C.* The atriotomy is closed with a continuous suture. (From Cooley DA, Hallman GL: Surgical Treatment of Congenital Heart Disease. Philadelphia, Lea & Febiger, 1966. Used with permission.)

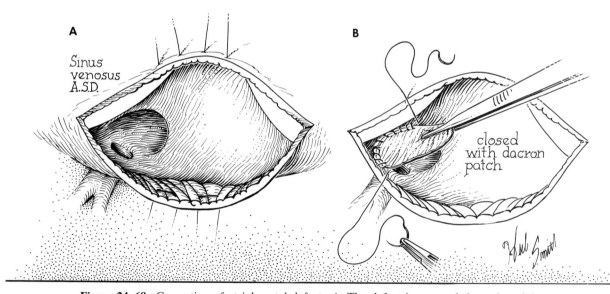

Figure 24–68. Correction of atrial septal defect. *A.* The defect is exposed through a right atriotomy. Retraction sutures are placed in either wall of the atrium. *B.* The defect is closed using a Dacron patch. (From Cooley DA, Hallman GL: Surgical Treatment of Congenital Heart Disease. Philadelphia, Lea & Febiger, 1966. Used with permission.)

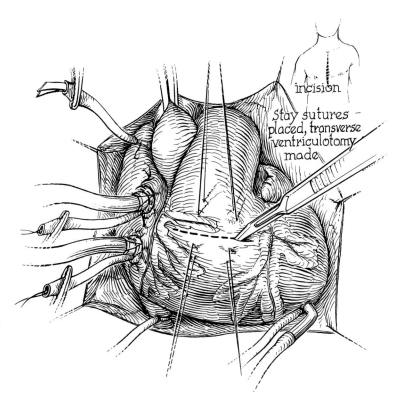

Figure 24–69. Closure of ventricular septal defect. Cannulation for total cardiopulmonary bypass is accomplished. The aorta is occluded. An incision is made with a No. 11 knife blade in the right ventricle. Sutures are placed through the ventricular wall of the incision for retraction to allow exposure of the ventricular septal defect. (From Cooley DA, Hallman GL: Surgical Treatment of Congenital Heart Disease. Philadelphia, Lea & Febiger, 1966. Used with permission.)

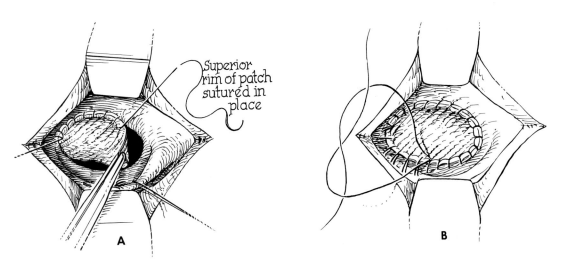

Figure 24–70. Closure of ventricular septal defect. *A.* An appropriate size patch is sutured along the edges of the defect with a continuous suture. *B.* The defect is closed and the suture is securely tied after all air is evacuated from the left ventricle. (From Cooley DA, Hallman GL: Surgical Treatment of Congenital Heart Disease. Philadelphia, Lea & Febiger, 1966. Used with permission.)

may be used. The surgeon then lowers the patch into position and secures it by tying all sutures. Before the final suture is tied, air is evacuated from the left ventricle by allowing it to fill with blood.

The surgeon removes the aortic clamp and closes the ventricle with a continuous suture, such as size 3-0 or 4-0 Prolene. Teflon pledgets may be used to reinforce the suture line. Cardiopulmonary bypass is discontinued and the surgeon performs decannulation, as described for a pulmonary valvulotomy. A temporary pacemaker lead may be sutured to the right ventricle and right atrium in standard fashion. Chest tubes are then inserted and the median sternotomy is closed, as described for a pulmonary valvulotomy.

Total Correction of Tetralogy of Fallot

Definition

This is the surgical repair of a congenital anomaly of the heart known as the tetralogy of Fallot. The four features of this anomaly are pulmonary stenosis, ventricular septal defect, right ventricular hypertrophy, and overriding of the aorta. The surgical correction of pulmonary stenosis alleviates cyanosis. Closure of the ventricular septal defect prevents heart failure.

It is desirable to correct the tetralogy of Fallot totally in early infancy. However, some infants may not be candidates for early correction because they are in critical condition and could not tolerate such extensive surgery. In addition, surgery is easier to perform when the anatomic structures are larger. Therefore, a systemic-pulmonary shunt is performed to increase blood flow to the lungs. This improves oxygenation of the blood and body tissues and allows the infant to survive and grow to a stage at which total correction is possible.

Highlights

1. A median sternotomy is performed.
2. Cannulation for total cardiopulmonary bypass is performed.
3. The aorta is occluded, and the coronary arteries are perfused with cardioplegic solution.
4. A right ventriculotomy is performed, the infundibular muscle is resected, and a pulmonary valvulotomy is performed.
5. The ventricular septal defect is closed, and the ventricle is closed using a patch.
6. Cardiopulmonary bypass is discontinued.
7. A temporary pacemaker lead is sutured to the heart.
8. Chest tubes are inserted, and the wound is closed.

Description

The type of incision used for total correction depends on the nature and type of shunt operation performed previously. A description of systemic-pulmonary shunts is beyond the scope of this chapter, but the four most common types are the Blalock shunt (subclavian artery to pulmonary artery), the Potts shunt (descending tho-

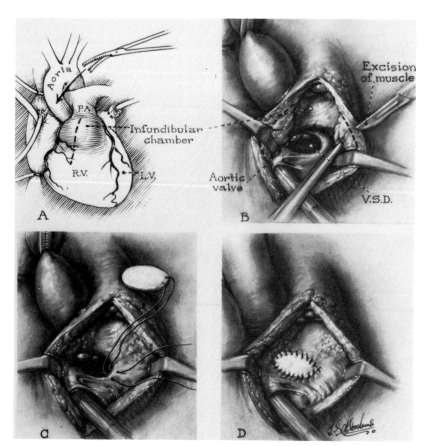

Figure 24–71. Correction of tetralogy of Fallot. *A.* Total cardiopulmonary bypass is achieved. The ascending aorta is occluded. An incision is made into the right ventricle and extended into the pulmonary artery. *B.* The infundibular muscle is excised with a knife and scissors. *C.* The ventricular septal defect is exposed and an appropriate size patch is sutured in place. *D.* The defect is completely closed. The pulmonary artery and right ventricle are then closed. (From Sabiston DC Jr, Spencer FC [eds]: Gibbons' Surgery of the Chest, 3rd ed. Philadelphia, WB Saunders, 1976.)

racic aorta to pulmonary artery), the Waterston shunt (ascending aorta to pulmonary artery), and the Glenn shunt (vena cava to pulmonary artery). The technologist is urged to become familiar with the techniques used and the anatomy involved in the shunt procedures.

Total correction, in the absence of a previous shunt, is performed through a median sternotomy. The surgeon performs the median sternotomy and cannulates for total cardiopulmonary bypass, as described for a pulmonary valvulotomy. The aorta is occluded, and the coronary arteries are perfused with cardioplegic solution.

The surgeon performs a right ventriculotomy using the deep knife and curved Mayo scissors. U.S. Army or Sauerbruch retractors are inserted, which are then held by the assistant to expose the intraventricular cavity.

The surgeon excises a portion of the infundibular muscle with Metzenbaum scissors and DeBakey or Russian tissue forceps to relieve the obstruction of blood flowing out of the ventricle. The technologist should wipe all tissue from these instruments after each use with a moist laparotomy sponge to prevent the formation of an embolus from tissue that has fallen into the ventricle.

The surgeon performs a pulmonary valvulotomy and closes the ventricular septal defect, as previously described. After air is evacuated from the left ventricle, the clamp is removed from the aorta.

The surgeon closes the ventricle with running sutures, such as size 4-0 Prolene. A patch of woven Dacron or Teflon is commonly used to enlarge the right ventricular outflow tract (area beneath the pulmonary valve). The pulmonary artery may also be enlarged with a patch, using a smaller size suture. Figure 24–71 illustrates the technique used to correct the tetralogy of Fallot.

The surgeon measures the pressures in the pulmonary artery and right ventricle using a 20-gauge spinal needle attached to an 8-foot-long pressure line connected to a pressure transducer. These pressures are measured to be certain that the obstruction to blood flow has been relieved sufficiently by the surgical procedure. The technologist should pay strict attention to the results of these pressure determinations because additional surgery may be necessary, requiring additional supplies such as patch material and sutures. Recannulation will be necessary if decannulation was performed before the pressures were measured.

As soon as satisfactory pressure readings are obtained, cardiopulmonary bypass is discontinued and the surgeon performs decannulation. A temporary pacemaker lead is sutured to the right ventricle or right atrium in standard fashion. Chest tubes are then inserted and the median sternotomy is closed, as described for a pulmonary valvulotomy.

Insertion and Removal of Intra-aortic Balloon Catheter

Definition

This is the insertion of a helium-filled balloon catheter into the descending thoracic aorta to assist circulation

when the patient is unable to come off cardiopulmonary bypass or has suffered a serious myocardial infarction. The pumping action of the balloon catheter decreases the workload, thus allowing the heart muscle to rest and recuperate from the injury caused by the surgery or infarction. It also provides more oxygen to the heart by increasing coronary blood flow during diastole. The balloon catheter in the aorta is shown in Figure 24–72.

The intra-aortic balloon catheter functions by counterpulsation. When the ventricle contracts, the balloon deflates, creating a vacuum that lowers the pressure in the aorta. The left ventricle need not work as hard to eject the blood when the aortic pressure is lowered. When the ventricle relaxes, the balloon inflates, bringing an increased volume of blood into the coronary arteries. This allows the heart to function with greater efficiency.

The size of the balloon catheter is determined by the size of the femoral artery. The average size for an adult is a 40-mL balloon. A description of the operation of the balloon pump is beyond the scope of this chapter. Although the technologist is normally not responsible for operating the pump, he or she should be familiar with the basic concepts. The balloon pump is shown in Figure 24–73, and the balloon catheter is shown in Figure 24–74.

As soon as the heart muscle has fully recuperated, the balloon catheter may be removed, either in the operating room or at the patient's bedside.

Highlights

Insertion

1. An incision is made in the groin.
2. The femoral artery and its branches are exposed and isolated with umbilical tapes.
3. A segment of prosthetic graft is placed over the balloon catheter.
4. A heavy silk suture is tied around the balloon catheter to mark the level of insertion.
5. The femoral artery and its branches are occluded.
6. The balloon catheter is inserted into the artery.
7. The graft is anastomosed to the femoral artery.
8. The open end of the graft is occluded with a heavy silk suture.
9. The femoral artery is unclamped, and the wound is closed.

Removal

1. The original groin incision is reopened.
2. The femoral artery is isolated with umbilical tapes.
3. The heavy silk sutures are removed from around the graft.
4. The balloon catheter is withdrawn.
5. The femoral artery is occluded.
6. The excess graft is trimmed.
7. The remaining segment of graft is oversewn.
8. The femoral artery is unclamped and the wound is closed.

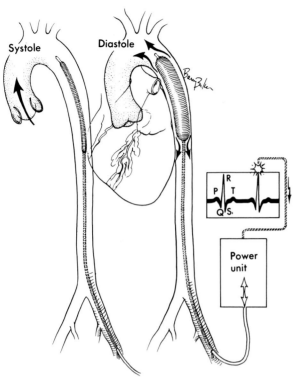

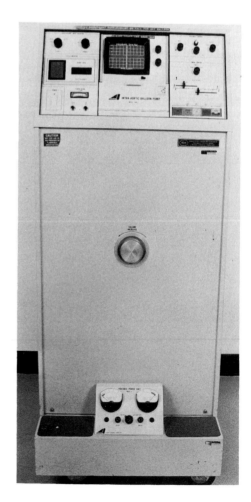

Figure 24–72. Intra-aortic balloon catheterization. The intra-aortic balloon catheter is placed in the descending thoracic aorta. The tip of the balloon catheter is below the level of the left subclavian artery. The balloon inflates during diastole and deflates during systole. The action of the balloon is triggered by the R wave of the electrocardiogram. (From DeBakey ME, Diethrich EB: Ventricular assistive devices, present and future. In Burford TH, Ferguson TB [eds]: Cardiovascular Surgery, Current Practice, vol 1. St. Louis, CV Mosby, 1969.)

Figure 24–73. Intra-aortic balloon pump. (Courtesy of Long Beach Memorial Medical Center, Long Beach, CA.)

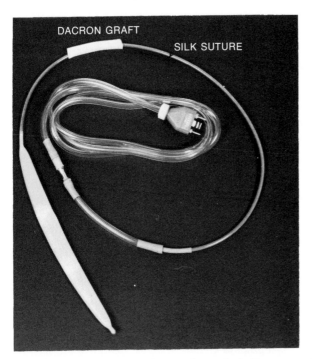

Figure 24–74. Intra-aortic balloon catheter, including segment of Dacron tube graft and silk suture to level of subclavian artery. (Courtesy of Long Beach Memorial Medical Center, Long Beach, CA.)

Description

Insertion

The procedure is often performed under local anesthesia for patients who have suffered a serious myocardial infarction. The patient is in critical condition and cannot tolerate a general anesthetic or a lengthy surgical procedure. The surgical team must perform with speed and efficiency.

With the patient in the supine position, both groins are prepped and draped, since the first attempt to insert the balloon catheter into the femoral artery may be unsuccessful owing to stenosis or occlusion of the vessel. If so, that femoral artery is closed and the surgeon attempts to insert the balloon catheter into the opposite femoral artery. (Patients who require the balloon catheter to come off bypass are already prepped and draped. Consequently the technologist uses the same instrument set-up as that used for the cardiac procedure.)

The surgeon makes an incision in the groin with the skin knife. The subcutaneous and fascial tissue layers are divided with Metzenbaum scissors, and hemostasis is maintained with the electrocautery pencil or by clamping and tying the vessels with silk or catgut sutures. A self-retaining retractor, such as a Gelpi or Weitlaner retractor, is used to retract the tissue layers.

The surgeon performs sharp dissection with Metzenbaum scissors and smooth forceps to expose the common femoral artery and its major branches. The arterial branches are encircled with moistened umbilical tapes secured in the jaws of a right-angled clamp. The assistant brings the tapes through bolsters and places a hemostatic clamp across the ends of the tapes.

The technologist obtains the balloon catheter from the circulator or technician in charge of operating the balloon pump. He or she then places the segment of graft (usually No. 10 woven Dacron graft) over the catheter. The surgeon holds the catheter next to the femoral artery with the tip of the balloon below the level of the patient's left subclavian artery. The assistant ties a heavy silk suture around the catheter at the level of the femoral artery. The silk tie on the catheter is used as a marker to ensure that the catheter is not introduced beyond the left subclavian artery, where it could obstruct the blood flow to the left arm. The technologist then hands the plug end of the catheter to the pump technician, who attaches a syringe to it and deflates the balloon during the insertion.

The surgeon occludes the femoral arteries with vascular clamps, such as Glover or DeBakey peripheral vascular clamps, or he or she forms tourniquets by snaring down on the umbilical tapes. An incision is made in the common femoral artery using a No. 11 knife, and it is extended with Potts scissors.

The technologist moistens the balloon with saline solution to facilitate its passage through the artery. The assistant removes the proximal clamp from the artery as the surgeon inserts the catheter and introduces it into the descending thoracic aorta up to the level of the heavy silk on the catheter. The assistant controls the bleeding by keeping tension on the umbilical tape; it is tightened securely around the artery when the catheter is in place.

The surgeon then joins the graft to the artery with a running suture, such as size 5-0 Prolene or 4-0 Ti-Cron. The technologist opens the air hole along the catheter by sliding back the rubber covering. The pump technician evacuates the atmospheric air from the catheter by filling it with helium. He or she then directs the technologist to cover the hole, and balloon pumping is begun.

The surgeon completes the anastomosis and then ties several heavy silk sutures around the graft to prevent leakage of blood when all clamps or tourniquets are removed from the arteries. The anastomosis is inspected and additional sutures are placed or a topical hemostatic agent, such as Surgicel, is applied to control bleeding.

The surgeon then trims any excess graft using straight Mayo scissors and secures the balloon catheter to the leg with a size 2-0 silk suture. The wound is irrigated with an antibiotic solution, such as Bacitracin, to reduce the possibility of infection.

The surgeon reapproximates the fascial and subcutaneous tissue layers over the graft with an absorbable suture, such as size 3-0 Dexon or chromic catgut. The skin is closed in the surgeon's preferred manner. Some surgeons do not close the skin; instead the wound is packed with iodine-soaked gauze sponges and closed at a later date. A pressure dressing is then applied to prevent hematoma formation.

Removal

The surgeon reopens the original groin incision and inserts a self-retaining retractor. The femoral artery is then isolated, as previously described. The sutures are removed from around the graft and the catheter is slowly withdrawn after the balloon is deflated by the pump technician. The assistant occludes the femoral artery, as previously described, or may use a small Cooley partially occluding vascular clamp. The surgeon trims off the graft, leaving approximately ½ inch remaining on the artery. The end of the graft is then oversewn with a running suture, such as size 4-0 Ti-Cron. Large ligature clips may be used instead of a suture. The surgeon removes the clamp(s) from the femoral artery, maintains hemostasis, and closes the wound as previously described.

Occasionally, a femoral embolectomy is necessary if the pedal pulse cannot be palpated by the circulating nurse or if there is poor retrograde blood flow from the artery. The surgeon immediately performs the embolectomy. The technologist should obtain the appropriate size embolectomy catheter.

Ventricular Assist Device

A ventricular assist device (VAD) is used to wean patients from cardiopulmonary bypass when other means are ineffective. The VAD maintains perfusion and consists of a polyurethane blood sac, flexible diaphragm, and pump assembly. The device provides continuity with the heart through cannulae that are placed into the different chambers of the heart, according to the type of assist needed and the placement of the outflow cannula. During *left ventricular assistance,* blood is directed from the left atrium into the assist device and returned to the ascending aorta. During *right ventricular assistance,* blood is directed from the right atrium, into the pump, and into the right atrium. The outflow cannula is sutured to the pulmonary artery. During *biventricular assistance,* both left ventricular and right ventricular devices support both ventricles simultaneously.

An extracorporal VAD is used for temporary, short-term assistance, and its power is derived from a pneumatic, compressed air, or electrical pump. This pump is connected to inflow and outflow cannulae that are passed into the thoracic cavity through the chest wall. The pump itself is secured to the outer chest wall and covered with an occlusive dressing.

Implantable VAD is used for long-term support and utilizes an electric pump that is implanted into the patient's abdomen. The battery pack for this type of support device is external and its cannulae passed through the diaphragm.

Bibliography

Ashworth PM: Cardiovascular Disorders: Patient Care. Baltimore, Williams & Wilkins, 1973.

Cooley DA, Norman JC: Techniques in Cardiac Surgery. Houston, Medical Press, 1975.

Gardner E, Gray D, O'Rahilly R: Anatomy: A Regional Study of Human Structure, 4th ed. Philadelphia, WB Saunders, 1984.

Jacob S, Francone C, Lossow WJ: Structure and Function in Man, 5th ed. Philadelphia, WB Saunders, 1982.

Lindskog GE, Liebow AA, Glenn WWL: Thoracic and Cardiovascular Surgery with Related Physiology. Norwalk, CT, Appleton-Century-Crofts, 1975.

McVay C: Surgical Anatomy, 6th ed. Philadelphia, WB Saunders, 1984.

Ochsner JL, Mills NL: Coronary Artery Surgery. Philadelphia, Lea & Febiger, 1978.

Sabiston DC Jr, Spencer FC (eds): Gibbon's Surgery of the Chest, 5th ed. Philadelphia, WB Saunders, 1990.

Walter JB: An Introduction to the Principles of Disease, 3rd ed. Philadelphia, WB Saunders, 1992.

Peripheral Vascular Surgery

Peripheral vascular surgery encompasses procedures of the arteries and veins, excluding those in or near the heart. Many surgical procedures of the vascular system are performed to treat arteriosclerotic or thromboembolic disease. In many cases the diseased vessel is completely bypassed with a synthetic or bovine graft (actual vessels removed from cattle and preserved in alcohol solution) or autograft (taken from the patient). Alternatively, the vessel may be opened and arteriosclerotic plaque removed (endarterectomy). Many vascular procedures must be performed quickly, particularly when major arteries are temporarily occluded. An orderly arrangement of instruments on the instrument table will aid the technologist in keeping pace with the surgeons.

SURGICAL ANATOMY

The peripheral vascular system is a complex network of vessels whose function is to carry blood to all parts of the body. The major components of the vascular system are veins and arteries.

An *artery* (Fig. 25–1) is a vessel that carries oxygenated blood from the lungs to the rest of the body. It is composed of three distinct structural layers: the *tunica intima,* or inner layer; the *tunica media,* or middle layer; and the *tunica adventitia,* or outer layer. Arteries are under considerable internal pressure from the pumping of the heart and are therefore much thicker than their corresponding vessels, the veins.

The arterial system is a branching network whose vessels decrease in size as they traverse the body. Beginning with the largest artery, the aorta, each branches into smaller and smaller tubules until the cellular level is reached where the artery is only slightly larger than a single red blood cell. At this level the artery is called an *arteriole.* Still smaller is the *capillary,* which is the smallest artery and the vessel that connects the arterial system with the venous system. Each capillary is anastomosed to a *venule,* the smallest vessel of the venous network.

Veins (Fig. 25–1) are vessels that carry deoxygenated blood from body tissues to the heart. Veins also have three layers, but the middle layer, composed of smooth muscle, is much thinner because the flow of venous blood does not depend on the action of this muscle layer. Venous blood is moved about the body by a series of mechanisms. The most significant of these mechanisms is the "massaging" action of the skeletal muscles of the body by a series of valves located within the lumens of the veins. These valves are one way and prevent blood from backing up and pooling in the vessels (Fig. 25–2).

The structure of each type of blood vessel is described in Table 25–1.

SPECIAL EQUIPMENT

Instrumentation includes small and large vascular clamps and forceps that are designed to grasp vessels securely without causing trauma. Right-angled (Mixter) clamps are needed for all procedures. DeMartel and Potts (right-angled) scissors are used frequently during

527

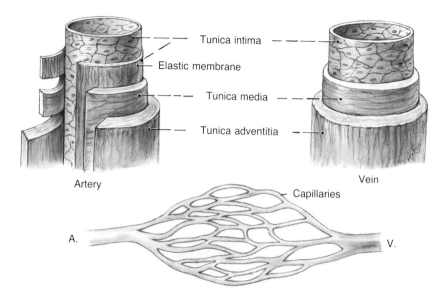

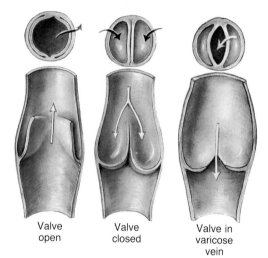

Figure 25–1. Tissue layers of artery and vein. Capillary transition between the two systems. (From Jacob S, Francone C, Lossow WJ: Structure and Function in Man, 5th ed. Philadelphia, WB Saunders, 1982.)

Figure 25–2. Valve system within veins. Valves open in one direction only to prevent backflow of blood and subsequent pooling. (From Jacob S, Francone C, Lossow WJ: Structure and Function in Man, 5th ed. Philadelphia, WB Saunders, 1982.)

Valve open   Valve closed   Valve in varicose vein

Table 25–1. STRUCTURE OF BLOOD VESSELS

Vessel	Outer Layer: Tunica Adventitia	Middle Layer: Tunica Media	Inner Layer: Tunica Intima
Large arteries (elastic)	Relatively thin layer, consisting of connective tissue	Layer consists largely of elastic fibers with some smooth muscle	Inner surface of endothelium, outer zone an elastic lamina, connective tissue matrix components and small number of smooth muscle cells in between
Medium and small arteries (muscular)	Thick layer, consisting of connective tissue	Fewer elastic fibers, more smooth muscle	Similar to large arteries, but elastic lamina more distinct
Arterioles	Thin	Consists of muscular tissue	Layer composed mainly of endothelium
Capillaries	Absent	Absent	Endothelial layer one cell thick
Veins	Layer of connective tissue	Thin; little muscle and few elastic fibers	Endothelial lining with scant connective tissue matrix components

From Jacob S, Francone C, Lossow WJ: Structure and Function in Man, 5th ed. Philadelphia, WB Saunders, 1982.

endarterectomy procedures. Suction should be available during all procedures. If the operation involves large vessels of the abdomen, a tonsil (Yankauer) or Andrews suction tip should be available. A Frazier suction tip is commonly used during operations on small vessels.

To prevent thrombosis (clotting) at the wound site, the surgeon irrigates the open vessel with a heparin and normal saline solution. Heparinized saline solution should be supplied to the surgeons by the technologist in a large syringe fitted with a catheter adapter (Fig. 25–3).

Hemostatic agents such as Surgicel and Avitene (see Chapter 13) are used to control oozing at the site of vessel anastomoses. A variety of suture materials such as Tevdek, Ti-Cron, Ethiflex, Prolene, and silk are commonly used.

Dacron vessel grafts are available in any length and in various diameters. They may be straight or bifurcated (Y-shaped). Because the grafts are costly, they should be handled with care. Most grafts must be preclotted by the technologist; this is done just before the insertion of the graft. Approximately 30 mL of the patient's blood is collected in a small basin from the wound site. The graft is then placed in the blood and the blood is worked gently through the fibers of the graft. Bovine grafts must be thoroughly rinsed before their insertion into the body to remove all traces of alcohol. This is done by rinsing the graft several times in three or four separate basins of normal saline solution. The basins should then be removed from the field to prevent their being used accidentally for irrigation in the wound, since they now contain traces of alcohol. The technologist should always read the manufacturer's directions before preparing any vascular graft, whether it is of synthetic or natural material.

The *Doppler* is a monitoring instrument that is used during most procedures on the vascular system. It is used to determine the rate of blood flow through an artery. This diagnostic tool is particularly important when the patient's circulatory system is depressed or compromised. When the sensing probe is placed over an artery, high-frequency sound waves generated by the probe are reflected back from the blood cells. Specific pitches, generated by the blood flowing through the artery, are associated with velocity, and these are easily interpreted by the surgeon. During vascular surgery, the nonsterile sending probe can be used at various locations away from the wound site to determine the patency of

blood vessels. The sterile probe can be used within the wound site to determine vascular competency.

DIAGNOSTIC PROCEDURES

Arteriography

Definition

This is the injection of radiopaque dye directly into an artery to obtain radiographs of the vessel and its tributaries. Arteriography is an important diagnostic tool for the vascular surgeon. Through the use of radiographs, the surgeon can determine the exact location and nature of an arterial disease or obstruction. Arteriography may also be performed during vascular surgery to determine whether the procedure has been successful in restoring circulation. The technique of femoral arteriography, similar to all other types of arteriography, is described here.

Highlights

1. The artery is injected with dye.
2. Radiographs are taken.

Description

When arteriography is performed as a diagnostic procedure before surgery, the patient is given a local anesthetic at the site of the arterial puncture. The patient should be warned, however, that the dye causes a burning sensation as it courses through the arteries. For this reason, a general or regional anesthetic is sometimes used.

The patient is placed in the supine position on the operating or x-ray table. All team members should remember to don a lead apron before scrubbing. The patient's groin is briefly prepped with antiseptic solution. The technologist should have several 30- or 50-mL syringes, an 18-gauge spinal needle or Cournand needle, small basins, and medicine cups available (Fig. 25–4). The circulator distributes contrast medium to the technologist, who then draws it into two syringes. A third syringe of saline solution is also prepared to flush the dye through after radiographs are taken. The technologist attaches the arteriogram needle to a short length of vinyl tubing and attaches the other end to one syringe of dye. All air bubbles must be removed from both the syringe and tubing. A Kelly or Mayo hemostat placed across the tubing will prevent air from backing into it. Alternatively, a stopcock may be attached to the tubing to prevent air bubbles from forming.

The surgeon injects a small amount of local anesthetic at the puncture site and then inserts the arteriogram needle into the femoral artery. The dye is injected while radiographs are taken. Some operating rooms are equipped with an image intensifier, which gives a continuous x-ray view of the vessels. Selected spot films are then taken to serve as a graphic record of the patient's

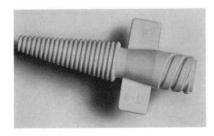

Figure 25–3. Catheter adapter. When fitted to a large syringe, it is used to provide irrigation during vascular surgery. (Courtesy of Becton-Dickinson & Company, Rochelle Park, NJ.)

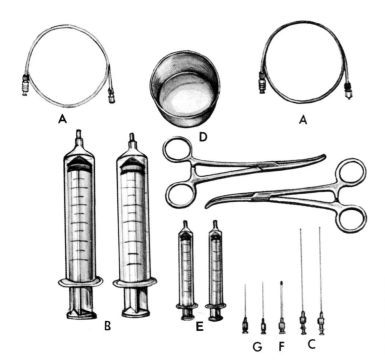

Figure 25–4. Equipment needed for arteriography: A, plastic catheters; B, 50-ml syringes; C, 18-gauge spinal needles; D, small basin; E, 30-ml syringes; F, 16-gauge needle; G, 22-gauge needles for infiltration of local anesthetic. (From Linton R: Atlas of Vascular Surgery. Philadelphia, WB Saunders, 1973.)

arterial system. Special arteriography catheters may be inserted into specific branches through a particular major artery, and dye is injected.

Following the procedure, the arterial needle or catheter is removed. The surgeon or technologist applies pressure over the puncture site for several minutes to control bleeding. The puncture site is then dressed with a small pressure dressing.

SURGICAL PROCEDURES

Most bypass procedures closely resemble each other from the technologist's point of view, except for their different locations in the body. Once the technologist has learned the basic principles of vascular surgery, he or she should be able to apply this knowledge to the various procedures.

Carotid Endarterectomy

Definition

This is the removal of arteriosclerotic plaque from an obstructed carotid artery. There are several sites in the body where arteriosclerotic plaque commonly forms. These areas are usually just above and below the bifurcation of a major artery. Obstruction of the carotid usually occurs at the point at which the common carotid artery divides into the internal and external carotids. The occlusion causes restricted blood flow to the brain and subsequent neurologic symptoms. The goal of surgical treatment is to remove the arteriosclerotic plaque and restore circulation.

Highlights

1. The neck is incised.
2. The common, external, and internal carotid arteries are mobilized and clamped.
3. The common carotid artery is incised.
4. The plaque is removed.
5. The artery is closed.
6. The wound is closed.

Description

During carotid endarterectomy, the surgeon works very swiftly to minimize the time during which the major arteries are clamped. The technologist should keep the instrument table and Mayo stand neatly organized to ensure maximum efficiency during the procedure. Attention to the wound site is extremely important during the procedure.

The patient is placed in the supine position, and the head is turned away from the affected side. A small sandbag or rolled towel is placed under the shoulders to hyperextend the neck. The scrub prep extends from the face to the axillary line. Draping is similar to that used for a thyroidectomy.

The surgeon begins the procedure by incising the neck (Fig. 25–5). The incision is carried deeper with the electrocautery pencil and Metzenbaum scissors. The technologist should have a variety of retractors available, including two Weitlaners, small rakes, and U.S. Army retractors. The rake retractors should have *dull* rather than sharp teeth to avoid trauma to the large vessels that lie in close proximity. The surgeon uses small sponge dissectors to divide the tissue layers in the incision. The incision is carried to the level of the carotid

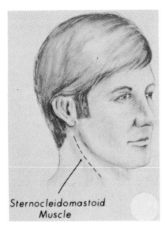

Figure 25–5. Carotid endarterectomy. Line of incision. (From Schwartz SI, et al: Principles of Surgery, 2nd ed. New York, McGraw-Hill, 1974. Used with the permission of McGraw-Hill Book Company.)

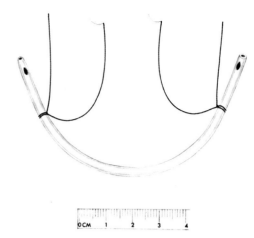

Figure 25–6. Shunt used for bypass during endarterectomy. (From Linton RR: Atlas of Vascular Surgery. Philadelphia, WB Saunders, 1973.)

artery and its bifurcation. The carotid and both branches are then mobilized with fine vascular tissue forceps and Metzenbaum scissors.

To apply traction to the artery and its branches, the surgeon may place a long narrow strip of cotton umbilical tape around the vessels. The technologist should moisten the tapes and mount them on a passer (right-angled or Schnidt clamp) before handing them to the surgeon. Mosquito or Kelly hemostats are used to clamp the two ends of the tape together. Some surgeons slip a small section of rubber tubing (bolster) over the two ends so that they can be snugged down on the vessel to act as a tourniquet. In place of umbilical tapes, the surgeon may prefer to use commercially prepared "loops," which resemble a severed rubber band.

Before beginning the endarterectomy, some surgeons prepare an internal shunt (bypass) to insert into the artery. This allows the blood to continue circulating during the procedure and thus permits the surgeon to proceed more slowly. The shunt is fashioned from a short (2 to 3 inch) length of vinyl tubing cut from a pediatric feeding tube or suction catheter. Some surgeons allow an experienced technologist to prepare the shunt, while others may wish to prepare it themselves. The shunt is prepared by tying two lengths of size 1 or 0 silk at each end of the tube to serve as traction devices (Fig. 25–6). Commercially prepared shunts (Javid shunts) are also available.

Before making the arterial incision, the surgeon requests that heparin be given to the patient intravenously. In addition, he or she may inject the artery with lidocaine to prevent arterial spasm during the procedure. The surgeon waits several minutes to allow the heparin to take effect. This time can be used by the technologist to make sure that all the proper instruments needed for the endarterectomy have been assembled, since timing is often critical after the procedure begins. A No. 11 knife blade, Potts and DeMartel scissors, a small nasal or neurosurgical elevator (Penfield or Freer type), and a straight hemostat will be needed. Some surgeons prefer that tonsil (Yankauer) suction also be available,

in case of sudden massive hemorrhage. Most surgeons will indicate which vascular clamps they intend to use during the procedure. All other vascular clamps can be set aside.

To begin the endarterectomy, the surgeon clamps the artery above and below the bifurcation. He or she notifies the anesthesiologist that the artery is clamped so that it can be noted on the anesthesia record. The surgeon then makes a small incision into the carotid with a No. 11 knife blade. The incision is extended with Potts or DeMartel scissors.

Arterial plaque is identified as a thick, yellow, rubbery material adhering to the lumen of the artery. The surgeon grasps the edge of the plaque with a straight hemostatic clamp and carefully dissects the plaque from the artery using one of the elevators described earlier (Fig. 25–7). The plaque is dissected free and passed to

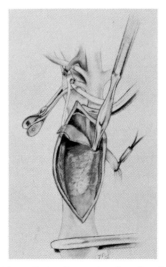

Figure 25–7. Dissection of arteriosclerotic plaque from the walls of the carotid artery. (From Schwartz SI, et al: Principles of Surgery, 2nd ed. New York, McGraw-Hill, 1974. Used with the permission of McGraw-Hill Book Company.)

the technologist as a specimen. The arterial lumen is then flushed with heparinized saline solution. The arterial incision is closed with size 5-0 or 6-0 cardiovascular sutures (Fig. 25–8).

When the incision is closed the surgeon removes the clamps to test for leaks in the suture line. These are repaired with additional sutures. The technologist should have a topical hemostatic agent, such as Gelfoam soaked in thrombin or Surgicel gauze, available at this time to control oozing from the suture line. When hemostasis is complete, the surgeon irrigates the wound with normal saline solution and closes it in layers with fine silk or Dexon sutures.

Resection of Abdominal Aortic Aneurysm and Aortic Femoral Bypass

Definition

This is the removal of an abdominal aortic aneurysm and the insertion of a bifurcated vessel prosthesis. An aortic aneurysm is a saclike bulging or weakening in the wall of the aorta, which may be the result of arteriosclerotic disease, trauma, syphilis, infection, or congenital defect in the artery. As the weakened area in the aorta fills with blood, its walls become distended and may burst, causing death. If the aneurysm is ruptured or is a *dissecting* aneurysm (one in which blood flows between the layers of the vessel rather than through its lumen), emergency surgery is performed. (A complete discussion of the different types of aortic aneurysms is found in Chapter 24).

Highlights

1. The abdomen is entered.
2. The posterior peritoneum is incised.

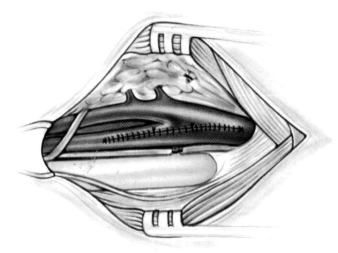

Figure 25–8. Carotid artery closed with fine sutures. (From Linton RR: Atlas of Vascular Surgery. Philadelphia, WB Saunders, 1973.)

3. The aorta and iliac arteries are clamped.
4. The aneurysm is opened and partially resected.
5. A graft is implanted.
6. The wound is closed.

Description

The patient is placed in the supine position, catheterized with a Foley catheter, prepped, and draped for a midline incision that extends from the xiphoid to the pubis. The surgeon enters the abdomen in routine fashion into the peritoneal cavity. Before incising the posterior peritoneum, the intestines are placed in a special plastic wound protector (Fig. 25–9). This protects them from injury during the procedure and also keeps them moist. The technologist should place a small amount of saline solution in the bag before passing it to the surgeon. The surgeon incises the posterior peritoneum over the aneurysm with the deep knife. The incision is extended with long Metzenbaum scissors (Fig. 25–10). The technologist should prepare at least four cotton umbilical tapes by moistening them in saline solution and tagging them with mosquito clamps. The surgeon slings these around the aorta, just above the aneurysm. The iliac arteries are mobilized using Metzenbaum scissors and small sponge dissectors. The arteries are then slung with umbilical tapes.

At this point the surgeon routinely requests that the anesthesiologist administer heparin to the patient. After a few minutes have elapsed, the surgeon is ready to incise the aneurysm. The aorta is cross-clamped with a large vascular clamp, such as a Satinsky or Craoord clamp. Both iliac arteries are also clamped with small vascular clamps of the surgeon's choice. The anesthesiologist is alerted that the aorta is clamped. The surgeon then incises the aneurysm with the knife. Suction must be immediately available to clear the wound site of blood that was trapped within the aneurysm. In cases in which the aneurysm sac is almost completely filled with plaque, the surgeon may remove the debris manually. The technologist should place a small basin on the field to collect the plaque. The surgeon completes the dissection of plaque and removes the anterior portion of the sac with dissecting scissors. The back (posterior) side of the aneurysm is left intact (Fig. 25–11). This is to prevent injury to the vena cava, which in many cases adheres to the aorta.

The technologist must prepare a bifurcated graft according to the manufacturer's instructions. If the graft is to be preclotted, the technologist supplies the surgeon with a 30- or 50-mL syringe. The surgeon withdraws approximately 30 mL of the patient's blood into the syringe and passes it to the technologist. The technologist then places the graft in the basin and saturates it with blood. This is done a few minutes before the graft is needed.

Using running sutures of size 3-0 vascular suture, the surgeon secures the upper end of the graft to the aorta (Fig. 25–12). When this anastomosis is completed, the iliac arteries are anastomosed to the bifurcated ends of the graft (Fig. 25–13). During the anastomosis, the

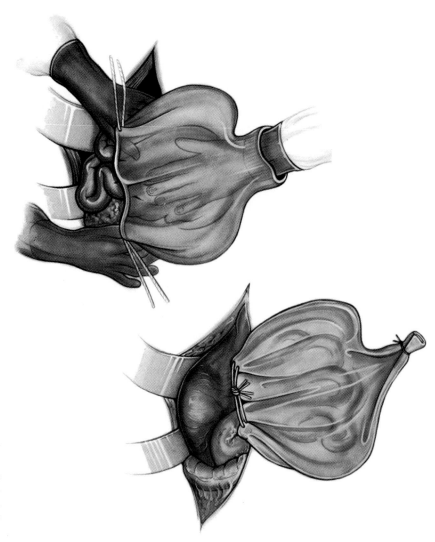

Figure 25–9. Resection of abdominal aortic aneurysm. Special intestinal bag used to protect the intestines during surgery. (From Linton RR: Atlas of Vascular Surgery. Philadelphia, WB Saunders, 1973.)

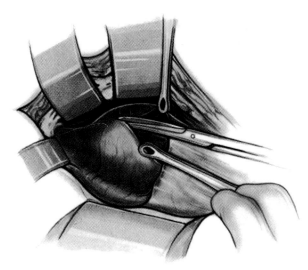

Figure 25–10. Resection of abdominal aortic aneurysm. Incision over aneurysm. (From Linton RR: Atlas of Vascular Surgery. Philadelphia, WB Saunders, 1973.)

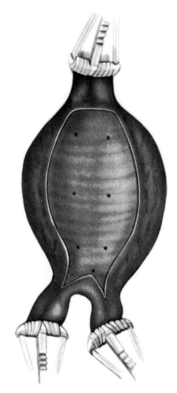

Figure 25–11. Resection of abdominal aortic aneurysm. The surgeon has dissected the anterior portion of the aneurysm free. The posterior portion is left intact, since it adheres to the vena cava in many cases. (From Linton RR: Atlas of Vascular Surgery. Philadelphia, WB Saunders, 1973.)

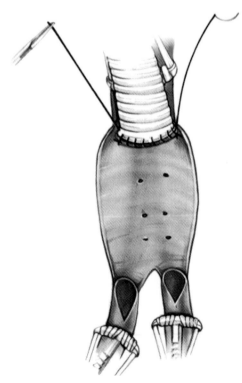

Figure 25–12. Resection of abdominal aortic aneurysm. Insertion of Dacron graft into the upper portion of the aorta. (From Linton RR: Atlas of Vascular Surgery. Philadelphia, WB Saunders, 1973.)

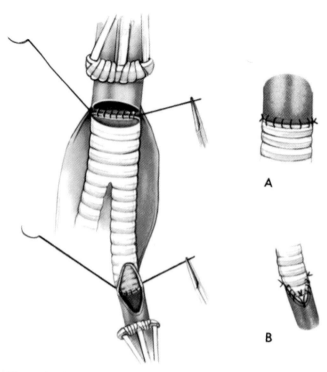

Figure 25–13. Resection of abdominal aortic aneurysm. The lower limbs of the graft are sutured to the iliac arteries. (From Linton RR: Atlas of Vascular Surgery. Philadelphia, WB Saunders, 1973.)

surgeon irrigates the wound frequently with heparinized saline solution. To test the suture lines, the surgeon slowly releases the vascular clamps. If leaks occur, they are repaired with additional vascular sutures. When bleeding is controlled, the surgeon irrigates the wound and closes it in routine fashion.

Femoral Popliteal Bypass

Definition

This is the implantation of an artificial or autogenous graft into the femoral and popliteal arteries for treatment of arteriosclerotic disease of the femoral artery.

Highlights

1. The groin is entered.
2. The femoral artery is mobilized.
3. The leg is incised, and the popliteal artery is mobilized.
4. The graft is implanted.
5. The wounds are closed.

Description

The patient is placed in the supine position, prepped, and draped with the affected leg and groin exposed. The surgeon incises the groin area and then deepens the incision to the level of the femoral artery with Metzenbaum scissors and small sponge dissectors (Fig. 25–14). A Weitlaner or Gelpi retractor is placed in the wound.

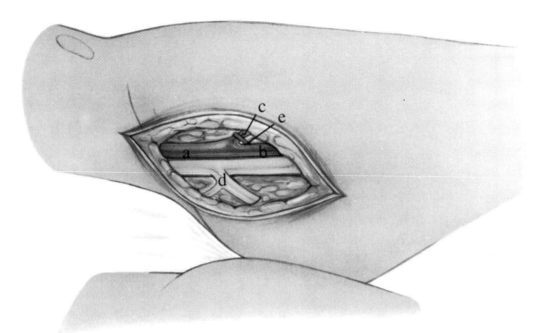

Figure 25–14. Exposure of the femoral artery during femoral popliteal bypass. a, Common femoral artery; b, superficial femoris; c, profunda femoris; d, saphenous vein; e, tributary of femoral vein. (From Linton RR: Atlas of Vascular Surgery. Philadelphia, WB Saunders, 1973.)

The femoral artery is mobilized with careful dissection and slung with a moistened cotton umbilical tape. A second incision is made on the medial side of the knee. The surgeon dissects the subcutaneous, fascial, and muscle layers using both sharp and blunt dissection. A Beckman self-retaining retractor is useful in exposing the vessels of the popliteal space (Fig. 25–15).

An appropriate size graft is chosen by the surgeon. If the graft is to be preclotted, the technologist does so at this time. Rather than using a Dacron graft, the surgeon may remove the greater saphenous vein (see Chapter 24) and use this as a graft.

To perform the anastomosis, the surgeon first places a vascular clamp across the femoral artery. A small incision is made in the artery with a No. 11 knife blade or vascular scissors. Using running sutures of size 5-0 or 6-0 cardiovascular suture, the surgeon performs the anastomosis between the femoral artery and graft. To bring the other end of the graft into the popliteal space, he or she inserts a Péan or sponge clamp into the leg incision. The clamp is advanced through the leg, and the end of the graft is grasped. The graft may then be drawn back easily into the popliteal space. The popliteal anastomosis is performed in the same manner as the femoral anastomosis. During both anastomoses, the technologist should have heparinized saline solution available for irrigation.

The surgeon may wish to take one or more radiographs at this time. If so, the technologist should assemble the equipment needed, as described for an arteriography. After the radiographs have been taken, the surgeon irrigates the wound and closes it in layers in routine fashion.

Related Procedures

Femoral peroneal bypass
Popliteal peroneal bypass
Femoral crossover (Fig. 25–16)
Axillary femoral bypass (Fig. 25–17)

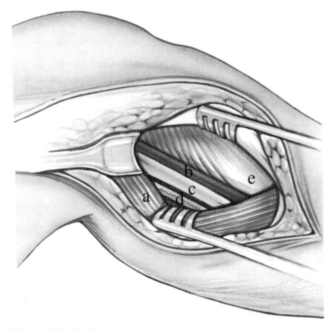

Figure 25–15. Femoral popliteal bypass. Exposure of the popliteal space. a, Gastrocnemius muscle; b, popliteal artery; c, popliteal vein; d, posterior tibial nerve; e, popliteus muscle. (From Linton RR: Atlas of Vascular Surgery. Philadelphia, WB Saunders, 1973.)

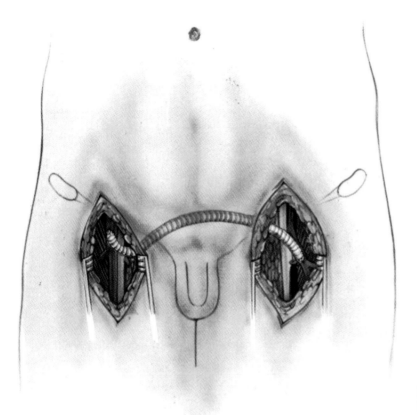

Figure 25–16. Femoral crossover bypass. (From Linton RR: Atlas of Vascular Surgery. Philadelphia, WB Saunders, 1973.)

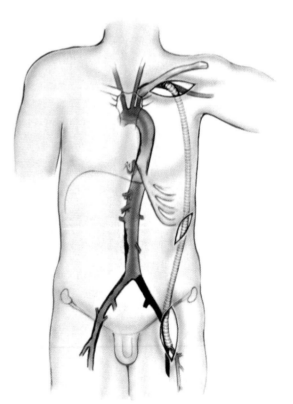

Figure 25–17. Axillary femoral bypass. (From Linton RR: Atlas of Vascular Surgery. Philadelphia, WB Saunders, 1973.)

Femoral Embolectomy

Definition

This is the removal of a blood clot from the femoral popliteal system. An embolus may be caused by a foreign body, tumor, or trauma to the vessels. The goal of surgery is to remove the clot and restore circulation to the limb.

Highlights

1. The groin is entered.
2. The embolus is removed.
3. The wound is closed.

Description

The patient is placed in the supine position, prepped, and draped for a groin incision. The surgeon incises the groin and carries the incision deeper with Metzenbaum scissors and cautery. When the wound is completely open, two Weitlaner or Gelpi retractors are placed. The surgeon identifies and mobilizes the femoral artery.

A moistened umbilical tape is placed around the artery for traction. Before the surgeon incises the artery, the technologist should have suction available. Heparinized saline solution will also be needed. The surgeon uses a small vascular clamp to occlude the vessel and then makes a small incision in the artery using a No. 11 knife blade or Potts scissors.

A common method of embolectomy uses a balloon embolectomy catheter (Fogarty catheter; Fig. 25–18). These catheters are available in a variety of sizes. The catheter is threaded into the artery and advanced beyond the clot. The balloon is then inflated with a tuberculin syringe and the catheter is withdrawn. The balloon forces the clot from the artery, which is immediately clamped to prevent the backflow of blood. In some instances the artery must be dilated to make it large enough to accept the catheter. The surgeon performs the dilatation using vascular dilators.

When the embolectomy is complete, the surgeon irrigates the wound with heparinized saline solution and closes the arterial incision with size 5-0 or 6-0 vascular sutures. A small piece of hemostatic agent is sometimes placed over the suture line to control oozing. The surgeon then irrigates the wound with normal saline solution and closes it in layers in routine fashion.

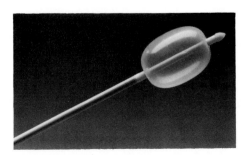

Figure 25–18. Embolectomy catheter. (Courtesy of Edwards Laboratories.)

Related Procedure

Surgical creation of a direct passageway between an artery and a vein, performed prior to dialysis.

Portacaval Shunt

Definition

This is the anastomosis of the portal vein to the vena cava to treat portal hypertension. In the normal liver, blood flows through the portal vein toward the liver. Within the liver itself, this blood travels through tiny capillaries and small sinusoids and then circulates out to continue its flow through the body. If the liver is diseased, scarring and obstruction can occur in the sinusoids and prevent portal circulation. The blood that would normally course through the liver backs up into the gastrointestinal system from which it came. The overload of blood causes veins in the digestive system to dilate, distending their walls. These distended veins are called *varices*. The veins of the esophagus are particularly prone to distention and subsequent rupture, which is a life-threatening occurrence. Portal hypertension can be caused by anatomic obstruction of the portal vein, infection, or alcoholic cirrhosis (which ranks as the fourth leading cause of death in patients older than 40 years of age in the United States).

The goal of portacaval shunting is to route the portal blood into the vena cava and bypass the liver. The procedure is performed only on selected patients. Those who suffer from alcoholic cirrhosis are carefully evaluated preoperatively to be certain that they can be rehabilitated from alcoholism postoperatively, thus allowing the surgery to be of subsequent benefit to the patient.

Highlights

1. The abdomen is entered.
2. The portal vein and vena cava are mobilized.
3. The portal vein and vena cava are anastomosed.
4. The wound is closed.

Description

The patient is placed in the supine position with the right side of the chest slightly elevated on sandbags or rolled bath towels. The patient is then prepped and draped for a right subcostal incision (Fig. 25–19).

The surgeon enters the upper right abdomen in routine fashion. If the chest is entered, a rib may be resected, as described for a flank incision (see Chapter 22). Moist lap sponges and a Balfour retractor are placed in the wound. The surgeon identifies the portal vein as it emerges from the liver (Fig. 25–20). The vein is mobilized using sharp and blunt dissection. The vena cava is mobilized in similar fashion. Penrose drains are slung around both vessels for traction.

The surgeon places a large right-angled vascular clamp over the portal vein. The vein is then ligated with a suture ligature of size 3-0 silk. A partially occluding vascular clamp is placed over the vena cava, and a small

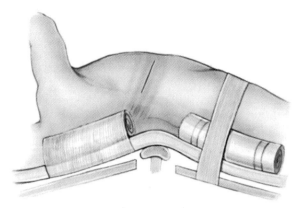

Figure 25–19. Portacaval shunt. Position of the patient and incisional line. (From Linton RR: Atlas of Vascular Surgery. Philadelphia, WB Saunders, 1973.)

disk of vessel tissue is removed with scissors (Fig. 25–21). The assistant brings the portal vein close to the excised vena cava, and the surgeon begins the anastomosis (Fig. 25–22). The anastomosis is performed with interrupted sutures of size 4-0 or 5-0 vascular suture. The completed anastomosis is shown in Figure 25–23.

Venous pressures are usually measured before and after completion of the anastomosis. The wound is then closed in routine fashion.

Related Procedures

Side-to-side anastomosis (Fig. 25–24)
Splenorenal shunt
Warren shunt (distal splenorenal shunt)
Drapanas shunt (mesocaval interposition shunt)

Ligation of the Vena Cava

Definition

This is the surgical interruption of circulation through the vena cava to treat thrombosis of the venous system. It may be caused by chronic infection, heart disease, pelvic trauma, or cancer. The condition of pulmonary embolism (occlusion of the pulmonary vascular system) occurs when a blood clot enters the pulmonary artery or one of its branches and interrupts the blood supply to the lungs. Patients who are not successfully treated with anticoagulant therapy are candidates for vena cava ligation to correct pulmonary embolism. Patients who are too ill to undergo radical surgery may be treated with an umbrella (Mobin-Uddin) filter, which is introduced into the vena cava through the jugular vein under local anesthetic. The filter does not stop the flow of blood through the vena cava, but it is successful in filtering large emboli.

Highlights

1. The flank is entered.
2. The vena cava is ligated.
3. The wound is closed.

Description

The patient is placed in the supine position. Rolled blankets or small sandbags are placed under the right flank to elevate it. The patient is prepped for a right flank incision. Some surgeons prefer to enter the wound through a low abdominal incision; however, the flank incision is more commonly used.

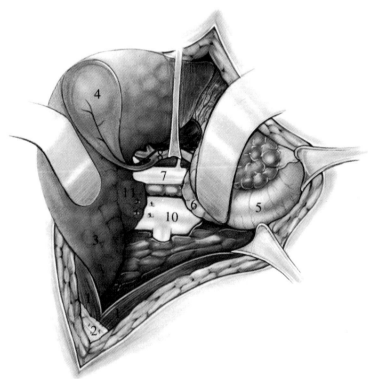

Figure 25–20. Portacaval shunt. Exposure of the portal vein: 1, diaphragm; 2, lung; 3, liver; 4, gallbladder; 5, duodenum; 6, pancreas; 7, portal vein; 8, common bile duct; 9, hepatic artery; 10, vena cava. (From Linton RR: Atlas of Vascular Surgery. Philadelphia, WB Saunders, 1973.)

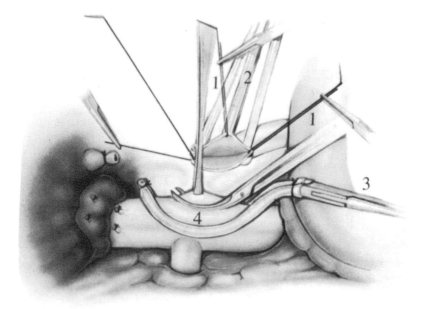

Figure 25–21. Portacaval shunt. The assistant brings the portal vein in close approximation to the vena cava. A small section of tissue is cut from the vena cava. 1, Traction sutures; 2, tourniquet clamp; 3, partially occluding clamp; 4, vena cava. (From Linton RR: Atlas of Vascular Surgery. Philadelphia, WB Saunders, 1973.)

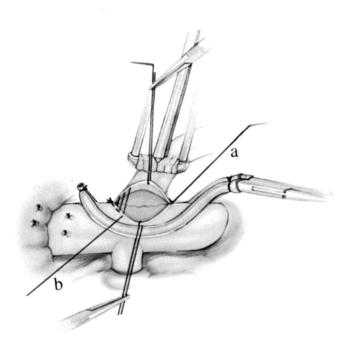

Figure 25–22. Portacaval shunt. Anastomosis of the portal vein and vena cava: a, posterior suture; b, anterior suture. (From Linton RR: Atlas of Vascular Surgery. Philadelphia, WB Saunders, 1973.)

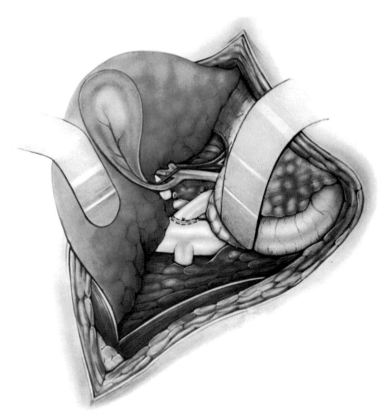

Figure 25–23. Portacaval shunt. Completed anastomosis. (From Linton RR: Atlas of Vascular Surgery. Philadelphia, WB Saunders, 1973.)

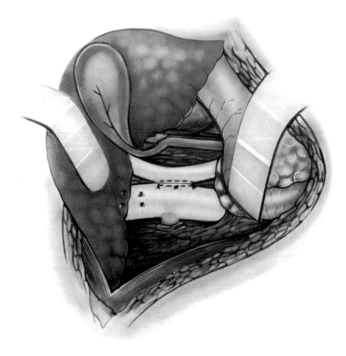

Figure 25–24. Side-to-side anastomosis. (From Linton RR: Atlas of Vascular Surgery. Philadelphia, WB Saunders, 1973.)

The surgeon begins the surgery by incising the flank and dividing the muscle layers by blunt dissection. Bleeders are coagulated or clamped with hemostats and ligated with fine absorbable sutures. The retroperitoneal space is entered, as described for a flank incision.

The surgeon places moist lap sponges in the wound and the assistant retracts the wound edges with a Deaver retractor. The technologist should have stick sponges, right-angled clamps, and Schnidt clamps available. Several heavy silk sutures should be mounted on right-angled clamps in preparation for the vena caval ligation.

The surgeon passes two sutures around the vessel with the aid of right-angled clamps and tags them with two small hemostats (Fig. 25–25). The sutures are tied close together (Fig. 25–26), and the wound is then closed in routine fashion.

Internal Vein Stripping

Definition

This is the surgical removal of the saphenous vein and its branches to treat varicosities of the leg. Varicose veins result in nonfunctioning valves in the veins, causing blood in the veins to pool and thus distend the vessels (Fig. 25–27). Patients whose occupations require long hours of standing are prone to varicose veins. There can also be a genetic predisposition to the condition. The veins and tributaries can be surgically removed to relieve the patient of pain and prevent ulceration and bleeding.

Highlights

1. The groin is entered.
2. The saphenous vein is identified and mobilized.
3. An internal vein stripper is placed into the lumen of the vein.
4. The stripper is advanced through the vein.
5. Tributaries are ligated and removed through separate incisions.
6. The saphenous vein is removed.
7. The wounds are closed.

Description

The patient is placed in the supine position, prepped, and draped with the affected leg and groin exposed. The surgeon makes an incision in the groin, over the saphenous vein. The incision is carried to the level of the vein with sharp and blunt dissection (Fig. 25–28). A self-retaining Weitlaner or Gelpi retractor is placed in the wound.

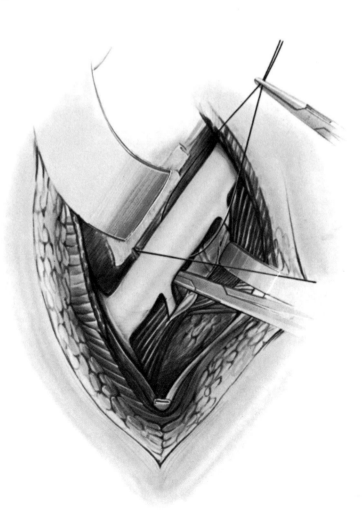

Figure 25–25. Ligation of the vena cava. Two sutures are passed around the vessel. (From Linton RR: Atlas of Vascular Surgery. Philadelphia, WB Saunders, 1973.)

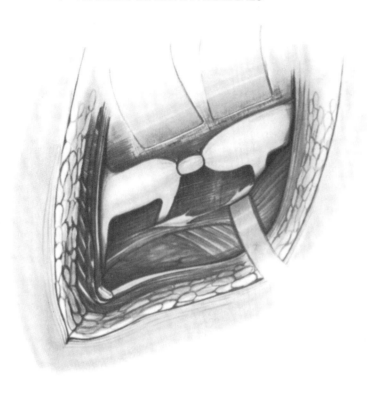

Figure 25–26. Ligation of the vena cava. The sutures are tied close together. (From Linton RR: Atlas of Vascular Surgery. Philadelphia, WB Saunders, 1973.)

The surgeon mobilizes the vein with Metzenbaum scissors and places two Mayo clamps across it. The vein is then divided with scissors or knife. The proximal end of the vein is ligated with a suture ligature of size 0 or 2-0 silk.

Internal or external vein strippers are used to remove the vein. The internal stripper (Fig. 25–29), used more commonly, is a length of stainless steel cable or disposable plastic. (Flat ribbon-like internal strippers are also available.) Solid metal "bullets" are attached to the ends of the stripper. To remove the vein, the surgeon threads the stripper into the lumen of the vessel and advances it until resistance is felt. The resistance is usually due to a tributary that has crossed the vein (called a "perforator"). The surgeon makes a small incision over the area of resistance to expose the end of the stripper. Small rake (Senn) retractors are used to help expose the stripper. The surgeon secures the distal end of the saphenous vein to the stripper with a length of heavy silk suture, size 0 or 2-0. A small hemostat is placed across the vein below the stripper, and the vein is divided at the end of the stripper. As the surgeon gently pulls the stripper back out, the vein inverts over the stripper and is thus removed (Fig. 25–30).

While the surgeon is stripping the vein, the assistant, using folded towel pads, puts pressure over the area to decrease bleeding from small branches that are literally torn free during the stripping. The surgeon passes the stripper to the technologist, who must remove the vein so that the stripper is available for immediate use. This is best done by cutting the suture from the stripper. The vein will then slide off the instrument easily.

The procedure is repeated until the entire saphenous vein has been removed. Other small veins are removed by dissection over the vein, division of the vein with knife or scissors, and ligation.

All incisions are closed in layers. Subcutaneous tissue is closed with size 3-0 chromic catgut or Dexon. Skin is usually closed with silk or nylon, size 4-0 (Fig. 25–31). The leg is wrapped in cotton flannel batting and a wide Ace or similar type of pressure bandage (Fig. 25–32).

Above-Knee Amputation

Definition

This is the surgical removal of the leg. Although amputation may not be considered strictly a vascular procedure, the operation is commonly performed when vascular insufficiency due to arteriosclerotic or thromboembolic disease causes the lower limb to necrose. Above-knee rather than below-knee amputation is chosen when the vascular supply in the lower limb is insufficient for proper healing at the amputation site. The procedures closely resemble each other.

Highlights

1. The leg is incised circumferentially.
2. The incision is carried to the femur.
3. The femur is severed.
4. The popliteal vessels are ligated.
5. The sciatic nerve is ligated.
6. The wound is closed.

Description

The patient is placed in the supine position and the affected leg is prepped. Many surgeons prefer to place the gangrenous foot in a plastic bag to protect the

Text continued on page 548

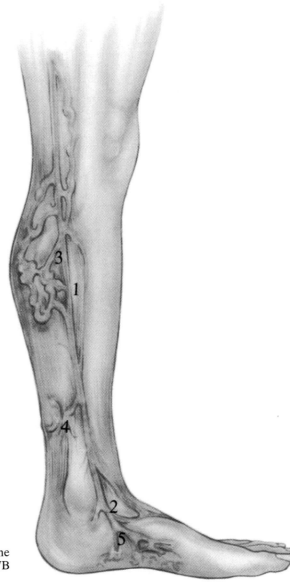

Figure 25–27. Varicose veins, resulting from defective valves within the veins. (From Linton RR: Atlas of Vascular Surgery. Philadelphia, WB Saunders, 1973.)

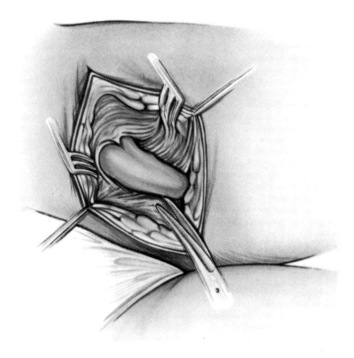

Figure 25–28. Internal vein stripping. Exposure of the saphenous vein. (From Linton RR: Atlas of Vascular Surgery. Philadelphia, WB Saunders, 1973.)

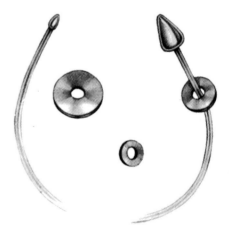

Figure 25–29. Internal vein stripper. Note "bullets" at each end. (From Linton RR: Atlas of Vascular Surgery. Philadelphia, WB Saunders, 1973.)

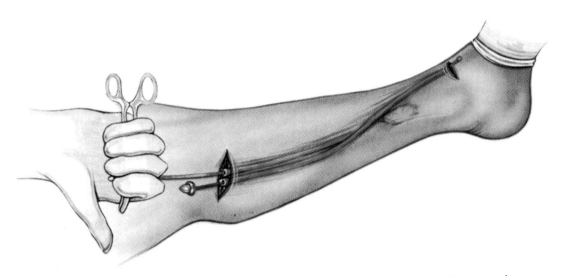

Figure 25–30. Method of vein stripping. The stripper is threaded into the vein, secured, and pulled back out, bringing the vein with it. (From Linton RR: Atlas of Vascular Surgery. Philadelphia, WB Saunders, 1973.)

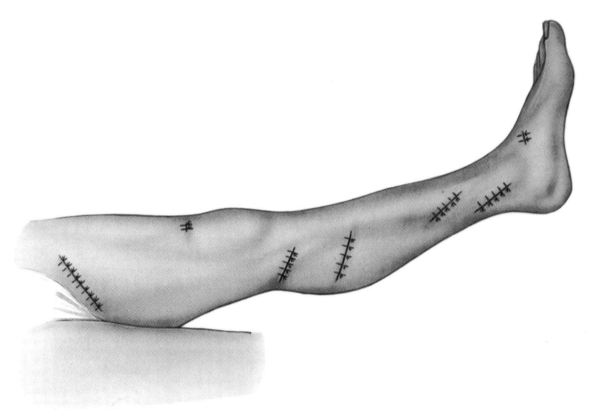

Figure 25–31. Internal vein stripping. After small tributaries have been removed through separate incisions, the wounds are closed with fine interrupted sutures. (From Linton RR: Atlas of Vascular Surgery. Philadelphia, WB Saunders, 1973.)

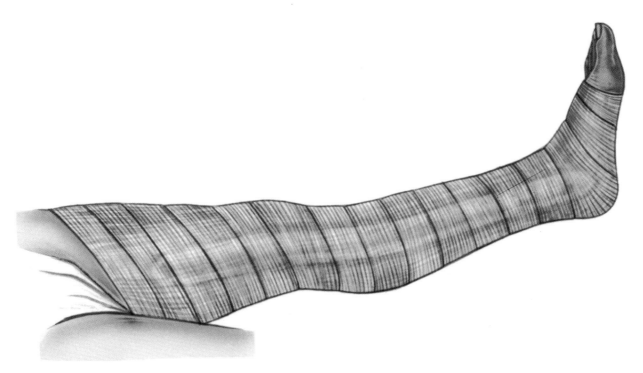

Figure 25–32. Internal vein stripping. The leg is dressed with gauze or plastic adhesive bandages and a compression type bandage. (From Linton RR: Atlas of Vascular Surgery. Philadelphia, WB Saunders, 1973.)

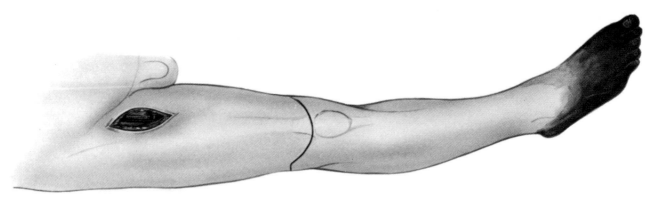

Figure 25–33. Above-knee amputation. Area of incision. (From Linton RR: Atlas of Vascular Surgery. Philadelphia, WB Saunders, 1973.)

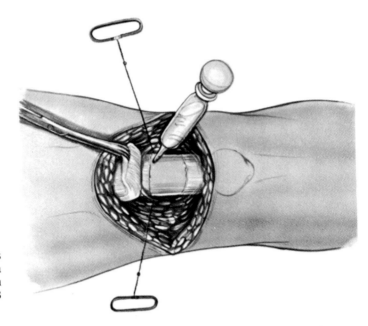

Figure 25–34. Above-knee amputation. The surgeon severs the femur with a Gigli saw. The technologist should drip a thin stream of saline over the saw to prevent friction. (From Linton RR: Atlas of Vascular Surgery. Philadelphia, WB Saunders, 1973.)

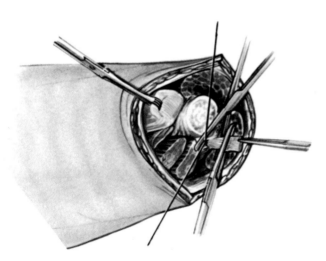

Figure 25–35. Above-knee amputation. The sciatic nerve is crushed and ligated, and the end is excised. It is then allowed to retract back into the femoral stump. This prevents the formation of a neuroma on the end of the nerve. (From Linton RR: Atlas of Vascular Surgery. Philadelphia, WB Saunders, 1973.)

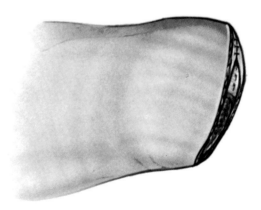

Figure 25–36. Above-knee amputation. The stump is closed in layers. Skin is usually closed with heavy nylon or stainless steel sutures. (From Linton RR: Atlas of Vascular Surgery. Philadelphia, WB Saunders, 1973.)

wound site from possible contamination. The foot is then excluded from the scrub prep.

To begin the procedure, the surgeon incises the leg (Fig. 25–33). The incision is carried through the subcutaneous, muscle, and fascial layers with the deep knife, heavy scissors, or electrocautery pencil. Large rake retractors are often useful in drawing the wound edges back to expose the femur. The surgeon may sever the femur with the Gigli saw (Fig. 25–34) or with an amputation saw, such as the Satterlee saw.

Once the femur is severed, the surgeon completes the amputation by severing the soft tissues that lie on the posterior side of the femur. The technologist removes the limb from the field and may pass it directly to the circulator. The surgeon ligates the popliteal artery and vein and grasps the sciatic nerve with a Kocher or other heavy clamp. The end of the nerve is crushed with the clamp to prevent the formation of a neuroma (tumor at the end of the nerve). It is then ligated with a suture ligature, size 0 or 2-0 (Fig. 25–35). The end of the nerve is cut with the knife or scissors and allowed to retract back into the femoral stump.

The stump is closed in layers with Dexon or other absorbable sutures, size 0 or 2-0 (Fig. 25–36). The skin is sutured with the surgeon's choice of material and dressed with bulky gauze.

Bibliography

Barker WF: Peripheral Vascular Disease, 2nd ed. Philadelphia, WB Saunders, 1975.

Cooley D, Wukasch D: Techniques in Vascular Surgery. Philadelphia, WB Saunders, 1979.

Gardner E, Gray D, O'Rahilly R: Anatomy: A Regional Study of Human Structure, 4th ed. Philadelphia, WB Saunders, 1984.

Haimovici H: Vascular Surgery: Principles and Techniques. New York, McGraw-Hill, 1976.

Jacob S, Francone C, Lossow WJ: Structure and Function in Man, 5th ed. Philadelphia, WB Saunders, 1982.

Linton RR: Atlas of Vascular Surgery. Philadelphia, WB Saunders, 1973.

McVay C: Surgical Anatomy, 6th ed. Philadelphia, WB Saunders, 1984.

Rutherford R: Vascular Surgery, 3rd ed. Philadelphia, WB Saunders, 1989.

Sabiston DC Jr (ed): Textbook of Surgery, 14th ed. Philadelphia, WB Saunders, 1991.

Walter JB: An Introduction to the Principles of Disease, 3rd ed. Philadelphia, WB Saunders, 1992.

Neurosurgery

Neurosurgical procedures are performed to remove pathologic lesions, relieve pressure on the brain due to disease or injury, relieve pain, and repair injured or diseased peripheral nerves. Neurosurgery is a highly specialized area of surgery, and many hospitals reserve a special team to assist the neurosurgeon. In some craniotomy procedures, two circulators may be needed.

SURGICAL ANATOMY

The nervous system is divided into two parts: the *central nervous system*, which includes the brain and spinal cord, and the *peripheral nervous system*, which includes the cranial and spinal nerves and their branches.

Central Nervous System

Skull

The skull is the protective housing of the brain. It is composed of 24 bones, each connected by a thin membrane called a *suture*. The skull is covered by the *scalp*, which is a multilayered vascular tissue. Directly superficial to the skull is the *pericranium*, the periosteum of the skull bones. This is followed by the occipitofrontalis muscle and the *galea*, which is a tough fibrous tissue sheet. Directly over the galea lies the subcutaneous tissue, which contains a highly vascular layer that bleeds profusely when cut. The *skin* of the scalp is very thick and covered with hair.

Meninges

Directly beneath the skull lie the three protective coverings of the brain, the *meninges*. The outermost layer, the *dura mater,* is composed of very dense fibrous tissue. The middle layer is the *arachnoid*. This is a very delicate serous membrane that has the appearance of a spider web. Beneath the arachnoid is the *subarachnoid* space, which is filled with cerebrospinal fluid. The *pia mater* is the layer closest to the brain. This is a vascular membrane that contains portions of areolar connective tissue. This membrane dips down into the various crevices and convolutions of the brain. The layers of the scalp, superficial brain, and associated structures are illustrated in Figure 26–1.

Ventricles

The *ventricles* are the spaces of the brain. These spaces lie between the various sections of the brain and are filled with cerebrospinal fluid, which bathes and nourishes it. There are four ventricles that lie within the brain. Two *lateral ventricles* occupy the two halves of the cerebrum. These are connected to each other by the *interventricular foramen*, which leads to the *third ventricle*. This ventricle opens into a narrow path called the *cerebral aqueduct*, which leads directly into the *fourth ventricle* lying near the base of the brain. Cerebrospinal fluid leaves the fourth ventricle through three openings, where it then circulates around the brain stem and cord. The ventricles are illustrated in Figure 26–2.

Brain

The brain itself is broken down into three main sections, and these sections are further divided into subdivisions as follows:

Forebrain
  Cerebrum

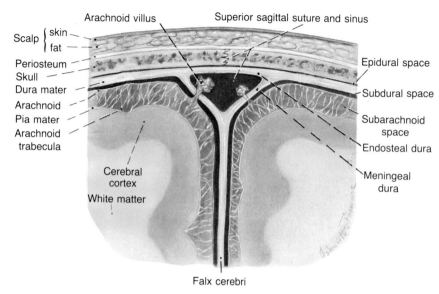

Figure 26–1. Cross section of skull, brain, and meninges. (From Jacob S, Francone C, Lossow WJ: Structure and Function in Man, 5th ed. Philadelphia, WB Saunders, 1982.)

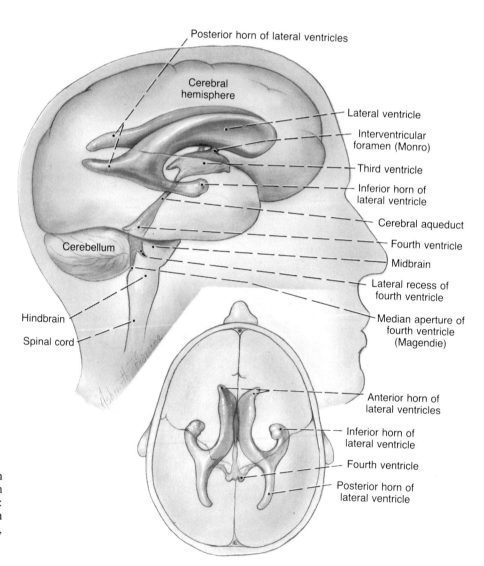

Figure 26–2. Ventricles of the brain with lateral and superior views. (From Jacob S, Francone C, Lossow WJ: Structure and Function in Man, 5th ed. Philadelphia, WB Saunders, 1982.)

Midbrain
  Corpora quadrigemina
  Cerebral peduncles
Hindbrain
  Cerebellum
  Pons
  Medulla oblongata

Forebrain

Cerebrum. The *cerebrum* governs all motor activities and sensory impulses. This section of the forebrain is also responsible for memory, intelligence, and reason. The cerebrum is the largest portion of the brain, occupying seven eighths of the total weight of the organ. The surface of the cerebrum is convoluted with small bulges that occur throughout its surface. These bulges are called *gyri* (singular, *gyrus*). Between the bulges are shallow indentations called *sulci.* Larger, deeper furrows in this area are known as *fissures.*

The cerebrum is divided into two distinct halves, which are separated by the *longitudinal fissure.* Each half is referred to as a *cerebral hemisphere.*

The outer tissue layer of the cerebrum is known as the *cerebral cortex.* This layer is composed of gray tissue matter and is divided into lobes, which receive their names from the bones that lie over them. The lobes include the *frontal lobe, parietal lobe, temporal lobe,* and *occipital lobe.* The location of these lobes is illustrated in Figure 26–3.

Midbrain

The midbrain is situated between the forebrain and the hindbrain. The cerebral aqueduct, which was previously mentioned, courses through the middle of the midbrain. On the ventral side of this portion of the brain are two masses of white matter called the *cerebral peduncles.* These peduncles carry impulses to and from the cerebrum. On the dorsal side are four rounded tissue masses called the *corpora quadrigemina.* This section is responsible for relaying auditory and visual impulses.

Hindbrain

Cerebellum. The *cerebellum* (Fig. 26–4) lies in the posterior cranial fossa and closely resembles the cerebrum in structure. Like the cerebrum, it is covered by a cortex composed of gray matter and is divided into lobes by fissures. The cerebellar lobes include the anterior, posterior, and flocculonodular. The first two, the anterior and posterior lobes, help control coordination and movement. The flocculonodular lobe helps control equilibrium.

Pons. The *pons* (see Fig. 26–4) lies between the midbrain and the medulla, in front of the cerebellum. It consists mainly of white matter and serves as a relay between the medulla and the cerebral peduncles. The fifth, sixth, seventh, and eighth cranial nerves have their origin in this portion of the hindbrain.

Medulla Oblongata. The *medulla oblongata* (see Fig. 26–4) is a continuous connection between the spinal

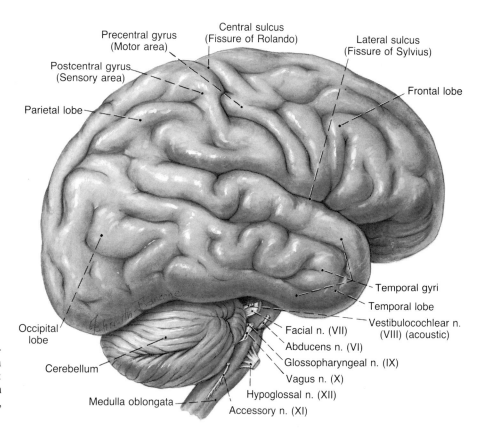

Figure 26–3. Side view of brain showing cerebral lobes and gyri. (From Jacob S, Francone C, Lossow WJ: Structure and Function in Man, 5th ed. Philadelphia, WB Saunders, 1982.)

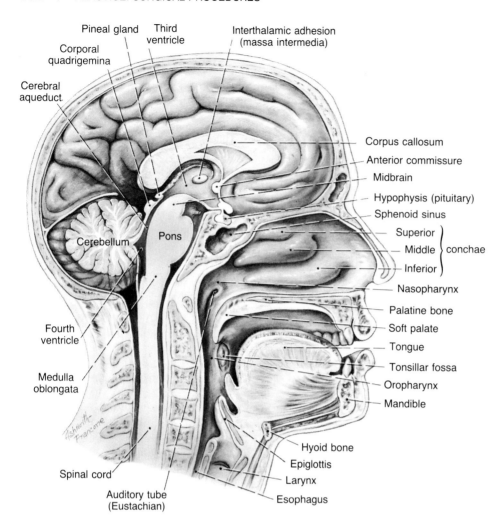

Pineal gland
Third ventricle
Interthalamic adhesion (massa intermedia)
Corporal quadrigemina
Cerebral aqueduct
Cerebellum
Pons
Fourth ventricle
Medulla oblongata
Spinal cord
Auditory tube (Eustachian)
Corpus callosum
Anterior commissure
Midbrain
Hypophysis (pituitary)
Sphenoid sinus
Superior
Middle } conchae
Inferior
Nasopharynx
Palatine bone
Soft palate
Tongue
Tonsillar fossa
Oropharynx
Mandible
Hyoid bone
Epiglottis
Larynx
Esophagus

Figure 26–4. Sagittal section through head showing components of the brain, anatomic location of the spinal cord, and structures of the throat and neck area. (From Jacob S, Francone C, Lossow WJ: Structure and Function in Man, 5th ed. Philadelphia, WB Saunders, 1982.)

cord and the pons. It is made up primarily of gray matter and closely resembles the spinal cord in internal structure except that it is much thicker. Lines of white matter are interspersed within the gray matter, and all impulses into and out of the spinal cord are located here. The medulla is responsible for vital functions such as control of the circulatory system, respiration, and heart rate.

Spinal Cord

The spinal cord is located within the vertebral canal (Fig. 26–5) and is continuous with the medulla oblongata of the hindbrain. The cord commences at the foramen magnum, a large foramen at the base of the skull, and terminates at the first and second lumbar vertebrae. Structurally, the spinal cord is somewhat flat on the dorsoventral side and contains an outer layer of white matter and an inner body of gray matter. A cross section of the cord reveals the gray matter to form a rough "H" shape. The two dorsal portions of the "H" are called the *dorsal horns,* and the two ventral portions are called the *ventral horns.* The cross portion of the "H" is called the *gray commissure,* and this portion encompasses a canal that traverses the length of the cord. The cord is surrounded by the meninges down to the level of the second or third sacral vertebra (Fig. 26–6).

Peripheral Nervous System

Cranial Nerves

The cranial nerves are 12 pairs of nerves that originate in the brain and are responsible for sensory and motor functions of the body. Each of the 12 pairs has a separate name and function:

1. *Olfactory:* Responsible for the sense of smell.
2. *Optic:* Conveys impulses for sight.
3. *Oculomotor:* Controls muscles that move the eye and iris.
4. *Trochlear:* Controls the oblique muscle of the eye.
5. *Trigeminal:* Sensory nerve controlling the sensations of the face, forehead, mouth, nose, and top of the head.
6. *Abducens:* Controls lateral movement of the eye.
7. *Facial:* A motor nerve that is responsible for the muscles in the face and scalp; also controls tears and salivation.
8. *Acoustic:* Controls hearing and equilibrium.
9. *Glossopharyngeal:* Serves the sense of taste and pharyngeal movement. This nerve also controls the parotid gland and salivation.

Table 26–1. CRANIAL NERVES

Number	Name	Superficial Origin	Exit From Skull	Function
I	Olfactory	(Extends from nasal mucosa to olfactory bulb)	Cribriform plate of ethmoid	Sensory: olfactory (smell)
II	Optic	(Extends from retina to optic chiasm)	Optic foramen	Sensory: vision
III	Oculomotor	Midbrain	Superior orbital fissure	Motor: external muscles of eyes except lateral rectus and superior oblique; levator palpebrae superioris Parasympathetic: sphincter of pupil and ciliary muscle of lens
IV	Trochlear	Roof of midbrain	Superior orbital fissure	Motor: superior oblique muscle
V	Trigeminal			
	Ophthalmic branch	Ventral surface of pons	Superior orbital fissure	Sensory: cornea; nasal mucous membrane; skin of face and scalp
	Maxillary branch	Ventral surface of pons	Foramen rotundum	Sensory: skin of face; mucous membrane of mouth and nose; teeth
	Mandibular branch	Ventral surface of pons	Foramen ovale	Motor: muscles of mastication Sensory: skin of face; mucous membrane of mouth; teeth
VI	Abducens	Lower margin of pons	Superior orbital fissure	Motor: lateral rectus muscle
VII	Facial	Lower margin of pons	Stylomastoid foramen	Motor: muscles of facial expression Sensory: taste, anterior two thirds of tongue Parasympathetic: lacrimal, submandibular, and sublingual glands
VIII	Vestibulocochlear			
	Vestibular	Groove between pons and medulla oblongata	Internal auditory meatus	Sensory: equilibrium
	Cochlear	Groove between pons and medulla oblongata	Internal auditory meatus	Sensory: hearing
IX	Glossopharyngeal	Medulla oblongata	Jugular foramen	Motor: stylopharyngeus muscle Sensory: taste, posterior one third of tongue; pharynx; branch of the carotid sinus and carotid body Parasympathetic; parotid gland
X	Vagus	Medulla oblongata	Jugular foramen	Sensory: external meatus, pharynx, larynx, aortic sinus, and thoracic and abdominal viscera Motor: pharynx and larynx Parasympathetic: thoracic and abdominal viscera
XI	Accessory	Medulla oblongata and upper five cervical segments of spinal cord	Jugular foramen	Motor: trapezius and sternocleidomastoid muscles; muscles of pharynx and larynx
XII	Hypoglossal	Anterior lateral sulcus between olive and pyramid	Hypoglossal canal	Motor: muscles of tongue

From Jacob S, Francone C, Lossow WJ: Structure and Function in Man, 5th ed. Philadelphia, WB Saunders, 1982.

10. *Vagus:* Innervates the pharyngeal and laryngeal muscles, the heart, pancreas, lungs, and digestive systems. This nerve also controls the sensory paths of the abdominal viscera, the pleura, and the thoracic viscera.

11. *Accessory:* Contains two parts: a cranial and a spinal portion. The cranial portion joins the vagus nerve to help control the pharyngeal and laryngeal muscles. The spinal portion controls the trapezius and sternocleidomastoid muscles.

12. *Hypoglossal:* Innervates the muscles of the tongue.

The cranial nerves and their origins, exit points, and functions are listed in Table 26–1.

Spinal Nerves

There are 31 pairs of spinal nerves that originate from the cord and are attached at various points along the length of the entire cord. These nerves exit the spinal column through the *vertebral foramina.* Each nerve is composed of small bundles of nerve fibers called *fascicles,* which are surrounded by a sheath called the *endoneurium.* The *perineurium,* fibers of connective tissue,

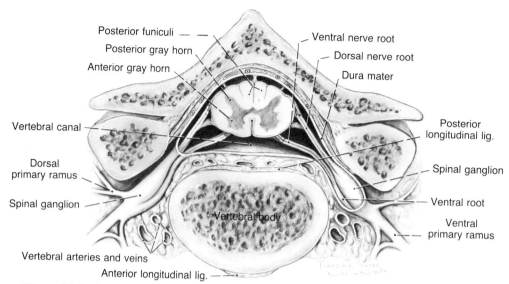

Figure 26–5. Anatomic relation between the spinal cord and the vertebrae. (From Jacob S, Francone C, Lossow WJ: Structure and Function in Man, 5th ed. Philadelphia, WB Saunders, 1982.)

extend within the spaces between each nerve fiber and bind them together. The nerve unit is then bound together by the *epineurium.*

The 31 pairs of spinal nerves correspond to the same number of *spinal segments,* each segment containing one pair of nerves. There are 8 cervical pairs, 12 thoracic, 5 lumbar, 5 sacral, and 1 coccygeal. Each spinal nerve has two roots: one dorsal and one ventral. The dorsal root contains an area of enlargement called the *dorsal root ganglion.* Each spinal nerve forms two branches; these are called *rami.*

POSITIONING, PREPPING, AND DRAPING

The patient may be placed in one of several positions, depending on the procedure. In most cases, the neurosurgeon is available to direct and assist in positioning the patient. The supine position may be used for many craniotomy and anterior cervical spine procedures and for the repair of peripheral nerves. A modified Fowler position (see Chapter 10) may be used for selected

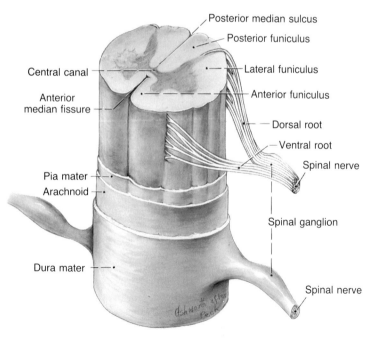

Figure 26–6. Section of spinal cord showing meninges, spinal nerve, and spinal ganglion. (From Jacob S, Francone C, Lossow WJ: Structure and Function in Man, 5th ed. Philadelphia, WB Saunders, 1982.)

craniotomy procedures and for posterior cervical spine operations. Laminectomy procedures are performed with the patient in the laminectomy position, with or without the use of a special laminectomy brace that elevates the thorax. A complete description of these positions and related safety precautions can be found in Chapter 10.

When prepping the patient for a craniotomy procedure, the hair is first shaved with electric clippers (this should be done outside the operating room suite) and then with a razor, as described in Chapter 11. The patient's hair must be saved and returned to the patient as personal property. In preparation for cervical spine procedures, the surgeon may order the patient's nape to be shaved to the level of the ears. If the patient's hair is quite long, it should be secured to the top of the head with an elastic band.

Because most surgeries involving the brain require complex draping routines, the surgeons may direct and complete the draping themselves. Drapes may be sewn directly to the scalp with silk sutures, or adhesive drapes may be used. In any case involving the head, it is wise to have extra drapes available to secure a large sterile field. (See Chapter 11 for a complete discussion of draping techniques.)

SPECIAL EQUIPMENT

In neurosurgical procedures involving the brain, special equipment should be available according to the surgeon's preference or specific need.

The *microscope* (see Chapter 27) is frequently used when microsurgical techniques are employed. It may be needed for cranial, spinal, or peripheral nerve procedures. When less magnification is needed, the surgeon may choose to wear *surgical loupes* (Fig. 26–7) and a *headlight* (Fig. 26–8).

The *electrosurgical unit* and *biopolar unit* are used frequently during cranial procedures. It is important to note that once the skull flap has been created and the brain is exposed, the *cutting* selection on the electrosurgical unit should be turned off to avoid inadvertent injury to the delicate brain tissue.

A special overhead table (*Mayfield table;* Fig. 26–9) is used in place of the Mayo stand during craniotomy procedures. With the surgeons standing at the patient's head, the table can be positioned, raised, or lowered to afford the optimum location from which instruments and supplies can be passed. The table offers the technologist ample working area on which to arrange the many supplies and solutions needed during a craniotomy procedure. In many cases, the Mayfield table is draped continuously with the patient to provide one large sterile field (see Fig. 11–16).

Drills and perforators (powered instruments used to penetrate the skull) are used for all brain procedures. A typical drill (craniotome) and perforator with special attachments to prevent injury to the brain tissues are shown in Figure 26–10. These specialized instruments

vary according to manufacturer, and the technologist and nurse should become familiar with those used in his or her operating room.

The patient's head is maintained in a fixed position during craniotomy or cervical spine procedures by a *head rest* that attaches to the operating table. There are many different types of head rests available, some designed with detachable pins that can be sterilized and then placed into the patient's skull. The patient is positioned with the head rest in place and the pins are then reattached to the head rest to immobilize the head completely. Three types of head rests are shown in Figure 26–11.

The Cavitron Ultrasonic Surgical Aspirator (CUSA) (Valleylab, Inc.) (Fig. 26–12) is a system that provides a console and a hand-held device that removes body tissue by fragmentation, irrigation, and suction. The CUSA is used in the removal of certain brain tumors. The sterile handpiece held by the surgeon contains an electrical device that causes the tip to vibrate in and out 23,000 times per second. The vibrating tip fragments tissue that it touches, and an irrigation solution flowing from a source near the tip suspends the fragmented tissue so it can be aspirated through the tip and transported to a reservoir in the console unit.

At least one surgical technologist or nurse from each hospital in which the unit is used is required to attend an in-service program given by the system's manufacturer. This program ensures that the system is set up and operated properly.

The CUSA system must be stored in an area that is free of dirt, blood, and water. It must be drained before storage, and the handpiece should be stored in its case.

Suction and irrigation are essential in every craniotomy procedure. Because the skull does not expand to accommodate an increase in tissue fluid or blood, it is vital that the wound be kept free of bleeding vessels. Otherwise, increased intracranial pressure caused by the accumulation of blood or fluid may damage the delicate nerve tissue and cause irreparable damage. Two separate suction tubes and tips should be available on the sterile field at all times. Frazier suction tips (see Fig.

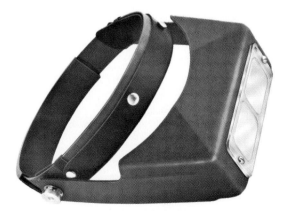

Figure 26–7. Surgical loupes. (Courtesy of Edward Weck & Company, Inc.)

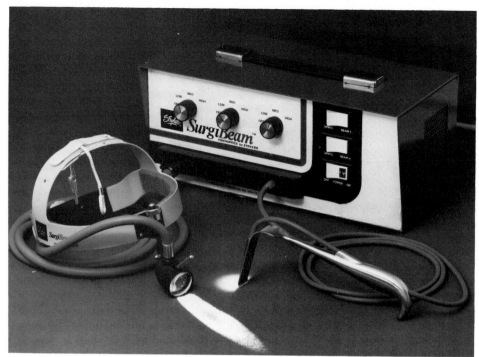

Figure 26–8. Surgeon's headlight. (Courtesy of the Stryker Corporation, Kalamazoo, MI.)

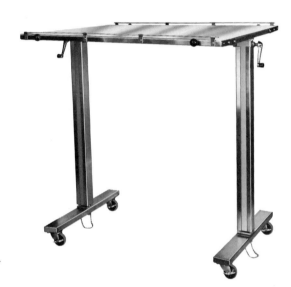

Figure 26–9. Mayfield overhead table used during cranial procedures. (Courtesy of Codman and Shurtleff, Inc., Randolph, MA.)

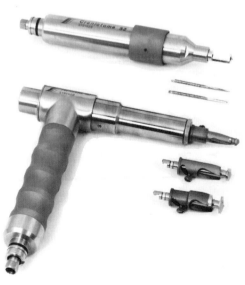

Figure 26–10. *Top.* Craniotome with dural guard. *Bottom.* Perforator used to create bur holes in the skull. (Courtesy of the Stryker Corporation, Kalamazoo, MI.)

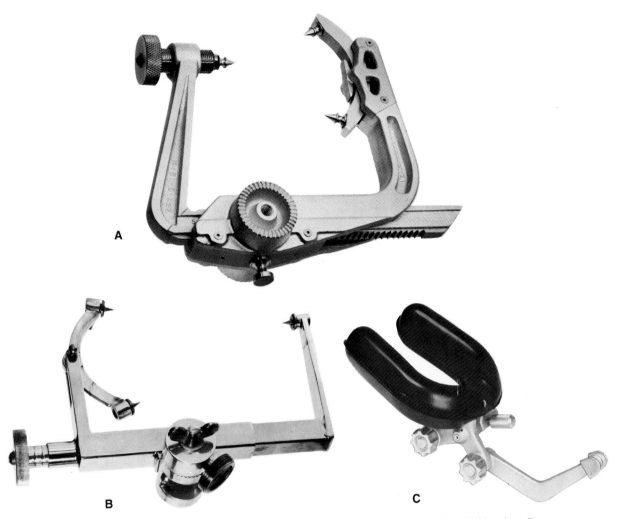

Figure 26–11. Neurosurgical head rests. *A.* Mayfield skull clamp with detachable pins. *B.* Gardner skull clamp with detachable pins. *C.* Mayfield horseshoe head rest. (Courtesy of Codman and Shurtleff, Randolph, MA.)

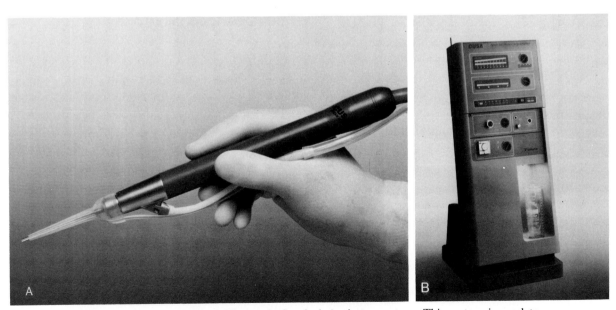

Figure 26–12. Cavitational Ultrasonic Surgical Aspirator system. This system is used to fragment, irrigate, and aspirate body tissue. Its application in neurosurgery is in the removal of certain types of brain tumors. *A.* Sterile handpiece. *B.* Control unit. (Courtesy of Valleylab, Inc., Stamford, CT.)

15–29) are commonly used. A suction tip equipped with a fiberoptic light at the end, if available, is also useful. In addition to removing fluid, the suction tip may also be used to evacuate tumor material, aid in dissection, or aspirate necrotic tissue, pus, or cystic matter. Irrigation solutions that help the surgeon identify bleeding and clear the wound of debris should be available at all times. Lactated Ringer's solution and physiologic saline solution are commonly used. The technologist should have two bulb syringes containing the surgeon's preferred solution filled at all times and readily available to the surgeons. Irrigation solutions are kept between 105°F and 115°F at all times. Fluid that exceeds 120°F causes cell damage to the cortex and must never be used.

Special *neurosurgical sponges* (see Chapter 13) are used during cranial and spinal procedures. These may be in the form of flattened radiopaque squares of feltlike material or cotton balls to which a string is attached. They are offered to the surgeon on a flat metal plate (or ribbon retractor, if a plate is not available) and should be moistened with saline solution before use. All sponges should be accounted for in the usual manner. Routine 4 × 4-inch sponges are used *only* when the brain is not exposed, since their rough texture can damage delicate brain tissues.

DRUGS USED IN NEUROSURGERY

Drugs used specifically during cranial procedures may be classified as hemostatics, diuretics, and antibiotics. As pointed out previously, hemostasis is one of the critical concerns during any cranial procedure. Agents commonly used are bone wax (applied to the skull), Gelfoam, Surgicel, topical thrombin, Avitene (microfibrillar collagen), and hydrogen peroxide. The technologist should cut the Gelfoam into several different sizes before use, unless otherwise directed by the surgeon. These pieces may or may not be soaked in topical thrombin, according to the surgeon's preference. Surgicel and Avitene are both supplied to the surgeon in their *dry* state. Avitene should be offered to the surgeon with a *dry* thumb forceps for placement in the wound; otherwise, the Avitene could stick to the forceps.

Intravenous diuretics are administered to the patient before, during, and after any cranial procedure to prevent the brain from swelling as the result of surgery. Consequently, the likelihood of increased intracranial pressure and subsequent tissue damage is reduced. Mannitol is a commonly used diuretic.

Most neurosurgeons use an antibiotic solution as a final wound irrigant in cranial procedures and in some peripheral nerve repairs. The choice of antibiotic varies according to the surgeon's preference.

Anesthesia

Brain tissue itself is insensitive to pain. Only the scalp, extracranial arteries, and portions of the dura mater are sensitive to pain. Local anesthetic injected into the incisional area of the scalp aids in hemostasis of this highly vascular area. When the procedure is performed under a general anesthetic, the level of anesthesia can be much lighter and therefore safer.

DIAGNOSTIC PROCEDURES

There are numerous neurologic diagnostic procedures that may or may not involve surgical personnel but with which the technologist and nurse should be familiar. If any of the procedures have been performed before surgery, the results should be readily available during surgery.

Angiography

During angiography a contrast medium such as diatrizoate compound (see Chapter 14) is injected into the vessels of the cranium to reveal aneurysms, certain tumors, or other vascular lesions. Once the dye is injected, radiographs are taken in rapid succession.

Myelography

Myelography, a procedure similar to angiography, employs a contrast medium that is injected into the subarachnoid space of the spinal canal. Radiographs may reveal lesions such as a herniated disk, spinal cord tumor, or other anomaly. Fluoroscopy is employed to visualize affected areas. The radiologist then takes spot films, which become a permanent record of the patient's condition.

Pneumoencephalography

During pneumoencephalography a lumbar puncture needle is introduced into the subarachnoid space and air is injected. Radiographs are then taken to determine the outline of the ventricular system and subarachnoid cisterns.

Ventriculography

During ventriculography air or contrast medium is substituted for cerebrospinal fluid. This study is particularly useful in diagnosing tumors. The procedure is performed when there is an obstruction between the ventricular system and the spinal canal. The ventricular fluid is aspirated, air is introduced through small bur holes, and radiographs are then taken.

Echoencephalography

This study utilizes ultrasonic waves for the identification of brain abscesses, tumors, and hematomas. The procedure is most commonly used in an emergency situation.

Computed Axial Tomography

Computed axial tomography produces radiographs of the brain (or other areas of the body) represented in cross section. The pictorial radiographs outline the ventricles of the brain, nerves, blood vessels, tumors, or other structures. The tissues are depicted according to their relative absorption coefficient for radiographs.

SURGICAL PROCEDURES

Peripheral Nerve Repair (Neurorrhaphy)

Definition

This is the anastomosis of a severed nerve, usually in the hand or forearm, to restore function. Peripheral nerve injuries may be caused by an industrial or other type of accident. Successful repair depends on the age of the patient, extent of injury to adjacent tissue, and type of injury to the nerve. Two different types are a clean cut, such as that caused by glass, or an injury that causes the nerve to shatter. If the nerve is severely damaged, it may be replaced by a nerve graft taken from another location in the body, usually the leg (sural nerve).

Highlights

1. The extent of the injury is evaluated.
2. The nerve is trimmed, if necessary.
3. The nerve is anastomosed.
4. The wound is closed and dressed with supportive material.

Description

The operation to repair a severed peripheral nerve is usually performed as an emergency procedure. If nerve repair is delayed, the possibility of full recovery is decreased. There are two common methods of peripheral nerve repair—the *funicular* suture technique and the *epineural* suture technique. In the funicular technique, the funiculi (fibers that make up the nerve) are joined together individually. In the epineural technique, the epineurium (component of connective tissue that surrounds the nerve) is anastomosed and the individual funiculi are not sutured together.

In preparation for peripheral nerve repair, the technologist should have microinstruments or eye instruments available. In addition, the microscope or surgical loupes, bipolar coagulation unit, physiologic saline solution such as that used in eye surgery, and a pneumatic tourniquet should be available. Fine sutures of sizes 10-0, 7-0, and 6-0 swaged to small cutting needles are also

needed. The choice of suture material and size depends on the surgeon's preference, but monofilament nylon is commonly used.

The patient should lie in the supine position with the affected arm or hand resting on an arm board or hand table, such as the one described in Chapter 23 for orthopedic surgery. If there has been extensive damage to the limb, the surgeon may want to débride (excise any devitalized or ragged tissue) before beginning the nerve repair. The débridement usually takes place in conjunction with the skin prep or immediately following it. If the surgeon wishes to perform the skin prep and débridement, the technologist or circulator should supply him or her with copious amounts of sterile saline solution, sponges, antiseptic soap, a fine scalpel, tissue forceps, and dissecting scissors.

Once débridement has been completed, the limb is draped in routine fashion. Some surgeons drape the limb first and then perform the débridement. The first step of the actual procedure is the mobilization of the injured nerve. The surgeon gently frees the severed nerve from its surrounding tissue using fine dissecting scissors and thumb forceps.

Before beginning the anastomosis, the jagged ends of the nerve must be severed. Two fine traction sutures are placed through each end of the nerve and are used to bring the nerve ends into approximation. To sever the nerve ends, the surgeon may use a scalpel or a razor blade breaker (commonly called a "blade breaker"). A moistened wooden tongue blade is useful in providing a firm surface on which to place the nerve. The technologist should have one or two new razor blades available. The surgeon then breaks a corner from the blade and uses it to sever the nerve ends. The nerve ends are cut serially in 1-mm slices until the ends appear satisfactory for anastomosis.

In the epineural technique, the surgeon places several sutures of size 6-0 or 7-0 nylon, one through each quadrant of the nerve (Fig. 26–13). For funicular repair, each individual funiculus is joined with interrupted sutures of size 10-0 nylon (Fig. 26–14). During the anastomosis, the technologist should irrigate the nerve frequently with balanced saline solution such as that used in eye surgery to prevent it from drying out.

Following the repair, the tissue layers are approximated with fine interrupted sutures. A dressing of cotton gauze and plaster of Paris or other casting material is used to immobilize the limb until healing is complete.

Sympathectomy

Definition

This is the interruption of the sympathetic nerve fibers and ganglia of the autonomic nervous system. In particular, lumbar sympathectomy is commonly performed to relieve arterial spasm due to vascular disease. A sympathectomy may be done in other locations along the spinal column to treat intractable pain due to advanced carcinoma or to increase vascular circulation. A *lumbar sympathectomy* is described below.

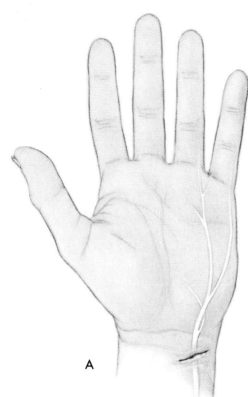

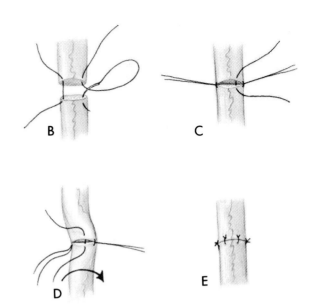

Figure 26–13. Epineural technique for peripheral nerve repair. *A.* Severed nerve. *B.* Two traction sutures applied. *C.* Third quadrant suture. *D.* Fourth quadrant suture. *E.* Completed anastomosis. (From Boyes JH: Suture Technics for Wounds of the Hand. Somerville, NJ, Ethicon, 1970. Courtesy of Ethicon, Inc.)

Highlights

1. The retroperitoneal space is entered.
2. The nerves are grasped and divided, and clips are applied.
3. The wound is closed.

Description

The patient may be placed in the Sims or supine position, depending on the approach the surgeon wishes to take. The sympathetic chain may be reached through a flank incision or transperitoneally through a paramedian incision. The flank incision is more commonly used. The surgeon enters the retroperitoneal space through this incision, as described in Chapter 22. The technologist should have deep hand-held retractors available, such as a Harrington, wide Deaver, or wide ribbon retractor. The assistant places these in the wound along with several moist lap sponges to help expose the sympathetic chain and associated ganglia.

Once the chain is exposed, the surgeon elevates it using a long nerve hook (Smithwick hook). The technologist should have two long ligating clip appliers available at this time. The surgeon clips the chain in several places and divides it using long Metzenbaum scissors. The wound is then closed in layers, as discussed in Chapter 22.

Related Procedures

Rhizotomy
Cordotomy
Thoracic sympathectomy
Cervical sympathectomy

Lumbar Laminectomy

Definition

This is the creation of an opening in the lamina to expose the spinal cord and/or disk. There are four common indications for a laminectomy. These are to remove a herniated disk, spinal cord tumor, or aneurysm or to repair the spinal cord injured by trauma such as that created by a bullet wound. The operating micro-

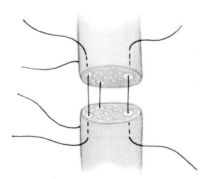

Figure 26–14. Technique of funicular repair of peripheral nerve. (From Boyes JH: Suture Technics for Wounds of the Hand. Somerville, NJ, Ethicon, 1970. Courtesy of Ethicon, Inc.)

scope is used for aneurysms or tumors or whenever fine dissection is required. The microscope is brought into the surgical field when the surgeon reaches the spinal cord dura, and microsurgical instruments are used to repair the defect. A lumbar laminectomy for the removal of a herniated disk is described here.

Highlights

1. The back is incised over the affected disk.
2. A cavity in the lamina is created.
3. The disk is removed piece by piece.
4. The wound is closed.

Description

The patient is placed in the laminectomy position onto a laminectomy brace (see Chapter 10) *after* induction. Alternatively, the patient may be placed on sandbags and rolled bath blankets to elevate the chest. (A complete description of proper padding and positioning is presented in Chapter 10.) The back is then prepped in routine fashion.

To begin the procedure, the surgeon may inject the incisional site with a small amount of local anesthetic with epinephrine added to aid in hemostasis. A midline vertical incision is made over the spine using a No. 20 knife blade (Fig. 26–15). The surgeon deepens the wound with the knife or cautery penicil to the level of the fascia and incises the fascia with toothed forceps and the cautery pencil (Fig. 26–16A). Two angled Weitlaner retractors are inserted into the wound for better exposure. The technologist should have a large number of unfolded 4 × 4-inch gauze sponges available at this time. The surgeon packs the sponges along the vertebra with periosteal elevators. This is done both to aid in hemostasis and to expose the vertebrae by retracting the larger back muscles (Fig. 26–16B).

Because the wound is now deep, the surgeon may replace the Weitlaner retractors with Adson-Beckman retractors, or Taylor retractors may be used. If Taylor retractors are used, the technologist should supply the surgeon with roller gauze. The surgeon wraps the gauze around the tail of the retractor and drops the opposite end to the circulator, who secures it to the table frame or a sandbag to keep the retractors in place (Fig. 26–16C).

The surgeon uses a large rongeur to bite off the protruding bony spinous process and expose the lamina. Up-biting and down-biting Kerrison rongeurs are then used to excise the lamina and create access to the disk. It is the technologist's responsibility to clean the end of the rongeur as the surgeon makes each small bite into the bone. This is best done with a moist 4 × 4-inch sponge. These bits of bone must be retained as specimens. Once the lamina has been reduced, cottonoid sponges are used instead of 4 × 4-inch sponges. To prevent the dura from tearing, the surgeon uses a dental probe or Freer type elevator to loosen any dura attached to the lamina. At this time the technologist may offer the surgeon bone wax on the end of a Penfield elevator or on the edge of a small medicine glass to aid in hemostasis.

The surgeon now identifies the yellowish ligamentum flavum (ligament that connects each vertebra to the next) and incises it with a No. 15 knife blade mounted on a No. 7 handle (Fig. 26–17). Down-biting Kerrison rongeurs may be used to remove any ligament that obstructs the surgeon's view of the disk. The disk is now approachable.

The assistant retracts the vertebral nerve using a Love or similar nerve root retractor as the surgeon snips off pieces of the bulging disk with a Takahashi or pituitary rongeur. As the disk is removed, the surgeon may use a curette for further evacuation (Fig. 26–18). The technologist must clean the tips of the instrument with each bite, as with the bits of lamina, and retain the bits of disk as specimens. These should be kept separate from the bone fragments previously retrieved. It is critical that the technologist remain alert during this maneuver, since the surgeon cannot turn his or her head away from the wound (the risk of spinal cord damage is great).

Once the herniated disk has been removed, the surgeon closes the wound. The fascial layer is usually closed with absorbable synthetic sutures mounted or swaged to a large cutting needle. Size 0 suture is commonly used. Before closing the muscle layer, the surgeon may inject a local anesthetic to help alleviate postoperative pain. The muscle and subcutaneous layers are closed with size 2-0 synthetic absorbable suture. The skin is closed according to the surgeon's preference (a variety of materials may be used), and the wound is dressed in routine fashion.

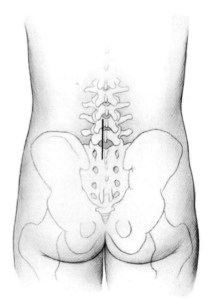

Figure 26–15. Area of incision for lumbar laminectomy. (From Jannetta PJ: Lumbar Hemilaminotomy and Disc Excision. Somerville, NJ, Ethicon, 1977. Courtesy of Ethicon, Inc.)

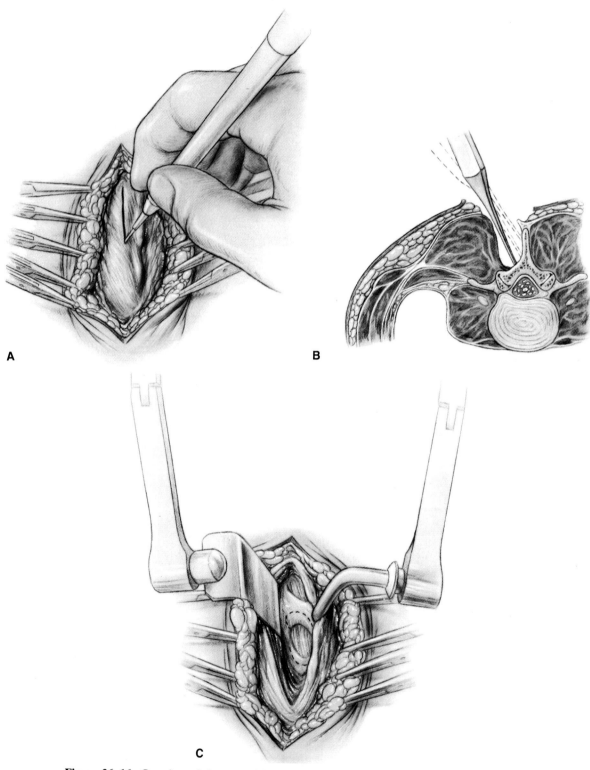

Figure 26–16. Opening of the wound for lumbar laminectomy. *A.* Fascia is incised with the cautery pencil. *B.* Muscles are retracted with a periosteal elevator and sponges. *C.* Deep retractor in place. (From Jannetta PJ: Lumbar Hemilaminotomy and Disc Excision. Somerville, NJ, Ethicon, 1977. Courtesy of Ethicon, Inc.)

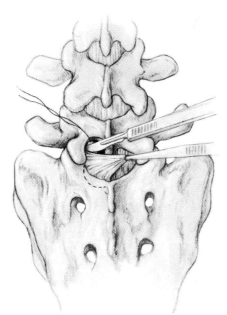

Figure 26–17. Lumbar laminectomy. The ligamentum flavum is incised with a No. 15 knife blade. (From Jannetta PJ: Lumbar Hemilaminotomy and Disc Excision. Somerville, NJ, Ethicon, 1977. Courtesy of Ethicon, Inc.)

Anterior Cervical Fusion

Definition

This is the excision of one or more herniated cervical intervertebral disks and the placement of bone grafts between the vertebra to fuse them together. The patient with a herniated cervical disk experiences pain in the shoulders and/or arms, accompanied with numbness and weakness in the hands and arms.

In addition to basic laminectomy instruments, the technologist should have Cloward bone-grafting instruments, a bipolar coagulation unit, osteotomes, curettes, and a Hudson brace available. The surgeon may also elect to use the operating microscope or surgical loupes for magnification of the operative site.

Highlights

1. The neck is incised.
2. The cervical vertebra is exposed.
3. The herniated disk is removed.
4. A bone graft is taken from the iliac crest and placed in the vertebral interspace.
5. The wounds are closed.

Description

There are two approaches to the diseased cervical vertebra, the anterior and the posterior. The approach used depends on the location of the diseased disk. When the posterior approach is used, the patient is placed in Fowler position. For an anterior approach, the patient is placed in the supine position with the head turned to

the left and the right hip elevated on a sandbag or rolled bath blanket. This facilitates exposure to the iliac crest from which the bone graft is taken. Both operative sites are prepped and draped in routine fashion. The exposed iliac crest can be covered with a sterile towel following draping until the surgeon is ready to take the bone graft.

The surgeon may mark the cervical incision with a knife blade and may inject the incisional site with a local anesthetic. A transverse incision is made in the skin crease of the neck at the level of the cricoid cartilage. The surgeon then deepens the wound with the deep knife, Metzenbaum scissors, or cautery pencil, severing the platysma muscle. A small self-retaining retractor is then placed in the wound. Hemostasis is maintained with the cautery unit or with fine ligatures of absorbable suture. The surgeon identifies the carotid artery digitally and incises the muscle fibers lying medially to expose the vertebrae. A layer of fascia lying over the vertebra is incised with a No. 15 knife blade mounted on a No. 7 handle. A U.S. Army or small Deaver retractor may be needed to help expose the vertebra. The surgeon then incises and removes the anterior longitudinal ligament. With the disk now clearly visible, the surgeon may put a hypodermic needle into it and request that radiographs be taken of the disk. This determines the level of the disk to ensure that it is indeed the diseased one.

The bone graft may be taken at this time or after the surgeons have removed the diseased disk. A Cloward self-retaining retractor is placed in the wound. The surgeon then incises the disk with a No. 15 knife blade. To remove the disk, the surgeon uses pituitary rongeurs and fine curettes (Fig. 26–19A). The disk is removed piece by piece, as in a laminectomy, and the technologist must retrieve the bits of disk from the rongeur or curette in the same manner as for a laminectomy. The surgeon may use a Cloward intervertebral spreader to expose the disk further. A small drill bit or bur may be used to

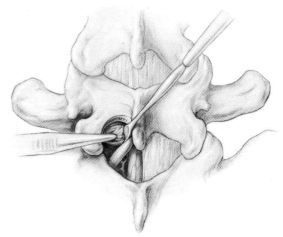

Figure 26–18. Lumbar laminectomy. The surgeon removes deeper portions of the interspace with a small curette. (From Jannetta PJ: Lumbar Hemilaminotomy and Disc Excision. Somerville, NJ, Ethicon, 1977. Courtesy of Ethicon, Inc.)

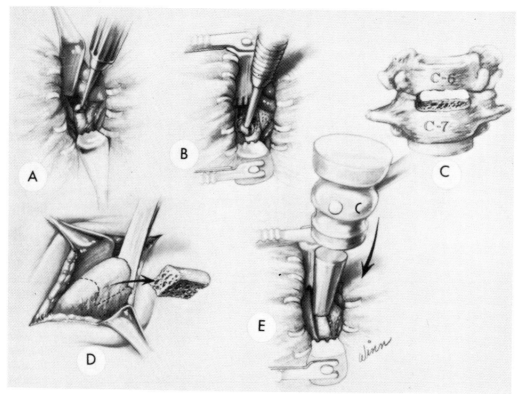

Figure 26–19. Method of anterior cervical fusion. *A.* Disk is removed with a curette. *B.* Power drill is used to remove small bits of bone from the interspace. *C.* Bone is completely excised. *D.* Bone graft is taken from the iliac crest with osteotome. *E.* Graft is impacted into the previously prepared vertebral interspace. (From Youmans J: Neurological Surgery, 2nd ed. Philadelphia, WB Saunders, 1982.)

expose the dura within the interspace (Fig. 26–19*B*). The dura is then elevated with a sharp nerve hook or dura hook and incised with a No. 15 knife blade. When the interspace has been adequately enlarged and all traces of disk have been removed (Fig. 26–19*C*), the bone graft is taken (if it has not been taken before the disk removal). While the graft is excised, the neck wound should be covered with a towel to protect it.

There are two methods used to take the bone graft. The Cloward method uses a special dowel cutter that creates a "plug" of bone from the iliac crest. Alternatively, an osteotome and mallet can be used to shear the surface of the iliac crest and create short slivers of bone for the graft (Fig. 26–19*D*). The surgeon incises the iliac crest and deepens the incision with the cautery pencil. Once the bone is exposed, a self-retaining retractor is placed in the wound. The surgeon then uses a periosteal elevator to strip the crest of periosteum. The graft is taken by one of the methods previously discussed. The technologist may be required to trim the bone graft with a rongeur. The graft is then placed in a basin; it may be moistened with saline solution or left dry (some surgeons believe that the saline solution destroys some of the bone cells). Bleeding vessels on the surface of the iliac are controlled with bone wax, and the surface is smoothed over with a rasp or rongeur.

The surgeon examines the graft and cuts it to the appropriate size to fit in the vertebral interspace. Any extra bits of bone from the graft must be saved, since they may be used later to fill the interspace. The surgeon places the graft in the interspace and taps it so that it fits snugly between the vertebrae (Fig. 26–19*E*). If the Cloward dowel cutter has been used, the Cloward impactor is used to place the graft.

The wound is then irrigated. Bleeding vessels are controlled with the cautery pencil or a topical hemostatic agent. The iliac wound and neck wound can be closed simultaneously, one by the surgeon and the other by the assistant. The iliac wound is closed with heavy absorbable suture, such as Dexon or Vicryl, mounted on cutting needles. The cervical incision is closed in layers with fine absorbable sutures, such as Dexon or silk. Both wounds are dressed in routine fashion.

When the patient is moved from the operating table to the stretcher, particular care is taken to keep the head in alignment with the body to prevent the graft from dislodging.

Craniotomy

Definition

This is an opening made in the skull to expose the brain and intracranial structures, usually a diseased or injured portion of the brain. Craniotomies are classified according to their location, such as anterior, middle, or posterior fossa; a craniotomy may also be classified as frontal, parietal, temporal, or occipital, depending on where the incision is to be made. In performing a craniotomy, a bone flap is created. When a bone flap is created, the bone may be left attached to muscle and turned back with the soft tissue to which it is attached, or it may be removed as a free bone flap. If bone is removed instead of a flap being created, the procedure is termed a *craniectomy*. In the event of intracranial hemorrhage, holes (bur holes) are drilled into the skull to relieve the pressure of blood against the brain.

Highlights

1. An incision is made in the scalp.
2. A bone flap is created.
3. The diseased or injured portion of the brain is exposed.
4. The pathologic condition is removed or repaired.
5. The bone flap is reattached, and the incision is closed.

Description

Depending on the location and size of the diseased portion of brain, the surgeon may request a microscope. If the pathology is superficial, however, the surgeon may choose to wear magnifying loupes only. It is wise for the technologist or circulator to check with the surgeon on this point before the procedure is begun.

The patient is positioned on the operating table with the head stabilized on a head rest. The surgeon usually assists in positioning the patient so as to ensure that it facilitates maximum exposure to the lesion. The skull is prepped and draped in routine fashion. Before beginning the procedure, the surgeon may mark the incision site with a needle, scalpel blade, or marking pen, particularly if the incision is long, since this aids in proper approximation of skin at the close of the procedure.

To aid in hemostasis, the surgeon may inject the scalp with local anesthetic combined with epinephrine. The incision is made with a No. 20 knife blade. Once the initial incision has been made, the surgeon uses numerous 4 × 4-inch sponges and digital pressure to maintain hemostasis. Raney clips or Kolodney clamps are then applied to the tissue edges. These will remain in place throughout the procedure (Fig. 26–20). The galea (tough fibrous layer of tissue around the skull) and pericranium are incised with the electrocautery pencil, thus exposing the skull itself. Two small, angled Weitlaner retractors are placed at either end of the incision, and the assistant may use a Cushing or similar retractor to aid in holding back the skin flap. The surgeon then uses a periosteal elevator to strip the pericranium farther from the skull so that it can be drilled. Two or more bur holes are made in the skull with the Hudson brace with perforator, Black and Decker battery-operated drill, or Hall craniotome (Fig. 26–21). After each bur hole is made, the surgeon curettes the bone debris and dust and enlarges

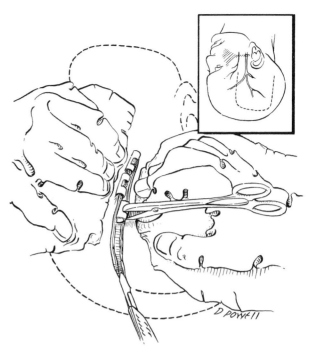

Figure 26–20. Craniotomy. Application of scalp clips for hemostasis. (From Youmans J: Neurological Surgery, 2nd ed. Philadelphia, WB Saunders, 1982.)

the holes. Kerrison rongeurs may be used to excise more bone, if necessary. The technologist should have bone wax available at this time to aid in hemostasis.

The surgeon then uses a Penfield No. 3 or Sachs dura separator to loosen the dura from the skull. A Gigli saw guide and wire or Hall Neurairtome is used to cut the skull between the bur holes, thus creating the skull flap. The surgeon then wedges two periosteal elevators under the flap to lift it from the dura (Fig. 26–22). If any dura remains attached to the skull flap, a joker elevator may be used to release it. To retract and protect the flap, the surgeon may wrap it in wet 4 × 4-inch sponges, turn it back, and suture it to the scalp. The Weitlaner retractors are removed and replaced with Gelpi retractors. At this time Gelfoam and cottonoid sponges may be placed at the periphery of the open dura.

In preparation for entry into the brain tissue, the technologist should have a bipolar cautery unit and a No. 6 Frazier suction tip available. The surgeon may request the microscope at this time, as previously discussed. The surgeon uses a dura hook to lift the dura away from the brain and incises it with a No. 15 knife blade mounted on a No. 7 handle (Fig. 26–23). The incision is lengthened with Frazier dura or Lahey-Metzenbaum scissors and toothed Adson or Cushings tissue forceps. The technologist should have traction sutures available, size 4-0 Ethibond or silk, swaged to a fine needle or threaded in French-eye needles. These are used to retract and tack the dura away from the wound. The brain is now exposed.

In the event of tumor or other pathologic lesion, the surgeon uses brain spoons, curettes, and delicate rongeurs to remove the diseased tissue. The technologist

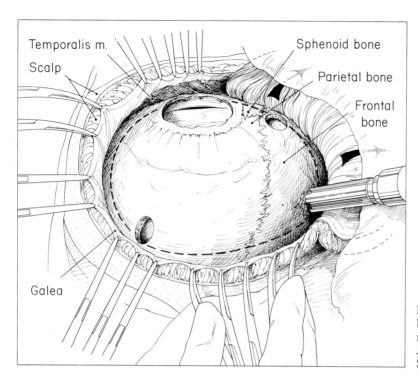

Figure 26–21. Craniotomy. A bone flap is created by drilling several bur holes, which are then "connected" with the saw or rongeur. (From Youmans J: Neurological Surgery, 2nd ed. Philadelphia, WB Saunders, 1982.)

should have irrigation available at all times during the procedure. A 30- or 50-mL syringe is used to contain the irrigation fluid. A variety of cottonoid sponges and topical hemostatic material should also be readily available to surgeons throughout the dissection of the brain tissue.

Following the removal of the lesion, the surgeon

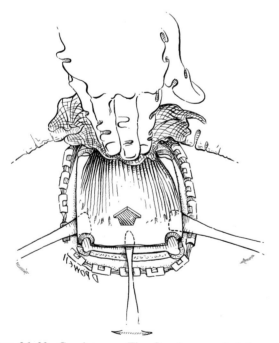

Figure 26–22. Craniotomy. The flap is separated from the dura mater with periosteal elevators and a joker elevator. (From Youmans J: Neurological Surgery, 2nd ed. Philadelphia, WB Saunders, 1982.)

irrigates the wound with antibiotic solution. The dura is then closed with fine Ethibond or silk sutures, although some surgeons prefer to leave the dura open. The surgeon then uses the craniotome to drill small holes in the bone flap and edges of the skull through which short lengths of No. 28 steel wire are passed, thereby reattaching the flap to the skull. A wire twister is used to snug the ends of the wire against the bone. Bur hole covers made of silicone, rubber, or metal are now applied over the previously made bur holes. The surgeon attaches the loose pericranium and galea over the bur holes and bone flap using No. 2-0 Vicryl or silk. The Raney clips or Kolodney clamps are then removed, and the muscle and subcutaneous layers are approximated with size 3-0 Vicryl, Dexon, or silk sutures. The skin is closed with size 4-0 synthetic suture (Ethiflex, silk, or other Dacron suture) mounted on a cutting needle.

Intracranial Aneurysm

An intracranial aneurysm is the outpocketing of an artery whose origin is the internal carotid or mid cerebral artery. The so-called berry aneurysm is located near the base of the brain at the circle of Willis, the most common site of an intracranial aneurysm.

Aneurysms are caused by a weakening of the arterial wall, usually due to a congenital defect. These aneurysms can range from the size of a pea to that of a baseball. As blood flows past the weakened area, it pushes on the vessel wall and causes subsequent thinning of the area. Sudden rupture and hemorrhage is the life-threatening result.

The aneurysm is approached through a standard suboccipital or subfrontal craniotomy, as previously de-

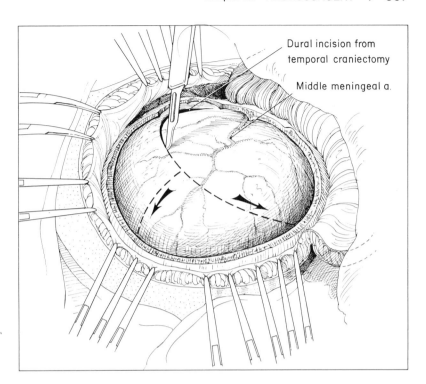

Figure 26–23. Craniotomy. The dura is incised with a No. 15 knife. (From Youmans J: Neurological Surgery, 2nd ed. Philadelphia, WB Saunders, 1982.)

scribed. The operating microscope is often used to locate the area of the aneurysm and to complete the procedure. Once the arachnoid tissues have been freed with delicate sharp dissection, the base of the aneurysm and often its "parent" or subbranches are occluded.

Occlusion is achieved with the use of aneurysm clips such as those illustrated in Figure 26–24 or by suture ligation. In some cases, methyl methacrylate or similiar epoxy is used to wrap the aneurytic area.

Intracranial Microneurosurgery

Advanced technology in lighting and magnification, afforded by the operating microscope, allows the neurosurgeon to perform intracranial microneurosurgery. A number of microprocedures have been developed.

Excision of an Acoustic Neuroma

Although removal of an acoustic neuroma through the middle fossa or labyrinth of the ear is performed by the otologist, the neurosurgeon can resect an acoustic

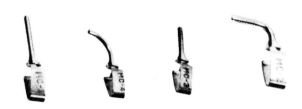

Figure 26–24. Aneurysm clips. (Courtesy of Codman and Shurtleff, Inc., Randolph, MA.)

neuroma that extends into the posterior fossa of the cranial cavity.

Decompression of Cranial Nerves

Microvascular decompression (release of pressure) of cranial nerves is performed to treat trigeminal neuralgia, glossopharyngeal neuralgia, and acoustic nerve dysfunction. In these conditions, an artery or small tumor may cause extreme pain or dysfunction.

During decompression surgery, a retromastoid (behind the mastoid bone) incision is used. The artery or vein that is the cause of some types of compression is freed from the nerve, or a small piece of Silastic sponge can be placed between the nerve and artery. If no decompression is found, the nerve may be removed to relieve pain.

Cerebral Revascularization

This is the anastomosis of an extracranial artery to an intracranial artery to bypass a stricture or blockage below the bifurcation of the common carotid artery. This bypass establishes increased blood flow to the cerebral circulation. An artery in the scalp is anastomosed to a branch of the middle cerebral artery. This procedure prevents a major stroke. If the diseased artery is blocked with plaque, the surgeon can remove the material from the cerebral artery rather than bypassing the artery altogether.

Excision of Arteriovenous Malformation

An arteriovenous malformation is an abnormal communication between the arteries and veins (called a fistula). As the connections become larger, under pressure, blood is diverted from surrounding brain tissue. When this occurs, multiple hemorrhages from the dilated blood vessels can cause seizures and subarachnoid hemorrhage. The goal of surgery is to resect the fistulas by coagulation or by application of ligation clips.

Bur Holes

The creation of bur holes is one of the steps performed during a craniotomy but can be a separate operative procedure. This procedure includes an incision of the scalp and underlying tissue and the creation of one or more holes in the skull, with possible entry into the tissues that lie directly beneath it.

The bur hole procedure is most commonly performed to treat brain abscess or subdural hematoma. Because the brain is encased in a rigid housing (the skull), any pressure exerted from within can potentially cause damage to the brain itself. Following traumatic head injury, one or more ruptured blood vessels may cause a hematoma to form under the dura. The goal, then, of bur hole surgery is to locate the hematoma, remove it, and thereby relieve the pressure.

The procedure is carried out as for a craniotomy to the level of the dura. If a hematoma is suspected, the technologist should have suction available and ample irrigation fluid to help clear the traumatized area of blood and tissue debris so that the bleeding area can be located and controlled. A typical subdural hematoma near the temporal lobe is illustrated in Figure 26–25.

Cranioplasty

Definition

This is the replacement of an area of bone in the skull with a methyl methacrylate plate, autograft, or metal prosthesis. Deformities in the skull resulting from trauma or disease may leave a portion of the brain and dura mater exposed. In these instances a prosthesis is used to cover the exposed area, protect it from injury, and improve the appearance. The use of methyl methacrylate is described below. Cranioplasty before and after surgery is illustrated in Figures 26–26 and 26–27.

Highlights

1. The scalp is incised.
2. If present, bone fragments are trimmed away.
3. A plate of methyl methacrylate is formed.
4. The plate is drilled and wired in place.
5. The wound is closed.

Description

The patient is positioned, prepped, and draped for access to a particular area of the skull. The scalp is incised over the defect, as for a craniotomy. Depending on the nature of the previous injury or disease, there may or may not be remnants of bone in the affected area. If bone fragments exist, the surgeon may use a rongeur to trim away the fragments. If the affected area is completely devoid of bone, the surgeon trims the

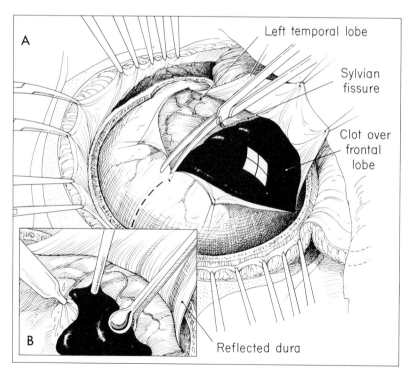

Figure 26–25. *A.* Subdural hematoma. *B.* After the dura is incised, the clot is gently removed by irrigation and suction. (From Youmans J: Neurological Surgery, 2nd ed. Philadelphia, WB Saunders, 1982.)

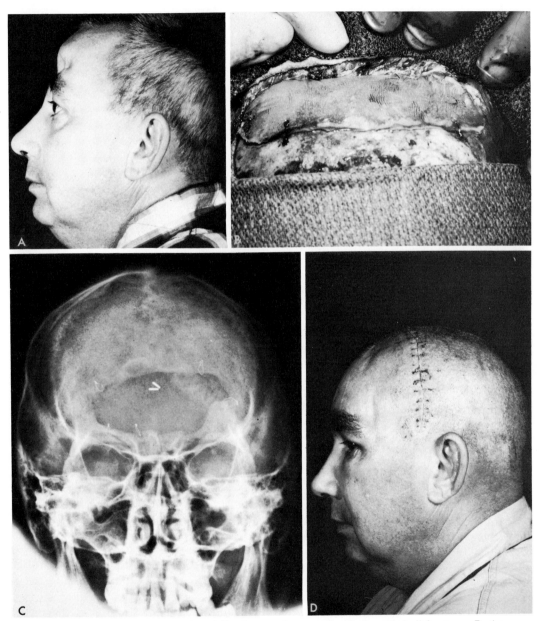

Figure 26–26. *A.* Frontal defect following craniectomy for depressed skull fracture. *B.* An acrylic plate has been wired into the defect (patient facing upward). *C.* Postoperative radiograph. *D.* Postoperative appearance of patient. (From Youmans J: Neurological Surgery, 2nd ed. Philadelphia, WB Saunders, 1982.)

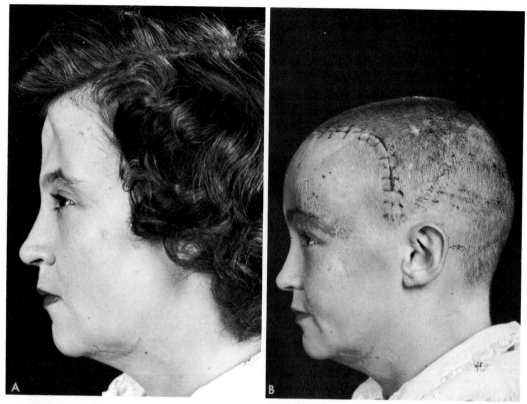

Figure 26–27. *A.* Frontal defect. *B.* Postoperative appearance after cranioplasty. (From Youmans J: Neurological Surgery, 2nd ed. Philadelphia, WB Saunders, 1982.)

periphery of the area with rongeurs to form a saucer-like ledge. This prevents the prosthesis from slipping below the level of the skull and aids in seating it in place. The technologist should retain all the bits of bone that are trimmed as specimen. Once the surgeon has completed this procedure, the wound is irrigated with warm saline solution. An antibiotic irrigant may also be used at this time.

The technologist prepares the methyl methacrylate, as described in Chapter 23. While the cement is still doughy, the surgeon may place it in a plastic bag. The mass is flattened out and molded over the cranial defect until it fits. The surgeon then removes the cement from the defect to allow it to harden. While the cement is drying and hardening, the technologist should prepare a dental or similar drill and fine drill point. Once the plate has hardened, the surgeon drills several holes in its edge. Similar holes are drilled at the periphery of the skull defect. Any rough spots in the plate are smoothed with the use of a large bur attached to a power drill or craniotome. The surgeon then fits the plate into the defect and secures it by passing fine stainless steel wires through the holes. The wound is then irrigated and closed in routine fashion.

Shunting Procedures

Definition

This is the diversion of cerebrospinal fluid away from the ventricles of the brain to another location in the body. The condition of *hydrocephalus* is a congenital anomaly that results in an increased amount of cerebrospinal fluid in the ventricles. This may be the result of overproduction of the fluid, or it may be a condition that interferes with the normal absorption of fluid. In selected cases, surgical intervention is aimed toward removing the excess fluid to relieve pressure on the brain.

Description

There are many different techniques employed in shunting procedures. The distal shunt may be placed in the atrium of the heart (ventriculoatrial shunt) or in the peritoneal cavity (ventriculoperitoneal shunt). The shunt may or may not contain a reservoir or flushing valve. Because of the many different types of shunts available from each manufacturer and, therefore, the different techniques associated with their use, it is best to read the manufacturer's specifications before the actual procedure is performed. As with all Silastic or other implant materials, the shunt should be handled carefully and protected from contamination by lint, dust, or glove powder. Specific guidelines on handling implant material are presented in Chapter 29.

Ventriculoatrial Shunt

During ventriculoatrial shunting, the proximal end of the shunt is positioned in the ventricle through a frontal bur hole. A second incision is made in the postauricular

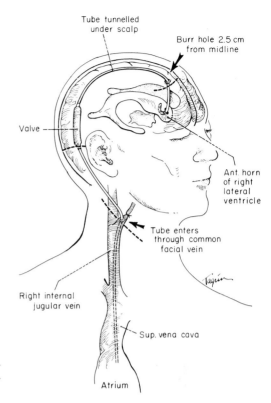

Figure 26–28. Insertion of ventriculoatrial shunt. Note three separate incisions—craniotomy, postauricular, and jugular. (From Youmans J: Neurological Surgery, 2nd ed. Philadelphia, WB Saunders, 1982.)

area, and the shunt is guided to the internal jugular vein (Fig. 26–28). The shunt is then threaded into the vein through a small incision and advanced to the atrium under fluoroscopy (the shunt is radiopaque).

Ventriculoperitoneal Shunt

During ventriculoperitoneal shunting, the proximal end of the shunt is placed in the peritoneal cavity, usually near the liver, through a tunnel made in the subcutaneous tissue. The tunnel may be made with uterine packing forceps or a tunneler, such as the one used during vascular surgery. All types of shunts may be revised as the patient grows and may require additional repair because of obstruction or mechanical failure.

Bibliography

Gardner E, Gray DJ, O'Rahilly R: Anatomy: A Regional Study of Human Structure, 4th ed. Philadelphia, WB Saunders, 1975.

Guyton AC: Basic Human Neurophysiology, 3rd ed. Philadelphia, WB Saunders, 1981.

Jacob S, Francone C, Lossow WJ: Structure and Function in Man, 5th ed. Philadelphia, WB Saunders, 1982.

McVay C: Surgical Anatomy, 6th ed. Philadelphia, WB Saunders, 1984.

Pleasants D: Managing hydrocephalus with a ventricular shunt. AORN J 35(5), 885–892, 1982.

Sabiston DC Jr (ed): Textbook of Surgery, 14th ed. Philadelphia, WB Saunders, 1991.

Williams RW: Surgical Techniques: Microlumbar Discectomy. Randolph, MA, Codman & Shurtleff, 1976.

Youmans J (ed): Neurological Surgery: A Comprehensive Reference Guide to the Diagnosis and Management of Neurosurgical Problems, 2nd ed. Philadelphia, WB Saunders, 1982.

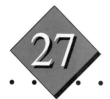

Eye Surgery

The goal of ophthalmic surgery is to restore vision lost from disease, injury, or congenital defect and to provide good cosmetic effect. Eye procedures are delicate and precise. In most cases surgeons prefer that talking and movement be kept to an absolute minimum during surgery. The patient about to undergo eye surgery may need extra comfort and emotional support if he or she is partially blind. Because most eye procedures are performed under a local anesthetic, the patient's physical comfort is of utmost importance. The technologist and nurse should pay strict attention to the position of the patient on the operating table to ensure that he or she does not become restless because of discomfort during the procedure.

SURGICAL ANATOMY

External Structures of the Eye

The external structures of the eye include the bony orbit, the ocular muscles, the eyelids, the conjunctiva, and the lacrimal apparatus.

The Bony Orbit

The *bony orbit* (also called the *orbital cavity*) (Fig. 27–1) houses the eye. It is situated in the front of the skull in the frontal bone. The cavity is lined with fatty tissue to provide cushioning for the eye. Although most of the orbit is composed of thin bone tissue, the *rim* is particularly thick and therefore more protective.

The Ocular Muscles

Six muscles attached to the sclera and the bony orbit move the eyeball around various axes and allow us to focus both eyes on one object. Each eye contains four *rectus* muscles—the superior, inferior, lateral, and medial—and two *oblique* muscles—the superior and inferior. The position of these muscles is shown in Figure 27–2.

The Eyelids

The eyelids are two plates of skin-covered tissue that open or close over the eye to protect it from injury, light, and dust. The space or interval between the upper and lower lids is called the *palpebral fissure*. At the inner corner, or *canthus*, lies a small pink mass of tissue called the *lacrimal caruncle*. This tissue contains sebaceous glands, which secrete oils. Along the free edge of the eyelids extends the *tarsal plate*, a fibrous tissue that gives the eyelids their characteristic shape. The *eyelashes*, which extend along the tarsus, protect the eye from dust and other pollutants and prevent perspiration from entering the eye from the forehead.

The Conjunctiva

The *conjunctiva* is a thin mucous membrane that lines each eyelid and is doubled back over the eyeball to protect it.

The Lacrimal Apparatus

The *lacrimal apparatus* (Fig. 27–3) is the eye's tear system. It is composed of several parts. The *lacrimal*

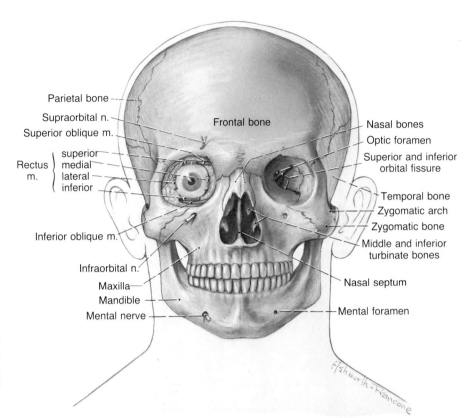

Figure 27–1. Anterior view of the skull showing bony orbit and relation of eye muscles to skull. (From Jacob S, Francone C, Lossow WJ: Structure and Function in Man, 5th ed. Philadelphia, WB Saunders, 1983.)

gland, located within the frontal bone at each angle of the orbit, secretes tears. The gland contains about 12 separate ducts, which supply tears to the conjunctiva. The *lacrimal ducts* (also called *lacrimal canaliculi*) extend from the inner canthus to the lacrimal sac. The opening of each duct is called the *lacrimal punctum.* The *lacrimal sac* is a large opening at the upper end of the *nasolacrimal duct,* which is a passageway between the lacrimal sac and the inferior meatus of the nose.

Internal Structures of the Eye

External Layers of the Eyeball

The eyeball contains several outer protective layers (Fig. 27–4): the sclera, cornea, ciliary body, choroid, and iris. The *sclera* is a thick white fibrous tissue that encompasses about three fourths of the eyeball. It is the external supportive structure of the eyeball and is continuous with the cornea, which covers the front of the eye.

The *cornea* is a fine, *transparent* membrane that covers the front of the eyeball. This layer contains no blood vessels and is the tissue that refracts light rays as they enter the eye.

The *choroid* layer is situated beneath the sclera and is a highly vascular, darkly pigmented tissue. The primary function of the choroid is to prevent the reflection of light within the eyeball. An extension of the choroid layer, the *ciliary body,* is located at the periphery of the anterior portion of the choroid. It consists of smooth muscle tissue from which suspensory ligaments are attached. These ligaments hold the lens in place. In addition, the *ciliary processes,* folds of tissue that attach to the internal portion of the ciliary body on the anterior side, produce *aqueous humor.* This is a fluid that fills the anterior and posterior chambers of the eye.

The *iris* or colored part of the eye is composed mainly of muscle tissue. The iris is circular and can close down or open up to exclude or admit light into the inner eye. The *pupil* lies at the center of the iris and may appear dilated or constricted according to the action of the iris.

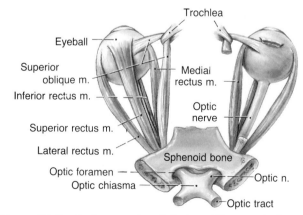

Figure 27–2. Ocular muscles (inferior oblique not shown). (From Jacob S, Francone C, Lossow WJ: Structure and Function in Man, 5th ed. Philadelphia, WB Saunders, 1982.)

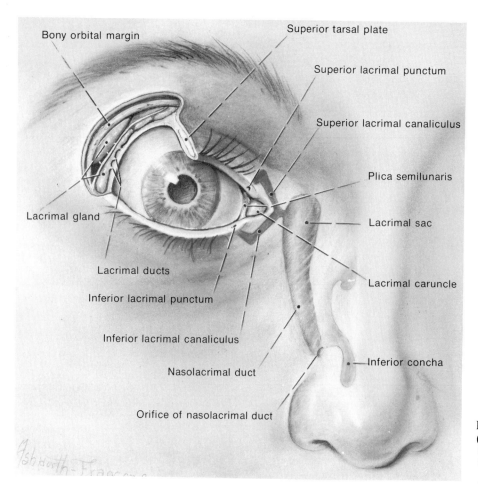

Bony orbital margin

Superior tarsal plate

Superior lacrimal punctum

Superior lacrimal canaliculus

Plica semilunaris

Lacrimal gland

Lacrimal sac

Lacrimal ducts

Lacrimal caruncle

Inferior lacrimal punctum

Inferior lacrimal canaliculus

Inferior concha

Nasolacrimal duct

Orifice of nasolacrimal duct

Figure 27–3. Lacrimal apparatus. (From Jacob S, Francone C, Lossow WJ: Structure and Function in Man, 5th ed. Philadelphia, WB Saunders, 1982.)

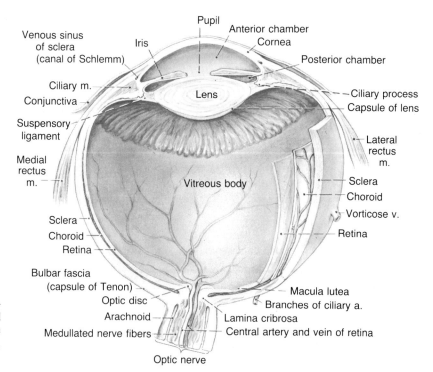

Venous sinus of sclera (canal of Schlemm)

Iris

Pupil

Anterior chamber

Cornea

Posterior chamber

Ciliary m.

Conjunctiva

Lens

Ciliary process

Capsule of lens

Suspensory ligament

Lateral rectus m.

Medial rectus m.

Vitreous body

Sclera

Choroid

Vorticose v.

Sclera

Choroid

Retina

Retina

Bulbar fascia (capsule of Tenon)

Optic disc

Arachnoid

Medullated nerve fibers

Macula lutea

Branches of ciliary a.

Lamina cribrosa

Central artery and vein of retina

Optic nerve

Figure 27–4. Midsagittal section through eyeball showing protective and visual layers and associated structures. (From Jacob S, Francone C, Lossow WJ: Structure and Function in Man, 5th ed. Philadelphia, WB Saunders, 1982.)

The inner layer of the eye is called the *retina*. This is the so-called photoreceptive layer of the eye. It lies on the inside posterior wall of the eyeball. Light is reflected onto the retina through the front of the eye where it is transmitted into nervous impulses, creating sight.

The Eye's Chambers

The eye contains several chambers that are filled with nourishing fluids. The iris divides two chambers that lie in front of the lens. The *anterior chamber* lies directly *in* front of the iris, whereas the *posterior chamber* lies directly behind the iris. Both of these chambers are filled with aqueous humor (Fig. 27–5), which is secreted by the ciliary processes. Because this fluid is continually produced, it must have an exit route from the internal eye. The *canal of Schlemm* is this exit. This canal is located within the sclera and shunts the fluid directly into the venous system.

The large posterior cavity of the eyeball, located behind the lens, is filled with a jelly-like substance called *vitreous humor*. This substance is vital to maintaining the shape of the eyeball.

The Lens

The *lens* lies directly behind the iris and is a biconvex clear structure that is encompassed by a transparent *capsule*. It is held in place by suspensory ligaments attached to the capsule. This area of suspension is the junction where the ciliary body and the choroid meet. The suspensory ligaments change the shape of the lens to bend light that passes through it and to focus images projected onto the retina.

SPECIAL EQUIPMENT

The Operating Microscope

The operating microscope (Fig. 27–6) allows the surgeon to operate on structures too small to be viewed effectively with the naked eye. Certain components of the microscope are important to understand because surgical personnel are responsible for their care and assembly.

The microscope's optical system has two main components—the *objective* lens and the *ocular* lens. The objective lens is closest to the object being viewed. The ocular lens magnifies the image on the objective lens. In the operating microscope there are two ocular lenses, one for each eye; thus, it is a *binocular* system. Each ocular lens is called an *eyepiece*. The total magnification of the subject can be calculated by multiplying the magnification of the ocular lens by that of the objective lens. To provide a range of magnification, the operating microscope has *interchangeable ocular* and *objective lenses*. Most operating microscopes have a *zoom lens*. This is a set of lenses that lie between the ocular lenses (eyepieces) and the objective lens that allows the surgeon to increase or decrease the magnification within the ranges allowed by the ocular and objective lenses.

The source of light used by the operating microscope can be fiberoptic, halogen, or tungsten. When the system is fiberoptic, the intense light is cool. Other sources of light require a *filter* in the system to prevent tissue burn. The light generated by the microscope is focused on the subject in the same way that the image is focused. The surgeon operates the microscope's focusing system by a foot pedal or by hand.

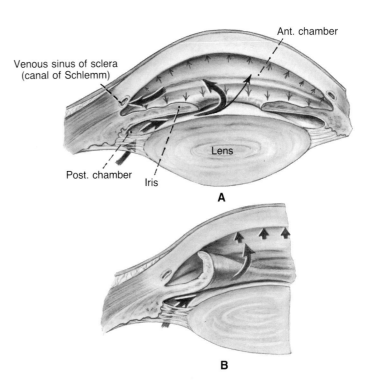

Figure 27–5. *A.* Normal flow of aqueous humor through eye. *B.* Blockage of flow, causing acute glaucoma. (From Jacob S, Francone C, Lossow WJ: Structure and Function in Man, 5th ed. Philadelphia, WB Saunders, 1982.)

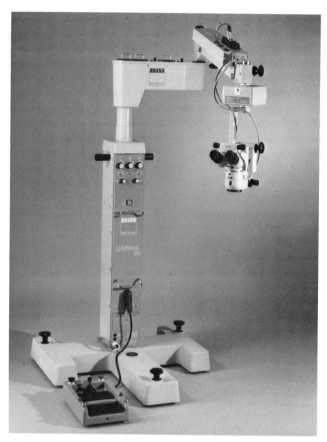

Figure 27–6. The new OPMI MDO for the Ultimate Red Reflex. (Courtesy of Carl Zeiss, Inc., Thornwood, NY.)

Accessory Equipment

The *assistant binoculars* contain a separate ocular system that is not connected to the motorized focus control. This second set of lenses allows the surgical assistant to view the subject and to assist appropriately.

The *foot pedals* allow the surgeon to adjust the focus, zoom mechanism, and angle of view.

The *laser adapter* allows the laser to be used in conjunction with the microscope. The microscope and laser head couplings must be securely and exactly aligned. The adapter's lens must be compatible with that of the microscope.

Draping the microscope is accomplished with single-use, nonwoven drapes that are lint free, heat resistant, and transparent. Sterile lens covers that secure the drape to the ocular lens are available.

Care and Handling

Lenses

The microscope lenses are made of high-quality ground glass and must be carefully handled. When changing or cleaning the lenses, the technologist should avoid touching the lens surface with any object that might scratch or mar it. To prevent skin oils from soiling the lens surface, the lens should be handled by the edges only. Lens should be cleaned only with an agent recommended by the manufacturer and should be stored properly in their case when not in use.

Electrical Components

Cords, plugs, and electrical adapters should be checked before the microscope is used. Power cords should be protected from pressure and stored in a loose coil when not in use. Spare lamps and fuses should be available during all procedures. The power source should be turned off when light bulbs are being changed.

Changing the Observation Tubes and Eyepieces

The observation tube should always be carried with both hands so that it is not dropped. When the eyepieces are changed, the eyepiece should be fit in slowly. If the fitting is threaded, it should be turned gently to avoid stripping the threads. An eyepiece must never be jammed in place because this could severely damage it.

Cleaning and Storage

The microscope housing should be damp-dusted before each procedure. A cleaning product recommended by the manufacturer should be used. When not in use, the microscope should be protected with a dust cover and stored with all protective coverings and caps in place in an area that is free of excessive traffic.

Sutures

Eye sutures are available in a wide range of materials in sizes from 4-0 to 12-0. These delicate sutures must be handled gently and carefully, since they are costly to the patient. The sutures should be handled as little as possible, and the points should be protected from injury. Eye suture-needle combinations are available as *single-arm* (one needle swaged to a strand of suture) or *double-arm* (one needle attached to each end of the suture length). The surgeon will specify a preference for single- or double-arm suture, either verbally or on the surgeon's preference card (see Chapter 16).

Sponges

Ophthalmic sponges (Fig. 27–7) are spear shaped and are made of lint-free cellulose material. These are available mounted on a plastic rod, or the technologist may be required to mount them on a mosquito hemostat for use. During surgery they are used to wipe away excess fluids or blood.

Cautery Unit

The ophthalmic cautery unit (Fig. 27–8) is a hand-held single-use item powered by household batteries.

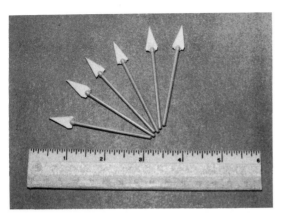

Figure 27–7. Cellulose sponges used in eye surgery. (Scale shown is in inches.)

Note that the unit must *not* be resterilized and used again unless the manufacturer specifies that it is safe to do so. The unit could malfunction after sterilization and cause injury to the patient.

Ophthalmic Instruments

Instruments used during eye surgery are delicate and costly. Special care must be taken by all surgical personnel to ensure that the edges and tips are not dulled or damaged from careless handling. In most operating rooms, the instruments should be cleaned individually by hand, a practice that is discouraged for other types of instruments. Ideally, the instruments should be gas sterilized to preserve the sharp and delicate edges. However, this may not be practical because many eye surgeons bring their own personal instruments to surgery and, in such cases, the instruments must be flash sterilized before surgery. During surgery the instruments can be placed on a rolled towel on the Mayo stand to protect the tips. The following are instruments that are usually included in a basic eye tray:

Speculums
Medicine glasses
Iris retractors
Muscle hooks
Lens scoop and spoon spatula
Needle holders
Irrigation tips
Corneal forceps
Tying forceps
Curved and straight iris scissors
Curved and straight tenotomy scissors
Corneal scissors, right and left
Olive-tip needle
30-gauge irrigating needle
Toothed and smooth Bishop-Harmon
    forceps
Scleral forceps
Van Ness iridotomy scissors
Suture scissors

Nos. 3 and 7 knife handles
Assorted Luer-Lok glass syringes

SPECIAL MEDICATIONS

During eye surgery there are a variety of medications used. These include anesthetics, antibiotics, anti-inflammatory agents, diagnostic agents, enzymatics, irrigants, mitotics (agents that constrict the pupil), and mydriatics (agents that dilate the pupil). A list of these agents and their uses is presented in Table 27–1.

SURGICAL PROCEDURES

The surgeons operate while seated at the patient's head. The technologist should sit to the right or left of the surgeon with the Mayo stand positioned over the patient's chest. *Care must be taken that the Mayo tray does not come in contact with the patient.* It is most important for the field to be kept free of lint, particularly the instruments themselves. Many surgeons prefer the use of nonfabric drapes to minimize the presence of lint. Also, a soft moist chamois should be available for wiping the instruments clean during surgery.

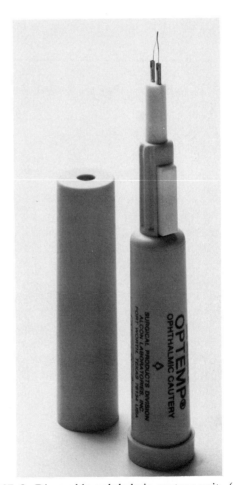

Figure 27–8. Disposable ophthalmic cautery unit. (Courtesy of Alcon Laboratories, Inc., Fort Worth, TX.)

Table 27–1. DRUGS USED IN OPHTHALMIC SURGERY

Generic Name	Trade Name	Action/Use
Anesthetics		
Lidocaine hydrochloride	Xylocaine	Local anesthetic for infiltration
Procaine hydrochloride	Novocain	Local anesthetic for infiltration
Proparacaine hydrochloride	Ophthaine	Topical anesthetic
Tetracaine hydrochloride	Pontocaine	Topical anesthetic
Antibiotics		
Chloramphenicol	Chloromycetin	All used to prevent or treat infection
Neomycin	Mycifradin	
Polymyxin B-neomycin-bacitracin	Neosporin	
Polymyxin B sulfate	Aerosporin	
Sulfisoxazole	Gantrisin	
Anti-Inflammatory Agents		
Betamethasone	Celestan	All reduce inflammation and help prevent edema
Dexamethasone	Decasone	
Fludrocortisone acetate	Scherofluron	
Diagnostic		
Fluorescein sodium	Fluorescein	Used to stain the cornea. Any interruption in the normal surface of the cornea is revealed under ultraviolet light.
Enzymatic		
Chymotrypsin	Quimotrase Zolyse Alpha-Chymar	Used during cataract surgery to dissolve the zonules that attach to the lens of the eye
Hyaluronidase	Wydase	Mixed with anesthetic solution to increase diffusion of anesthetic through tissue and improve efficacy of nerve block
Irrigants		
Balanced saline solution	Tis-U-Sol	Used to keep eye tissue moist during surgery
Lactated Ringer's solution		
Lubricant		
Sodium hyaluronate	Healon Amvisc Viscot	Used as a lubricant and as a viscoelastic support to maintain separation between tissues. During intraocular procedures it protects corneal endothelium. During retina and vitreous procedures it is used as a tamponade and vitreous substitute.
Mitotics		
Acetylcholine chloride, intraocular	Miochol	Used to constrict the pupil to reduce intraocular pressure; in cataract surgery used to help prevent loss of vitreous
Pilocarpine hydrochloride	Almocarpine	
Mydriatics		
Atropine sulfate	Atropisol	Cause the pupil to dilate; facilitate examination of the retina and lens removal
Cyclopentolate hydrochloride	Cyclogyl	
Phenylephrine hydrochloride	Neo-Synephrine	
Tropicamide	Mydriacyl	

Excision of Pterygium

Definition

This is the removal of elastic degenerative tissue that slowly proliferates from the conjunctiva to the front of the cornea. A pterygium originates from a pinguecula (inherited benign elastic nodule) in response to irritation. All pterygia need not be removed surgically—only those that show documented growth, periodic inflammation, a marked cosmetic defect, induction of progressive astigmatism, interference with vision, or interference with motility of the globe.

Highlights

1. The neck of the pterygium is incised.
2. The conjunctiva is incised, and scar tissue is removed.
3. The head of the pterygium is dissected.
4. The conjunctiva is closed.

Description

The patient is usually brought into the hospital the morning of surgery and the procedure is performed as a "come and go" case. This means that the patient is only mildly sedated and may leave the hospital a few hours after surgery, without being admitted to the hospital.

The patient is placed in the supine position with the head stabilized on a head rest. The circulator instills tetracaine ophthalmic anesthetic drops to the operative eye. The eye prep (discussed in Chapter 11) extends from the hairline to the mouth and from the nose to the ear. The eye is draped as described in Chapter 11.

The surgeon inserts an eye speculum and administers local anesthetic directly into the conjunctival tissue around the pterygium using 1% lidocaine with epinephrine in a 3-mL syringe fitted with a ½-inch 27-gauge needle. The surgeon may or may not utilize a bridle (traction) suture for immobilization. The technologist should pass toothed tissue forceps and Westcott scissors to the surgeon. The surgeon then incises the neck of the pterygium parallel to the limbus (Fig. 27–9A). The conjunctiva is then incised along both sides of the pterygium (Fig. 27–9B), and any scar tissue is dissected and removed. The technologist retains the scar tissue as a specimen. The surgeon then dissects the base of the pterygium, taking special care to avoid cutting into the medial rectus muscle, which is just beneath the scar tissue (Fig. 27–9C). Using a No. 3 knife handle with a No. 15 blade or a Beaver handle with a No. 64 blade, the surgeon dissects the head of the pterygium from the cornea and scrapes the denuded area with the blade exactly horizontal to the cornea (Fig. 27–9D). The conjunctiva is pulled over the exposed area (Fig. 27–9E) and secured with interrupted sutures of size 5-0 Dexon or 6-0 silk, according to the surgeon's preference.

The speculum and bridle suture (if used) are removed, and an antibiotic ointment such as polymyxin B-bacitracin-neomycin (Neosporin) is applied to the eye. Many patients receive postoperative beta radiation on the site to prevent the reoccurrence of a pterygium.

Repair of Entropion

Definition

Entropion is the abnormal inversion of the lower eyelid. This causes the eyelashes to rub on the cornea, resulting in irritation and pain. The condition is caused by injury or the aging process.

Highlights

1. The lid is retracted.
2. A triangular incision is made into the lid.
3. The lid is sutured closed.

Description

In preparation for this procedure, the technologist should have chalazion clamps, dye marking pen, calipers, and a metal ruler available. A large package of sterile cotton-tipped applicators is necessary, along with a basic eye soft tissue set. The procedure is commonly performed under local anesthesia. A solution of 1% lidocaine with epinephrine is usually injected with a 5-mL syringe and a ½-inch 27-gauge needle.

The patient is placed in the supine position with the head stabilized on a doughnut-type head rest. Before the procedure begins, the circulator instills tetracaine ophthalmic drops to the operative eye. The eye is then prepped and draped, as discussed previously (see Chapter 11).

The surgeon usually sits on the side of the operative eye. If both eyes are operated on, he or she switches sides when the first side has been completed.

The most common and successful surgical procedure for the treatment of entropion is the excision of a base-down tarsoconjunctival triangle (Fig. 27–10A). The surgeon retracts the lid with a chalazion clamp (Fig. 27–10A). The surgeon may wish to mark out the triangle with a dye marking pen before making the incision. The incision is made with a No. 15 Bard Parker blade mounted on a No. 3 handle. Straight iris scissors may be used to free the tissue excised by the scalpel. Small bleeders are controlled with the electrocautery pencil.

During the procedure the technologist is usually asked to dry the site when necessary with a cotton-tipped applicator. He or she may also be required to irrigate the cornea to prevent it from drying out. Because the surgeon is busy with the surgery, the technologist should be conscious of the need for this and should irrigate when necessary.

Once the triangle has been excised, the technologist should pass three or four interrupted absorbable sutures size 5-0 or 6-0 swaged to spatula-type needles to the surgeon. The surgeon places each suture one at a time with the aid of smooth tissue forceps and leaves the suture ends untied (see Fig. 27–10B). When the last suture is placed, the technologist should pass tying forceps so that the surgeon can tie the sutures in place (see Fig. 27–10C). The technologist may be required to cut the knots very short to prevent any further irritation to the cornea.

When hemostasis is maintained, the surgeon releases the chalazion clamp and instills an antibiotic ointment to the eye. The eye is dressed with a cotton eye patch, which is then taped in place.

Repair of Ectropion

Definition

Ectropion is the abnormal sagging of the lower eyelid away from the eye. A major concern for the patient with ectropion is the overflow of tears down the patient's face. In addition, the exposed conjunctiva may become irritated. The goal of surgical treatment is to provide proper tear drainage and good cosmetic appearance.

Highlights

1. A triangular tissue specimen is removed from the lower lid.
2. The lid is closed.

Description

As for repair of entropion, the technologist should have a basic soft tissue eye set, cotton-tipped applicators, metal ruler, caliper, and marking pen available. The eye prep, draping, and anesthetic are the same as for entropion repair.

To begin the procedure, the surgeon usually marks the area of incision in the lid with a marking pen (Fig. 27–11A). The technologist should pass a fine-toothed forcep and either a No. 15 knife blade or a straight tenotomy scissor. The surgeon then excises the tissue (Fig. 27–11B) and cauterizes any small bleeding vessels with the hand-held cautery unit. The technologist is

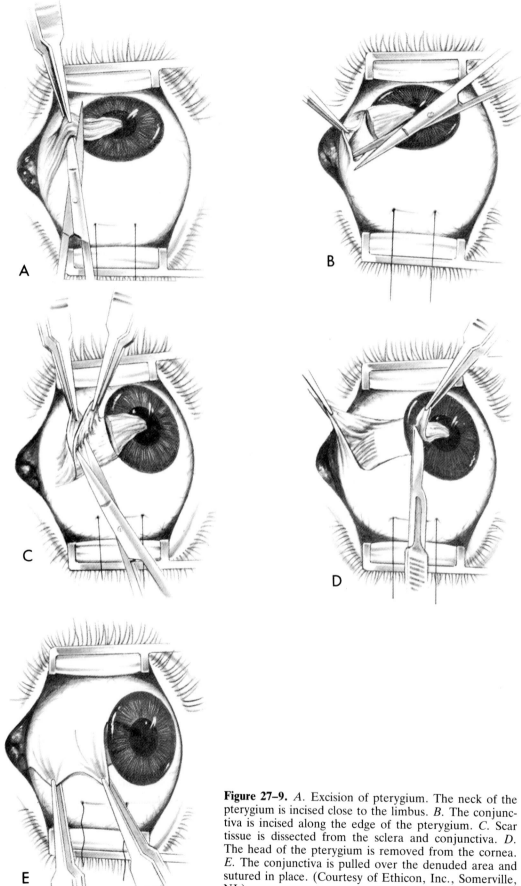

Figure 27–9. *A.* Excision of pterygium. The neck of the pterygium is incised close to the limbus. *B.* The conjunctiva is incised along the edge of the pterygium. *C.* Scar tissue is dissected from the sclera and conjunctiva. *D.* The head of the pterygium is removed from the cornea. *E.* The conjunctiva is pulled over the denuded area and sutured in place. (Courtesy of Ethicon, Inc., Somerville, NJ.)

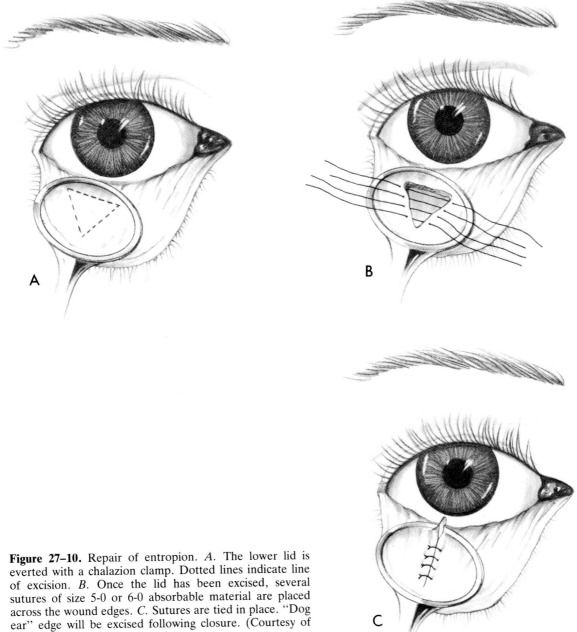

Figure 27–10. Repair of entropion. *A.* The lower lid is everted with a chalazion clamp. Dotted lines indicate line of excision. *B.* Once the lid has been excised, several sutures of size 5-0 or 6-0 absorbable material are placed across the wound edges. *C.* Sutures are tied in place. "Dog ear" edge will be excised following closure. (Courtesy of Ethicon, Inc., Somerville, NJ.)

required to irrigate the cornea and blot any excess blood or irrigation fluid as necessary.

To begin the closure, the surgeon places one or more sutures of size 4-0 absorbable suture swaged to a spatula-type needle through the tarsal plate and canthal ligament. This prevents the ectropion from recurrence (Fig. 27–11*C*). The surgeon then closes the deep tissue layers with several size 4-0 or 5-0 absorbable sutures (Fig. 27–11*D*). After the deeper layers are closed, the technologist should pass several interrupted sutures of size 5-0 or 6-0 silk swaged to cutting needles for skin closure (Fig. 27–11*E*). Fine-toothed tissue forceps are used in skin closure. At the completion of the procedure, the surgeon instills antibiotic ophthalmic ointment to the eye. The surgeon may or may not wish to patch the eye.

Note: There are many procedures and techniques for ectropion surgery, and the technologist should study the particular techniques used by his or her surgeons.

External Levator Resection for Ptosis

Definition

Ptosis is the abnormal drooping of the upper eyelid. This condition may be caused by deficient nerve stimulation, lack of muscle strength, or paralysis of the levator palpebrae muscle. The goal of ptosis surgery is to resect the levator tissues to correct the patient's vision and to produce good cosmetic effect.

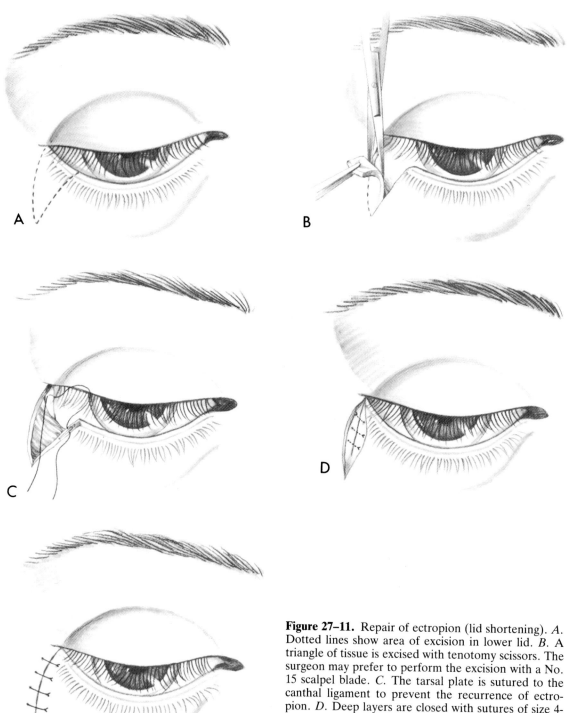

Figure 27–11. Repair of ectropion (lid shortening). *A.* Dotted lines show area of excision in lower lid. *B.* A triangle of tissue is excised with tenotomy scissors. The surgeon may prefer to perform the excision with a No. 15 scalpel blade. *C.* The tarsal plate is sutured to the canthal ligament to prevent the recurrence of ectropion. *D.* Deep layers are closed with sutures of size 4-0 synthetic absorbable suture or catgut. *E.* Skin is closed with size 5-0 or 6-0 silk or nylon. (Courtesy of Ethicon, Inc., Somerville, NJ.)

Highlights

1. A skin incision is made just below the upper tarsal border.
2. The levator muscle is exposed and clamped.
3. The muscle is incised.
4. The conjunctiva is separated from the muscle and sutured to the tarsus.
5. The levator muscle is sutured to the tarsus.
6. The skin incision is closed.

Description

In preparation for this procedure, the technologist should have available a basic eye muscle tray, skin hooks, selected muscle clamps, a caliper, a metal ruler, cotton-tipped applicators, and surgical loupes for the surgeon (if requested).

The patient is placed in the supine position with the head stabilized on a head rest. The operative eye is prepped and draped in routine fashion. A general anesthetic may be administered, although local anesthesia may be used on selected patients.

To begin the procedure, the surgeon places two skin hooks just above the eyelashes. The assistant uses these to retract the lid. When an assistant is *not* available, the technologist is required to retract during the procedure. If this is the case, the Mayo tray should be neatly organized with all instruments readily available so that the surgeon may locate them. The surgeon then incises the upper eyelid (Fig. 27–12*A*) from canthus to canthus. Straight tenotomy scissors and fine-toothed forceps are used to separate the pretarsal levator fibers from the fascia (Fig. 12–12*B*). The technologist is required to irrigate the surgical site frequently so that the anatomy is clearly visible to the surgeon. The cautery unit and cotton-tipped applicators are used to control excess bleeding.

The dissection is continued to expose the orbital fat. The surgeon then places a muscle clamp across the levator muscle (Fig. 27–12*C*). The muscle is then released from its attachments with the scalpel (Fig. 27–12*D*). The surgeon separates the conjunctiva from Müller's muscle using tenotomy scissors. With the use of a continuous suture of Dexon, size 5-0 or 6-0, Müller's muscle is sutured to the upper portion of the tarsus (Fig. 27–12*E*).

The technologist now passes a double-arm silk suture, size 5-0 to 6-0, which the surgeon uses to suture the levator to the tarsus (Fig. 27–12*F*). Additional sutures of the same material are now placed in the levator to secure it to the tarsus, and the excess levator is resected

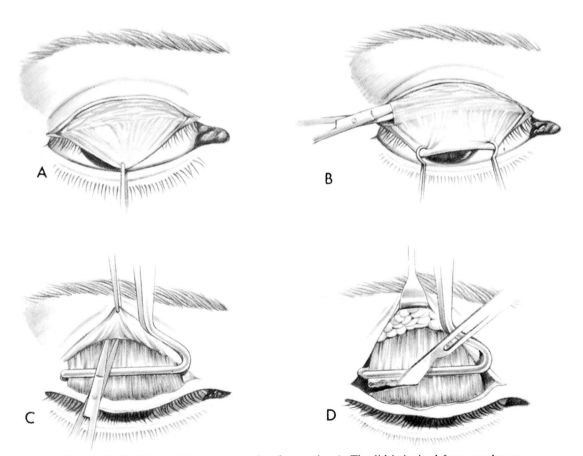

Figure 27–12. External levator resection for ptosis. *A.* The lid is incised from canthus to canthus. *B.* Tenotomy scissors are used to separate the pretarsal levator fibers from the fascia. *C.* A muscle clamp or ptosis clamp is placed across the muscle. *D.* The muscle is released from its attachment with the scalpel.

Illustration continued on following page

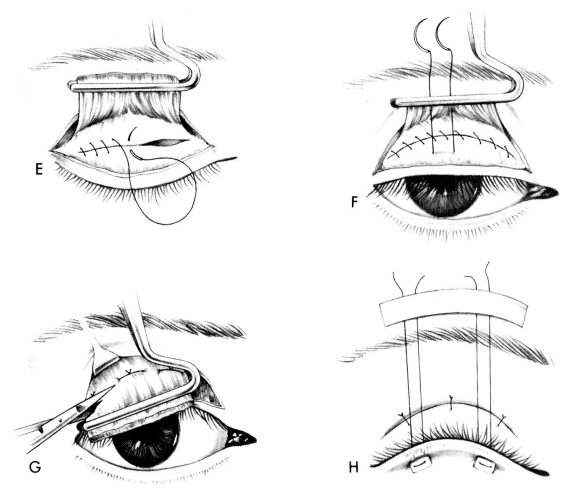

Figure 27–12 *Continued. E.* The conjunctiva is separated from Müller's muscle, and the muscle is sutured to the tarsus. *F.* A double-arm suture is used to suture the levator muscle to the tarsus. *G.* The excess levator muscle is resected. *H.* Additional sutures are placed in the lid and taped to the patient's forehead to prevent stress on the lid. (Courtesy of Ethicon, Inc., Somerville, NJ.)

(Fig. 27–12*G*). The muscle specimen is retained by the technologist as a specimen.

The skin incision is closed with silk or nylon sutures, size 5-0 to 8-0, according to the surgeon's preference. The surgeon may place two temporary fine silk sutures through the lid margin and tape the ends to the patient's forehead to prevent stress on the lid for a short time after surgery (Fig. 27–12*H*). An antibiotic ointment is then instilled, and the eye is closed and dressed with a cotton eye pad and metal Fox shield. A Telfa dressing may be placed over the skin incision and taped in place.

Muscle Surgery: Lateral Rectus Resection and Medial Rectus Recession

Definition

Muscle surgery is performed to correct a condition called *strabismus* in which the eye (or eyes) cannot focus on an object because the muscles lack coordination.

One eye (the fixing eye) looks directly at the object of attention; the other eye (the deviating eye) does not. There are two surgical procedures commonly performed to treat strabismus. In lateral rectus *resection,* a portion of the muscle is excised and the severed end is reattached at the original point of insertion. In medial rectus *recession,* the muscle is severed at the point of insertion and sutured to a point farther back. This allows the eye to move further laterally.

In preparation for either type of muscle surgery, the technologist should have some special instruments available. These include calipers, a metal ruler to check the accuracy of the caliper, at least four muscle hooks of the surgeon's choice, a marking pen, two straight mosquito hemostats, two curved mosquito hemostats, assorted muscle clamps, and a large pack of cotton-tipped applicators.

Highlights: Lateral Rectus Resection

1. The conjunctiva is incised.
2. A portion of the lateral rectus muscle is excised,

and the severed end is attached at the point of its original insertion.

3. The conjunctiva is closed.

Description: Lateral Rectus Resection

The patient is placed in the supine position, and the head is stabilized on a head rest. Before the prep, the circulator instills tetracaine ophthalmic drops to the operative eye. Following the administration of a general anesthetic, the eye is prepped and draped in routine fashion. The surgeon may wish to use a retrobulbar injection (see the discussion of enucleation) in addition to the general anesthetic. The surgeon usually sits on the operative side facing the assistant.

To begin the procedure, the surgeon inserts an eye speculum. To expose the lateral rectus muscle, he or she makes an incision in the conjunctiva at the limbus with Westcott scissors and Bishop forceps. The assistant

grasps the eye with a scleral biting forcep and rotates it as far medially as possible for better exposure. The surgeon may place two size 4-0 silk traction sutures in the conjunctiva at this time.

The conjunctiva is freed from the underlying tissue by blunt and sharp dissection and is carried back over the muscle. The surgeon then locates the muscle insertion and passes a muscle hook under it to ensure that it is free of adhesions. During the procedure the technologist must occasionally irrigate the eye and wipe away any excess fluids with cotton-tipped applicators. The surgeon then uses a caliper that has previously been adjusted to measure the amount of muscle to be excised (Fig. 27–13A). A muscle clamp is placed over the rectus muscle, and the measured portion is excised with straight tenotomy scissors. The portion of muscle is passed to the technologist, who retains it as a specimen.

The surgeon then reattaches the end of the muscle to the original insertion point with a double-arm suture of

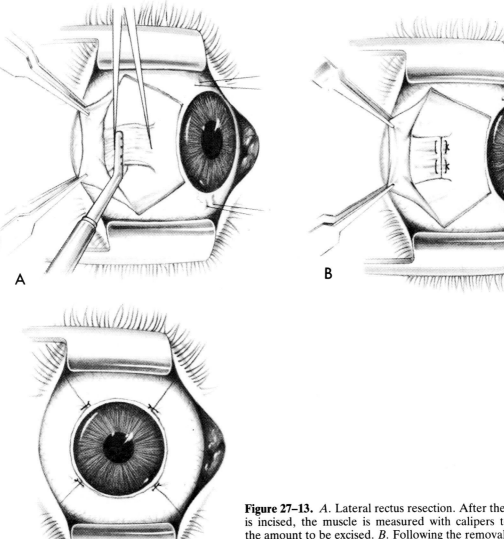

Figure 27–13. *A.* Lateral rectus resection. After the conjunctiva is incised, the muscle is measured with calipers to determine the amount to be excised. *B.* Following the removal of a section of muscle, the end of the muscle is reattached at the original insertion point. *C.* The conjunctival incisions are closed with absorbable sutures. (Courtesy of Ethicon, Inc., Somerville, NJ.)

size 5-0 or 6-0 Dexon, chromic catgut, or Vicryl (Fig. 27–13*B*). After all bleeding vessels have been controlled with the cautery pencil, the conjunctival incision is closed with size 5-0 or 6-0 absorbable suture of the surgeon's choice (Fig. 27–13*C*). An antibiotic ophthalmic ointment is instilled and the eye is dressed with a cotton eye pad and metal Fox shield.

Highlights: Medial Rectus Recession

1. The conjunctiva is incised.
2. The medial rectus muscle is detached from its insertion, moved posteriorly, and reattached.
3. The conjunctiva is closed.

Description: Medial Rectus Recession

The procedure for medial rectus recession is identical to that for lateral rectus resection to the point of the conjunctival incision (Fig. 27–14*A*). The surgeon uses tenotomy scissors to undermine the conjunctiva. Using a previously adjusted caliper, the surgeon measures the distance from the original insertion point to its new one. The surgeon may wish to mark the new insertion point with a marking pen.

The surgeon now places two sutures of size 5-0 or 6-0 absorbable material at the end of the muscle but does not tie them (Fig. 27–14*B*). A straight mosquito hemostat may be placed across the muscle between the sutures and the insertion point. The clamp is allowed to remain on the muscle for up to 3 minutes. This crushes tiny vessels that would otherwise bleed profusely when the muscle is severed. The clamp is removed and the technologist passes a muscle hook, which the surgeon places under the muscle to elevate it away from the globe. The surgeon then incises the muscle with a straight iris scissor. At this point the cautery pencil may be necessary to ensure hemostasis.

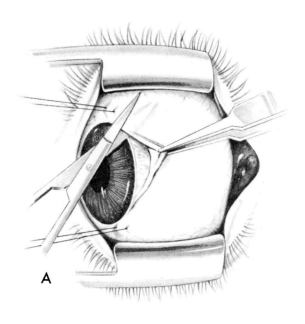

A

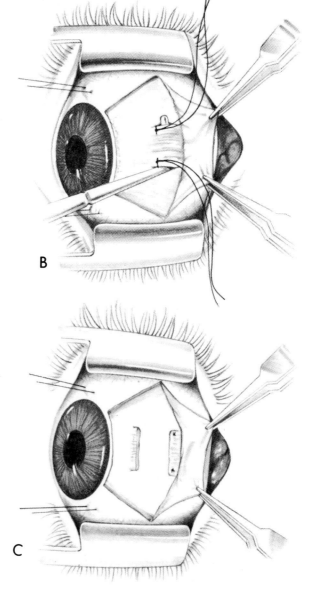

B

C

Figure 27–14. *A.* Medial rectus resection. The conjunctiva is incised close to the limbus to expose the medial rectus muscle. *B.* A muscle hook is placed beneath the muscle, and two sutures are placed at the borders. *C.* The muscle is attached to a premeasured location further back on the globe. (Courtesy of Ethicon, Inc., Somerville, NJ.)

The technologist now passes an empty needle holder and smooth tissue forceps to the surgeon, who moves the muscle back to the dye marks and sutures it at its new location with the previously placed muscle sutures (Fig. 27–14C). The conjunctival incision is closed with size 5-0 or 6-0 absorbable sutures swaged to a spatula needle. An antibiotic ophthalmic ointment is instilled, and the eye is dressed with a cotton eye pad and metal Fox shield.

Dacryocystorhinostomy for Lacrimal Blockage

Definition

This is the creation of a new, larger opening between the lacrimal sac and the nasal sinus. Candidates for this procedure are those who suffer from chronic dacryocystitis and have not responded to the clinical treatments of lacrimal probing and irrigation. The goal of surgery is to create a permanent opening in the tear duct for the drainage of tears. Many surgeons are assisted during this surgery by an ear, nose, and throat surgeon because the nasal structures are involved.

Highlights

1. The skin is incised over the lacrimal sac.
2. The lacrimal sac is exposed.
3. The lacrimal bone is penetrated.
4. The lacrimal sac flaps are sutured to the nasal mucosa.
5. A petrolatum pack is placed in the nasal passage and into the bony antrum.
6. The incisions are closed.

Description

In preparation for this procedure, the technologist should have the following instruments available:

Basic soft tissue instruments
Freer elevators
Power drill, such as the Hall or Stryker drill
Bayonet forceps
Small Kerrison rongeurs
Nos. 3 and 7 knife handles with Nos. 15 and 11 blades
Irrigation tips and assorted syringes, sizes 3, 5, and 10mL
A hand-held cautery unit
Frazier suction tips
Small rake retractors, such as Senn retractors
Lacrimal probes and dilators
A nasal speculum
Small malleable (ribbon) retractors

The patient is placed in the supine position with the head stabilized on a small doughnut head rest. Before the patient prep, the surgeon usually packs the nasal airway with gauze packing that has been impregnated with Neo-Synephrine. This packing helps to maintain hemostasis during the procedure. The circulator then preps the patient's entire face from the hairline to the chin and from ear to ear. The operative eye is then draped, as described in Chapter 11.

To begin the procedure, the surgeon makes a small incision over the lacrimal sac using a No. 15 knife blade (Fig. 27–15A). Small bleeding vessels are cauterized. The periosteum is then incised, and the surgeon uses a Freer elevator to elevate the periosteum, exposing the sac. Small rake retractors are placed at the wound edge (Fig. 27–15B). The lacrimal sac is elevated from its bed with the elevator and retracted back with a small malleable retractor. The technologist should then pass the power drill with a medium-sized ball bur to the surgeon and a bulb syringe filled with irrigation fluid to the assistant. The technologist may be asked to suction bits of bone with the Frazier suction tip while the surgeon drills the anterior lacrimal crest.

The surgeon then removes the nasal packing, using bayonet forceps. A Kerrison rongeur is used to enlarge the hole made by the drill. The surgeon then makes an H-shaped incision in the nasal mucosa. This may cause brisk bleeding, which is controlled by repacking the nasal passage with Neo-Synephrine impregnated gauze. A No. 7 knife handle with a No. 11 blade is used to create the same size H incision in the lacrimal sac. The surgeon then approximates the lacrimal sac flaps to the nasal mucous flaps using size 4-0 Dexon sutures swaged to a taper needle.

Before closing the skin and subcutaneous layers, the surgeon packs the nasal passage with petrolatum gauze using bayonet forceps. The subcutaneous tissue is closed with sutures of size 4-0 Dexon and the skin is closed with size 5-0 or 6-0 silk or nylon (Fig. 27–15C). Antibiotic ointment is spread on the skin incision and a Telfa dressing is applied.

Note: Some surgeons pass a silicone tube through the punctum into the lacrimal sac for postoperative irrigation.

Corneal Transplant (Penetrating Keratoplasty)

Definition

This is the replacement of a full thickness corneal button 7 to 8 mm in diameter with a donor graft. Corneal transplant procedures may be performed in cases of corneal injury or disease. The donor graft is obtained from one of several eye banks in the United States. Grafts are commonly preserved by a process called *cryopreservation*.

Highlights

1. The donor cornea is prepared with antibiotic solution and wrapped in moist gauze.
2. The donor graft is taken with a trephine.

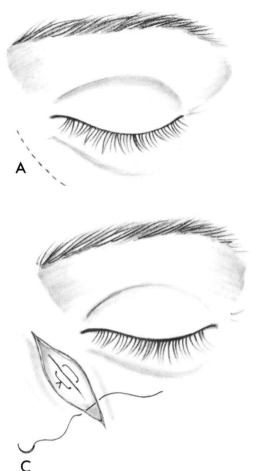

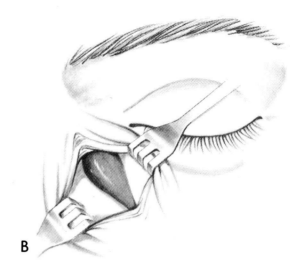

Figure 27–15. Dacryocystorhinostomy for lacrimal blockage. *A.* Skin incision over the lacrimal sac. *B.* Small rake retractors are used to expose the lacrimal sac. *C.* The wound is closed in layers with size 5-0 or 6-0 interrupted sutures. (Courtesy of Ethicon, Inc., Somerville, NJ.)

3. The donor graft is placed in a container with physiologic saline solution until needed.

4. A corneal trephination is performed on the operative eye.

5. The donor graft is positioned and sutured in place.

Description

In preparation for the procedure, the technologist should have the following instruments available along with those especially requested by the surgeon:

Basic eye tray
Trephine
Haab knife
No. 3 knife handle with Nos. 15 and 11 blades
Curved and straight iris scissors
Needle holders

In addition to these instruments, the surgeon uses the operating microscope to suture the corneal graft in place.

The patient is placed in the supine position with the head stabilized on a doughnut-type head rest. A rolled towel or bath blanket is placed under the patient's shoulders to hyper-extend the neck. If the procedure is to be performed with the patient under local anesthesia, a pillow can be placed under the patient's knees to relieve any back discomfort. Before beginning the patient prep, the circulator positions the microscope above the patient and the surgeon adjusts it to his or her needs. The microscope is then locked into position and rotated out of the field.

The circulator instills tetracaine ophthalmic drops to the operative eye. The eye is then prepped in routine fashion. If a local anesthetic is employed during the procedure, the postauricular area is also prepped. Drapes are then applied, as described in Chapter 11.

The surgeon administers a Nadbath injection as described for enucleation. An optic nerve block is then performed using a muscle hook for exposure and a 3-mL syringe fitted with a 25-gauge ½-inch needle. The surgeon may need a 4×4-inch sponge, which is placed over the eye while finger pressure is applied to aid in infiltration of the anesthetic.

After allowing a few minutes for the anesthesia to take effect, the technologist should pass a trephine and the donor eye to the surgeon. The surgeon then performs a *trephination* (excision of a circular portion of the cornea) on the donor eye. After the graft is taken, the technologist places it in a container of physiologic saline solution, with the *endothelial side facing upward,* and covers the container. The graft should be placed on the back table for safe keeping until the surgeon is ready to insert it.

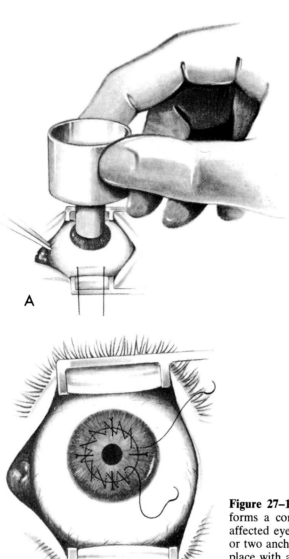

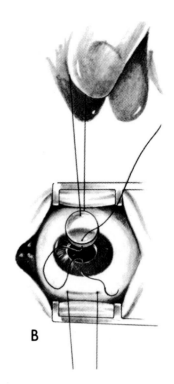

Figure 27–16. Corneal transplant. *A.* The surgeon performs a corneal trephination (circular excision) on the affected eye. *B.* The donor cornea is stabilized with one or two anchor sutures. *C.* The donor cornea is sutured in place with a double-arm continuous suture of size 9-0 to 12-0 silk or nylon, according to the surgeon's preference. (Courtesy of Ethicon, Inc., Somerville, NJ.)

The surgeon places a lid speculum in the eye and rotates the microscope over the eye. With the use of a scleral biting forcep and the trephine, a corneal trephination on the operative eye is completed (Fig. 27–16A). The trephined tissue is passed to the technologist, who retains it as a specimen. The technologist should then pass the donor graft *in its container* to the surgeon, who gently removes it with Calibri forceps. To stabilize the donor tissue in place, the surgeon places two or three sutures of silk, size 9-0 to 12-0 (Fig. 27–16B). Many interrupted sutures are then placed circumferentially around the transplant, using size 9-0 to 12-0 silk or nylon swaged to a cutting needle. Some surgeons prefer to use one running suture to encircle the edges of the transplant (Fig. 27–16C).

Before the last suture is tied, the surgeon fills the anterior chamber with balanced saline solution using a 3-mL syringe fitted with a cannulated needle. At the completion of the procedure, the surgeon instills an antibiotic ophthalmic ointment and patches the eye with a cotton eye pad and metal Fox shield.

Enucleation

Definition

This is the removal of the entire globe (eyeball). Indications for enucleation include intraocular malignancy, penetrating ocular wound, painful blind eye, and an eye that is blind and painless but disfigured. An artificial prosthesis may be inserted to replace the globe.

Highlights

1. Traction sutures are placed in the upper and lower eyelids.

2. The conjunctiva is incised.
3. The eye muscles are severed.
4. The recti and inferior oblique muscles are anastomosed.
5. The optic nerve is severed.
6. The globe is removed.
7. A sphere is introduced into the socket.
8. The conjunctiva and Tenon's capsule are sutured over the sphere.

Description

In this procedure a general anesthetic is preferred over local anesthesia because of the psychological effects of the surgery. In addition to the general anesthetic, a retrobulbar (behind the eyeball) anesthetic solution is injected to block the oculocardiac reflex that is produced by manipulation of the extraocular muscles. This injection is usually 1% lidocaine with epinephrine added and is administered with a 5-mL syringe fitted with a 1½-inch needle.

The patient is placed in the supine position with the head stabilized on a doughnut-type head rest. After the general anesthetic and retrobulbar injection have been administered, the circulator preps the patient from hairline to mouth and from nose to ear on the operative side. The eye is then draped in routine fashion (see Chapter 11).

To begin the procedure, the surgeon places a suture of size 4-0 silk on a fine cutting needle through the upper eyelid and tags it with a fine hemostat. A second suture is placed in the lower eyelid. These sutures aid in retracting the levator muscles away from the area of dissection and prevent their injury. The surgeon then makes a 350-degree incision around the cornea in the conjunctiva as close to the limbus as possible (Fig. 27–17A). This conserves as much conjunctiva as possible for closure later in the procedure. The incision is made with a No. 15 Bard-Parker blade or delicate scissors, such as iris scissors. Using the iris scissors, the surgeon undermines the conjunctiva and Tenon's capsule and then prepares to sever the recti and oblique muscles from the globe.

Because the recti muscles will be sutured to the inferior oblique muscle, both muscles are tagged with sutures of silk or Dexon, size 4-0 or 5-0. The superior oblique muscle is severed and allowed to retract back. The surgeon then severs the previously tagged inferior oblique muscle, secures it to the lateral rectus muscle with sutures of size 4-0 silk, and pulls the globe anteriorly (forward).

The technologist should have a muscle hook available at this time. The surgeon passes the hook around the globe to ensure that all connections except the optic nerve have been severed. The surgeon places a Mayo clamp across the optic nerve for 30 to 60 seconds to effect hemostasis. The clamp is then removed and curved enucleation scissors are used to sever the optic nerve across the area crushed by the Mayo clamp. This frees the globe, which is passed to the technologist as a specimen. If any intraocular contents have been ex-

truded into the socket, they must be cleaned out with irrigation solution and 4×4-inch gauze sponges. (Occasionally remnants of the iris escape from the globe into the socket and appear as a sooty material, which must be removed.)

Insertion of Intraorbital Implant and Conformer

Once the globe has been removed, an implant must be placed and sutured to the socket to shape the socket (Fig. 27–17B). This implant is called a *sphere*, over which a *conformer* is placed. This implant covers the surface of the implanted sphere and will eventually be replaced by an artificial eye. The technologist should have several sizes of implant spheres available from which the surgeon may choose. The sizes for an adult usually range from 14 to 18 mm. Rarely is it necessary to have a sphere larger than 18 mm available.

The surgeon selects the implant and conformer, and the sphere is introduced into the orbit. Some surgeons use a sphere introducer to insert the implant (see Chapter 15). The technologist passes a suture of size 4-0 Dexon to the surgeon, along with scleral biting forceps. Tenon's capsule is pulled over the sphere and sutured in place (Fig. 27–17C). The recti muscles are sutured to their appropriate positions on the sphere with size 4-0 or 5-0 Dexon sutures. The conjunctiva is closed with size 5-0 Dexon sutures. The technologist then passes the conformer to the surgeon for insertion. The silk retraction sutures are removed, and the surgeon instills an antibiotic ophthalmic ointment. The area is patched with a cotton eye pad and secured with tape.

A prosthesis may be fitted 4 to 6 weeks after surgery (this is not a surgical procedure). The prosthesis is shaped in very much the same way as the conformer it is replacing, and the patient can remove and insert it himself.

Intracapsular Cataract Extraction

Definition

This is the removal of an opaque lens. A cataract may be a congenital defect or may be caused by trauma or certain medications. However, it is most commonly due to the aging process. Cataract is one of the most common causes of gradual, painless loss of vision. The process may not become severe for several years. Surgical intervention is indicated only for advanced cataracts, at which time the patient no longer has satisfactory vision. The goal of surgical intervention is to remove the opaque lens and restore vision by means of eyeglasses, contact lenses, or an intraocular lens (artificial prosthesis that takes the place of the lens).

Highlights

1. The conjunctiva is incised.
2. The cornea is incised at the limbus.
3. Closing sutures are placed but not tied.

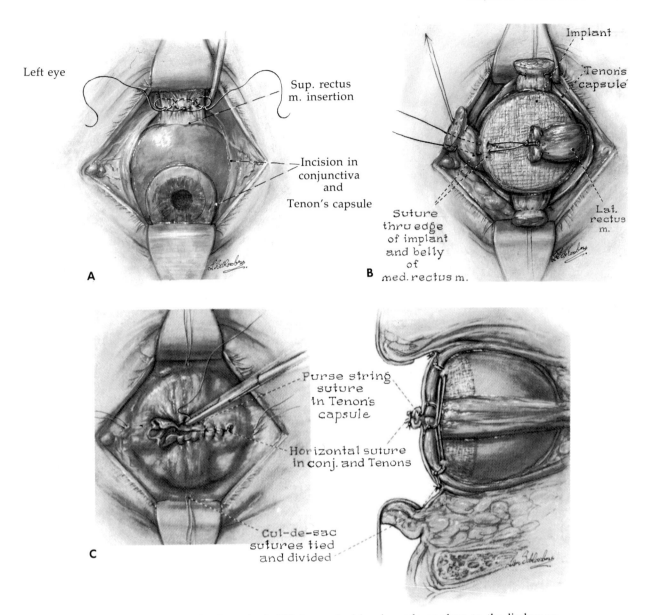

Figure 27–17. Enucleation. *A.* A 350-degree incision is made as close to the limbus as possible. *B.* The implant sphere is sutured in place. *C.* Tenon's capsule is closed over the sphere. (From Iliff E, Iliff WJ, Iliff NT: Oculoplastic Surgery. Philadelphia, WB Saunders, 1979.)

4. An iridotomy is performed, and the lens is removed.

5. The corneal incision is sutured.

6. The conjunctiva is sutured.

Description

Most cataract procedures are performed under a local anesthetic. In these cases the patient arrives in surgery sufficiently sedated to be completely relaxed but alert enough to respond to the surgeon. A special Nadbath anesthetic block placed behind the ear may be used. In preparation for a cataract procedure, the technologist should have the following instruments available (modified according to the surgeon's preference):

Basic eye tray
Westcott scissors
Tenotomy scissors
Fixation forceps
Beaver handle with No. 64 blade
No. 3 knife handle with No. 15 blade
Ziegler knife
Mosquito forceps (for use as a sponge carrier)
Cotton-tipped applicators.

In addition, a hand-held cautery unit, cellulose sponges, and several syringes should be included in the set-up. Many surgeons operate with the microscope or with surgical loupes. Various medications are used throughout the procedure, and these are discussed below.

The patient is placed in the supine position with the head placed on a "doughnut" or similar type of head rest for stability. A small rolled towel may be placed under the shoulders to hyperextend the neck. The patient's comfort is of utmost importance, since he or she must be as still as possible during the procedure. Because most cataract patients are elderly and may experience some back discomfort while lying on the operating table, a pillow may be placed under the knees to relieve this stress.

Before the eye prep, the circulator or technologist positions the microscope above the patient. The surgeon is usually available at this time to focus it according to his or her needs. The microscope is then locked into position and rotated just out of the field to allow for the prep and draping.

Just before the prep, the circulator instills tetracaine ophthalmic anesthetic drops to the operative eye. The eye prep (see Chapter 11) extends from hairline to mouth and from nose to ear. The postauricular area is also prepped for the Nadbath anesthetic block. The eye is then draped. Many surgeons prefer to use paper drapes during cataract surgery to minimize the presence of lint on the operative field.

The surgeon administers the Nadbath block with a 10-mL syringe fitted with a 27-gauge ½-inch Luer-Lok needle. Using scleral biting forceps, a muscle hook, and a 3-mL syringe fitted with a 1½-inch 25-gauge needle, the surgeon then performs the optic nerve block. A folded 4 × 4-inch sponge may have to be placed over the eye for finger pressure to be applied and to aid in infiltration of the anesthetic.

After allowing a few minutes for the anesthetic to take effect, the surgeon positions the microscope and places a bridle (traction) suture using a muscle hook and scleral biting forceps. The bridle suture (size 3-0 or 4-0 silk swaged to a tapered intestinal needle) is placed in the superior sclera; this aids in immobilizing and positioning the eye during the procedure.

After placing a lid speculum in the eye, the surgeon uses conjunctival (Westcott) scissors to dissect the conjunctiva from the superior cornea at the 3 o'clock to 9 o'clock position (Fig. 27–18A). The cornea is then incised with a No. 64 Beaver blade or Ziegler knife (Fig. 27–18B). The incision is lengthened with right and left corneal scissors. Small bleeding vessels are cauterized with the hand-held cautery unit. At this time, the surgeon may place the closing corneal sutures. Sutures of size 9-0 or 10-0 silk swaged to a micropoint spatula needle are commonly used. Approximately six sutures are placed (Fig. 27–18C).

After the corneal sutures are placed, the surgeon performs an iridotomy (incision in the iris) using Calibri forceps and Van Ness scissors. The assisting surgeon retracts the cornea with smooth forceps by holding the central corneal suture. During the entire procedure, the assistant or technologist should irrigate the surface of the cornea frequently with ophthalmic saline solution and sponge the excess solution away lightly. While the surgeon performs the iridotomy (Fig. 27–18D), the technologist should prepare a solution of α-chymotryp-sin, which is used to dissolve the zonules that hold the lens in place. The surgeon irrigates the anterior chamber of the eye with this solution using an olive tip needle or Troutman cannula. After 3 minutes, the lens is ready to be removed.

While waiting for the α-chymotrypsin to take effect, the technologist should prepare acetylcholine (Miochol) solution in a syringe fitted with a 27-gauge cannulated irrigation needle. Miochol solution is used to constrict the pupil to prevent vitreous loss. This will be injected as soon as the corneal flap is approximated.

Note: The Miochol solution must be used within 15 minutes after preparation. If complications arise, new solution should be prepared.

The technologist should pass smooth forceps, an eye sponge, and saline solution to the assistant and a corneal retractor and cryoextractor to the surgeon. The type of cryoextractor used depends on the surgeon's preference. Either a hand-held single-use extractor such as the one shown in Figure 27–19 or a larger table model with an attaching hand component may be used (Fig. 27–20). Both function in the same manner. The tip of the unit maintains a very low freezing temperature, and, when the surgeon touches the lens with the tip, the lens adheres to it and can be slowly withdrawn from the eye (Fig. 27–21A). The technologist must receive the lens and retain it as a specimen.

Using two tying forceps, the surgeon closes the corneal incision. After all preplaced sutures are tied and cut, the surgeon may place two or three additional sutures of size 12-0 nylon between the preplaced sutures (Fig. 27–21B). The anterior chamber is then filled with saline solution to normal fluid pressure (Fig. 27–21C). The surgeon pulls the conjunctiva over the corneal incision and places interrupted or running sutures of size 6-0 silk or synthetic absorbable sutures at the 3 o'clock and 9 o'clock positions (Fig. 27–21D). The bridle suture is then cut and the speculum is removed.

The surgeon dresses the eye with ophthalmic ointment of his or her choice, an oval eye pad, and a metal Fox shield (see Fig. 15–41U). At the completion of the case it is vital for the patient to be transported to the post-anesthesia care unit with as little jarring as possible.

Related Procedure

Phacoemulsification and Intraocular Implantation

In this procedure, extracapsular cataract extraction is performed by *phacoemulsification*. This is the emulsification of a mature cataract with ultrasonic vibration and the extraction of the lens by irrigation and aspiration. During this procedure, only a small initial incision is necessary. The high-frequency probe fragments the lens into many small pieces so that it can be emulsified and aspirated. The rims of the anterior capsule and posterior capsule remain intact. After the procedure, a very small intraocular lens is implanted to restore vision.

Because of the complex nature of the equipment used during this procedure, the novice scrub assistant must

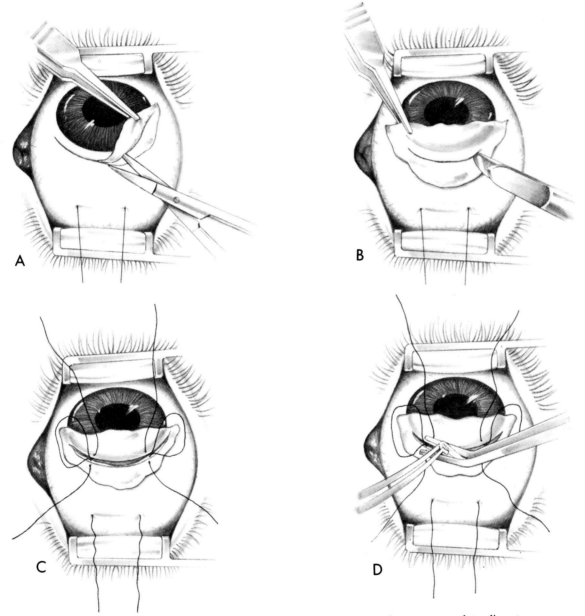

Figure 27–18. Intracapsular cataract extraction. *A.* Westcott scissors are used to dissect the conjunctiva from the superior cornea. *B.* The cornea is incised with a No. 64 Beaver blade or Ziegler knife. *C.* The closing corneal sutures are placed before the extraction of the lens. *D.* A peripheral iridectomy is performed. (Courtesy of Ethicon, Inc., Somerville, NJ.)

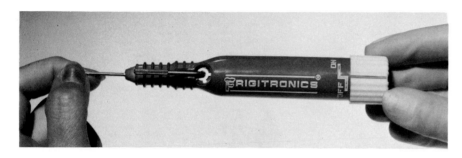

Figure 27–19. Hand-held (disposable) cryoextractor used for extraction of the opaque lens. (Courtesy of Frigitronics, Inc., Shelton, CT.)

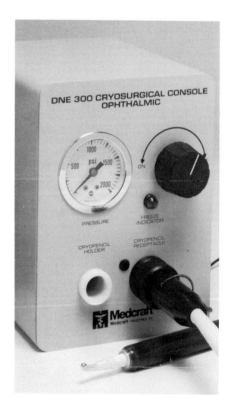

Figure 27–20. Table model cryounit. Note pencil attachment that is sterilized prior to use. (Courtesy of Medcraft Industries, Inc., Darien, CT.)

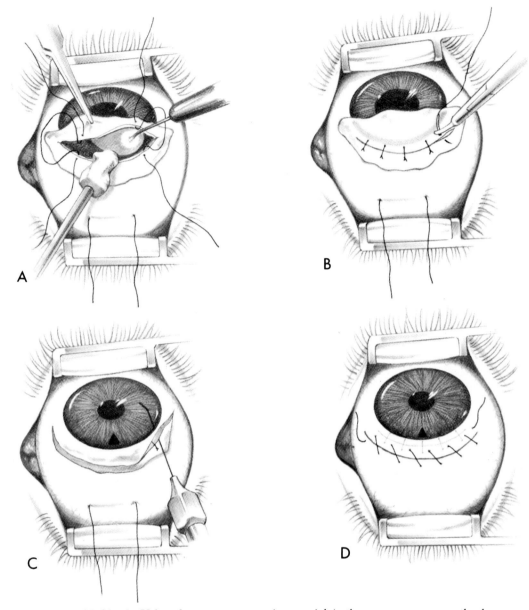

Figure 27–21. *A.* Using the cryoextractor *(upper right),* the surgeon removes the lens. Because the closing sutures were preplaced, the incision can be closed very quickly. *B.* The aligning sutures are tied. Additional sutures are placed as needed. *C.* The anterior chamber is pressurized with normal saline solution. A Troutman cannula is commonly used to fill the chamber. *D.* The conjunctiva is closed with a size 6-0 running suture of the surgeon's preference. (Courtesy of Ethicon, Inc., Somerville, NJ.)

work with trained personnel to master the techniques used.

Insertion of Intraocular Lens with Intracapsular Cataract Extraction

Definition

The intraocular lens is a prosthesis that replaces the lens after its extraction during cataract surgery. This allows the patient almost immediate postoperative vision. Even though this vision is not perfect, the procedure is much more beneficial than conventional cataract extraction. When an intraocular lens is not inserted, the patient may wait up to 3 months postoperatively before he or she can be fitted with a prescription contact lens.

There are many types of intraocular lenses available, much too numerous to describe here. There are, however, four basic types of intraocular lenses used:

1. Anterior chamber
2. Iris plane
3. Iridocapsular
4. Posterior chamber

Some commonly used intraocular lenses are illustrated in Figure 27–22.

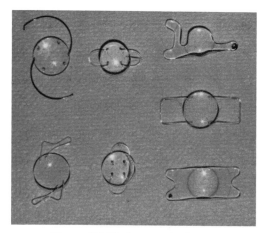

Figure 27–22. Intraocular lenses.

Highlights

1. The lens implant is prepared.
2. The cataract is removed.
3. The lens is implanted and may be sutured in place.
4. The wound is closed.

Description

The procedure for implantation of an intraocular lens begins as soon as the cataract has been extracted, as described previously for intracapsular cataract extraction. However, the technologist must prepare the lens before the procedure for cataract extraction is begun. After the back table and Mayo stand set-up are complete, the technologist should inspect the field for any extraneous lint, which must be removed before the intraocular lens is removed from its container. The technologist then removes the intraocular lens from the container and places it in the neutralizing solution provided with it. It is then rinsed with saline solution and stored in a covered container containing balanced saline solution until the surgeon is ready to insert it.

As soon as the cataract is extracted, the technologist brings the intraocular lens to the Mayo stand. The surgeon grasps it with smooth tissue forceps and inserts it as the assistant elevates the cornea by elevating one of the preplaced sutures (Fig. 27–23). The technologist should then immediately pass to the surgeon a 3-mL syringe fitted with an irrigation cannula and filled with balanced saline solution. The anterior chamber is filled with the solution as the assistant lowers the cornea to prevent the intraocular lens from contacting the endothelial side of the cornea.

At this time the surgeon may suture the implant in place (note that not all intraocular lenses require sutures). If the implant does require sutures, the surgeon may use one or two of size 12-0 nylon.

The remainder of the procedure is identical to that followed in routine cataract extraction (see Fig. 27–21).

Retinal Detachment

Definition

Under certain circumstances, the sensory retina may become detached from the pigmented layer, and this is called *retinal detachment*. Causes include hemorrhage, tumor, or inflammatory reaction. The most common cause of retinal detachment is a thinning of the retina due to the aging process. The patient suffers from flashing lights and progressive shadowing or darkening of the visual field, which may lead to complete blindness.

Description

There are numerous techniques used in the treatment of retinal detachment. To describe each technique in detail is beyond the scope of this text. However, the goals of nearly all the techniques are to bind the two retinal layers together. In *cryothermy*, the sclera is undermined and a diathermy electrode is used to dot the area of retinal detachment. The diathermy electrode produces a high-frequency electrical current that warms but does not damage the tissue (Fig. 27–24*A*). This treatment causes small adhesions that bind the two retinal layers together. The sclera is then approximated with sizes 4-0 or 5-0 sutures of the surgeon's preferred material (Fig. 27–24*B*).

In *laser therapy*, a similar technique is employed with laser beams directed toward the area of detachment. An alternative technique is with the use of a thin Silastic band (or "buckle"), which the surgeon places over the area of detachment following diathermy to assist in the binding of the retinal layers.

The technologist is urged to study new techniques to be completely familiar with the techniques and materials used by the surgeons.

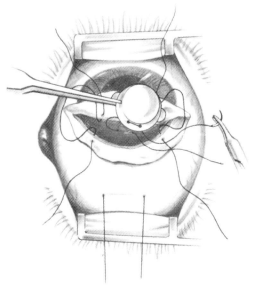

Figure 27–23. Insertion of intraocular lens. Following the removal of the cataract, the surgeon implants the artificial lens. In some cases, the lens is sutured in place. (Courtesy of Ethicon, Inc., Somerville, NJ.)

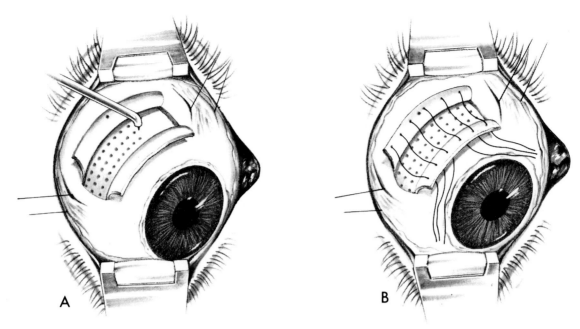

Figure 27–24. *A.* Procedures for retinal detachment. The diathermy unit is used to dot the area of detachment. *B.* Fine sutures are placed over the treated area. (Courtesy of Ethicon, Inc., Somerville, NJ.)

Filtering Procedure for Glaucoma

Definition

Glaucoma is a condition in which intraocular pressure is increased. There may be a number of causes for the condition, such as an accompanying disease or trauma. In all cases the aqueous humor is prevented from flowing from the anterior chamber to the limbal area where it is normally excreted. The aqueous humor is continuously produced and causes severe intraocular pressure if not excreted. This pressure, if unchecked, pushes on the optic nerve and retina, causing progressive loss of vision, which in most cases is never fully restored. The goal of surgical intervention is to provide an adequate channel from which the aqueous humor may drain out of the anterior chamber.

Highlights

1. The conjunctiva is incised.
2. The limbus is incised.
3. An iridectomy is performed.
4. The limbus incision is cauterized.
5. The conjunctiva is closed.

Description

In preparation for the procedure, the technologist should have the following instruments available:

Hand-held cautery unit eye sponges
Cotton-tipped applicators
No. 3 knife handle
Nos. 15 and 11 scalpel blades
Corneal scissors (left and right)
Van Ness scissors
Westcott scissors
Calibri forceps
Scleral biting forceps
Burch eye pick
Needle holders
Iris spatula
Lid speculum
Assorted irrigation tips and needles
Assorted glass syringes (3, 5, and 10 mL)

The patient is placed in the supine position, the head is stabilized on a head rest, and the operative eye is prepped and draped in routine fashion.

To begin the procedure, the surgeon inserts a speculum and incises the conjunctiva using toothed forceps, such as Bishop-Harmon forceps, and tenotomy scissors. The incision is made about 5 to 10 mm back from the limbus and directed toward the limbus, creating a flap. Bleeding vessels are cauterized. Before making the limbal incision, the surgeon may cauterize the limbal area. The technologist then passes a Burch pick, which is used to stabilize the eye while the limbus is incised. The surgeon then incises the limbus to enter the anterior chamber. The incision is made with the scalpel and may be extended with corneal scissors. The edge of the incision is cauterized to prevent closure.

The iridotomy is then performed. The surgeon makes the incision in the iris with Van Ness scissors and Calibri forceps. The technologist may be required to hold the Burch pick in the absence of an assistant. Likewise, if there is no assistant, the technologist is required to irrigate the eye frequently and sponge away any excess fluid.

The conjunctiva is then closed. The surgeon uses interrupted sutures of silk or nylon, size 6-0 to 9-0 according to preference, to close the incision. Just before the last suture is placed, the surgeon repressurizes the anterior chamber with balanced saline solution. An antibiotic ophthalmic ointment is then instilled, and the eye is dressed with a cotton eye pad and metal Fox shield.

Closed Vitrectomy

Definition

This is the surgical removal of the vitreous humor contained in the posterior globe of the eye, behind the lens. A vitrectomy is performed when the vitreous is opaque because of hemorrhage, amyloidosis, or inflammatory cells. Vitreous hemorrhage due to proliferative diabetic retinopathy is the most common indication for vitrectomy. Other causes are Eales' disease, sickle cell retinopathy, and trauma.

Highlights

1. Two incisions are made into the cornea.
2. Two incisions are made into the vitreous body.
3. A cutting-suction-infusion cannula is inserted.
4. Intraocular scissors are introduced.
5. The vitreous is aspirated as the vitreous body is refilled with fluid.
6. The incisions are closed.

Description

The patient is placed in the supine position with the head on a doughnut-type head rest, prepped, and draped, as previously described. The patient is administered a general anesthetic. During the procedure the surgeon uses the microscope along with a corneal contact lens for better visualization. The technologist should have the following instruments available:

Vitreous infusion suction
Intraocular scissors and forceps
No. 3 knife handle
Nos. 15 and 11 scalpel blades
Hand-held cautery unit
Cotton-tipped applicators and eye sponges
Toothed and smooth tissue forceps
Curved and straight iris scissors
Suture scissors
Needle holders

Additionally, any instruments especially requested by the surgeon should be available.

The surgeon inserts a lid speculum and then receives a contact lens from the technologist. The circulator should be available to drop sterile contact lens lubricant onto the contact lens. The surgeon then applies the lens to the patient's cornea.

Using iris scissors and toothed tissue forceps, the surgeon makes two conjunctival incisions (Fig. 27–25A). Bleeding vessels are cauterized, and two stab incisions are made through the sclera with a No. 11 scalpel blade. The surgeon now inserts the vitreous infusion suction cannula and the intraocular scissors through the two incisions (Fig. 27–25B). The vitreous is aspirated and replaced with fluid at the same time.

When the vitreous is removed, the instruments are withdrawn and the scleral incisions are closed with sutures of size 8-0 to 10-0 nylon on cutting needles. The conjunctiva is then closed with size 6-0 to 9-0 synthetic absorbable sutures swaged to taper needles (Fig. 27–25C). An antibiotic ophthalmic ointment is instilled, and

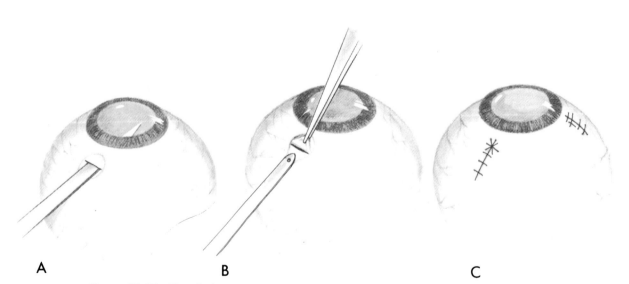

Figure 27–25. Closed vitrectomy. *A.* Two incisions are made in the conjunctiva. *B.* A cutting suction infusion cannula is inserted into the wound to aspirate the vitreous. *C.* The wounds are closed with interrupted synthetic absorbable sutures of nylon, Dexon, or Vicryl. (Courtesy of Ethicon, Inc., Somerville, NJ.)

the eye is patched with a cotton eye pad and metal Fox shield.

Bibliography

Audrey F et al: ECCE with phacoemulsification and flexible IOL implantation. Todays OR Nurse 10:6, 1988.

Dorland's Illustrated Medical Dictionary, 27th ed. Philadelphia, WB Saunders, 1988.

Ethicon, Inc: Suture Use Manual: Use and Handling of Sutures and Needles. Somerville, NJ, Ethicon, Inc, 1978.

Gardner E, Gray D, O'Rahilly R: Anatomy: A Regional Study of Human Structure, 5th ed. Philadelphia, WB Saunders, 1986.

Jacob S, Francone C, Lossow WJ: Structure and Function in Man, 5th ed. Philadelphia, WB Saunders, 1984.

McVay C: Surgical Anatomy, 6th ed. Philadelphia, WB Saunders, 1984.

Paparella M, et al: Otolaryngology, 3rd ed. Philadelphia, WB Saunders, 1991.

Saunders WH, et al: Nursing Care in Eye, Ear, Nose, and Throat Disorders, 4th ed. St. Louis, CV Mosby, 1979.

Scheie HG, Albert DM: Textbook of Ophthalmology, 9th ed. Philadelphia, WB Saunders, 1977.

Shambaugh GE, Glasscock ME: Surgery of the Ear, 3rd ed. Philadelphia, WB Saunders, 1980.

Sheridan E, Patterson HR, Gustafson EA: Falconer's The Drug, The Nurse, The Patient, 7th ed. Philadelphia, WB Saunders, 1985.

Trischank HL: Intraocular lens implant. AORN J 39(5): 1984.

Walter JB: An Introduction to the Principles of Disease, 3rd ed. Philadelphia, WB Saunders, 1992.

Ear, Nose, Throat, and Mouth Surgery

Part I ◆ EAR SURGERY

Operations of the middle and inner ear are performed to restore the patient's hearing. Hearing loss may be due to disease or injury and is classified as *conductive* (mechanical obstruction of the external or middle ear such as that caused by a tumor or fixation of the ear bones) or *sensorineural* (deafness caused by a lesion in the nerve tissue or sensory paths to the brain).

SURGICAL ANATOMY

The ear (Fig. 28–1) is divided into three distinct parts: the external, middle, and internal ear. The external ear consists of the auricle, the large rigid skin flap that surrounds the opening of the ear canal, and the external acoustic meatus. The middle ear spans the end of the external meatus at the tympanic membrane, or eardrum, to the tympanic cavity. The inner ear encompasses the labyrinth, a complex series of fluid-filled spaces.

External Ear

The structures of the external ear are the *auricle* and the *external acoustic meatus*. The auricle (also called the ear flap) is a skin-covered cartilaginous structure that captures sound waves. At the center of the auricle lies the opening of the external acoustic meatus. This is a canal lined with small glands that secrete a waxy sub-

stance known as *cerumen*. The acoustic meatus is approximately 2½ inches long and terminates at the tympanic membrane (eardrum).

Middle Ear

The *middle ear*, or *tympanic cavity*, lies within the temporal bone of the skull. It is lined with mucous membrane and contains the three bones of the ear, which transmit sound to the mastoid air cells beyond. These bones or ossicles are the malleus, incus, and stapes. The mucous membrane of the cavity wraps around these bones collectively. The first of the bones, the *malleus* (or hammer bone), is partially embedded in the tympanic membrane. The *incus* (or anvil) is the middle bone, whose body articulates with the malleus. The *stapes* (or stirrup) communicates with the oval window, the entrance to the inner ear. The *eustachian tube* allows air to enter the middle ear through the nasopharynx to equalize pressure between the outside of the body and the middle ear. The opening of the eustachian tube (or auditory tube) is situated near the oval window.

Inner Ear

The inner ear is composed of a series of tunnels called *labyrinths* (Fig. 28–2). These labyrinths are responsible

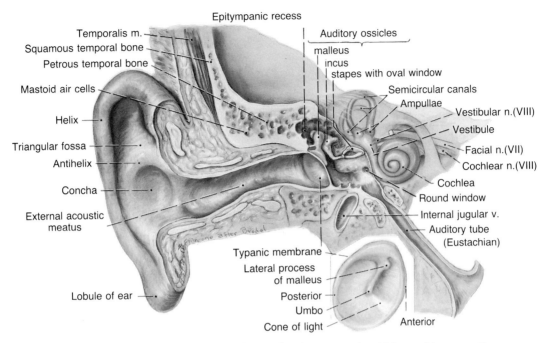

Figure 28–1. Frontal section through the ear showing external, middle, and inner portions. (From Jacob S, Francone C, Lossow WJ: Structure and Function in Man, 5th ed. Philadelphia, WB Saunders, 1982. p. 341)

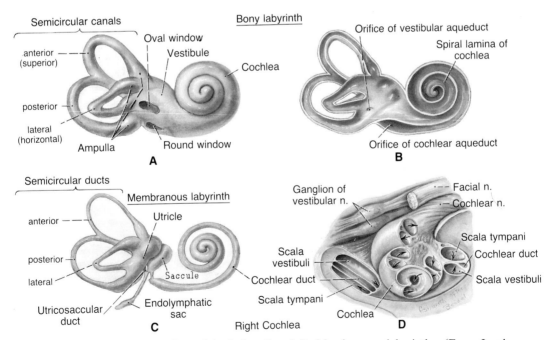

Figure 28–2. *A* and *B*. Bony labyrinths. *C* and *D*. Membranous labyrinths. (From Jacob S, Francone C, Lossow WJ: Structure and Function in Man, 5th ed. Philadelphia, WB Saunders, 1982.)

for the body's equilibrium and for the final reception of sound waves. The *bony labyrinth* is a series of canals hollowed out of the temporal bone. It consists of the *cochlea,* a snail-shaped structure that contains the *organ of Corti,* the organ of hearing. Within the bony labyrinth lies the membranous labyrinth. The bony labyrinth contains a fluid called *perilymph,* and the membranous labyrinth contains *endolymph.* In addition to the cochlea, the bony labyrinth also contains a structure called the *vestibule.* This in turn contains two other structures, the *utriculus* and the *sacculus,* which function along with the *semicircular canals* to control equilibrium and the body's ability to sense its position.

SPECIAL EQUIPMENT

Power Drills

Power drills are needed during many ear procedures to remove bony tissue. These are used in conjunction with small burs, such as those shown in Figure 28–3. Whenever bone is drilled, the technologist is usually required to irrigate the area lightly during drilling. Two drills commonly used in ear surgery are the Jordan-Day drill (Fig. 28–4) and the Stryker drill (Fig. 28–5).

Microscope

The microscope is used during all surgery of the middle and inner ear (see Chapter 27).

Suction-Irrigation

A special suction-irrigation tip (Fig. 28–6) is used during ear surgery. This instrument allows the surgeon to irrigate and suction the wound of fluids and tissue debris simultaneously. It is the technologist's and circulator's responsibility to assemble the suction-irrigation tip before the start of surgery. Lactated Ringer's solution is frequently used for irrigation.

Sponges

In addition to 4×4-inch sponges, many surgeons use cotton dental pledgets and cottonoids (those used during

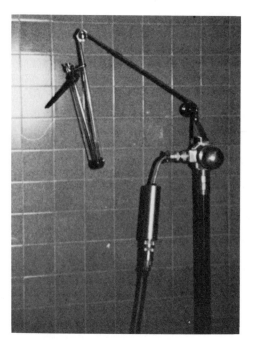

Figure 28–4. Jordan-Day drill. This drill may also be used during dental surgery.

neurosurgical cases). All sponges are accounted for before, during, and after the procedure.

Speculum Holder

The speculum holder (Fig. 28–7) is used to retain the ear speculum in place, thus freeing the surgeon's hands during the procedure.

Dressings

Two types of dressing are used following ear surgery. The ear canal may simply be packed with ¼- or ½-inch gauze, usually impregnated with antibiotic ointment, or a *mastoid dressing* (Fig. 28–8) may be necessary for more complicated procedures. This dressing consists of fluffed gauze, which is placed over the affected ear and roller gauze (Kerlix or Kling) placed over the fluffs and around the head to hold the dressing in place.

Instruments

In addition to the basic ear instruments included in Chapter 15, there are a number of special microsurgical instruments used during ear surgery. These include fine forceps, knives, picks, probes, and curettes. Some basic microsurgical instruments are illustrated in Figures 28–9 through 28–13. A standard instrument set-up for the back table is shown in Figure 28–14.

Text continued on page 608

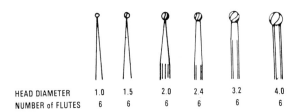

HEAD DIAMETER	1.0	1.5	2.0	2.4	3.2	4.0
NUMBER of FLUTES	6	6	6	6	6	6

Figure 28–3. Assorted burs used to clear bone from the middle and inner ear.

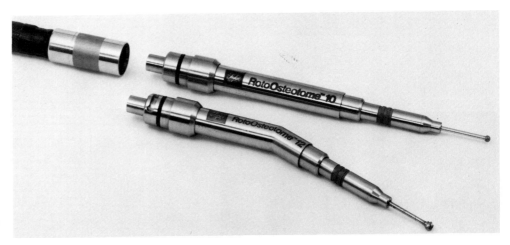

Figure 28–5. Stryker drill. (Courtesy of the Stryker Corporation, Kalamazoo, MI.)

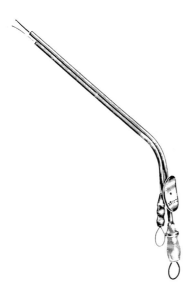

Figure 28–6. Suction-irrigation tip. (Courtesy of the Storz Instrument Company, St. Louis, MO.)

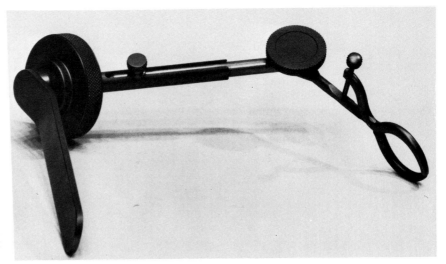

Figure 28–7. Speculum holder. Used mainly during mastoid procedures, the speculum holder frees the surgeon's hands during ear surgery. (Courtesy of the Storz Instrument Company, St. Louis, MO.)

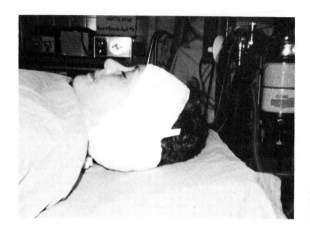

Figure 28–8. Mastoid dressing in place. This ear dressing consists of fluffed gauze, with roller gauze to hold the dressing in place and protect the affected ear.

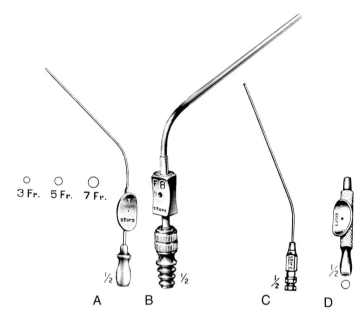

Figure 28–9. Suction tips. *A.* Baron suction tip. *B.* Frazier suction tip. *C.* Rosen suction tip. *D.* Suction adapter. (Courtesy of the Storz Instrument Company, St. Louis, MO.)

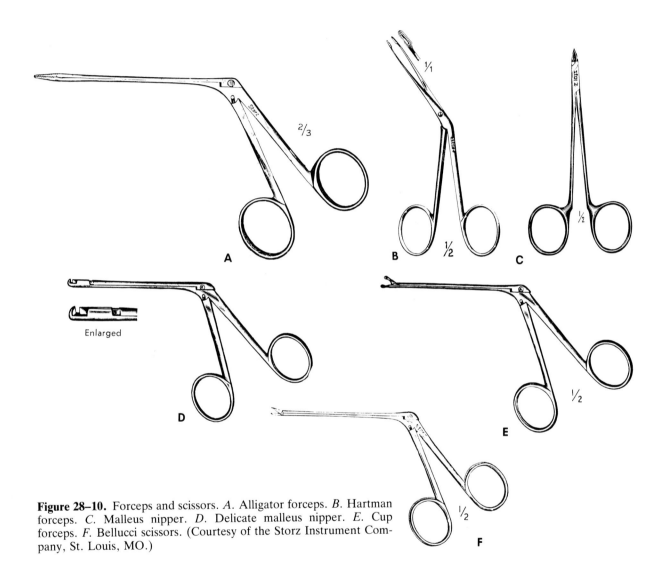

Figure 28–10. Forceps and scissors. *A.* Alligator forceps. *B.* Hartman forceps. *C.* Malleus nipper. *D.* Delicate malleus nipper. *E.* Cup forceps. *F.* Bellucci scissors. (Courtesy of the Storz Instrument Company, St. Louis, MO.)

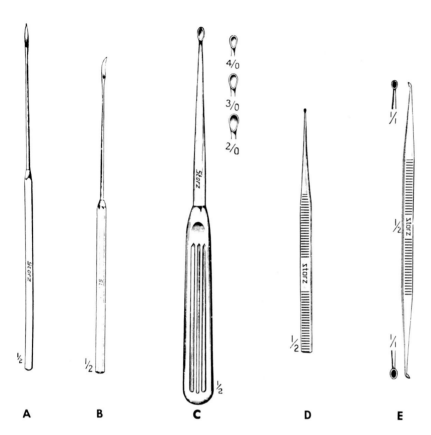

Figure 28–11. Knives and curettes. *A.* Myringotomy knife. *B.* Curved myringotomy knife. *C.* Lempert curette. *D.* Small bone curette. *E.* House double-ended curette. (Courtesy of the Storz Instrument Company, St. Louis, MO.)

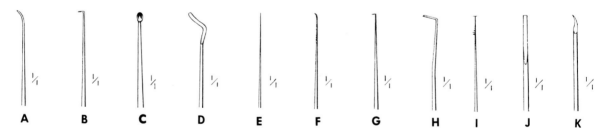

Figure 28–12. Delicate sharps. *A.* Duckbill knife-elevator. *B.* Right-angle elevator. *C.* Oval curette. *D.* Excavator. *E.* Heavy needle. *F.* Pick, 45. *G.* Pick, 90. *H.* Attic dissector. *I.* Strut caliper. *J.* Straight chisel. *K.* Sickle knife. (Courtesy of the Storz Instrument Company, St. Louis, MO.)

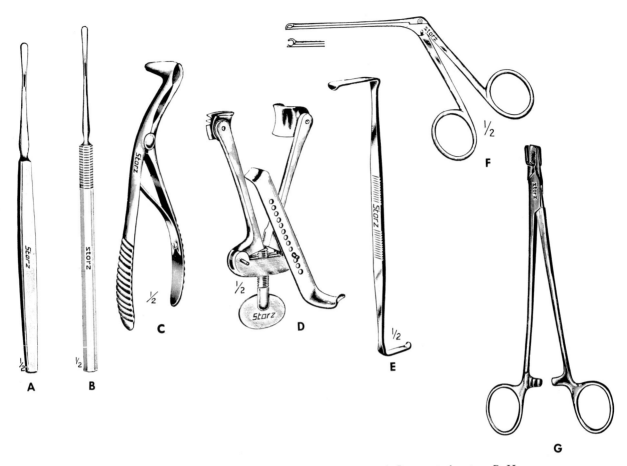

Figure 28–13. Miscellaneous microsurgical instruments. *A.* Lempert elevator. *B.* House elevator. *C.* Endaural speculum. *D.* Endaural retractor. *E.* House retractor. *F.* Crimper. *G.* Fascia press. (Courtesy of the Storz Instrument Company, St. Louis, MO.)

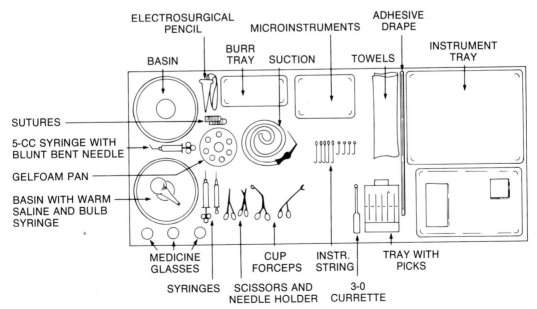

Figure 28–14. Standard back table set-up for ear surgery.

Medications

There are three major categories of medications used during ear surgery: anesthetics, hemostatic agents, and irrigation fluids. A local anesthetic with epinephrine is often the surgeon's choice, since the epinephrine acts as a vasoconstrictor and prevents oozing in the wound. Epinephrine-soaked pledgets are also used to control bleeding. A hemostatic agent such as Gelfoam is routinely used during most ear procedures.

SURGICAL PROCEDURES

During ear surgery, it is necessary to move some of the furniture in the suite to accommodate the position of the operating table, microscope, and anesthesia equipment. The patient is usually positioned with the head resting at the foot end of the table for the surgeon to operate while seated (most tables cannot accommodate the microscope and the surgeon's knees and feet at the head of the table). The positions of the surgeon, anesthesiologist, technologist or scrub nurse, back table, and other equipment are shown in Figure 28–15.

The patient's comfort during surgery is of utmost importance, since most procedures are done under a local anesthetic. A patient who is uncomfortable may become restless, making it difficult for the surgeon to operate. To prevent back strain, a pillow can be placed under the patient's knees. With the patient in the supine position, the affected ear should face upward and the head should be placed as close to the edge of the operating table as possible. A small sandbag can be placed at the back of the patient's head for greater stability. The ear is prepped and draped as described in Chapter 11.

Myringotomy With Insertion of Drainage Tubes

Definition

This is the incision of the tympanic membrane and the insertion of a drainage tube in the myringotomy site. There are many types of drainage tubes available, but the most common is the "bobbin" type.

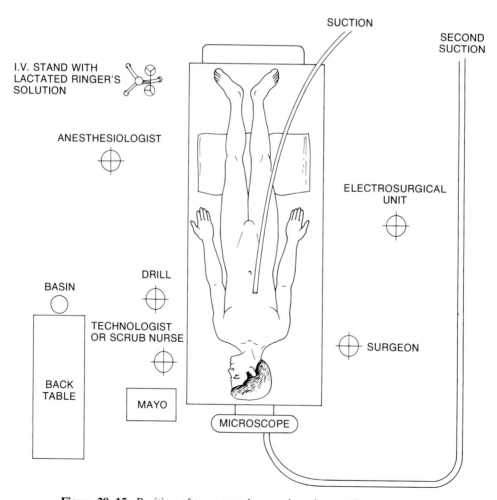

Figure 28–15. Position of team members and equipment for ear surgery.

Myringotomy is indicated in acute otitis media when infectious fluid builds up within the middle ear space, causing bulging of the tympanic membrane. Pain, fever, and/or hearing loss may also be present. Incision of the tympanic membrane releases pus or fluid and usually stops pain, restores hearing, and hastens recovery from infection. Drainage tubes are usually not placed when there is an acute infection.

In chronic serous otitis media there is no pain, fever, or bulging of the eardrum. The fluid is suctioned from the middle ear space after incising the tympanic membrane. Insertion of a drainage tube in the myringotomy site helps to prevent new fluid from forming.

Highlights

1. The tympanic membrane is incised.
2. If present, fluid or pus is suctioned.
3. If indicated, a drainage tube is inserted.

Description

The patient is placed in the supine position and the head is turned with the affected side up. The surgeon's preference determines whether a surgical prep and/or sterile gloves are used.

With the microscope in position, the surgeon inserts the proper size aural speculum into the ear canal. Any wax present in the ear canal is removed with a cerumen spoon or alligator forceps. The technologist should be ready to wipe the instrument tip to remove debris using a saline-moistened 4 × 4-inch sponge. Suction should also be available at this time. In acute cases, the surgeon uses a myringotomy knife to incise the posterior inferior quadrant of the pars tensa (Fig. 28–16). Occasionally

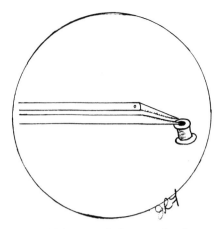

Figure 28–17. Bobbin-type drainage tube for myringotomy held with alligator forceps.

the surgeon may order a culture of the fluid to determine the causative organism. Fluid and pus are suctioned with a small Baron suction tip.

In cases of chronic serous otitis media, the incision site may be in the posterior inferior, anterior inferior, or anterior superior quadrants. If indicated, a drainage tube is inserted (Fig. 28–17). The technologist should grasp the drainage tube with microforceps to pass it to the surgeon. The ear canal may then be packed with a small amount of cotton.

Stapedectomy

Definition

This is the surgical removal of the stapes and the insertion of a prosthesis to re-establish the linkage between the incus and the oval window. The prosthesis may be an autologous vein graft taken from the dorsum of the hand or from fascia, a perichondrium graft taken from behind the ear, or an artificial prosthetic device. Many different types of prostheses are available, and the technologist should become familiar with the types used in his or her operating room (Fig. 28–18). A stapedectomy is indicated for patients with chronic progressive deafness due to otosclerosis (the formation of spongy bone within the ear).

Highlights

1. The tympanomeatal flap is created and elevated.
2. The annulus is identified and elevated.
3. Bone is curetted from the annulus.
4. The stapes superstructure is removed.
5. A prosthesis is inserted.

Description

The patient is placed in the supine position and the head is turned with the affected ear up. Sandbags can be placed on the opposite side of the head to ensure

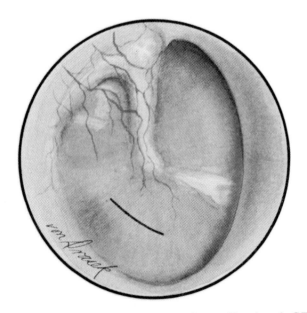

Figure 28–16. Site of myringotomy. (From Shambaugh GE, Jr: Surgery of the Ear, 2nd ed. Philadelphia, WB Saunders, 1967.)

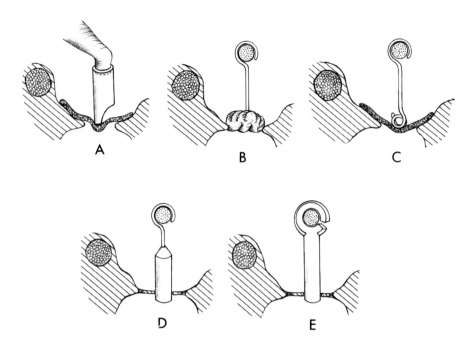

Figure 28–18. Stapedectomy prostheses. *A.* Vein-polyethylene strut (Shea). *B.* Wire fat (Schuknecht). *C.* Wire on compressed Gelfoam (House). *D.* Wire Teflon piston. *E.* Teflon piston (Shea). (From Paparella MM, Shumrick DA (eds): Otolaryngology, 2nd ed., vol II. Philadelphia, WB Saunders, 1980.)

that the position is stable. The patient is prepped and draped in the usual manner.

After draping the microscope, the technologist should have local anesthetic immediately available. A 27-gauge needle is commonly used. Anesthetic is used at the beginning of the procedure and also later, when the tympanic membrane has been elevated and the middle ear has been exposed.

The technologist offers several assorted sizes of endaural speculums to the surgeon. A speculum holder is used so that the surgeon can use both hands during the procedure.

The surgeon creates a tympanomeatal flap using a canal knife and ear suction. The incision is then completed with Bellucci scissors (Fig. 28–19*A*). A cotton pledget soaked in epinephrine is used to maintain hemostasis and also to protect the flap. The technologist should pass this to the surgeon on alligator forceps.

Next, the surgeon anesthetizes the middle ear with additional local anesthetic. The fibrous annulus is then identified and elevated (Fig. 28–19*B*). More cotton pledgets with epinephrine may be required for hemostasis. The surgeon uses a sharp curette to remove the bony annulus and to create a larger working space (Fig. 28–19*C*). The chorda tympani is then moved aside, or it may be cut with Bellucci scissors if necessary to expose the ossicles and oval window.

All bleeding is controlled before the stapes is approached. The surgeon uses an 18- or 20-gauge suction tip to clean all the bone chips and blood clots from the ear canal. The technologist should at this point change the suction tip to a size 24 so as not to traumatize the inner ear. The surgeon cuts the stapedial tendon (Fig. 28–19*D*) and uses an incudostapedial joint knife to separate the incus from the stapes. A fine needle is then used to fracture the crura from the footplate, and the stapes superstructure is removed with fine alligator or cup forceps (Fig. 28–19*E*). Stapes hooks are used to remove the fragments of the footplate.

To select a proper size piston prosthesis, the surgeon uses a measuring rod to determine the distance between the incus and the footplate level (Fig. 28–19*F*). The circulator then distributes the prosthesis to the technologist. (The prosthesis is not distributed until the surgeon determines the exact size needed, since it is very expensive.) Many surgeons place Gelfoam pledgets around the piston to help stabilize the prosthesis. If the footplate has been removed, a tissue graft is taken from a site determined by the type of tissue needed to cover the oval window, according to the surgeon's preference. Various sites include the temporalis fascia, ear lobe fat (Fig. 28–20), tragal perichondrium, and vein from the hand. The surgeon hooks the prosthesis onto the incus and positions it at the oval window. Microcrimpers are used to press the prosthesis onto the long process of the incus, thus securing it (Fig. 28–21). At the completion of the procedure, the surgeon uses a tuning fork to determine the patient's hearing status. The ear is then packed loosely with gauze or cotton.

Related Procedure

Reconstruction of the Incus

This is the reconstruction of the incus with an alloplastic implant that is assembled by the surgeon using a Middle Ear Reconstruction Kit (Ziv Middle Ear Reconstruction System, Dr. Moshe Ziv, Columbus, OH). The kit includes prosthetic materials that may be cut to fit the exact measurements of the new ossicle.

Radical Mastoidectomy

Definition

This is the surgical removal of the mastoid air cells, posterior and superior bony external auditory canal walls, tympanic membrane, and malleus and incus, if

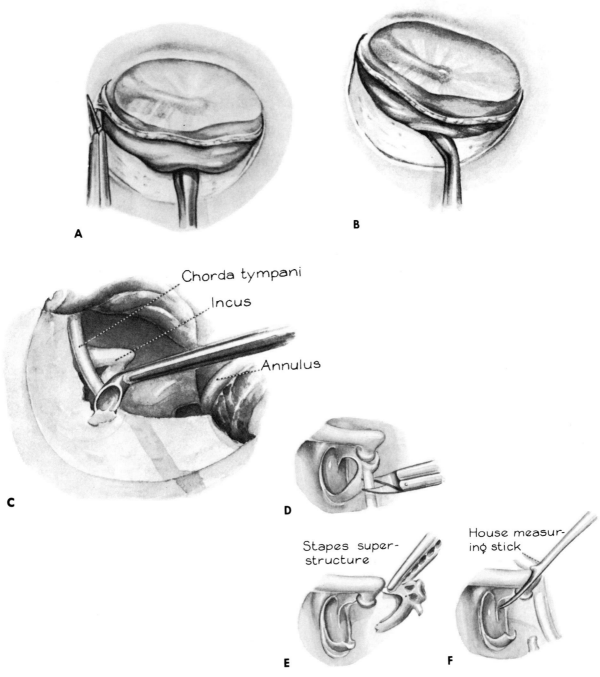

Figure 28–19. Stapedectomy. *A.* A tympanomeatal flap is created and the incision is completed with Bellucci scissors. *B.* The fibrous annulus is elevated. *C.* A curette is used to remove the bony annulus and to create a larger working space. *D.* The stapedial tendon is severed. *E.* The stapes superstructure is removed. *F.* A House measuring rod is used to determine the correct size prosthesis. (From Shambaugh, GE Jr: Surgery of the Ear, 2nd ed. Philadelphia, WB Saunders, 1967.)

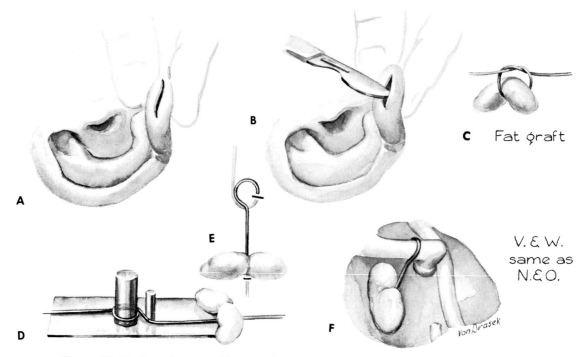

Figure 28–20. Stapedectomy. Tissue graft taken from the ear lobe. *A.* Incision site. *B.* The fat graft is freed. *C.* Wire tied to graft. *D.* Wire loop shaped. *E.* Excess wire cut. *F.* Fat and wire graft are inserted. (From Shambaugh GE, Jr: Surgery of the Ear, 2nd ed. Philadelphia, WB Saunders, 1967.)

present. The mastoid cavity is completely exteriorized and the external meatus of the auricle is usually enlarged so that any future accumulation of diseased tissue can be visualized and removed through the external meatus. During *modified* radical mastoidectomy, less bone is removed and the ossicles may or may not be removed, depending on the extent of disease.

A radical mastoidectomy is indicated for some patients with chronic middle ear and mastoid infection or for cholesteatoma, a condition in which a growth of skin in the middle ear acts as a foreign body and produces erosion. The radical mastoid operation, with certain modifications, may also be indicated for some cases of petrositis (inflammation of the petrous area of the temporal bone), removal of glomus jugular tumors of the middle ear, early carcinoma of the ear, decompression

and repair of the tympanic and mastoid portion of the facial nerve, and the fenestration operation.

Highlights

1. An endaural or postauricular incision is made.
2. The mastoid antrum is exposed.
3. The ossicles, facial nerve, and horizontal semicircular canal are identified.
4. The mastoid cavity is completely exenterated.
5. The wound is closed.

Description

The patient is placed in the supine position and the head is turned with the affected side up. After routine prepping and draping, the surgeon uses a No. 15 Bard-Parker knife to create an endaural and/or postauricular incision. Bleeding vessels are controlled with the electrocautery pencil or with fine ties. To make a connection between the auditory canal and the mastoid area, the surgeon incises the skin of the auditory canal with angled and straight canal knives. With the use of the scalpel, a meatal flap is created and the mastoid area is then exposed with a narrow periosteal elevator and curved scissors. A self-retaining endaural retractor is then placed in the wound.

The bony cortex, which lies superior and posterolateral to the antrum, and the posterior and superior osseous meatal walls are removed with a rongeur or

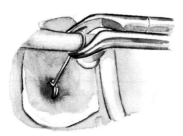

Figure 28–21. Stapedectomy. A microcrimper is used to secure the prosthesis on the long end of the incus. (From Shambaugh GE, Jr: Surgery of the Ear, 2nd ed. Philadelphia, WB Saunders, 1967.)

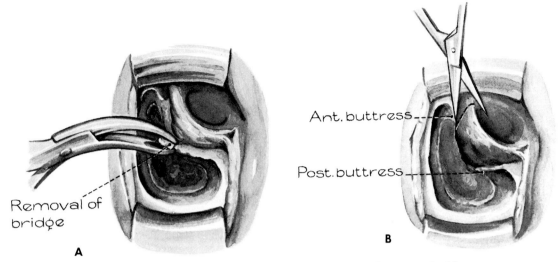

Figure 28–22. Radical mastoidectomy. *A.* Bony meatal wall is removed with a rongeur. *B.* The bridge is removed. (From Shambaugh GE, Jr: Surgery of the Ear, 2nd ed. Philadelphia, WB Saunders, 1967.)

electric drill and round cutting bur (Fig. 28–22A). Suction and continuous irrigation with lactated Ringer's solution are used when the surgeon is drilling. Many surgeons request that the technologist have bone wax and Gelfoam available for hemostasis at this time.

After the majority of mastoid air cells have been removed, the surgeon uses a small middle ear curette or an electric drill to remove the thin ridge of bone that comprises the posterior and superior external auditory canals (Fig. 28–22B). Fine hooks and ear picks are then used to excise the tympanic membrane. The malleus, incus, and mucoperiosteal lining of the middle ear cavity are excised with stapes instruments. At this point, the radical mastoidectomy is completed.

After identifying the horizontal semicircular canal, facial nerve, and stapes, the surgeon cleans out the tympanic cavity using a curette and/or an electric drill. The mastoid cavity is packed with a strip of ¼- or ½-inch gauze impregnated with an antibiotic ointment, which the technologist has prepared. The wound is then closed with subcutaneous sutures of size 4-0 catgut or Dexon and skin sutures of size 4-0 or 5-0 Nylon or Prolene.

An ear dressing consisting of several fluffed 8 × 4-inch gauze dressings is applied behind and around the affected ear and then covered by flat compresses. A gauze bandage is applied around the head to hold the dressings in place.

Tympanoplasty

Definition

This is the surgical restoration of a diseased or injured tympanic membrane and/or middle ear structure. Tympanoplasty is the operation performed to repair both the perforation in the tympanic membrane and the sound-transmitting mechanism. This procedure seals the middle ear and, in most cases, improves hearing.

Diseases that cause damage to the tympanic membrane and middle ear structures include chronic otitis media (infection of the middle ear) and cholesteatoma. There are five basic types of tympanoplasties (Fig. 28–23), each differing according to the extent of the disease or injury (Table 28–1). Various types of grafts may be used to replace the damaged tympanic membrane. An autograft taken from the patient's postauricular fascia (Fig. 28–24A) or a segment of vein from the arm are among the most common donor graft sites. When the middle ear structures are damaged (types II through V), surgery is performed to re-establish the connections from the sound-conducting structure and to protect the round window by the creation of an air pocket between the graft and round window.

Table 28–1. TYPES OF TYMPANOPLASTY

Type	Condition of Middle Ear	Repair and Graft Placement*
I	Ossicular chain intact and mobile Perforated tympanic membrane	Graft covers the defect in the tympanic membrane and is placed against the malleus.
II	Damaged malleus	Closure with graft primarily contacting the body of the incus.
III	Malleus and incus are missing with intact and mobile stapes.	Graft is depressed against the normal stapes.
IV	All ossicles are missing except a mobile stapes footplate.	Graft is invaginated tightly into the oval window.
V	Similar to type I, but the stapes footplate is not mobile.	Graft is invaginated into the oval window.

*Homograft tympanoplasty may be performed for any degree of ossicular damage. The homograft ossicle is used to bridge a defect between the oval window and tympanic membrane.

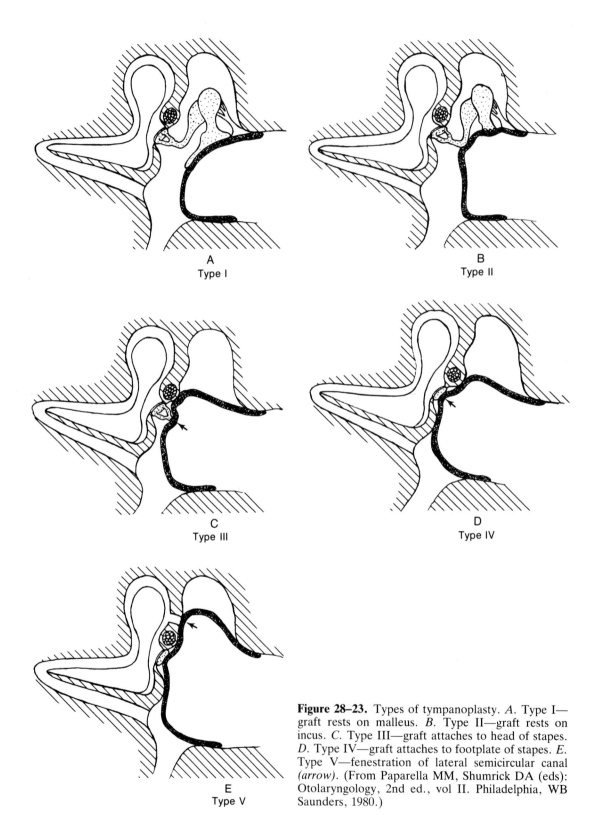

A
Type I

B
Type II

C
Type III

D
Type IV

E
Type V

Figure 28–23. Types of tympanoplasty. *A.* Type I—graft rests on malleus. *B.* Type II—graft rests on incus. *C.* Type III—graft attaches to head of stapes. *D.* Type IV—graft attaches to footplate of stapes. *E.* Type V—fenestration of lateral semicircular canal *(arrow).* (From Paparella MM, Shumrick DA (eds): Otolaryngology, 2nd ed., vol II. Philadelphia, WB Saunders, 1980.)

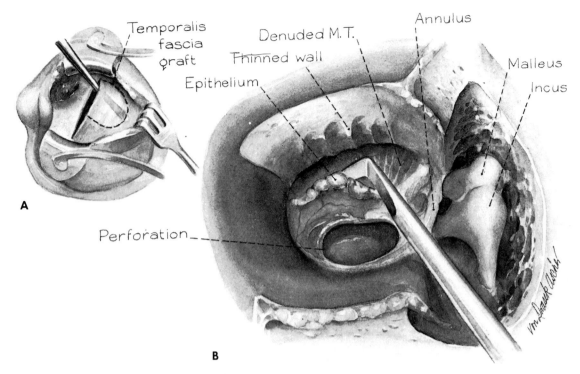

Figure 28-24. *A*. Graft taken from the patient's postauricular fascia. *B*. All or some of the tympanic membrane remnants are removed. (From Shambaugh GE, Jr: Surgery of the Ear, 2nd ed. Philadelphia, WB Saunders, 1967.)

In many cases, it is not possible to repair the sound-transmitting mechanism and the tympanic membrane during one operation. The tympanic membrane is repaired first, and, several months later, the sound-transmitting mechanism is reconstructed, when possible.

Description

The patient is placed in the supine position with the affected ear up. The ear is then prepped and draped in routine fashion. The surgeon may approach the ear through the canal, through a postauricular incision, or both. The exact steps of the procedure vary according to its type (see Table 28–1). However, some steps are basic to all types and are discussed here.

The graft may be taken before or after the initial ear procedure has begun. Once the graft is taken, the surgeon may smooth it out on a flat surface such as an overturned basin and allow it to dry, or the graft may be placed within a press. Pressing and drying make the graft easier to handle.

In the first basic steps of the procedure, the surgeon removes all or some of the tympanic membrane remnants (Fig. 28–24*B*). The technologist may be asked to save these remnants as a specimen. Next, depending on the nature and type of procedure to be performed, the surgeon may remove diseased tissue with middle ear curettes, picks, or a power drill and small bur. The technologist may be required to irrigate the area as the surgeon drills.

Before the graft is inserted, the surgeon trims the graft to the proper size using a No. 15 knife blade and/or small curved scissors. The middle ear is reconstructed by placing the graft in position using alligator forceps and fine picks. Small pledgets of Gelfoam or a paper patch may be used to hold the graft in position. The wound is then closed, and a mastoid dressing is applied.

Cochlear Implantation

This is the surgical implantation of an electronic hearing device in the cochlea. Patients who are able to speak but whose hearing has been lost to disease are candidates for implantation. Extensive patient auditory training is necessary postoperatively to teach the patient how to interpret the device's electronic signals.

The cochlear implant receives sound waves through a receiver that is implanted in the patient's mastoid cavity. Electrical impulses transmitted along the acoustic nerve are then received and interpreted in the temporal cortex.

Part II ◆ NOSE, THROAT, AND MOUTH SURGERY

Procedures of the nose and throat are generally performed by the surgeon specializing in otorhinolaryngology, although some general surgeons may perform a tonsillectomy or radical neck procedure. Nasal procedures, including the Caldwell-Luc procedure, are performed to establish a patent airway by removing and/or reconstructing bone and cartilage in the nasal cavity and sinuses. More extensive procedures, such as the radical neck dissection, are performed following tissue biopsy through the laryngoscope or by examination of suspect tumors in the neck and mouth area and are aimed at eradicating any cancerous tissue.

Dental procedures are logically placed in this section, even though performed by a dental surgeon rather than one specializing in ear, nose, and throat surgery.

SURGICAL ANATOMY

Nose

The nose serves as a passageway for air between the outside of the body and the lungs. As air is drawn in, the nose warms, humidifies, and filters it.

External Nose

The external nose is formed by two U-shaped cartilaginous structures called the *nares*. Within each naris is the *nostril*, the actual opening through the naris. The nares are formed by the *alar cartilage*. Another cartilaginous structure, the *septum*, separates the two nostrils (Fig. 28–25). The roof of the nose is formed by the *nasal bone*, which consists of portions of the ethmoid, sphenoid, and palatine bones. The floor of the nose is formed by the maxilla and palatine bones, and the lateral walls are formed by the *nasal conchae*, which divide the two nasal cavities into passageways called *meatuses*. The nasal cavity is lined with mucous membrane, which aids in the warming and humidifying process. Small hairs or *vibrissae* are also present, and these filter out large foreign material as the air passes over them. The *posterior nares*, the back portion of the passageways, open directly into the *pharynx* (discussed subsequently).

Paranasal Sinuses

The paranasal sinuses (Fig. 28–26) are located within the bones for which they are named: the *maxillary*, *frontal*, *ethmoid*, and *sphenoid*. These lighten the weight of the skull and also secrete mucus for lubricating and cleansing the nasal passages. In addition, the paranasal sinuses act as a "sounding board," which resonates during speech. The *nasolacrimal duct* opens into the sphenoid sinus, where tears are drained from the eye.

Throat

Pharynx

The pharynx (Fig. 28–27) is a passageway that leads from the base of the skull to the esophagus. This structure is divided into three separate sections. The *nasopharynx* is the uppermost portion. It lies directly behind the nasal sinuses above the soft palate of the mouth. The two openings to the eustachian tubes lie on each lateral wall, connecting the nasopharynx to the middle ear. At the upper end of the posterior wall of the nasopharynx lies the *adenoids*, also known as the *pharyngeal tonsils*. These are small masses of lymph tissue that are commonly removed during a tonsillectomy procedure on pediatric patients (the adenoids almost always recede in adult life).

The *oropharynx* is the second section of the pharynx. It extends from the soft palate to the level of the hyoid bone of the neck. The palatine tonsils ("tonsils") are located in this area on each lateral wall. The tonsils are soft masses composed of lymph tissue. They are suspended by a fold of tissue called the *pillar*.

The *laryngopharynx* is the lowest portion of the pharynx. It lies below the hyoid bone behind the larynx. At this level, the pharynx becomes continuous with the esophagus. Because the *larynx*, a continuation of the trachea, also lies in this area, the laryngopharynx is a cross point for both nutrients and air. During swallowing, food and liquid are pushed back into the esophagus posteriorly while air moves forward into the larynx.

Larynx

The larynx (Fig. 28–28), or so-called voice box, bridges the pharynx and the trachea. This passageway is located between the base of the tongue and the trachea, in front of the fourth, fifth, and sixth cervical vertebrae. It is composed of nine separate cartilages. The largest of the cartilages, the thyroid cartilage, is composed of two plates, which in turn form the Adam's apple. The smaller spoon-shaped cartilage, the epiglottic cartilage, has a rounded upper end, which results in the

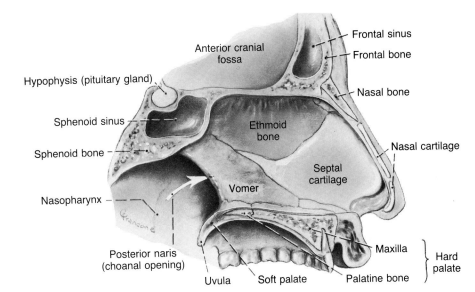

Figure 28–25. Sagittal section through the nose, illustrating the components of the nasal septum and the bones that surround it. (From Jacob S, Francone C, Lossow WJ: Structure and Function in Man, 5th ed. Philadelphia, WB Saunders, 1982.)

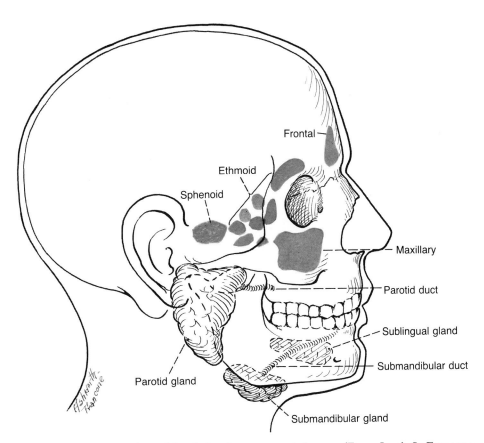

Figure 28–26. Lateral view of head showing paranasal sinuses. (From Jacob S, Francone C, Lossow WJ: Structure and Function in Man, 5th ed. Philadelphia, WB Saunders, 1982.)

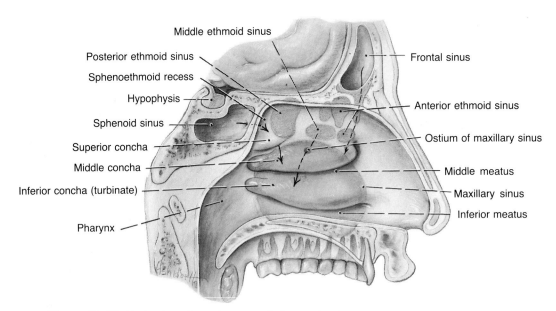

Figure 28–27. Sagittal section of nose and throat showing the location of the pharynx. (From Jacob S, Francone C, Lossow WJ: Structure and Function in Man, 5th ed. Philadelphia, WB Saunders, 1982.)

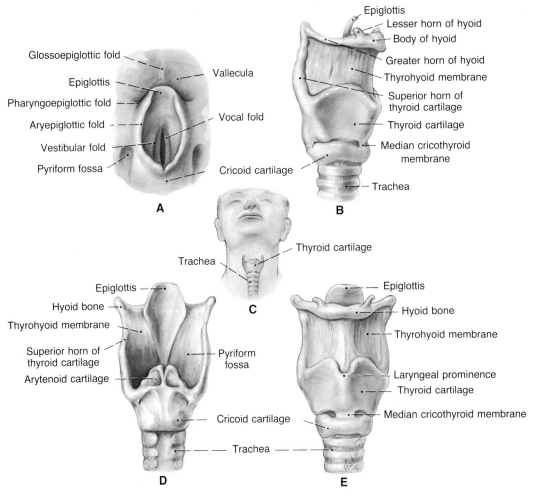

Figure 28–28. The larynx. *A.* As viewed from above. *B.* As viewed from the side. *C.* In relation to the head and neck. *D.* From behind. *E.* Frontal view. (From Jacob S, Francone C, Lossow WJ: Structure and Function in Man, 5th ed. Philadelphia, WB Saunders, 1982.)

epiglottis. The inferior portion of the larynx is bound by the cricoid cartilage. Within the laryngeal cavity lie a pair of *vocal folds,* which are the true vocal cords, and a pair of *ventricular folds,* which are the false vocal cords. As air is forced through the larynx, sound is produced by the vocal cords. *Speech,* however, is a function of the cavities above and below the larynx.

Trachea

The *trachea* (commonly called the "windpipe") is a rigid tube that extends about 4½ inches from the level of the sixth cervical vertebra to the fifth thoracic vertebra. Thus, half of the trachea lies in the neck (Fig. 28–29) whereas the other half is situated within the thoracic cavity. The trachea is composed of four layers of tissue: the mucosa (lining), the submucosa, a cartilaginous layer, and an outside connective tissue layer (the adventitia).

The main structure of the tracheal wall is composed of a series of C-shaped rings, varying in number between 16 and 20. Within the tracheal wall, cilia and mucous glands are present. These sweep pollutants out of the trachea and into the pharynx and also further warm and moisten air as it passes down into the lungs.

At the level of the second, third, and fourth tracheal rings lies the *thyroid gland* (see Fig. 28–29). This gland is situated on the anterior side of the trachea and is composed of two lobes, which are connected by a narrow bridge called the *isthmus.* The thyroid secretes hormones, which are stored within the follicles of the gland.

Mouth

The mouth is composed of the lips, cheeks, tongue, teeth, and salivary glands.

Lips

The lips are composed of skeletal muscle and fibroelastic connective tissue. They are covered by skin on the outer surface and mucous membrane on the inner surface.

Cheeks

The cheeks are composed of skeletal muscle and form the walls of the mouth. The buccinator muscles aid in mastication (chewing) by preventing food from escaping from between the teeth.

Tongue

The tongue (Fig. 28–30) is composed of two sets of muscles bound by fibroelastic tissue. It is a highly moveable structure that aids in swallowing, chewing, and speech. The base of the tongue is connected to the floor of the mouth by the *frenulum,* a fold of mucous membrane. The uppermost surface of the tongue contains many small projections called *papillae.* The taste buds are located on these projections.

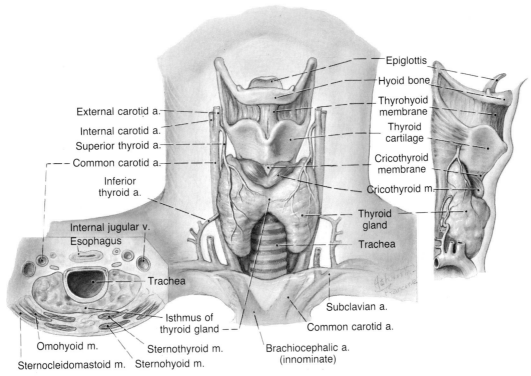

Figure 28–29. Location of trachea and thyroid gland. (From Jacob S, Francone C, Lossow WJ: Structure and Function in Man, 5th ed. Philadelphia, WB Saunders, 1982.)

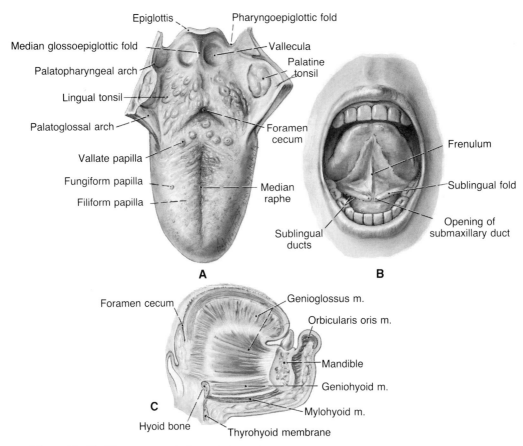

Figure 28–30. The tongue. *A.* Dorsal view. *B.* Anterior view of the mouth with the tongue raised. *C.* Midsagittal section through the tongue. (From Jacob S, Francone C, Lossow WJ: Structure and Function in Man, 5th ed. Philadelphia, WB Saunders, 1982.)

Teeth

At birth, there are two sets of teeth present in the jaws. The first set, the *deciduous* teeth, number 20. Between the ages of 6 and 12 years, the second set of teeth takes the place of the deciduous teeth. These teeth are called the *permanent* teeth. In each jaw are four incisor, two canine, four premolar, and six molar teeth. (The third molars, the wisdom teeth, erupt at 17 to 21 years of age.)

Each tooth (Fig. 28–31) is divided into two primary sections: the *crown*, or exposed part, and the *root*, or that portion that is embedded in the jaw (maxilla or mandible, depending on whether it is upper or lower). The crown is covered with *enamel*, which is a hard calcified material. Beneath the enamel is the *dentin*, which is composed mainly of calcium phosphate. Within the dentin is a small cavity called the *pulp cavity*, which is composed of an upper *pulp chamber* and a narrow *root canal*. At the base of the root canal lies the *apical foramen*, through which the blood vessels and nerves enter the pulp cavity. The root is covered by *cementum*, a bonelike substance. Between the cementum and the bone in which the tooth is embedded is a membrane called the *periodontal membrane*. The lower part of the crown is embedded in the *gingiva* or *gum*. This is a mucous membrane that surrounds the base of the crown and covers the bone.

Salivary Glands

There are three pairs of salivary glands: the *parotid, sublingual,* and *submaxillary*. The parotid glands are buried within the subcutaneous layer of the cheeks, below the ear. The submaxillary glands lie in the floor of the mouth, and the sublingual glands are situated under the tongue. Each gland has a separate duct that empties into the mouth region. The location of each gland is illustrated in Figure 28–26.

SURGICAL PROCEDURES

Nasal Septal Reconstruction

Definition

This is the excision and resection of the nasal cartilage. The procedure is performed to correct a deviated septum or other septal defect to restore an inadequate airway.

Highlights

1. The nasal mucosa is incised.
2. Nasal cartilage is removed.
3. The cartilage is reconstructed.
4. The incision is closed.

Description

There are many different techniques presently employed in nasal reconstruction, and the technologist is best prepared for assisting in nasal surgery by working with the same surgeons and learning their preferred techniques and instrumentation. For the novice, a thorough knowledge of nasal instruments will facilitate learning a given routine. The following description of the nasal septal reconstruction procedure is written as a broad guideline for the surgery.

The patient is placed in the supine position, and the operating table is tilted into a slight reverse Trendelenburg position. The face may be prepped, although the nose *is* considered a contaminated area.

Nasal surgery is commonly performed with the use of a local anesthetic unless the patient is very uncooperative. Before beginning the procedure, the technologist usually sets up a "local stand" on which the items needed for administration of the anesthetic are placed. Many surgeons swab the nasal cavity with cocaine solution or crystals before injecting the local anesthetic, so metal applicators and cotton will be needed for this. The surgeon usually prefers to prepare the swabs because, if the cotton swabs are improperly placed on the applicator, the swab can come loose within the patient's nose and lodge in the airway.

Once the patient has been anesthetized, the surgeon uses a columella retractor to pull the nasal septum downward. A small incision is then made in the mucoperichondrium with a No. 11 or No. 15 knife blade. Small skin hooks are placed at the wound edges to retract them (Fig. 28–32). The technologist may be required to retract. Only *gentle* traction is necessary; too much pressure on the hooks causes them to pierce the tissue and leads to unnecessary trauma. The surgeon deepens the incision with fine, sharp dissecting scissors.

The surgeon then elevates the mucoperichondrium from the septal cartilage using a fine elevator. A rongeur is used to remove any spurs from the septum or nasal bone. With the mucoperichondrium fully elevated, the surgeon removes the septal cartilage with a rongeur. All segments of cartilage are saved and preserved in saline solution on the instrument table. The technologist should have a small basin available to receive the segments. The surgeon may use fine osteotomes to remove any redundant bony tissue.

The septal tissue is now examined and reshaped for reinsertion into the nose. The surgeon may simply trim the cartilage with scissors or may place it in a special bone crusher and flatten the cartilage. The cartilage is then replaced within the nose (Fig. 28–33).

The incision is closed with fine absorbable sutures and the nasal cavity is packed with Adaptic or a similar packing material. Some surgeons use Silastic splints to hold the septum straight while healing takes place. Short strips of tape are placed over the bridge of the nose for stability.

Caldwell-Luc Procedure

Definition

This is the creation of a new passageway between the nasal sinuses to establish drainage. Chronic infection and sinusitis can cause extensive scarring within the nasal sinuses. The Caldwell-Luc procedure is performed to clear away the scar tissue and re-establish an opening or "window" to ensure drainage.

Highlights

1. The canine fossa is incised.
2. Bone and scar tissue are removed by sharp dissection.

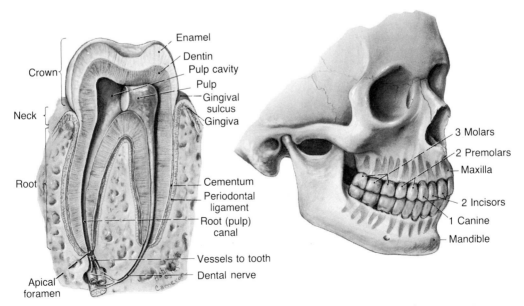

Figure 28–31. Cross section of a molar tooth and vertical position. (From Jacob S, Francone C, Lossow WJ: Structure and Function in Man, 5th ed. Philadelphia, WB Saunders, 1982.)

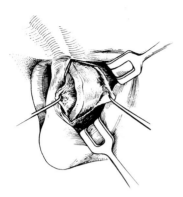

Figure 28–32. Nasal septal reconstruction. The mucoperichondrium is elevated. (From Paparella MM, Shumrick DA (eds): Otolaryngology, 2nd ed, vol III. Philadelphia, WB Saunders, 1980.)

3. The window is created.
4. The wound is closed.

Description

In preparation for this procedure, the technologist should have available a large selection of nasal instruments, including rongeurs, elevators, curettes, small osteotomes, and U.S. Army or similar retractors. The cutting instruments are used to remove small bits of bone or fibrous scar tissue that occlude the patient's sinuses. A small Frazier suction tip should also be available.

The patient is placed in the supine position and tipped into a slight reverse Trendelenburg position. The face may be prepped, although the mouth is exposed and is considered a contaminated area. A head drape and body sheet are applied.

To begin the procedure, the technologist retracts the patient's upper lip with a Caldwell-Luc or U.S. Army retractor. The surgeon then makes a small incision just above the patient's teeth, above the canine tooth and premolars (Fig. 28–34A). A No. 15 knife blade is used to make the incision. Once the gum has been incised,

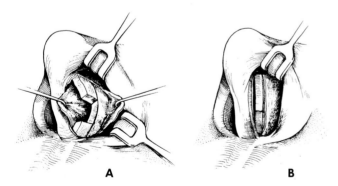

Figure 28–33. Nasal septal reconstruction. A. Segment of septum has been removed. B. The caudal septum is straightened after it has been repositioned. (From Paparella MM, Shumrick DA (eds): Otolaryngology, 2nd ed, vol III. Philadelphia, WB Saunders, 1980.)

the surgeon uses a periosteal elevator to strip the periosteum from the maxilla. A Frazier suction tip is used to clear the wound site of blood.

To gain access to the inner nasal sinuses, the surgeon perforates the bone with a chisel and mallet. The perforation is then enlarged bit by bit with small rongeurs. Once the sinus has been reached, the surgeon may use curettes to scrape away scar tissue from the sinus. Rongeurs (Kerrison, up-biting and down-biting) are used to create a passageway in the bone (Fig. 28–34B). Chisels and osteotomes may also be used to remove diseased tissue (Fig. 28–34C). During this time, the technologist continues to retract the patient's lip.

When adequate drainage has been established, the surgeon closes the gingival incision with plain catgut sutures (some surgeons prefer not to suture the wound). The nasal sinus may or may not be packed with Gelfoam or standard nasal packing, according to the surgeon's preference.

Polypectomy

Definition

Nasal polyps are edematous outgrowths of the sinus mucosa usually located in the middle meatus. Surgery is performed when the patient's airway is obstructed and/or if the sense of smell has been obliterated by the polyps.

Description

The patient is placed in supine position, and the operating table is tipped to a slight reverse Trendelenburg position. The procedure is usually performed with the patient under local anesthesia with the aid of combined topical cocaine solution and injectable local infiltration.

The nasal cavity may be packed with cotton gauze, and the polyps are removed with a polyp snare, similar to that used in a tonsillectomy procedure. Each polyp is recovered and retained as a specimen. The cotton gauze is then removed, and the nasal cavity is packed with Adaptic or other similar type petrolatum gauze.

Laryngoscopy

Definition

This is the visualization of the larynx through a fiberoptic *laryngoscope* (Fig. 28–35) to determine the presence of disease. Tissue biopsy specimens may also be taken through the laryngoscope.

Highlights

1. The laryngoscope is inserted.
2. Biopsy specimens are taken.
3. The scope is withdrawn.

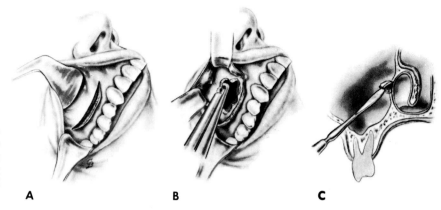

Figure 28–34. Caldwell-Luc procedure. *A.* An incision is made just above the canine tooth. *B.* Kerrison rongeurs are used to widen the fossa. *C.* The antral window is created. (From Paparella MM, Shumrick DA (eds): Otolaryngology, 2nd ed, vol III. Philadelphia, WB Saunders, 1980.)

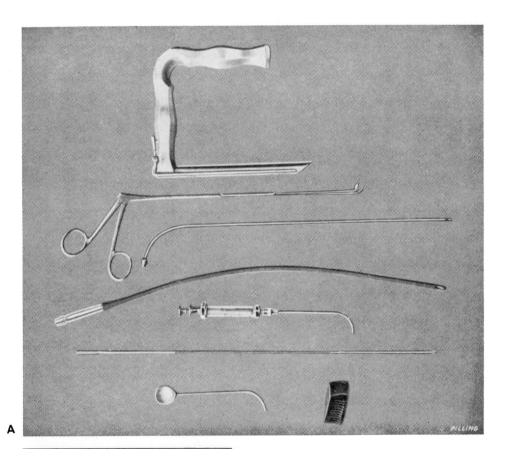

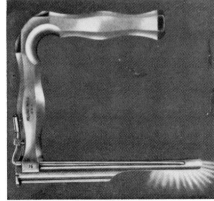

Figure 28–35. *A.* Jackson laryngoscope *(top)* and accessories, including biopsy forceps, suction, sponge carrier, aspirating tube, laryngeal syringe, and bite block. *B.* Laryngoscope (enlarged view). (From Jackson C, Jackson CL: Bronchoesophagology. Philadelphia, WB Saunders, 1950.)

Description

Patients undergoing laryngoscopy may be given a local or general anesthetic. The patient is placed in the supine position on the operating table. To facilitate passage of the laryngoscope, the technologist tilts the patient's head back and supports the neck with sandbags or rolled bath blankets. The patient is not prepped. The surgeon inserts the laryngoscope and views the larynx and associated structures. The technologist should stand by the surgeon, ready to pass the suction tip and biopsy forceps. It is convenient to work directly from the back table during laryngoscopy rather than from the Mayo stand. When suction is needed, the technologist assists the surgeon by directing the suction tip into the scope.

Biopsy samples are taken with the biopsy forceps. When the surgeon withdraws the forceps containing the biopsy tissue, he or she usually passes it directly to the technologist. The tissue can be retrieved from the forceps by dipping the tip into a small basin or by "picking" the tissue from the forceps with a hypodermic needle. All tissue specimens should be kept separate from each other unless the surgeon indicates otherwise.

Small sponges, should they be needed, are mounted on a sponge carrier. The technologist should be very careful to secure the sponge tightly so that it is not lost in the patient's larynx. Concluding the procedure, the surgeon withdraws the laryngoscope slowly to avoid trauma to the larynx and associated structures.

Tonsillectomy and Adenoidectomy

Definition

This is the excision of the tonsils and adenoids. Chronic tonsillitis, associated otitis media, and nasal obstruction due to enlarged adenoid glands are indications for a tonsillectomy and adenoidectomy. The adenoids are usually absent in the adult patient.

Highlights

1. The adenoids are curetted and removed.
2. The tonsils are excised by sharp and blunt dissection.
3. Bleeding is controlled.

Description

The patient is placed in the supine position on the operating table, and a small rolled bath blanket is placed under the shoulders to hyperextend the neck. Because the mouth is considered a contaminated area, the patient is usually not prepped.

In preparation for the case, the technologist should have available the surgeon's choice of mouth gag (usually indicated on the preference card), assorted hemostatic clamps (Schnidt and Murphy clamps are commonly used), a No. 12 scalpel blade mounted on a No. 7 handle, sponge sticks, a Hurd or similar elevator, dissecting scissors, tonsil snares, adenoid curettes, and a Yankauer suction tip.

The surgeon sits at the patient's head while operating. To begin the procedure, the surgeon inserts a mouth gag into the patient's mouth to retract it open. The Davis mouth gag attaches to the technologist's Mayo stand. If this particular gag is used, the technologist must be very careful not to lean on or jar the Mayo stand, since the patient's jaw can be fractured.

The surgeon first removes the adenoids by curetting them loose. When the surgeon deposits the adenoid tissue onto the Mayo stand, the technologist should gather the tissue in a small basin and retain it as a specimen.

The surgeon then grasps the tonsil with a small tenaculum or tonsil-seizing forceps. An incision is made around the tonsil with the scalpel (Fig. 28–36A and B). Suction should be immediately available. The technologist may be required to suction for the surgeon. Using a Hurd dissector or other elevator and dissecting scissors, the surgeon frees the tonsil from its fossa until only the tonsillar pillar remains to attach it (Fig. 28–36C). A tonsil snare is then looped over the tonsil and snapped over the pillar, thus releasing the tonsil (Fig. 28–36D). Bleeding is usually brisk at this time, and the surgeon may pack the fossa with a large dissecting sponge for a few moments to help control the bleeding. Many surgeons place one or two plain catgut sutures, size 3-0, over the tonsillar fossa. An alternate method of hemostasis is with a combined cautery-suction unit. The procedure is then repeated on the opposite tonsil. Note that whenever a snare is used for the procedure, the snare wire is used only once and must be replaced after each single use. When the second tonsil is removed, it is kept separate from the first and both tonsils are identified as left or right. A common method of identification is to place a safety pin through the right tonsil.

Following the procedure, the technologist may assist in cleaning any blood from the patient's face. It is vital that the suction tip and tubing not be dismantled *until the patient has left the operating suite* so that in the event of sudden bleeding from the fossa the surgeon can suction the blood and prevent the patient from aspirating it. The patient is placed on his or her side before transportation to the post-anesthesia care unit to help prevent the aspiration of blood.

Radical Neck Dissection

Definition

This is the en bloc removal of lymphatic chains and all nonvital structures of the neck. Radical neck dissection is indicated when the patient has had a previous tumor of the tongue, larynx, lip, or other area of the mouth removed and when near metastasis has occurred by way of the lymphatic system. Tumors of the head and neck grow slowly, and metastasis may occur months after the primary lesion has been identified and re-

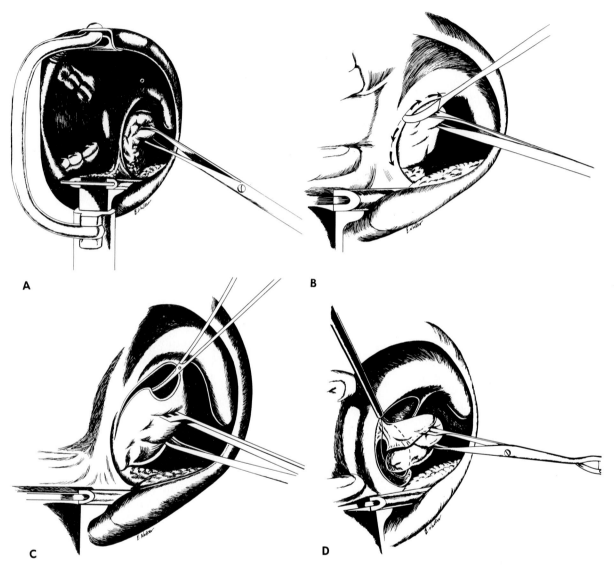

A

B

C

D

Figure 28–36. Tonsillectomy. *A.* The tonsil is grasped with a tenaculum. *B.* A circular incision is made around the tonsillar fossa. *C.* Dissecting scissors are used to separate the tonsil capsule from underlying tissue. *D.* The surgeon places a tonsil snare over the pillar and snaps it free. (From Paparella MM, Shumrick DA (eds): Otolaryngology, 3rd ed, vol III. Philadelphia, WB Saunders, 1991.)

moved. This procedure may also be performed in conjunction with removal of a primary lesion when near metastasis is suspected.

Highlights

1. The neck is incised and skin flaps are created.
2. Tissues and major structures of the neck are removed.
3. If necessary, a tracheostomy is performed.
4. The wound is closed.

Description

Numerous techniques are employed in radical neck surgery. The operation is not technically complicated for the surgical technologist because, while the surgery can be quite lengthy, it involves simply the removal of diseased and nondiseased tissues by sharp and blunt dissection and the ligation of major vessels. From the technologist's point of view, the surgery closely resembles a thyroidectomy.

The patient is placed in the supine position with the affected side of the neck facing upward. The neck is slightly hyperextended with a rolled bath blanket or towel. The patient is prepped to include the face, neck, and upper chest. During draping, a wide area of the neck is exposed. Sterile adhesive drapes may be used or the surgeon may wish to sew linen drapes at the periphery of the operative site.

To begin the procedure, the surgeon marks the incisional area with a skin marker. Various incisions are used, including H and Y shapes. Once the initial skin incision is made with the scalpel, most surgeons use the electrosurgical pencil to dissect the deeper tissues and to create skin flaps that are turned back with retractors. Moist lap sponges should be available throughout the dissection. Once the skin flaps are elevated, the technologist should have available at all times several ties of size 2-0 and 3-0 suture (surgeon's choice of material) mounted on passers. These will be used to ligate major vessels that are encountered during the procedure. In addition, many surgeons use a nerve locator to differentiate between nerves and vessels. The surgeon continues the dissection, removing tumor, lymph, and muscle tissues. In most cases the dissection is carried out with tissue forceps, Metzenbaum and Mayo scissors, a scalpel, and an electrocautery pencil (Fig. 28–37). Large rake (Israel) retractors are often useful for traction of the wound edges.

When the dissection is complete, the surgeon may elect to perform a tracheostomy. This is done particularly if extensive postoperative swelling is anticipated. At the completion of the procedure, the surgeon irrigates the wound thoroughly with warm saline solution and checks any oozing, since the wound must be as dry as possible before closure.

The wound is closed with absorbable sutures (Dexon or Vicryl are commonly used) and skin sutures or staples, according to the surgeon's preference. A bulky dressing is then applied to the skin.

Related Procedure

Laryngectomy (removal of the larynx, strap muscles, and hyoid bone)

DENTAL PROCEDURES

Under normal circumstances, the oral surgeon performs dental procedures in the office. However, if the patient wishes to have a general anesthetic or is otherwise very uncooperative, the surgeon may elect to perform the procedure in the operating room. In other instances, the patient may need to be monitored by the anesthesiologist because of his or her general physical condition.

In most cases the dentist brings his or her personal dental technician or dental assistant to assist in the surgery. This assistant then takes the place of the surgical technologist at the field. However, the surgical technologist may be required to scrub with the dental technician to help set up the back table, assist in gowning and gloving, and help with other routines that may be unfamiliar to the dental technician.

It is common practice for the dental surgeon to bring his or her own personal instruments to the operating room, where they are flash sterilized by operating room personnel. Many practicing surgical technologists are unfamiliar with the names of specific dental instruments because very few dental procedures are performed in the operating room. Therefore, after the surgeon has been gowned and gloved, and when a dental technician is *not* available to scrub on the case, the surgical technologist should ask the surgeon to identify the instruments he or she would like to have available on the Mayo stand. During the case, the surgeon usually picks up instruments directly from the Mayo stand. An exception to this is when a common instrument with which the technologist is familiar is needed, such as scissors, hemostat, or needle holder and suture.

A typical dental tray with assorted instruments used in dental extraction is shown in Figure 28–38. In addition to these instruments, the technologist should have a roll of throat packing, several small basins, and tonsil (Yankauer) suction available. Occasionally a power drill may also be necessary.

Dental Extraction

Definition

This is the removal of one or more teeth in the presence of gingival (gum) or tooth disease. If all the patient's teeth are to be removed, the procedure is referred to as a *full mouth extraction*.

Highlights

1. The throat is packed.
2. The gingiva is incised.
3. The tooth is loosened and removed.

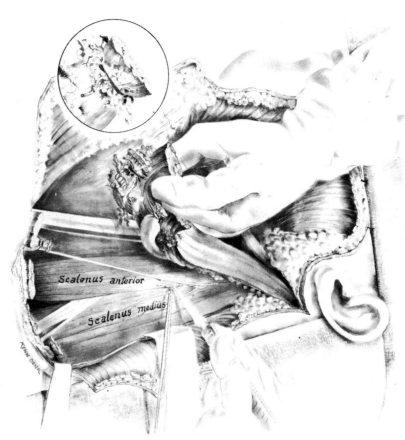

Figure 28–37. Radical neck dissection. Ligation of the large neuromusculovascular bundle with transfixion sutures. (From Paparella MM, Shumrick DA (eds): Otolaryngology, 3rd ed, vol III. Philadelphia, WB Saunders, 1991.)

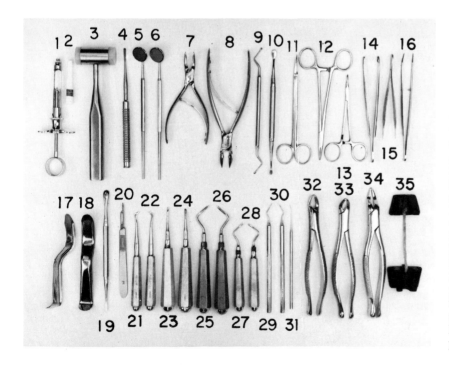

Figure 28–38. Instruments used for multiple tooth extraction: 1, syringe for local anesthetic; 2, hypodermic needle; 3, mallet; 4, single-bevel chisel; 5 and 6, mirrors; 7, rongeurs; 8, bone forceps; 9, curette; 10, bone file; 11, tissue scissors; 12, needle holder; 13, hemostat; 14, Russian tissue forceps; 15, Adson tissue forceps; 16, cotton pliers; 17 and 18, Minnesota retractors; 19, periosteal elevator; 20, scalpel; 21, No. 30 elevator; 22, No. 31 elevator; 23, No. 301 elevator; 24, No. 34 elevator; 25, No. 302 elevator; 26; No. 303 elevator; 27 and 28, apical elevators; 29 and 30, apical root picks; 31, Gilmore probe; 32, No. 150 forceps; 33, No. 151 forceps; 34, No. 286 forceps; 35, McKesson mouth props. (From Torres HO, Ehrlich A: Modern Dental Assisting, 4th ed. Philadelphia, WB Saunders, 1990.)

4. The wound is closed.
5. The throat packing is removed.

Description

The patient is placed in the supine position, draped as for a tonsillectomy and adenoidectomy, and tipped into a slight reverse Trendelenburg position. Following the administration of a general anesthetic, the technologist should provide the surgeon with a roll of throat packing (vaginal packing is commonly used) that has been dipped into saline solution and tightly wrung out. Using smooth tissue forceps, the surgeon packs the patient's throat with the packing. The packing prevents the aspiration or ingestion of blood. *It is critical that the packing be removed after the procedure.* For both the surgeon and technologist to remember to remove the packing after the operation, a hemostat can be clamped to the edge of the Mayo stand cover so that it hangs downward. This is done as soon as the packing is inserted and serves as a reminder that the packing is in place. Should the packing be left in place, the patient could aspirate it and suffocate postoperatively. It is the dual responsibility of the surgeon and technologist to be aware that the packing is in place.

To begin the procedure, the surgeon injects a small amount of local anesthetic combined with epinephrine in the area around the diseased tooth. This aids in hemostasis. Using a No. 15 knife blade, the surgeon makes a small incision at the base of the tooth. The technologist is responsible for suctioning any blood or secretions at this time and throughout the procedure. After incising the gum, the surgeon uses a fine periosteal elevator such as that used in nasal surgery to loosen the gingiva from the tooth. An extractor is then used to loosen the tooth and remove it from its socket. The technologist should place a small basin on the Mayo stand to receive the teeth as the surgeon removes them and to preserve them as specimens. After the teeth have been removed, the oral cavity is irrigated with warm saline solution and all fluid is suctioned away. The incision(s) are closed with interrupted sutures of size 3-0 plain catgut or silk swaged to a small cutting needle. The throat packing is then removed.

Bibliography

DeWeese DD, Saunders WH: Textbook of Otolaryngology, 6th ed. St. Louis, CV Mosby, 1982.

Dorland's Illustrated Medical Dictionary, 27th ed. Philadelphia, WB Saunders, 1988.

Ethicon, Inc: Suture Use Manual: Use and Handling of Sutures and Needles. Somerville, NJ, Ethicon, Inc, 1978.

Gardner E, Gray D, O'Rahilly R: Anatomy: A Regional Study of Human Structure, 5th ed. Philadelphia, WB Saunders, 1986.

Jacob S, Francone C, Lossow WJ: Structure and Function in Man, 5th ed. Philadelphia, WB Saunders, 1984.

McVay C: Surgical Anatomy, 6th ed. Philadelphia, WB Saunders, 1984.

Paparella M, et al: Otolaryngology, 3rd ed. Philadelphia, WB Saunders, 1991.

Saunders WH, et al: Nursing Care in Eye, Ear, Nose, and Throat Disorders, 4th ed. St. Louis, CV Mosby, 1979.

Shambaugh GE, Glasscock ME: Surgery of the Ear, 3rd ed. Philadelphia, WB Saunders, 1980.

Sheridan E, Patterson HR, Gustafson EA: Falconer's The Drug, The Nurse, The Patient, 7th ed. Philadelphia, WB Saunders, 1982.

Walter JB: An Introduction to the Principles of Disease, 3rd ed. Philadelphia, WB Saunders, 1992.

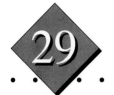

Plastic and Reconstructive Surgery

Plastic and reconstructive surgical procedures encompass operations to correct congenital defects or deformities due to disease or injury and to alter the patient's appearance for simple cosmetic purposes. Whether the patient arrives in surgery for an elective or nonelective procedure, special psychological needs must be met. The technologist or nurse should treat the patient in an honest and straightforward manner and should offer as much emotional support as possible. There has been a recent trend to perform many of the plastic surgeries (e.g., rhytidectomy, blepharoplasty, dermabrasion) on an outpatient basis or in the plastic surgeon's office. Consequently, in some geographic areas these procedures are seen in the operating room only occasionally.

SURGICAL ANATOMY

The skin (Fig. 29–1) covers nearly all outside surfaces of the body and is critical to temperature regulation and as a barrier against infection and injury to the inner surfaces of the body. The skin is composed of two layers: the *epidermis* and the *dermis*.

The Epidermis

The epidermis is the outermost layer of the skin. This layer contains five sublayers: the stratum corneum, stratum lucidum, stratum granulosum, stratum spinosum, and stratum germinativum.

The *stratum corneum* is a tough, somewhat transparent layer that is a barrier against water. This layer is composed of dead cells that are filled with a protein substance called *keratin.* The stratum corneum is thickest on those parts of the body that bear weight or friction such as the palms of the hands and the soles of the feet.

The *stratum lucidum,* which lies directly under the stratum corneum, is a very thin layer that is entirely absent in areas of the body where the skin is thin. This layer is only about five cells thick and is composed of fine transparent dead or dying cells.

The *stratum granulosum* is active in the keratinization of skin cells (the process whereby the cells manufacture keratin and take on their characteristic tough, durable appearance).

The *stratum spinosum* is composed of several rows of spiny cells. It is the middle layer of the epidermis and is often referred to as the *malpighian layer.*

The *stratum germinativum* is the regenerative layer of the epidermis. The cells of this layer give rise to all other layers of the epidermis. As the cells in the stratum germinativum go through mitosis and subsequent morphologic changes, they migrate to the upper surfaces of the epidermis. The skin pigment *melanin* is also formed here. Specialized cells called *melanocytes* form the melanin. The more active the melanocytes, the darker the skin.

The Dermis

The *dermis* (sometimes called the *corium*) is situated directly beneath the epidermis. It is this layer that contains blood vessels, nerve endings, hair follicles, and glands.

629

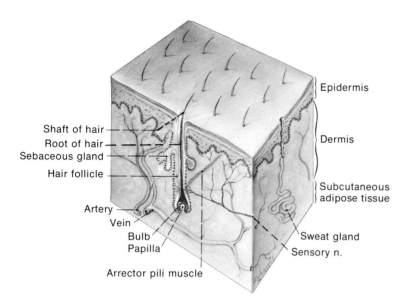

Figure 29–1. Three-dimensional view of the skin. (From Jacob S, Francone C, Lossow WJ: Structure and Function in Man, 5th ed. Philadelphia, WB Saunders, 1982.)

Skin appendages (Fig. 29–2) is a term given collectively to the hair, nails, and glands of the skin. *Hair,* found on nearly all surfaces of the body, contains several components. The *shaft* is the visible portion of the hair. That part of the hair that is embedded in the dermis is called the *root.* Surrounding the root is the *follicle.* The root is expanded at its base to form the *bulb.* The *papilla* is a portion of dermal tissue that extends into the bulb from below. The papilla contains nerve endings and blood vessels that supply the hair. *Nails,* present on the fingers and toes, are composed of hard keratin. The nail emerges from the *matrix* portion of the nail bed, which

lies beneath the nail itself. The *glands* of the skin include sebaceous glands and sweat glands. The sebaceous glands produce a substance called *sebum,* which is a lubricant for the skin. Sebaceous glands are generally, but not always, associated with the walls of hair follicles. *Sweat glands* are found in most areas of the body. They are most numerous in the soles of the feet and palms. At the base of the gland is the secretory portion, which is a blind, twisted tubular structure that leads to the excretory portion at the surface. Sweating is essential to the cooling system of the body and is also associated with the emotions.

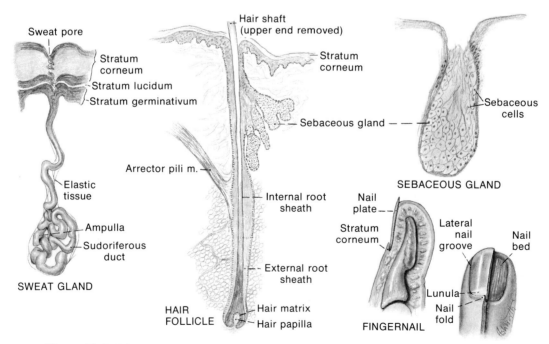

Figure 29–2. The skin appendages. (From Jacob S, Francone C, Lossow WJ: Structure and Function in Man, 5th ed. Philadelphia, WB Saunders, 1982.)

SPECIAL EQUIPMENT AND MATERIALS

Instruments

Because of the demands of plastic and reconstructive surgery, the instruments used are very fine. Most of these have been hand-honed and must be *carefully protected* from injury so that they provide maximum service to the surgeon. Delicate scissors, skin hooks, and forceps are particularly prone to injury and should never be placed with heavy blunt instruments, either for cleaning or sterilization. Many plastic surgeons prefer to bring their own instruments to the operating room rather than use the hospital's. The instruments may arrive in a wrapped sterile package or the technologist may have to flash sterilize them before the case. Particular care must be taken to ensure the safety of the physician's personal tools.

Suture

Most plastic surgery sutures are swaged to fine cutting needles. Size 5-0, 6-0, and 7-0 nylon, Prolene, and silk are commonly used. These fine sutures are very expensive and should be distributed onto the technologist's table only as needed.

Silastic and Teflon Materials

Many plastic and reconstructive procedures require the use of Silastic or Teflon implants. Even though these materials are very inert, they *are* foreign materials and special techniques must be used to prevent them from causing a foreign body reaction in the patient. The following are guidelines for their use:

1. If the materials are nonsterile when they arrive from the manufacturer, they should be washed in a mild soap (such as Ivory) and rinsed thoroughly before sterilization. The manufacturer's instructions for sterilization should be followed very carefully.
2. Silastic and Teflon tend to attract dust particles because of static electricity. Therefore, before and after sterilization they should be covered. Ideally, a sterile paper drape should be used to cover the implants because linen or towel drapes contain lint that could adhere to the implant.
3. The materials should never be handled with bare hands, since oil from the skin could rub off on the materials. This oil will remain on the implant after sterilization and could possibly cause a tissue reaction in the patient.
4. Implants should be handled as little as possible.

Miscellaneous Equipment

Dyes

Most plastic surgeons mark the skin with colored dye to indicate incisional lines or for geographic reference points before the procedure. *Sterile colored marking pens* are available for this purpose. If the operating room does not stock such items, the technologist can provide a "pen" by breaking a wooden cotton-tipped applicator in half. The surgeon can then dip the broken end of the applicator into a small amount of methylene blue or brilliant green dye contained in a medicine glass and use it to mark the skin.

Plaster

Plaster is commonly used to immobilize and protect the surgical site postoperatively. (See Chapter 23 for a complete discussion of plaster application.)

Sponges

Sponges used in fine plastic surgery should be smaller than standard 4×4-inch sponges. Square gauze sponges of the 2- or 3-inch size are used for very fine procedures.

Magnification

The surgeon often uses a headlight and surgical loupes or operating microscope (see Chapter 27) for magnification of the surgical site.

Electrocautery

The bipolar electrocautery unit is used for very fine work (see Chapter 13).

DRAPING

Most plastic and reconstructive procedures are performed with the patient in the supine or Fowler position. Head drapes are used for procedures of the face. Whenever there are multiple wound sites, such as for skin grafting, the technologist is sometimes required to "invent" a draping routine to fit the needs of the procedure.

SURGICAL PROCEDURES

Skin Grafts

Definition

A skin graft is a section of skin transplanted to an area of the body that has been denuded of skin. Skin grafting is necessary whenever the patient suffers loss of skin due to injury or disease. The graft may come from the patient's own body (autograft) or the skin bank (previously donated from another patient and preserved), or it may be a temporary dressing in the form of pigskin that has been freeze-dried (porcine graft).

A *full-thickness graft* is one that includes both the dermis and epidermis. A *split-thickness graft* contains the epidermis and a small portion of the dermis. A graft that contains other types of tissue in addition to skin, such as a graft composed of skin, subcutaneous tissue, and cartilage is called a *composite graft*.

Description

Split-Thickness Graft

The autograft donor site is chosen from a number of areas (Fig. 29–3). The abdomen and thigh are the sites most commonly used.

The instrument used to take the split thickness graft is called a *dermatome*. There are many types available; these may be manually operated or power-driven by compressed nitrogen, electricity, or a battery. The Brown dermatome (Fig. 29–4) is commonly used. The Reese or Padgett dermatome is used in conjunction with special glue that is painted over the surface of the donor site. The dermatome has a drum and a cutting sham that are rolled over the glued surface of the skin, cutting the graft away as it is rolled. For very small grafts, the Davol disposable head dermatome may be employed. The use of this dermatome, which is operated by a rechargeable battery, is illustrated in Figure 29–5. The technique for obtaining grafts with the Davol or Brown dermatome is the same.

To obtain a graft, the donor site is first lubricated with a light mineral oil, such as Muri-Lube. This oil allows the dermatome to slide easily over the skin. The technologist pulls the donor skin taut with the edge of a wooden tongue blade. The surgeon then operates the dermatome over the taut skin, applying enough pressure to obtain a graft of desired thickness. The technologist may be required to pick up the skin as it emerges from the dermatome to prevent it from bunching under the instrument. This is easily done with fine Adson forceps (see Fig. 29–5). When the surgeon has obtained the required amount of skin, he or she severs it from the donor site with scissors. A saline solution–soaked sponge may be placed on the donor site temporarily.

The technologist takes the graft from the surgeon and places it in a basin with a few drops of saline solution. The practice of placing the graft on a moistened sponge, as some surgeons prefer, can be hazardous. The surgeon or technologist might inadvertently throw the sponge into the kickbucket, thus contaminating the graft. The technologist should not immerse the graft in saline solution unless requested to do so by the surgeon.

The surgeon trims any devitalized tissue around the recipient site before applying the graft. This procedure is called *débridement* and is performed with scissors, scalpel, and toothed forceps.

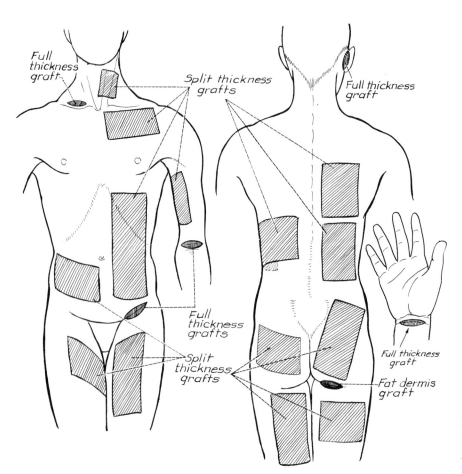

Figure 29–3. Sites for donor autografts. (From Converse JM (ed): Reconstructive Plastic Surgery, 2nd ed. Philadelphia, WB Saunders, 1977.)

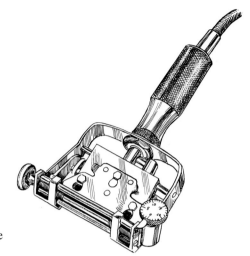

Figure 29–4. The Brown dermatome. (From Converse JM (ed): Reconstructive Plastic Surgery, 2nd ed. Philadelphia, WB Saunders, 1977.)

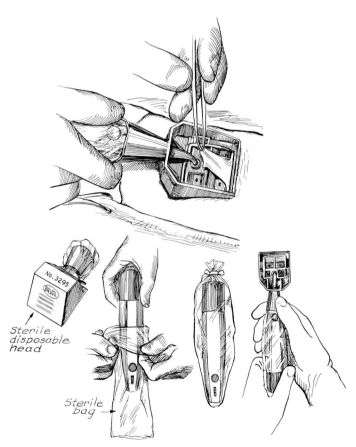

Figure 29–5. The Duval disposable head dermatome. *Top.* The assistant picks up the graft as it emerges from the instrument. *Bottom.* A method of receiving the nonsterile power unit from the circulator. (From Converse JM (ed): Reconstructive Plastic Surgery, 2nd ed. Philadelphia, WB Saunders, 1977.)

Before applying the graft, the surgeon compares the graft to the recipient site and trims it to fit. The technologist should save the trimmed pieces in case they are needed later. If the recipient site is very large (e.g., as with some burn patients), the surgeon may enlarge the graft by passing it through a skin graft mesher (Fig. 29–6A). The mesher cuts many tiny slits in the graft, which can then be stretched over the recipient site (Fig. 29–6B). Alternatively, the surgeon may cut the graft into many tiny pieces and place the pieces randomly over the recipient site. This is called a *pinch graft*.

The surgeon positions the graft over the recipient site and places many fine sutures around its edges, attaching it to the recipient tissue. The ends of the suture are left long. A small amount of saline solution–soaked cotton or gauze may be placed in the center of the graft and the sutures tied over the cotton. The resulting *stent* keeps the graft in contact with the recipient site during healing. Although the surgeon ties the sutures, the technologist is required to hold the first loop of the tie with a fine hemostat to prevent it from slipping loose while the second loop is tied. The technique of stenting is illustrated in Figure 29–7. Some surgeons do not apply a stent but use sterile tapes (Steri-Strips) rather than sutures to hold the graft in place. The donor site is dressed with gauze mesh impregnated with petrolatum and gauze squares (dry) or bandaging material, such as Kerlix or Kling bandage. The grafted recipient site may be dressed with a pressure dressing consisting of petrolatum-impregnated gauze and fluffy gauze padding.

Full-Thickness Graft

The full-thickness graft is generally very small as compared with the split-thickness graft. These grafts are commonly taken from the inner arm or groin (see Fig. 29–3). To take the graft, the surgeon simply incises the area with a scalpel and approximates the tissues of the donor site with interrupted sutures.

Pedicle Grafts

Definition

Pedicle grafts (also called flap grafts) are those that are raised from the donor site but are not immediately severed free. This type of graft is used when the recipient site requires tissue other than just skin (e.g., subcutaneous fat). Pedicle grafts are classified as either near or distant. A near graft is created in adjacent tissue (e.g., from the palm to the finger). Distant grafts are created from the trunk or other areas to a limb.

Description

The technique for pedicle grafts is the same regardless of the location of the graft. The graft is raised from the donor site with sharp dissection. This can be done in the same operation or in separate operations that allow the pedicle to increase its blood supply (when the pedicle is raised slowly over a period of time, its blood vessels actually increase in number and size). The pedicle is then sutured directly to the recipient site. The area left denuded from the donor site may be covered with a split-thickness graft or, if possible, the edges of the incision are sutured together. The technique of a distant graft from the abdomen to the forearm is illustrated in Figure 29–8. The graft is released from the donor site when it has acquired vascularization from the donor site, which usually takes place in 2 to 3 weeks. Often the surgeon may apply a plaster splint to the pedicle graft to keep it immobilized during the healing phase. A near graft from the palm to the finger is illustrated in Figure 29–9.

A *tube graft* is one in which a tube of tissue is formed by the technique illustrated in Figure 29–10. The end of the tube is transferred to the recipient site after 2 to 3 weeks (Fig. 29–11).

Scalp flaps are often used to transplant a hair-bearing area to an area of baldness (Fig. 29–12).

Rhytidectomy

Definition

This is the removal of excess skin in the face and neck area and the tightening of underlying support structures, such as muscle and superficial fascia. As aging takes place, the face and neck skin begins to lose tone and to sag. A rhytidectomy (facelift) is performed to improve the appearance of the patient. The cosmetic effect provides both emotional and social benefits for the patient.

Description

The patient is placed in a supine or semi-Fowler position. Before beginning the procedure, the surgeon marks the incisional lines with a surgical marking pen (Fig. 29–13). The incisions are made close to the hairline or in the hair so that the resulting scars are unnoticeable. A small amount of hair may be shaved from the hairline; in most cases this is done by the surgeon. The shaded portions of the face in Figure 29–13 indicate the area of *undermining* (separation of the skin and subcutaneous tissue from their attachments beneath). The surgeon may place a traction suture through the earlobe to aid in exposing the incision (Fig. 29–14). Once the skin has been partially undermined, small, very sharp skin hooks are placed on the edge of the incision for retraction. If the technologist is asked to retract, he or she must exert only gentle pressure on the hooks because of their tendency to tear through the skin (Fig. 29–15). When undermining is completed, small bleeding vessels are coagulated with the cautery pencil (Fig. 29–16).

The surgeon now pulls the skin back from the face toward the ear and scalp (Fig. 29–17). He or she judges the amount of skin to be left intact and trims the excess with dissecting scissors. The skin and hairline are approximated with fine interrupted sutures. Many surgeons

Text continued on page 641

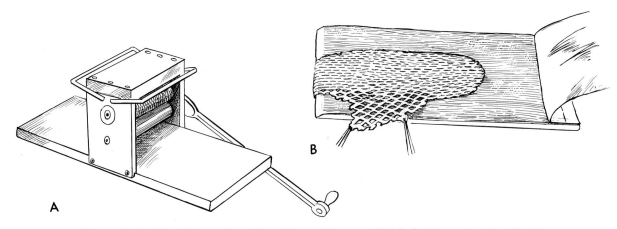

Figure 29–6. The skin graft mesher. (From Converse JM (ed): Reconstructive Plastic Surgery, 2nd ed. Philadelphia, WB Saunders, 1977.)

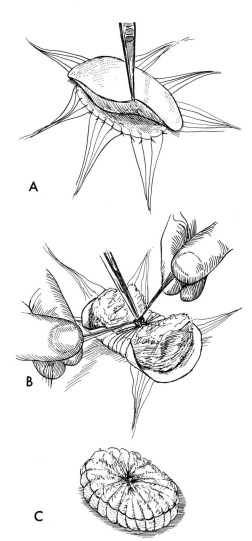

Figure 29–7. Method of stenting the skin graft. *A.* A small amount of saline-soaked cotton is placed over the graft. *B.* The previously placed sutures are secured over the cotton. *C.* Finished stent. (From Converse JM (ed): Reconstructive Plastic Surgery, 2nd ed. Philadelphia, WB Saunders, 1977.)

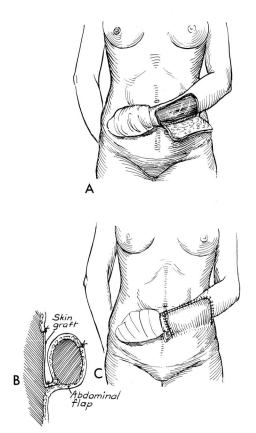

Figure 29–8. Flap graft from the abdomen to the forearm. (From Converse JM (ed): Reconstructive Plastic Surgery, 2nd ed. Philadelphia, WB Saunders, 1977.)

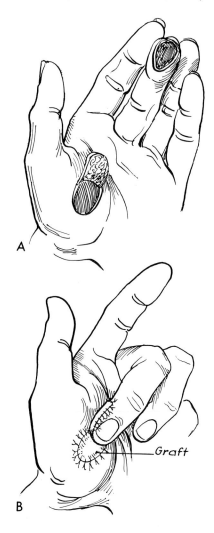

Figure 29–9. Flap graft from palm to finger. (From Converse JM (ed): Reconstructive Plastic Surgery, 2nd ed. Philadelphia, WB Saunders, 1977.)

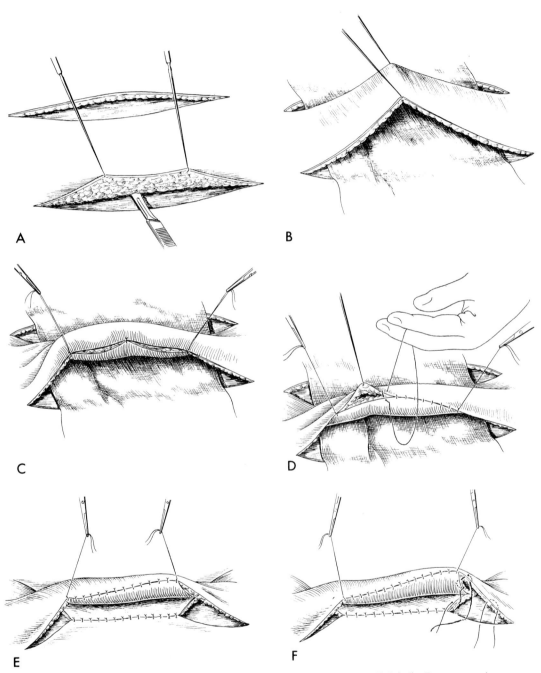

A

B

C

D

E

F

Figure 29–10. Method of creating a tube graft. (From Converse JM (ed): Reconstructive Plastic Surgery, 2nd ed. Philadelphia, WB Saunders, 1977.)

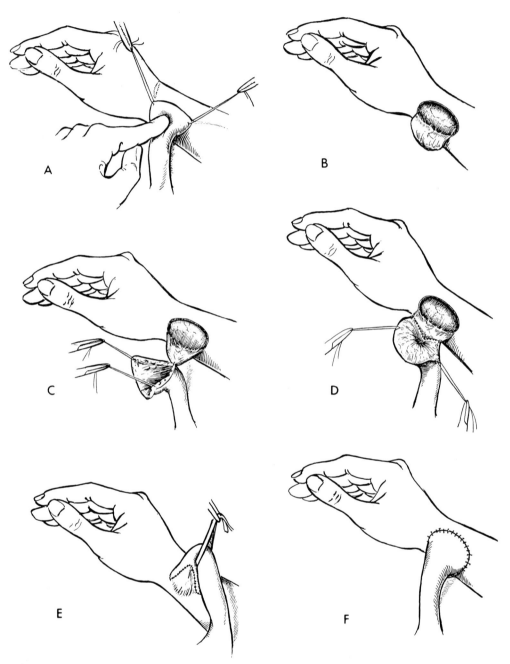

Figure 29–11. Method of transferring the tube graft to the recipient site. (From Converse JM (ed): Reconstructive Plastic Surgery, 2nd ed. Philadelphia, WB Saunders, 1977.)

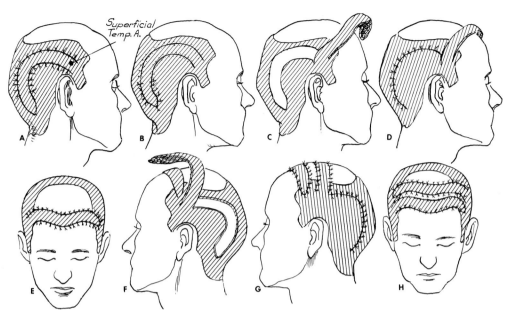

Figure 29–12. Scalp flaps, used to transfer hair-bearing tissue to an area of baldness. (From Converse JM (ed): Reconstructive Plastic Surgery, 2nd ed. Philadelphia, WB Saunders, 1977.)

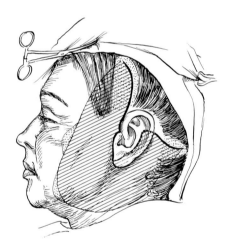

Figure 29–13. Incisional lines and area of undermining for rhytidectomy. (From Converse JM (ed): Reconstructive Plastic Surgery, 2nd ed. Philadelphia, WB Saunders, 1977.)

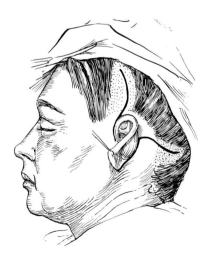

Figure 29–14. Rhytidectomy. Traction suture through ear lobe. (From Converse JM (ed): Reconstructive Plastic Surgery, 2nd ed. Philadelphia, WB Saunders, 1977.)

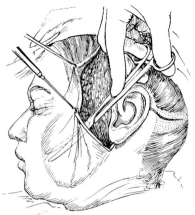

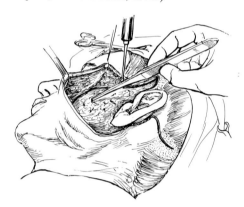

Figure 29–15. Rhytidectomy. Undermining the facial skin. (From Converse JM (ed): Reconstructive Plastic Surgery, 2nd ed. Philadelphia, WB Saunders, 1977.)

Figure 29–16. Rhytidectomy. Bleeders are coagulated. (From Converse JM (ed): Reconstructive Plastic Surgery, 2nd ed. Philadelphia, WB Saunders, 1977.)

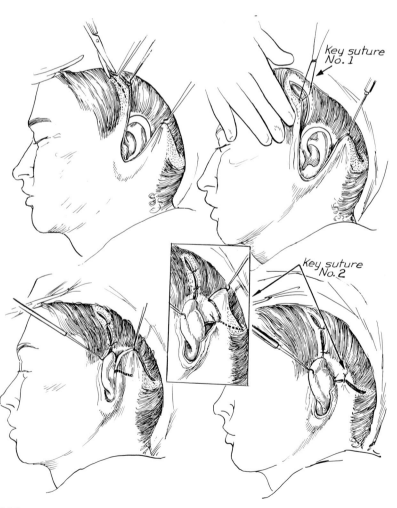

Figure 29–17. Rhytidectomy. The surgeon pulls the redundant skin toward the ear to judge the amount to trim. The excess skin is trimmed with scissors and the incision is closed. (From Converse JM (ed): Reconstructive Plastic Surgery, 2nd ed. Philadelphia, WB Saunders, 1977.)

tighten up the tissues underlying the skin with interrupted absorbable sutures. In some cases a Hemovac drain (Chapter 12) may be inserted before closure. A light pressure dressing is then applied.

Blepharoplasty

Definition

This is the removal of excess skin around the eyes. With age, the skin around the eyes becomes loose and begins to sag. Blepharoplasty is performed for both cosmetic and functional purposes. Sagging skin from the upper lids may interfere with the patient's eyesight.

Description

The patient is positioned in a slight reverse Trendelenburg position. Before beginning the procedure, the surgeon marks the incisional lines with a marking pen (Fig. 29–18A and B). A cotton-tipped applicator is helpful for stretching the skin while the incisional lines are drawn. Using a small scalpel blade or sharp dissecting scissors, the surgeon incises and removes the skin encompassed by the marked lines (Fig. 29–18C). Grasping the subcutaneous fatty tissue with fine tissue forceps, the surgeon gently teases a small amount free with dissecting scissors (Fig. 29–18D). Where small bleeding vessels occur, fine mosquito hemostats may be used to clamp them (Fig. 29–18E) and cautery is used to maintain hemostasis (Fig. 29–18F). The surgeon approximates the incisional lines with fine interrupted sutures (Fig. 29–18G). The procedure may be performed on the lower lids (Fig. 29–19). A topical antibacterial ointment or dressings are applied to the suture lines.

Dermabrasion

Definition

Dermabrasion is the physical "sanding" of skin with a rotary power-driven abrasive disk. The *dermabrader* (Fig. 29–20) is used to plane the skin where it has been scarred or pitted by diseases such as acne or pox or by trauma. Commercial tattoos may also be removed by dermabrasion.

Description

Dermabrasion may be performed over the entire face or over a small area. If the area to be treated is on or near the cheek, the surgeon may wish to pack the patient's mouth with gauze to stretch the skin taut. Before dermabrasion, the surgeon marks the center of any pitted scar so that he or she knows when the lowest level of the scar has been reached. The dermabrader in use is shown in Figure 29–21. After treatment, a light pressure dressing of Telfa or petrolatum-impregnated material and gauze is applied.

Chemical Peel

An alternative method of sanding the skin is through a procedure called *chemical peel*. In this procedure the face is painted with a solution of phenol (carbolic acid), which burns and erodes the areas to which it is applied. The effect is the same as any other type of burn except that the surgeon controls the depth of the burn by neutralizing the phenol with alcohol. The burned skin is then allowed to slough over a period of weeks and a new surface of epithelial tissue develops.

Microtia

Definition

Microtia is a congenital defect that results in the absence of all or part of the ear. The deformity also affects the inner ear, resulting in deafness. Two examples of microtia are shown in Figure 29–22. Reconstructive surgery is performed before the child reaches school age.

Description

Reconstruction of the ear is usually performed in multiple stages with several operations. The technique varies, depending on the type and severity of the defect. A common method of reconstruction is to elevate the skin where the ear would normally lie and insert either an artificial implant or a graft taken from the patient's costal cartilage. A Silastic ear implant is shown in Figure 29–23.

When an autograft is to be taken, the patient is placed in the supine position. The surgeon creates a template (pattern) for the graft by placing a sheet of transparent material over the *unaffected* ear and tracing its outline on the material (Fig. 29–24). The template is then placed over the affected ear and the ear remnants are traced on the template (Fig. 29–25).

The surgeon makes an incision over the seventh, eighth, or ninth intercostal space. The template is then placed over the costal cartilage and the tissue is excised, following the outline of the template (Fig. 29–26). The incision is closed in layers in routine fashion.

The surgeon may wish to carve the graft so that it resembles the shape of the ear more closely. This is done with a power drill and small bur attachments (Fig. 29–27). The surgeon outlines the postauricular area (behind the ear) where the graft will be inserted. The technique of undermining the skin and the insertion of the newly constructed graft are illustrated in Figure 29–28. The surgeon pulls the skin over the graft and sutures it in place. This completes the first stage of the reconstruction.

When the first stage has healed, subsequent operations are performed to raise the frame of the ear and to construct the folds and recesses of the outer ear. The surgeon accomplishes this by incising flaps of adjacent skin and shifting them into position. Fine sutures of

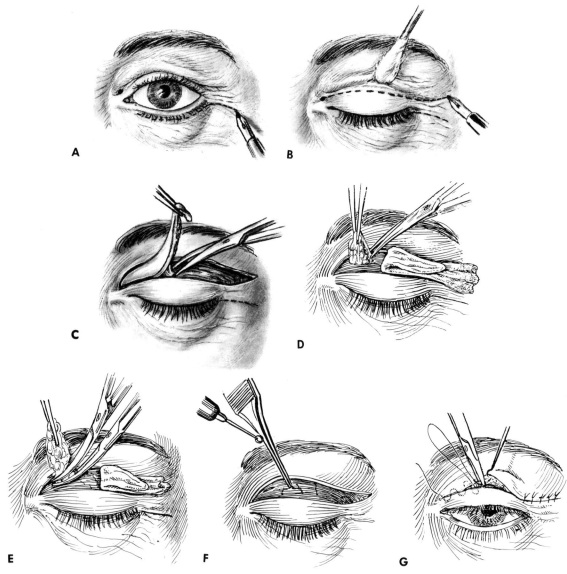

Figure 29–18. *A* and *B*. Blepharoplasty. Incisional lines are drawn with marking pen. *C*. Redundant skin is removed. *D*. A small amount of subcutaneous tissue is teased free. *E*. Bleeders are clamped with mosquito hemostats. *F*. Cautery is used to maintain hemostasis. *G*. The incision is closed. (From Converse JM (ed): Reconstructive Plastic Surgery, 2nd ed. Philadelphia, WB Saunders, 1977.)

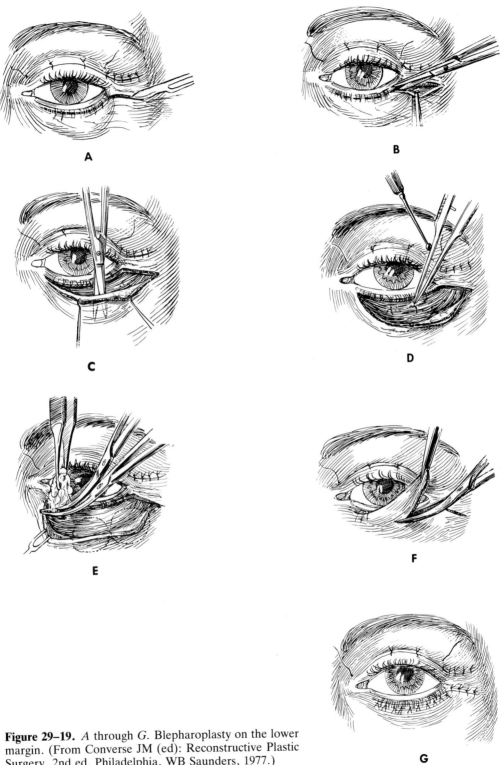

Figure 29–19. *A* through *G*. Blepharoplasty on the lower margin. (From Converse JM (ed): Reconstructive Plastic Surgery, 2nd ed. Philadelphia, WB Saunders, 1977.)

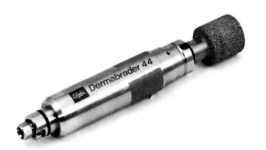

Figure 29–20. The dermabrader. (Courtesy of the Stryker Corporation, Kalamazoo, MI.)

nylon, Prolene, or other synthetic material are used to suture the flaps in place. Bulky dressings are employed after ear repair to protect it from injury during healing.

Correction of Lop Ears

Definition

Lop ear is a congenital defect that causes the ears to protrude noticeably from the head. This defect often leads to ridicule by a child's peers, so the correction is generally performed before the child reaches school age. The defect and the result of surgical correction are shown in Figure 29–29.

Description

There are a variety of operations performed to correct this defect. A common approach involves incising the skin on the posterior side of the concha. The patient is placed in the supine position with the affected ear up. The underlying cartilage is then incised or scored. The surgeon places interrupted absorbable or nonabsorbable sutures through the cartilage to tighten it. The resulting effect "pins" the ear closer to the head. The surgeon closes the skin incision with fine interrupted synthetic sutures (Fig. 29–30). At the close of the procedure, bulky gauze dressings are applied to the ear.

Rhinoplasty

Definition

This is reconstruction of the nose for cosmetic purposes.

Description

The technologist cannot visualize nasal operations once the initial incisions have been made. With the patient in the supine position, the surgeon operates from *within* the nose during most procedures and completes the reconstruction by feeling the shape of the tissues and by observing the cosmetic effect as he or she works.

Therefore, it is difficult for the technologist to anticipate instrumentation during this procedure. A step-by-step description of the procedure is not feasible here, since each nasal procedure differs according to the defects present. A workable approach for the technologist is to become completely familiar with all instrumentation and basic techniques of these operations.

The technologist's duties during nasal reconstruction are to retract when asked, to suction blood with a Frazier suction or similar suction tip, to pass instruments as directed, and to preserve any tissue specimens by keeping them moistened with saline solution. Many procedures require the removal of cartilage or bone. The tissue is then replaced in a different location in the nose. Therefore, all tissue is retained in a small basin on the instrument table.

Several techniques employed in nasal reconstruction are shown in Figures 29–31 through 29–33.

At the close of the procedure, extensive dressings are used to hold the nose in shape until healing takes place. The technologist may assist the surgeon in dressing the nose. The nasal cavity is usually packed with Gelfoam material or petrolatum-impregnated gauze. Splints may also be applied (plaster or other materials, such as dental compound, are commonly used). The surgeon then tapes the outside of the nose (Fig. 29–34).

Text continued on page 651

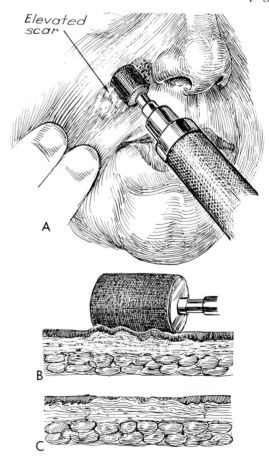

Figure 29–21. The dermabrader in use. (From Converse JM (ed): Reconstructive Plastic Surgery, 2nd ed. Philadelphia, WB Saunders, 1977.)

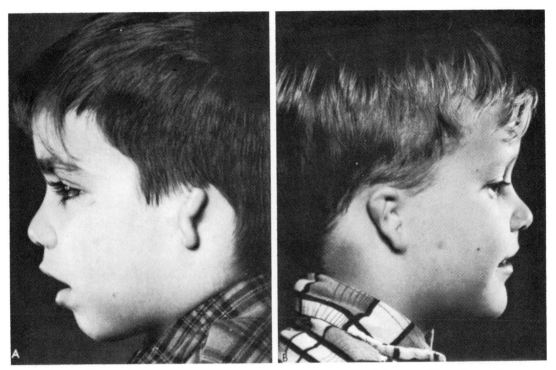

Figure 29–22. *A* and *B*. Microtia. The absence of all or part of the ear. (From Paparella MM, Shumrick DA (eds): Otolaryngology, vol 3. Philadelphia, WB Saunders, 1973.)

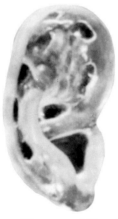

Figure 29–23. Silastic ear implant. (Courtesy of Dow Corning Wright, Arlington, TN.)

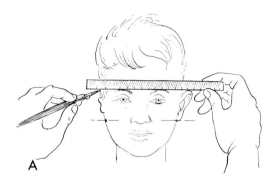

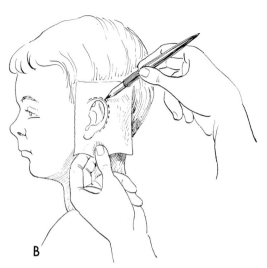

Figure 29–24. Correction of microtia. *A.* The surgeon measures the level of the unaffected ear. *B.* A template for the ear graft is formed. (From Paparella MM, Shumrick DA (eds): Otolaryngology, vol 3. Philadelphia, WB Saunders, 1973.)

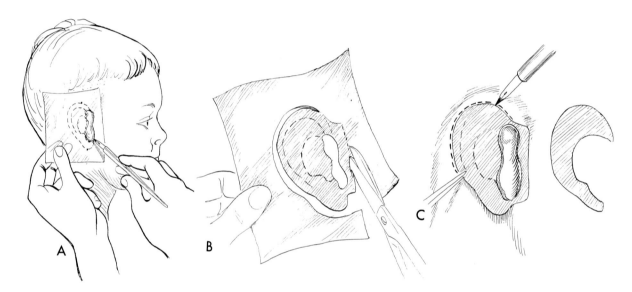

Figure 29–25. Correction of microtia. The surgeon places the template over the affected ear and traces the ear remnants on the template. (From Paparella MM, Shumrick DA (eds): Otolaryngology, vol 3. Philadelphia, WB Saunders, 1973.)

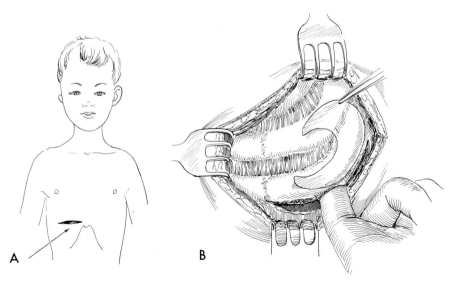

Figure 29–26. Correction of microtia. Taking a cartilage graft. *A.* Area of incision. *B.* The template is placed over the costal cartilage. (From Paparella MM, Shumrick DA (eds): Otolaryngology, vol 3. Philadelphia, WB Saunders, 1973.)

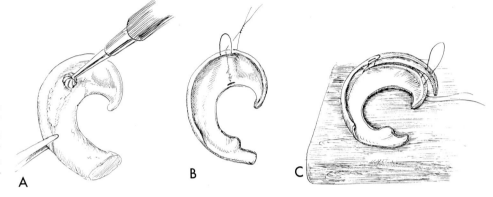

Figure 29–27. After the graft is taken, the surgeon carves it or pieces it together to resemble an ear. (From Paparella MM, Shumrick DA (eds): Otolaryngology, vol 3. Philadelphia, WB Saunders, 1973.)

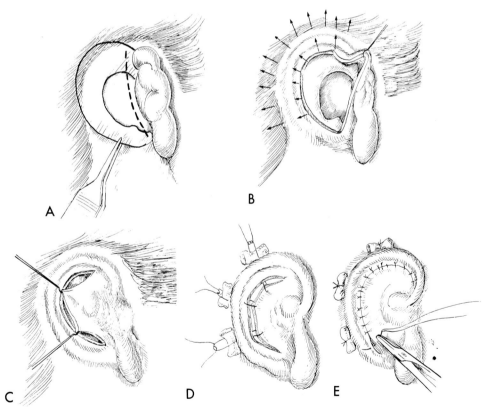

Figure 29–28. Method of inserting the graft. The skin is undermined, the graft inserted, and the incision closed. The ear will be elevated from the head in subsequent surgery. (From Paparella MM, Shumrick DA (eds): Otolaryngology, vol 3. Philadelphia, WB Saunders, 1973.)

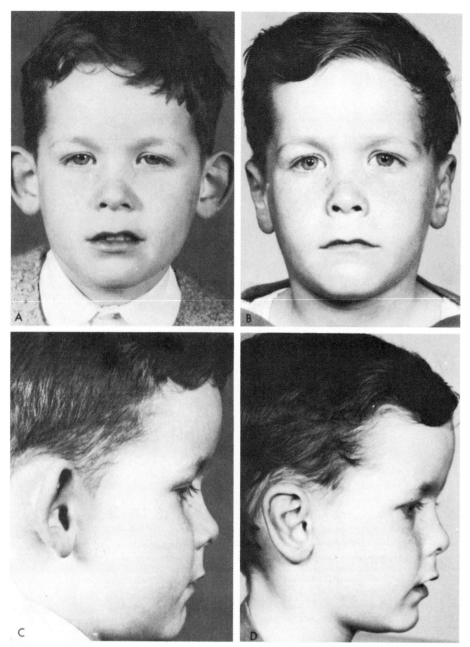

Figure 29–29. Lop ears before and after surgical correction. (From Paparella MM, Shumrick DA (eds): Otolaryngology, vol 3. Philadelphia, WB Saunders, 1973.)

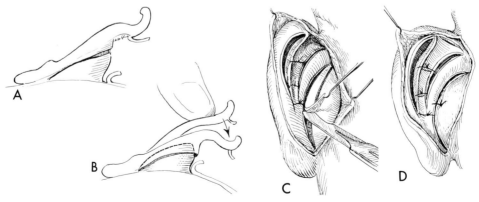

Figure 29–30. Correction of lop ears. *A.* Position of ear in relation to the head. *B.* The surgeon depresses the ear to demonstrate the line of incision. *C.* The ear is scored with the knife. *D.* The incisions are closed. (From Paparella MM, Shumrick DA (eds): Otolaryngology, vol 3. Philadelphia, WB Saunders, 1973.)

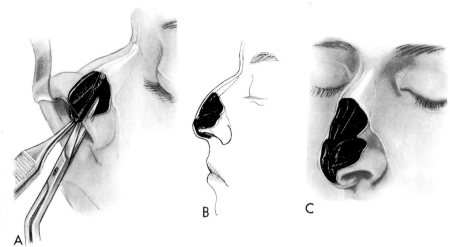

Figure 29–31. Nasal reconstruction. *A.* Trimming the lateral cartilage. *B.* Line indicates the postoperative profile. *C.* Appearance after the cartilage is removed. (From Paparella MM, Shumrick DA (eds): Otolaryngology, vol 3. Philadelphia, WB Saunders, 1973.)

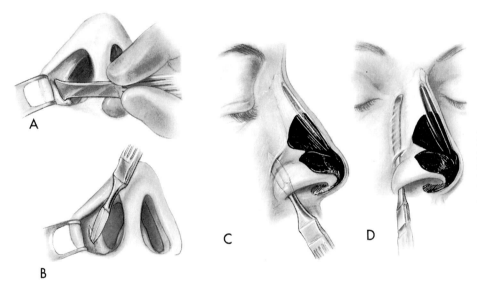

Figure 29–32. Nasal reconstruction. Reduction of the nasal bone on the lateral side. *A.* The surgeon palpates the lateral side of the nose with a blunt instrument. *B.* Incision. *C.* The incision is extended upward. *D.* A periosteal elevator is used to establish a tunnel. (From Paparella MM, Shumrick DA (eds): Otolaryngology, vol 3. Philadelphia, WB Saunders, 1973.)

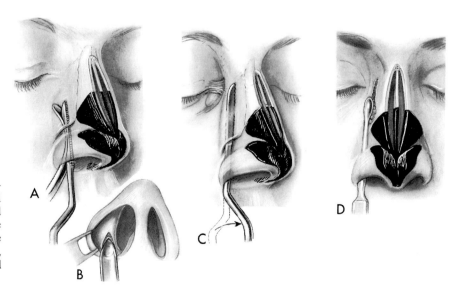

Figure 29–33. Nasal reconstruction. Reduction of the nasal bone on the lateral side. A saw guide is inserted in the tunnel and an angled saw is used to reduce the bone. A "sweeper" is used to remove the bone particles. (From Paparella MM, Shumrick DA (eds): Otolaryngology, vol 3. Philadelphia, WB Saunders, 1973.)

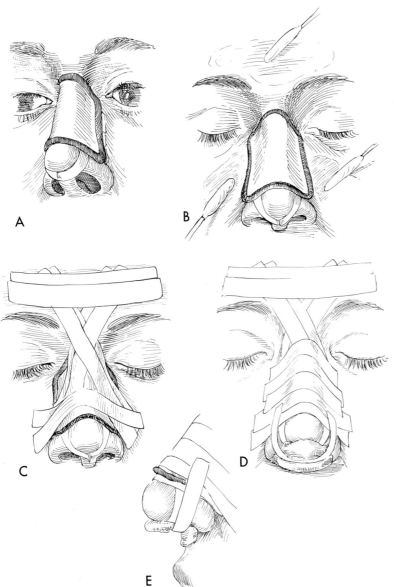

A

B

C

D

E

Figure 29–34. Dressing the nose following surgery. Tape and splints are used to keep the nose in proper shape. (From Converse JM (ed): Reconstructive Plastic Surgery, 2nd ed, vol 2. Philadelphia, WB Saunders, 1977.)

Repair of Cleft Palate

Definition

Cleft palate is a congenital deformity that results in a cleft (split) in the hard palate, soft palate, or both. This allows food and liquid to escape into the nasal cavity and is also associated with speech defects. Surgical repair of the cleft palate is performed when the patient is between 1 and 2 years of age.

Description

There are many different types of procedures for the repair of cleft palate. All procedures utilize flaps raised from adjacent mucosal tissue to close the defect. The patient is usually placed in the supine position for the procedure. A common technique for the repair of cleft palate is shown in Figure 29–35.

Repair of Cleft Lip

Definition

Cleft lip is a congenital deformity that results in a splitting of the upper lip, usually on one side or the other but rarely in the middle. The cleft may extend to include the palate and/or nose. Corrective surgery is performed when the patient is 3 or 4 months old.

Description

The patient is placed on the operating table in the supine position. To repair a simple defect, the surgeon makes incisions in the upper lip in a pattern that allows the lip to be approximated in a cosmetically appealing and functional manner. The incisions are carried through the full thickness of the lip. The surgeon then approximates the muscle, subcutaneous, and skin layers separately. Two methods of closure are shown in Figure 29–36.

Chin Implant

Definition

This is the insertion of a Silastic or Teflon prosthesis in the chin. The procedure is performed for the patient with a recessive mandible.

Description

The procedure for implantation of a chin prosthesis is illustrated and explained in Figure 29–37.

Application of Arch Bars

Definition

This is the application of metal bars and fixating wires to the upper and lower teeth to hold the jaws shut. The use of arch bars is indicated for mandibular or maxillary fractures. The bars keep the teeth occluded while the fracture heals. They are used by themselves to achieve successful fixation of the fracture site or may be applied in conjunction with open reduction procedures for a fractured mandible or maxilla.

Description

Metal arch bars (Fig. 29–38) are available in precut lengths. The surgeon bends the bar to fit the contour of the patient's maxillary and mandibular arches. The bars are attached by passing short lengths of 25- or 26-gauge stainless steel wire between the teeth and around the bar. Additional wires or small elastic bands are looped around the bars to occlude the jaw. At the completion of the procedure, it is crucial that wire cutters be sent with the patient to the post-anesthesia care unit in the event that the jaws must be freed in an emergency. The technique for applying arch bars is illustrated in Figure 29–39.

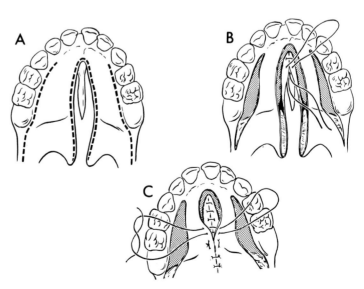

Figure 29–35. Repair of cleft palate. *A.* Incisions are made in the palate. *B* and *C.* The cleft is sutured. (From Sabiston DC Jr (ed): Davis-Christopher Textbook of Surgery, 11th ed. Philadelphia, WB Saunders, 1977.)

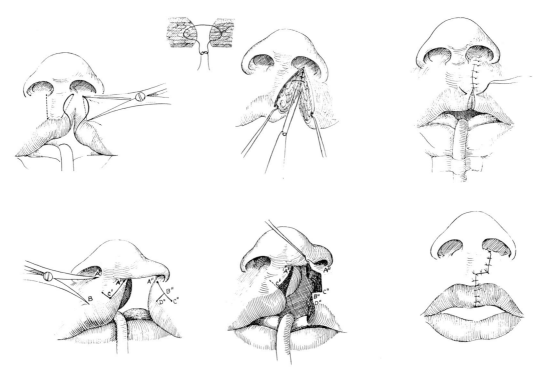

Figure 29–36. Two methods of correction of cleft lip. (From Sabiston DC Jr (ed): Davis-Christopher Textbook of Surgery, 11th ed. Philadelphia, WB Saunders, 1977.)

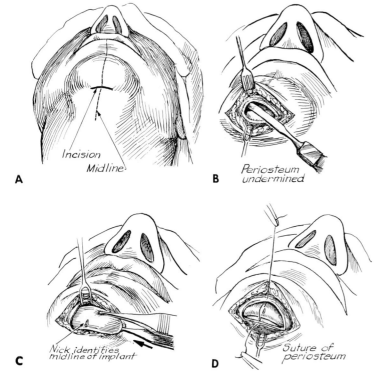

Figure 29–37. Method of inserting chin implant. *A.* A midline incision is made. *B.* The periosteum is undermined. *C.* The implant is inserted (note small nick that represents the midline). *D.* The wound is closed in layers. (From Converse JM (ed): Reconstructive Plastic Surgery, 2nd ed. Philadelphia, WB Saunders, 1977.)

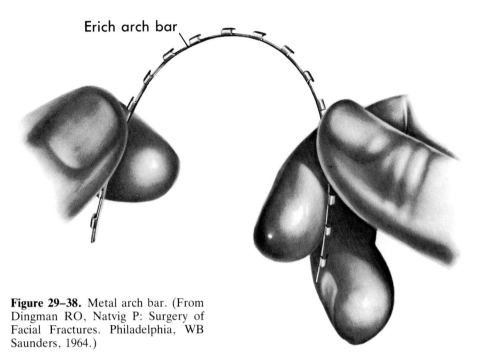

Erich arch bar

Figure 29–38. Metal arch bar. (From Dingman RO, Natvig P: Surgery of Facial Fractures. Philadelphia, WB Saunders, 1964.)

Repair of Fractured Mandible

Definition

This is the open reduction of a fractured mandible and internal fixation of the fracture with stainless steel wire.

Description

Repair of a fractured mandible, like all facial fracture repairs, requires a combination of dental, nasal, and orthopedic instruments. A large facial fracture instrument set-up is shown in Figure 29–40. This set-up is larger than most; the surgeon may use only a few of the instruments shown.

The surgeon gains access to the fracture site (Fig. 29–41A) by sharp dissection through the skin and muscle layers of the lower jaw. Small rake retractors are used to retract the wound edges (Fig. 29–41B). The surgeon applies one or two small bone-holding clamps to stabilize the fracture site. Using a small drill point mounted on a power-driven drill, the surgeon makes a small hole through each of the bone fragments (Fig. 29–41C). The surgeon may request that the technologist pour a slow trickle of saline solution over the drill point to prevent the build-up of heat from friction.

The surgeon then passes a 6- or 7-inch length of 25-gauge stainless steel wire through the holes. The wire is grasped with a blunt needle holder (wire twister; Fig. 29–41D). The wire is then twisted around to bring the fragments in close approximation, and the ends are cut with wire cutters (Fig. 29–41E). The completed fixation is shown in Figure 29–41F.

The periosteum and muscle layers are closed with interrupted absorbable sutures, size 2-0 or 3-0 (Fig. 29–

41G). The skin is closed with fine sutures of silk, Prolene, or nylon (Fig. 29–41H). Arch bars are applied, as previously described. The bars may be applied before the open reduction or after reduction and fixation.

Repair of Fractured Zygoma

Definition

This is the open reduction and internal fixation of a fractured zygoma with stainless steel wire.

Description

The technique of open reduction and internal fixation of a fractured zygoma is similar to that of the fractured mandible, previously discussed. This technique is illustrated in Figure 29–42.

Repair of Fractured Maxilla

Definition

This is the open reduction and internal fixation of the maxilla with stainless steel wires and arch bars.

Description

Techniques used for the open reduction and internal fixation of the maxilla are the same as those previously discussed, with one exception. Because the maxilla must be stabilized by an adjacent structure, the application of "sling wires" is necessary. Stainless steel wires are

Text continued on page 661

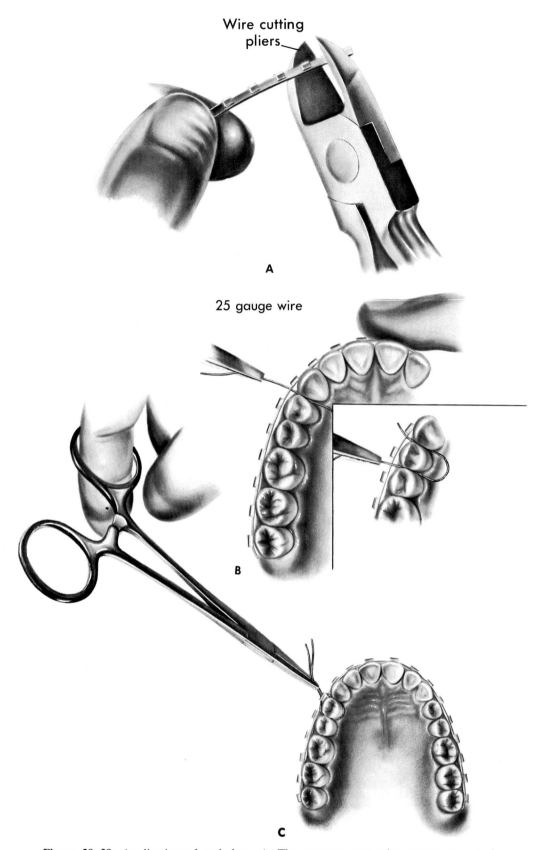

Wire cutting
pliers

A

25 gauge wire

B

C

Figure 29–39. Application of arch bar. *A.* The surgeon uses wire cutters to cut the appropriate length of bar. *B.* The bar is placed at the base of the teeth and secured with lengths of stainless steel wire that are passed around the teeth and the bar. *C.* The surgeon twists the wire to snug it around the arch bar.

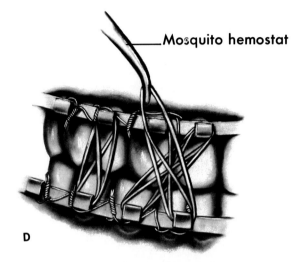

D

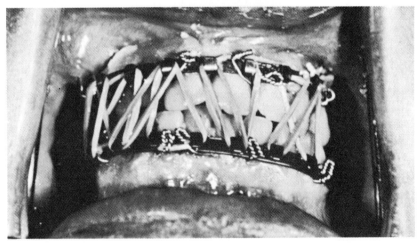

E

Figure 29–39 *Continued. D and E.* The completed procedure. (From Dingman RO, Natvig P: Surgery of Facial Fractures. Philadelphia, WB Saunders, 1964.)

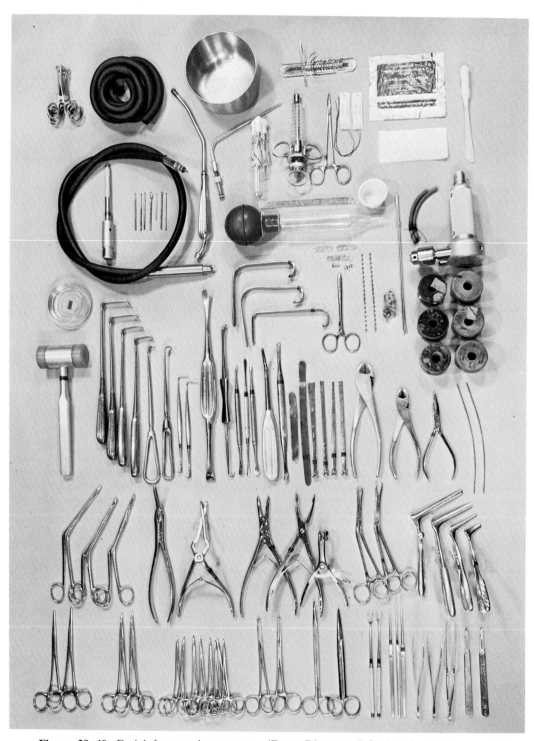

Figure 29–40. Facial fracture instruments. (From Dingman RO, Natvig P: Surgery of Facial Fractures. Philadelphia, WB Saunders, 1964.)

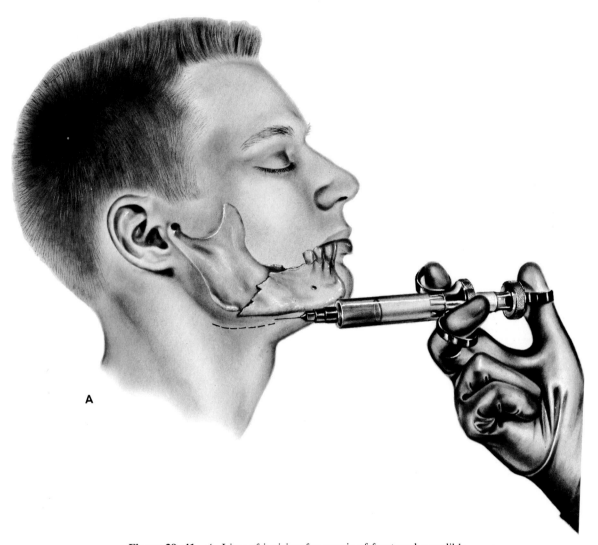

A

Figure 29–41. *A.* Line of incision for repair of fractured mandible.

Illustration continued on following page

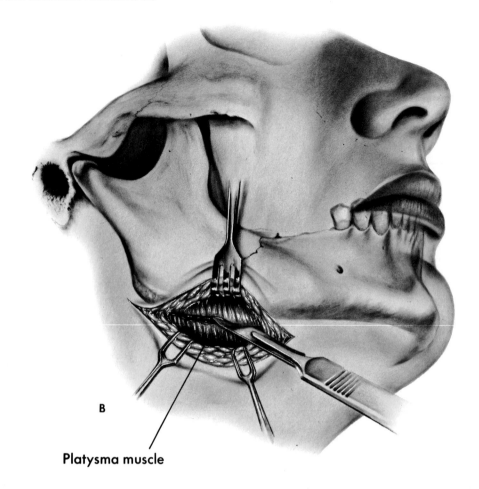

Platysma muscle

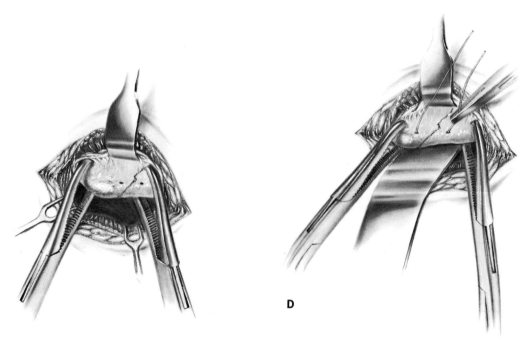

Figure 29–41 *Continued. B.* Sharp dissection through the tissues of the jaw. *C.* Bone clamps are used to bring the bone fragments together. *D.* The surgeon passes a length of stainless steel wire through the holes.

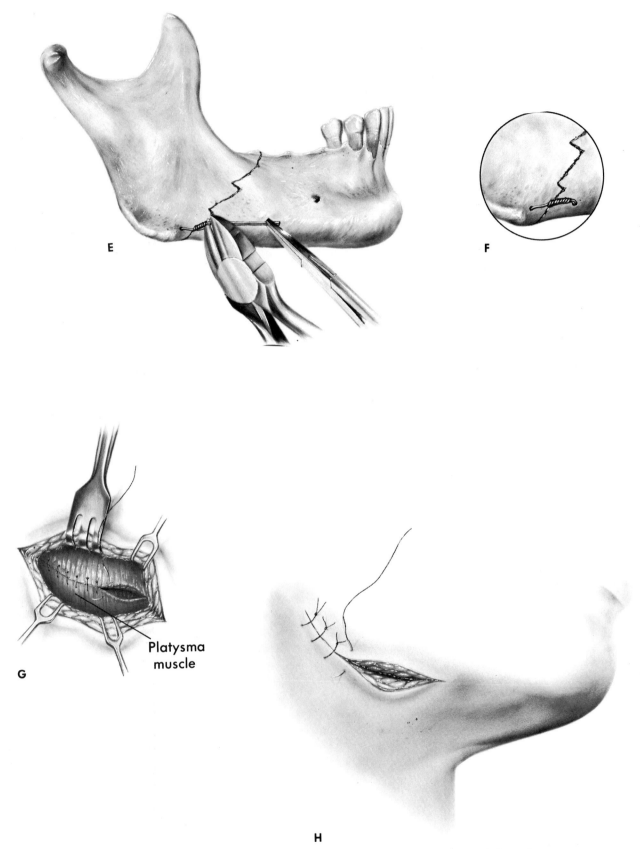

Figure 29–41 *Continued. E.* The ends of the wire are twisted together, and the ends are cut with wire cutters. *F.* The completed fixation. *G.* Muscle closure. *H.* The skin is closed with fine interrupted sutures. (From Dingman RO, Natvig P: Surgery of Facial Fractures. Philadelphia, WB Saunders, 1964.)

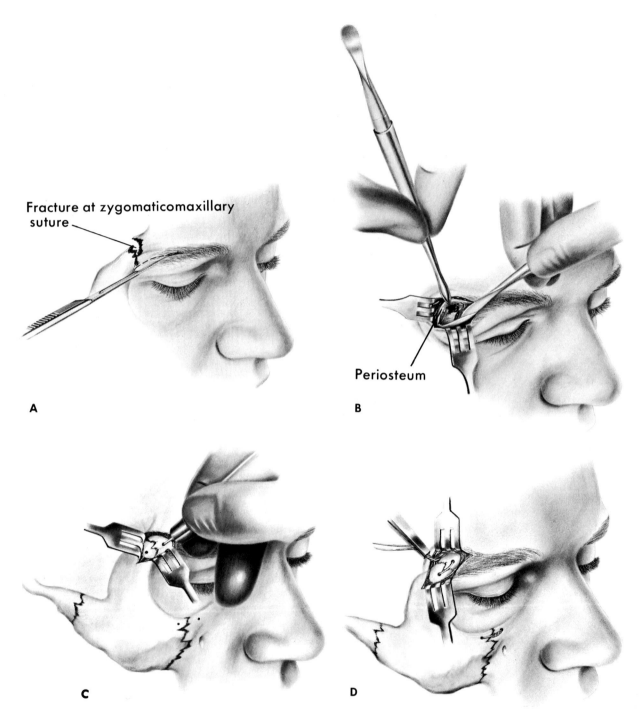

Figure 29–42. *A*. Fracture of the zygoma. *B*. The surgeon uses a fine periosteal elevator to lift the periosteum from the bone. *C*. Small holes are drilled in each fragment. *D*. A length of stainless steel wire is passed through the holes and twisted down. (From Dingman RO, Natvig P: Surgery of Facial Fractures. Philadelphia, WB Saunders, 1964.)

passed through the orbital rim of the zygoma and then attached to the previously applied arch bars. During the application of sling wires, it is wise to have a wire passer available. This instrument resembles an eyed needle but is very large and long. The technique is further described in Figure 29–43.

Reduction Mammoplasty

Definition

This is the surgical removal of excess breast and skin tissue. The patient with heavy, pendulous breasts suffers both socially and psychologically. In extreme cases the patient may suffer from backache because of the added weight that constantly pulls forward. The condition may affect one or both breasts.

Description

The patient is placed in a modified Fowler position and prepped from the neck to the lower abdomen. A wide variety of techniques are employed for reduction of the breast tissue. Most require that the surgeon remove a wedge from the breast with sharp dissection. Many surgeons use numerous towel clamps for traction on the breast tissue. The nipple may be removed and transplanted, or the surgeon may create a pedicle flap and simply transfer the nipple to its new location, thus retaining both its vascular and nerve supply.

Once the wedge has been removed, the edges of the subcutaneous and breast tissue are approximated with interrupted absorbable sutures. The surgeon may approximate the skin using a subcuticular suture or interrupted sutures of nylon, Prolene, or other synthetic materials. Breast closure once the wedge has been removed is shown in Figure 29–44. Some surgeons insert a Hemovac drain before closure. At the completion of the procedure, the breast is dressed with bulky gauze and tape and the patient is fitted with a supportive Surgi-Bra.

Augmentation Mammoplasty

Definition

This is the insertion of a Silastic implant behind the breast to increase its size. Augmentation may be performed after subcutaneous mastectomy or may be done on the patient whose breasts are asymmetric. The procedure may also be performed on the patient whose breasts are normal but smaller than desired.

Description

The patient is positioned on the operating table in a modified Fowler position and prepped from the neck to the abdomen. Before the procedure begins, the technologist should ask the surgeon what size and type of implant will be needed and also be certain that it is available in the operating room. Implants are available in a variety of sizes and shapes.

The surgeon creates a pocket for the implant by dissecting the breast through a small incision below or to one side of the nipple. The pocket lies behind or in front of the pectoralis muscle. The surgeon cauterizes small bleeding vessels or ligates them with fine absorbable sutures. The assistant retracts the upper surface of the pocket with a Deaver or fiberoptic retractor, and the surgeon places the implant within the pocket. The pocket is then closed with interrupted absorbable sutures. The surgeon may choose a subcuticular or interrupted skin closure. The wound is dressed with gauze squares, and the patient is fitted with a Surgi-Bra for support.

Trans–Rectus Abdominis Myocutaneous Flap

Definition

This is the implantation of a flap from the transverse rectus abdominis muscle to reconstruct the breast following mastectomy. This procedure offers an alternative to a Silastic implant. This is a single-stage reconstruction; however, most surgeons prefer to perform the nipple reconstruction at a later date.

In this procedure, the patient is placed in a supine position. The arms are extended on armboards. The entire abdominal, thoracic, and axillary areas are prepped and draped. A transverse lower pelvic incision is made, and the transverse abdominal muscle is freed from its attachments in the lower abdominal wall. The muscle is then tunneled under the abdominal and thoracic wall to its new location. It emerges from the site of the mastectomy scar, which is removed. The flap is then secured medially, and the thoracic wall skin is used to cover and construct the newly implanted muscle flap.

Burns

Definition

Burns are the result of heat transfer to the body from any one of several sources. Causes of burns include flame, scalding (water), electric current, radiation, and chemicals. The area of injury may be limited to the skin or it may involve other superficial tissues. Other systems such as the respiratory system, liver, or kidney may also be affected and lead to the patient's death.

Classification of Burns by Depth

One way of classifying burns is by the depth at which tissue destruction has occurred. This includes the following:

1. A *first-degree burn* involves only the outside layer of the epidermis, as seen in mild sunburn. This type of burn is characterized by pain and reddening of the skin and usually heals spontaneously within a few days.

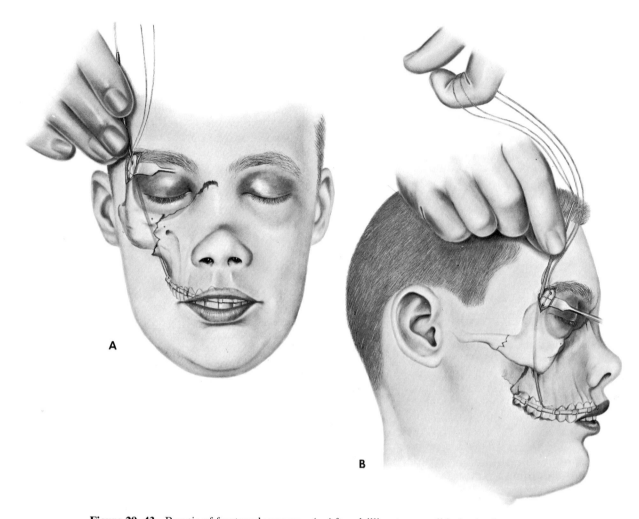

Figure 29–43. Repair of fractured zygoma. *A.* After drilling two small holes in the zygoma, the surgeon passes a long length of stainless steel suture through the holes. *B.* A passing needle is used to bring the wire down to the previously placed arch bar where it is secured. (From Dingman RO, Natvig P: Surgery of Facial Fractures. Philadelphia, WB Saunders, 1964.)

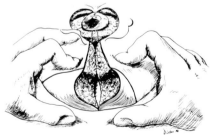

Figure 29–44. Closure of breast following wedge reduction. (From Schwartz SI, et al: Principles of Surgery, 2nd ed. New York, McGraw-Hill, 1974. Used with the permission of McGraw-Hill Book Company.)

2. A *second-degree burn* is the result of injury to the entire epidermis and a portion of the dermis. This type of burn is characterized by pain, blister formation, and a reddish-pink mottled discoloration. The area of destruction forms a brown crust, which separates from the underlying tissues within a few weeks as new epithelium begins to develop.

3. A *third-degree burn* results in the destruction of the entire skin thickness. The burn is dry and white and usually causes little pain. Within a few days, the burn area develops a thick, black, leathery crust called *eschar*. In this type of burn there is no possibility of spontaneous regeneration of the epithelium.

First- and second-degree burns are called *partial-thickness* burns, while third-degree burns are known as *full-thickness* burns.

Treatment

Basic treatment of the burn patient aims at replacing fluid loss and preventing infection, both of which are a major cause of mortality. The onset of infection is a *major* threat to the patient's life. Patients with third-degree burns may be brought to the operating room for débridement of the area and for dressing changes when the pain is so great that a general anesthetic is required. Once initial débridement and subsequent débridement have taken place, the patient is a candidate for skin grafting.

Bibliography

Converse JM (ed): Reconstructive Plastic Surgery: Principles and Procedures in Correction, Reconstruction, and Transplantation, 2nd ed. Philadelphia, WB Saunders, 1977.

Dingman RO, Natvig P: Surgery of Facial Fractures. Philadelphia, WB Saunders, 1964.

Dorland's Illustrated Medical Dictionary, 27th ed. Philadelphia, WB Saunders, 1988.

Gardner E, Gray D, O'Rahilly R: Anatomy: A Regional Study of Human Structure, 5th ed. Philadelphia, WB Saunders, 1986.

Jacob S, Francone C, Lossow WJ: Structure and Function in Man, 5th ed. Philadelphia, WB Saunders, 1984.

Journal of the Association of Operating Room Nurses: Proposed Recommended Practices for Storing, Preserving, and Maintaining Skin, Bone, Cartilage, and Blood Vessel Tissue. AORN J 35(5): 1982.

Walter JB: An Introduction to the Principles of Disease, 3rd ed. Philadelphia, WB Saunders, 1992.

Glossary

· ·

ablation: Removal by erosion or vaporization, usually due to intense heat.

abscess: A localized area of pus in the body.

absorbable suture: Any suture that is digested by body tissue.

aerobe: A microorganism that requires free oxygen in the environment for survival.

aerosol effect: The release of minute particles of liquid in the air. Liquid may harbor bacteria, which thus spread through the air droplets.

AIDS: Acquired immunodeficiency syndrome, a fatal disease transmitted by blood and body fluids.

alienation: The patient's emotional and physical separation from home, loved ones, work environment, and community.

amenorrhea: The absence of menstruation.

ampule: A small glass container that holds medication that has been sterilized.

anaerobe: A microorganism that can survive only in the absence of oxygen.

analgesia: The absence of pain.

anastomosis: The surgical formation of a passageway between two spaces, hollow organs, or lumens.

anesthetic: An agent that produces analgesia.

aneurysm: A saclike bulge in an artery, vein, or the heart often due to the accumulation of arteriosclerotic plaque within an artery.

animate surface: Living tissue.

anodized: Metal coated with a very thin layer of another metal, usually applied by electrolysis, used to give a colored or nonglare finish.

antibiotic: A drug that inhibits the growth of, or kills, microorganisms in living tissue.

antibody: A protein substance that destroys specific foreign bodies. Its production in the body is stimulated by an antigen.

anticoagulant: A drug that prolongs blood clotting time.

antisepsis: A process that destroys most pathogenic microorganisms from animate surfaces.

antiseptic: A chemical agent used on tissue that kills most, but not all, bacteria.

antiseptic solution: Antiseptic mixed with water.

appose: To bring two structures together.

approximate: To bring body parts or tissues together by sutures or other means.

armboard: Detachable extension on the operating table that accommodates the patient's arms.

asepsis: The prevention of contact with microorganisms; also used to refer to methods used in the operating room and other areas of the hospital to protect the environment from contamination by pathogens.

aseptic: Free of disease-producing microorganisms.

aseptic technique: Methods and practices that prevent cross-contamination in surgery.

aspirate: To withdraw fluids or gases by means of suction, as when removing fluid from the body with a syringe; also refers to the material thus obtained.

atelectasis: Incomplete expansion of the lungs at birth, or the collapse of an adult lung. Collapse may be caused by trauma or from pressure due to the presence of fluid on the lung.

atraumatic: Refers to a suture-needle combination that has no needle eye. The suture is swaged into the end of the needle shaft.

autoclave: Steam sterilizer.

autotransfusion: Transfusion using the patient's own blood.

autotroph: An organism that can ingest inorganic matter.

bacillus: A single, rod-shaped bacterial cell (plural: *bacilli*).

Bacillus stearothermophilus: A microorganism used as a biologic control in steam sterilization.

Bacillus subtilis: A microorganism used as a biologic control in gas sterilization.

bactericidal: Able to kill bacteria.

bacteriostatic: Capable of inhibiting the growth of bacteria, but not of killing them.

Bankart procedure: Operation of the shoulder girdle to treat recurrent shoulder dislocation.

barbiturate: Pharmaceutical agent that produces hypnosis and sedation.

bifurcated: Y-shaped; divided into two branches.

binary fission: Bacterial form of reproduction in which the cell splits to reproduce a copy of itself.

biologic control: A method that determines the presence

of pathogenic bacteria on objects subjected to a sterilization process.

biopsy: Removal of a small piece of tissue from a living body for microscopic examination.

bipolar: Refers to a type of electrosurgical unit in which the electrical current is localized at the tip of the electrocautery probe and does not pass through the patient.

bipolar coagulation: Electrosurgery that utilizes forceps rather than an electrosurgical pencil.

bleeder: A severed blood vessel.

blunt dissection: The separation of tissues or tissue planes with an instrument that has no cutting ability.

bolsters: Tubing through which retention sutures are threaded to prevent them from cutting into the patient's skin.

bone wax: Medical-grade beeswax used on bone tissue to control bleeding.

Bovie cleaner: Small, rough-surfaced pad used to clean the electrocautery tip during surgery.

box lock: The ratchet closure mechanism of many surgical instruments.

bradycardia: An abnormally slow heart rate or pulse rate.

Brown and Sharp (B & S) gauge: Sizing standard used to measure steel sutures.

bur: A round instrument with sharp cutting edges used for drilling holes in bone.

calculi: An abnormal accumulation of mineral salts; commonly called "stones."

capillary action: Refers to the absorption of liquids along the length of a suture.

cardiac tamponade: The inability of the heart to fill during diastole due to pressure from within the pericardial sac.

case assignments: Written schedule of each team member's assigned surgical cases for the day.

caudal: Toward the feet.

caudal anesthetic: An anesthetic agent introduced into the caudal canal to induce a type of epidural anesthesia.

cavitation: A process in which air pockets are imploded (burst inward), releasing particles of soil or tissue debris.

cephalopelvic disproportion: A condition in pregnancy in which the mother's pelvis is too small to accommodate the fetal head.

certification: Formal recognition by a private organization that a person has demonstrated certain skills or has received certain training.

chordee: A congenital defect that involves stricture of the fibrous tissue of the penis and that causes the penis to bow. This condition is often associated with hypospadias.

chromic salts: Chemicals used to treat surgical gut suture so that it resists digestion by body tissues.

circulator: Surgical team member who does not perform a surgical hand scrub or don sterile attire, and thus does not work within the sterile field.

clamp: Instrument that is designed to hold tissue, objects (such as surgical needles), or fabric (such as a towel clamp).

cleaning: A process that removes organic or inorganic debris.

cleft lip: A congenital defect that results in a split in the lip on one side or the other that may extend into the palate.

cleft palate: A congenital defect that results in a split of the hard and/or soft palate.

closed anesthesia system: In general anesthesia, the recirculation of anesthetic gases through the gas machine and back to the patient that prevents exposure of personnel to the gases.

closed gloving: Method of donning sterile gloves when a surgical gown is worn.

closed reduction: A process in which bone fragments are reduced manually, without surgical intervention.

coagulation: Clotting of blood.

cobalt 60 radiation: A method of sterilizing prepackaged equipment; ionizing radiation.

coccus: A spherical bacterial cell (plural: *cocci*).

code blue: Alert signal given during cardiopulmonary arrest anywhere in the hospital.

code red: Alert signal given when a fire occurs in the hospital.

communicate: When two structures or organs connect.

compassion: Expression of care and support given by surgical team members.

complaint: The legal document that begins a civil lawsuit and designates who is suing whom and why.

contaminated: Refers to any surface, living or nonliving, that is known to harbor organisms.

contrast medium: A radiopaque dye (not penetrated by x-rays) that is introduced into body cavities to outline their inside surfaces.

corticosteroid: One of a group of complex drugs that have many beneficial uses. In surgery these drugs are used to reduce inflammation.

critical items: In medicine, those items that must be sterile before their use on a patient; items that penetrate body tissues or the vascular system.

cross-contamination: A process in which infection or disease is spread from one source to another.

cryptorchidism: A developmental defect in which the testicles fail to descend into the scrotum at birth.

culture: To introduce tissue or fluid that is suspected of harboring pathogens onto a sterile test tube or plate containing growth medium. The organisms are allowed to grow and are later tested to determine their genus and species.

curette: A spoon-shaped instrument used to scrape tissue from a surface.

cutting instrument: Any instrument with a sharp edge.

cyanosis: A bluish-gray discoloration of body tissue due to a reduced oxygen level in the blood.

damages: Money awarded in a civil lawsuit to compensate the injured party.

dead space: An area lying between tissue layers or opposing them that the surgeon has not approximated. Dead space within a wound can lead to infection.

débridement: A process of removing dead skin, debris, or foreign bodies from a wound.

decontamination: A process of disinfection.

defamation: A derogatory statement concerning another person's skill, character, or reputation.

defendant: In a lawsuit, the person or corporation being sued. In a criminal case, the person being prosecuted.

defibrillator: A piece of equipment used to generate electrical impulses to the heart during cardiac arrest in an attempt to restart the heartbeat.

deflect: To peel or retract back and away but not detach.

dehiscence: The splitting apart of a surgical wound postoperatively.

delegate: To assign one's duties or tasks to another person.

deposition: A statement given by a witness, under oath, and transcribed by a court reporter during the pretrial phase of a civil lawsuit.

dermabrasion: The physical sanding of the skin to remove pockmarks and other scars.

desiccation: The drying up of a substance.

detritus: Dead epithelial tissue, such as that found on the surface of skin.

diaphoresis: Profuse sweating.

diastolic: One component of the patient's blood pressure that registers when the heart is dilating between beats.

dilators: Graduated, rodlike instruments used to enlarge the diameter of a channel or duct.

diplococci: Cocci that occur in pairs.

disinfectant: An agent that kills microorganisms on inanimate surfaces.

disinfection: A process by which most but not all pathogenic microorganisms are destroyed on inanimate objects.

dissector: A tiny sponge mounted on a clamp and used to perform blunt dissection.

distal: A point farther away from a given reference point; the opposite of proximal. For example, the foot is distal to the knee.

diuretic: A drug that draws fluid away from tissue.

divide: To cut or sever.

dormant: Refers to a living but inactive organism.

dorsal recumbent: Term synonymous with *supine;* position of the patient lying on his or her back.

drill bit: In orthopedics an instrument used in a drill to create a hole in bone to accommodate a screw.

dye: Any agent that stains tissues.

dysmenorrhea: Painful or difficult menstruation.

dystocia: Painful or difficult labor or childbirth.

ectopic pregnancy: A pregnancy that occurs when the fetus lodges in a location other than the uterus.

embolism: An obstruction in a blood vessel due to a foreign body, tumor, blood clot, or air.

emergence: The arousal from general anesthesia after cessation of the anesthetic agent.

endotoxin: Toxin released when a cell dies and breaks up.

endotracheal tube: Tube that is inserted into the patient's trachea for the administration of anesthetic gas.

endotracheal tube fire: A fire that occurs within the patient's endotracheal tube during laser surgery that causes immediate and severe trauma to the lungs.

epidural anesthetic: Type of anesthetic agent that is introduced into the epidural space of the spine.

Esmarch bandage: Rolled rubber bandage that is wrapped around the limb to force blood away from the surgical site before the application of a tourniquet.

ethylene oxide gas: Highly flammable, toxic gas that is capable of sterilizing an object.

etiology: The origin of a disease; its cause.

evisceration: In surgery, the splitting open of a surgical wound and subsequent spillage of its contents.

excise: To remove by cutting out.

excitement: The second stage of general anesthesia, in which the patient is sensitive to external stimuli.

exotoxin: Toxin released from living bacteria.

exposure: The anatomic area that the surgeon can see and thus operate on.

extractor: In orthopedics, an instrument used to remove a metal implant from bone.

facultative bacteria: Bacteria that can live with or without the presence of oxygen.

fallout contamination: Contamination of a sterile surface by particles arising from a source above it.

fiberoptic: A flexible material that carries light along its length; refers to fibers of glass or plastic that are bundled together to form the cables used for endoscopic examination.

first intention: A process by which a clean surgical wound heals directly, without granulation.

fistula: An abnormal passageway from a normal cavity to the outside of the body or another cavity.

fixation: In orthopedics, to hold bone fragments in place following a fracture. In *external* fixation, the fragments are held in alignment by an external device such as a plaster cast. In *internal* fixation, fragments are held in alignment with an appliance such as a rod, nail, or screw.

flaking: The tendency of some suture materials to release tiny particles of the suture in the wound.

flash autoclave: An autoclave used in surgery to sterilize equipment quickly by steam under pressure.

fomite: A substance that is capable of harboring and transmitting disease.

footboard: Section of the operating table at the foot end that can be removed or angled up or down.

four by four (4 × 4): Type of surgical sponge, consisting of loosely woven gauze squares.

Fowler position: Sitting position.

fracture: The breaking of a part, especially bone. Different types of fractures include: (1) *comminuted*—the bone is splintered into many small fragments; (2) *compound*—the fracture penetrates adjacent soft tissue and skin (also called an *open* fracture); (3) *greenstick*—extending only partway through the bone; incomplete, occurring in children; (4) *impacted*—a portion of the bone is traumatically driven into another bone or fragment; (5) *pathologic*—caused by disease rather than injury; (6) *spiral*—the fracture forms a spiral pattern; it has been twisted apart; (7) *transverse*—the fracture line lies perpendicular to the long axis of the bone.

free tie: A term used by the surgeon when he or she requests a length of suture for ligation.

French-eye: A delicate needle whose eye contains a spring.

friable: Refers to any tissue that is easily torn.

frozen section: A fine slice of frozen biopsy tissue that is microscopically examined for the presence of disease.

full length: Refers to the length of a suture strand. Full length is 54 or 60 inches.

gangrene: Necrosis (death) of tissue; usually due to inadequate blood supply.

gas: Matter in its least dense state; air at room temperature is a gas.

Gelfoam: Medical-grade gelatin that is used to control capillary bleeding.

general anesthetic: Type of anesthetic agent that causes unconsciousness.

glutaraldehyde: Chemical capable of rendering objects sterile.

Gram staining: A process in which microorganisms are classified according to whether they absorb a special dye; bacteria may be typed as *gram positive* or *gram negative.*

gravity displacement sterilizer: Type of sterilizer that removes air by gravity.

grounding cable: During electrosurgery, the cable connecting the control unit to the inactive electrode.

grounding pad: Gel-covered pad that grounds the patient during electrosurgery; inactive electrode.

gurney: Stretcher.

HBV: Hepatitis B virus.

headboard: Removable section of the operating table at the head end that can be angled up or down.

hematoma: A localized accumulation of blood in tissue.

hemorrhage: Heavy bleeding, usually arising from an artery.

hemostasis: The control of hemorrhage during surgery.

hemostat: An instrument used to clamp a blood vessel.

hemostatic agent: A drug that promotes blood coagulation.

heterotroph: An organism that ingests only organic matter.

high-level disinfection: Disinfection process that kills spores.

high vacuum sterilizer: Type of steam sterilizer that removes air in the chamber by vacuum.

HIV: Human immunodeficiency virus—the cause of AIDS.

hold: Indicates that the surgeon wishes to place a small clamp on the end of the suture rather than cut it.

host: Organism that provides nutrition for parasites.

hydrocele: A localized accumulation of fluid, especially in the scrotal wall.

hydronephrosis: A condition in which the ureter becomes obstructed and urine backs up into the renal pelvis.

hypospadias: A congenital defect in which the ureteral orifice is found abnormally on the undersurface of the penis.

imminent abortion: An abortion that is about to occur immediately.

impactor: In orthopedics, an instrument used to drive an implant into bone; may also be called a "driver."

inanimate: Nonliving.

incise: To cut or sever with a cutting instrument.

incomplete abortion: A condition in which only part of the products of conception have aborted.

induction: The first stage of general anesthesia, during which the patient's physiologic status is unstable.

inert: Refers to certain types of suture material, indicating that it causes little or no tissue reaction.

infection: The invasion of healthy tissue by pathogenic microorganisms.

inflammation: The localized, protective reaction of tissue to injury or disease.

inflammatory response: The body's reaction to injury or disease.

informed consent: Permission given with full knowledge of the risks involved.

infrared: That portion of the electromagnetic spectrum just below visible light. All warm objects give off infrared radiation.

infusion pump: Containment and monitoring equipment used when the patient receives intravenous solutions, including anesthetics.

insurance: A contract in which the insurance company agrees to defend the policyholder if he or she is sued for acts covered by the policy and to pay any damages.

intentional hypotension: During surgery, the intentional lowering of the patient's blood pressure to control hemorrhage.

intentional hypothermia: During surgery, the intentional lowering of the patient's core temperature to control bleeding.

Javid shunt: A commercially prepared length of plastic tubing used to bypass the carotid artery temporarily during carotid endarterectomy.

jaws: The working end of a surgical instrument.

JCAHO: Joint Commission on Accreditation of Healthcare Organizations.

Kerlix bandage: A rolled bandage made of soft, woven material.

Kraske position: Operative position used for procedures of the perianal area; also called "jackknife" position or "knee-chest" position. The patient lies in prone position, with the table broken at its midsection so that the head and feet are lower than the midsection.

laminectomy position: Operative position used for spinal surgery; a form of prone position.

laparotomy tape: Also called a "lap tape." The largest surgical sponge available, used during major surgery.

laser: *L*ight *a*mplification by *s*timulated *e*mission of *r*adiation; a device that generates a beam of extremely bright light of a single color.

lateral: Refers to a side. For example, the small toe lies on the lateral aspect of the foot.

lavage: Irrigation of body cavities. During malignant hyperthermia, cold saline is used to lower the patient's temperature.

leiomyoma: A benign tumor of smooth muscle, usually found in the uterus; also called "fibroid uterus."

leukocyte: A white blood cell that ingests foreign material such as bacteria.

liable: Legally responsible.

license: Governmental permission to perform an act or possess property.

ligate: To tie a length of suture around a vessel or duct and secure it with knots.

ligation clips: Sometimes referred to as "silver clips." Small V-shaped clips that are applied around blood vessels or ducts in place of a ligature.

local anesthetic: Type of anesthetic agent that causes loss of sensation or feeling to a localized area.

local infiltration: The anesthetic is injected directly into the operative tissue.

lop ears: A congenital defect that results in the exaggerated protrusion of the ears from the head.

lumen: Hollow tube.

malignant hyperthermia: Anesthetic-related phenomenon that causes the patient's temperature to rise suddenly and become critically high. Emergency procedures are initiated during this crisis.

malpractice: Negligence committed by a professional.

medial: Refers to the middle. For example, the large toe lies on the medial aspect of the foot.

medical practice acts: Laws that regulate the practice of physicians and surgeons.

memory: A suture's ability to "remember" its configuration during packaging (i.e., coiled or twisted).

menometrorrhagia: Excessive bleeding during menstruation and at irregular intervals.

metastasis: The spread of disease, usually cancer, to a location other than the primary lesion.

metrorrhagia: The presence of active uterine bleeding at times other than during menstruation.

microfibrillar collagen hemostat: Substance derived from collagen and used as a hemostatic agent.

microorganism: An organism that is visible only with the aid of a microscope.

microtia: A congenital defect that results in the absence of all or part of the external ear.

missed abortion: A condition in which the products of conception are nonliving and are retained in the uterus for over 2 months.

monitored anesthesia care: The patient receives an intravenous sedative anesthetic, which may be given in conjunction with a local anesthetic or by itself.

monofilament suture: Suture composed of a single, nonfibrous strand of material.

monopolar: Refers to a type of electrosurgical unit in which the electrical current passes through the patient and back to the control unit.

morphology: The study of structure and form.

multifilament suture: Suture composed of many fine strands of fiber that are twisted or braided together.

nanosecond: One billionth (10^{-9}) of 1 second.

necrotic: Refers to dead tissue.

negligence: The failure to exercise due care. See *tort.*

nerve block: Anesthesia of a large single nerve or nerves.

neuromuscular blocking agent: A pharmaceutical agent that causes paralysis during general anesthesia.

nonabsorbable suture: Suture that is never digested by tissue but becomes encapsulated by it.

nosocomial infection: An infection acquired while in the hospital or as a result of being in the hospital.

nuncupative will: A will given orally; also called a dying declaration.

nurse anesthetist: Registered nurse who administers anesthesia under the supervision of an anesthesiologist.

nurse practice acts: Laws that regulate the practice of nursing.

open gloving: Method of donning sterile surgical gloves when a gown is not worn.

open reduction: To reduce bone fragments with surgical instruments.

osteotome: A chisel-like instrument used with a mallet to cut bone.

oxidized cellulose: Medical-grade cellulose manufactured into mesh squares and used as a hemostatic agent.

oxytocic: A drug that causes uterine contractions.

PACU: Post-anesthesia care unit.

paraphimosis: A retraction of the prepuce, which causes a painful swelling of the glans.

parasites: Organisms that derive nutrients from a living source.

pathogenic: Disease-causing.

pathologist: Medical doctor who specializes in the identification of diseased tissue.

patient care plan: Extensive written plan that outlines the patient's physical, social, psychological, and spiritual needs.

patient fears: Fears shared by many surgical patients, including fear of death or mutilation and fear of anesthesia, pain, and exposure.

patty: A type of sponge used during neurosurgery.

peracetic acid: Chemical capable of rendering objects sterile.

perioperative nursing: Nursing care of the patient before, during, and after surgery.

personnel protective equipment: Special barrier attire worn to prevent the cross-communication of blood-borne diseases.

phagocytosis: The process by which white blood cells engulf bacteria.

phimosis: A condition in the uncircumcised male in which the prepuce will not retract from the glans.

photodynamic: Caused by the motion or influence of photons (light).

photon: The smallest particle of light. A photon is massless and travels at the speed of light.

physical restrictions: The patient's inability to move

freely in his or her environment. The patient is required to stay within the limits of his or her unit, room, and bed. These restrictions can be very distressing.

placenta abruptio: Premature separation of the placenta from the wall of the uterus.

placenta previa: A condition in which the placenta is abnormally implanted in the lower uterine segment.

plaintiff: In a civil lawsuit, the person filing the suit; the injured party.

points: The tips of a surgical instrument.

polyp: A protuding mass of mucous membrane or other membrane.

precut: Lengths of suture material that are cut to a standard length by the manufacturer.

presentation: The manner in which the fetus is positioned in relation to the cervix: (1) *breech*—the buttocks are presented; (2) *footling*—the feet are presented; (3) *transverse*—the fetus is presented crosswise; (4) *vertex*—the upper back of the head is presented.

probe: An instrument placed within a lumen to determine its length and direction.

prone: A position in which the patient lies face down.

prosthesis: Any artificial organ or body part.

proximal: A point nearest to a given reference point; opposite of distal. For example, the elbow lies proximal to the hand.

pursestring: A technique of suturing. A continuous strand is passed in and out around the circumference of a hollow structure and then is pulled tight like a drawstring.

pus: An accumulation of dead bacteria, necrotic tissue, tissue fluid, and white blood cells that forms at the site of an infection.

ratchets: Interlocking clasps that hold a finger ring instrument closed.

reamer: An instrument used in orthopedic surgery to create a hollow area in bone.

reduce: In orthopedics, to bring two bone fragments in alignment following their fracture.

reel: A continuous strand of suture mounted on a spool; used for ligation of many blood vessels in rapid succession.

relaxation: During general anesthesia, the operative phase.

reperitonealization: In gynecologic surgery, the replacement of the bladder flap with sutures after hysterectomy or cesarean section when it must be separated from the uterus.

resect: To cut out and remove a section of tissue.

resident flora: Bacteria that inhabit normal skin.

respondeat superior: A legal doctrine that states that an employer is legally responsible for the acts of its employees committed during the course of their employment.

retention suture: Heavy nonabsorbable sutures placed behind the skin sutures and underneath all tissue layers to give added strength to the closure.

retract: To pull tissues back or away to expose a structure or other tissue.

reverse Trendelenburg position: Operative position in which the patient lies in supine position, and the operating table is tilted so that the head is higher than the feet.

running suture: A method of suturing that uses one continuous suture that is passed over and under the tissue edges.

sanitation: A process that cleans an object.

saprophytes: Organisms that feed on dead or decaying material.

scope of practice: The limits of professional duties set by law, training, and experience.

second intention: A process involving granulation by which an infected wound heals without sutures.

seeding: The breaking away and implantation of cancer cells from the original tumor to a new site.

self-tapping: In orthopedics, a screw that creates its own hole in bone as it is being inserted.

semiconductor: A material, such as silicon, that is neither a conductor of electricity nor an insulator. Its electrical properties can be changed by adding minute amounts of other elements. Semiconductors are the basis of transistors and computer chips.

septic: Infectious. The term *septic* is now considered outdated.

shank: The area of a surgical instrument between the box lock and the finger ring.

sharp dissection: The use of a scalpel or other sharp instrument for the separation of tissues.

shelf life: The amount of time a wrapped object will remain sterile after it has been subjected to a sterilization process.

Sims position: Also called lateral position; position of the patient lying on his or her side.

sizer: A dummy or model of a prosthesis used to determine the correct size prosthesis needed during an operation.

slander: Spoken defamation.

solid: Matter in a rigid state, not liquid or gaseous.

solid-state: Using the electrical properties of solid components (such as transistors) instead of vacuum tubes.

specimen: Any tissue, foreign body, prosthesis, or fluid that is removed from the patient.

speculum: An instrument used for exposure of a body cavity, such as the nose.

sphygmomanometer: An instrument used for measuring the patient's blood pressure.

spirochetes: Bacteria that are corkscrew shaped.

sponge stick: A folded four by four mounted on a sponge clamp.

spore or endospore: Protective reproductive form of the bacterium that contains all the genetic material capable of becoming a living bacterial cell. Some are extremely difficult to destroy.

sporicidal: Able to kill spores.

staphylococci: Cocci that occur in irregular masses.

steam sterilizer: Sterilizer that exposes objects to high-pressure steam.

sterile: Completely free of living microorganisms.

sterile field: An area that encompasses draped equipment, scrubbed personnel, and the draped patient.

sterilization: A process by which all types of microorganisms are destroyed.

sterilization control monitor: Method of determining whether a sterilization process has been completed; it does not indicate whether the items subjected to that method are sterile.

stick tie: Name given to suture ligature—a suture-needle combination that is passed through a vessel or duct before ligation to prevent it from slipping off the edge of the structure.

streptococci: Cocci that occur as long chains.

strict aerobes: Bacteria that cannot survive without oxygen.

strict anaerobes: Bacteria that cannot survive in the presence of oxygen.

stricture: A narrowing in a body cavity due to infection, disease, or congenital defect.

strikethrough contamination: Contamination of a sterile surface by moisture that has originated from a non-sterile surface and penetrated the protective covering of the sterile item.

subpoena: A court order requiring its recipient to appear and testify at a trial or deposition.

subungual area: The space beneath the nails.

summons: A court-issued document that is received by a person being sued, notifying the person that he or she is a defendant in the lawsuit.

suppuration: The accumulation of bacterial cells, dead white blood cells, and cellular fluid.

surgeon's preference card: File card that contains information pertaining to suture materials, equipment, or special instruments used by a particular surgeon.

surgical drape: Sterile cloth or nonwoven material placed around the surgical site to create a sterile field.

surgical scrub: Precise method by which all team members who will be working in sterile attire scrub their hands and arms before performing an operation.

surgically clean: As clean as possible, but not sterile.

suture: A material used to bring tissues together by sewing; can also refer to a suture-needle combination.

suture ligature: A needle and suture combination used to tie a bleeding vessel and attach it to nearby tissue simultaneously, thus preventing the tie from slipping off the end of the vessel.

swage: Area of an atraumatic needle that holds the suture.

systemic infection: Infection that has spread from one area to other parts of the body through the bloodstream.

systolic: Refers to one component of the patient's blood pressure that registers when the heart contracts.

table breaks: Hinged sections of the operating table that can be folded up or down to create different postures.

tachycardia: An abnormally fast heart rate.

teamwork: Cooperation in working toward a common goal by giving the goal the highest priority.

tenaculum: An instrument used to grasp tissue.

tensile strength: The amount of stress a suture will withstand before breaking.

terminal disinfection: A process in which an area or object is rendered disinfected after contamination has occurred.

theft: Taking the property of another with the intention of keeping it.

tie-on-passer: A strand of suture material whose end is secured to the end of a long clamp; used to ligate deep vessels where exposure is limited.

tincture: Any agent that is mixed with alcohol.

topical anesthetic: A drug used on the surface of tissue such as the eye.

topical thrombin: Drug used in conjunction with gelatin sponges to halt capillary bleeding.

torsion: The twisting of an organ or structure upon itself that often causes diminished blood supply to the affected area.

tort: A wrongful act, other than a breach of contract, that can result in a lawsuit for money.

tourniquet: A device that prevents the flow of blood to the surgical wound.

toxigenicity: A bacterium's ability to release toxic substances.

transect: To cut *across* an organ or section of tissue.

transient flora: Bacteria that have been acquired from a contaminated source and inhabit skin.

Trendelenburg position: Operative position in which the patient lies in supine position with the operating table tilted such that the head is lower than the feet.

triage: Classification system used during major disasters such as earthquakes, air accidents, or industrial explosions. Victims are classified according to the severity of their condition and are treated in a corresponding order.

trocar: A spear-shaped instrument or needle.

ultrasonic cleaner: Equipment that cleans instruments through cavitation.

unit secretary: Secretary of the operating room.

Universal Precautions: Precautionary standards issued by the Occupational Safety and Health Administration and the Centers for Disease Control for the containment and isolation of blood and body fluids.

USP: United States Pharmacopoeia, the agency that regulates and issues standards of quality for medical products such as suture materials.

vasoconstriction: The constriction of a blood vessel.

vasoconstrictor: A drug that constricts blood vessels, used in conjunction with local anesthetics.

vector: An intermediate source that transmits bacteria from one surface to another.

viricidal: Able to kill viruses.

washer-sterilizer: Equipment that washes and sterilizes instruments following an operative procedure.

Webril: A soft, rolled cotton material used to pad a limb before the application of a plaster cast.

Index

. . . .

Page numbers in *italics* refer to illustrations; numbers followed by t indicate tables.

673